Medicine in the Practice of Anaesthesia

Edited by

Leon Kaufman
MD, FFARCS

Honorary Senior Lecturer, University College and
Middlesex School of Medicine;
Consultant Anaesthetist, University College Hospital, London

and

D. John Betteridge
BSc, PhD, MD, FRCP

Reader in Medicine, University College and
Middlesex School of Medicine;
Consultant Physician, University College Hospital, London

Edward Arnold
A division of Hodder & Stoughton
LONDON   MELBOURNE   AUCKLAND

© 1989 Edward Arnold

First published in Great Britain 1989

British Library Cataloguing in Publication Data
Medicine in the practice of anaesthesia.
 1. Man. Diseases — For anaesthesia
 I. Kaufman, L. (Leon) II. Betteridge, John
 616′.0024617

 ISBN 0-7131-4685-4

Whilst the advice and information in this book is believed to be true and accurate at the date of going to press, neither the authors nor the publisher can accept any legal responsibility or liability for any error or omissions made.

Typeset in 10/11 pt Times by Colset Private Limited, Singapore
Printed and bound in Great Britain for Edward Arnold,
the educational, academic and medical publishing division of Hodder and Stoughton Limited, 41 Bedford Square, London WC1B 3DQ by Butler & Tanner Ltd, Frome and London

Contributors

D. John Betteridge BSc, PhD, MD, FRCP
Reader in Medicine,
University College and Middlesex School of
Medicine;
Consultant Physician,
University College Hospital,
London

Allan Binder MRCP
Senior Registrar in Rheumatology,
Whittington Hospital,
London

Peter Bradbury MA, MRCP
Consultant Neurologist,
Broomfield Hospital,
Chelmsford,
Essex

Anthony Goldstone FRCP, FRCPath
Consultant Haematologist,
University College Hospital,
London

David Grant BSc(Hons), MRCP, FRCR
Consultant Radiologist,
Whittington Hospital,
London

John Gribben BSc (Hons), MRCP
Research Fellow and Honorary Senior Registrar,
University College and Middlesex School of
Medicine,
London

David Isenberg MD, MRCP
Consultant Rheumatologist and Honorary Senior
Lecturer,
University College Hospital,
London

Leon Kaufman MD, FFARCS
Honorary Senior Lecturer,
University College and Middlesex

School of Medicine
Consultant Anaesthetist,
University College Hospital,
London

Ian McNeil MA, MD, MRCP
Lecturer in Medicine,
University College and Middlesex School of
Medicine
London

Martyn Partridge MD, MRCP
Consultant Physician,
Whipps Cross Hospital,
London

Charles Singer BSc(Hons), MBChB, MRCP,
MRCPath
Consultant Haematologist,
Royal United Hospital,
Bath

Roderic Thomas MA, MD, FRCP
Consultant Cardiologist,
Royal United Hospital,
Combe Park,
Bath

Mark Vella MPhil, MRCP
Senior Registrar in Medicine,
Guy's Hospital,
London

Bryan Walton MB BS, FFARCS
Consultant Anaesthetist,
The London Hospital,
London

Gwyn Williams MD, FRCP
Consultant Nephrologist and Senior Lecturer in
Medicine,
Guy's Hospital,
London

Preface

Anaesthetists are well aware that pre-existing medical disorders exert a marked influence on the successful outcome of surgical operations. Although a knowledge of medicine and advances in therapy have become an essential prerequisite for the anaesthetist, it is surprising that it is only within the last 10 years that medical textbooks have been published specifically designed to cater for the interests of the speciality. A small book entitled *Medical Problems and the Anaesthetist* (in conjunction with Dr Edward Sumner) proved popular not only in this country but also in France, Italy, Germany, Spain, Japan and the United States. It has been reprinted and surprisingly continues to attract subscribers.

Although it was tempting to replace *Medical Problems and the Anaesthetist* with a larger volume written mostly by anaesthetists, we have been persuaded that advances in medicine and medical treatment would have made this an arduous and protracted task. We therefore succumbed to the need to invite specialist contributors, many of whom are intimately aware of the medical problems that confront anaesthetists. It is impossible to encompass the whole of medicine in a volume of this size, but we trust that the text will assist not only the examination candidates but also become a ready source of reference. Notes on taking a history, examining the patient and preoperative assessment are included as a guide not only to perioperative care but also to the provision of medical care in high dependency units. The interpretation of investigations are outlined as well as the rationale for medical treatment. The anaesthetist is often confronted with the ECG and chest X-ray for elucidation and thus these investigations are considered in some detail. Medical disorders and therapy may influence the use of anaesthetic agents and techniques while one must be aware of the possible hazards of pacemaker or surgical operations in patients who have had bypass surgery.

We are grateful to our contributors for their painstaking preparation of their chapters, which include also guides to further reading. Where relevant these have been replaced by lists of references. It is hoped to produce a multiple choice booklet based on this volume in the near future.

We acknowledge the assistance of our publishers, Edward Arnold, for their guidance in the preparation of this book as well as the many secretaries who produced the manuscripts with devotion, care, and with the assistance of the word processor.

London, 1989

LK
JB

Contents

1

Cardiovascular Disorders

Roderic Thomas

Introduction

Cardiovascular disease is the leading cause of death in developed countries. A thorough knowledge of its manifestations, diagnosis and treatment is therefore important. Though advances in cardiology have revolutionized many of its aspects the approach to patient management is unchanged. A careful history is usually the most rewarding source of information and this should be followed by a thorough clinical examination and laboratory tests if indicated.

Symptoms

In most patients the primary question will be 'is cardiovascular disease present?' If the answer is yes, 'how bad is the disease?', and 'will it affect the operation?' The history needs particular attention to breathlessness, fatigue (from low cardiac output), chest pain or tightness, and palpitations or syncope.

Signs

Examination of patients should include careful measurement of the height of the jugular venous pulse (JVP) above the sternal angle. The trunk can be raised or lowered to clarify this. The upper limit of normal is 3–4 cm (use a ruler a few times to see how most observers do not measure the height correctly). The blood pressure should be recorded carefully. The left ventricular impulse is often difficult to quantify; if it is felt over an area larger than 3 cm (or 1½ finger tips) then the left ventricle is enlarged. The presence of a third or fourth heart sound on auscultation may be the only sign of left ventricular disease. The third sound, an early diastolic filling sound, is most effectively heard with a stethoscope bell applied lightly to the apex with the patient on his or her left side. It is a normal physiological finding in young people (up to the age of 30), in pregnant women and is heard with the increased diastolic flow in mitral regurgitation. Otherwise, it is a good sign of abnormal left ventricular function from any cause. A fourth heart sound is never normal, and is a sign of an abnormal but not failing ventricle when there is vigorous atrial contraction filling a stiff or ischaemic left ventricle.

Heart murmurs are graded on a scale of 1–6. Grade 1 can only be heard after concentration (and never in a noisy ward), grade 2 is faint, grade 3 is moderately loud and grade 4 is loud, with a thrill. A grade 5 murmur is very loud and heard with the edge of a stethoscope and grade 6 is so loud that it can be heard with a stethoscope off the chest.

Cardiac risks in non-cardiac surgery

It is essential to try and assess the cardiac risks of non-cardiac surgery (Braunwald, 1984; Hurst, 1986 and Goldman, 1983). It is useful to consider this here because it highlights some of the areas of knowledge required and emphasizes features of preoperative assessment. The serious risks are of myocardial infarction, cardiac failure and arrhythmias.

Risk of myocardial infarction

Studies have shown that the risk of postoperative myocardial infarction in adults is between 0.1 and 0.4 per cent in patients with no evidence of previous infarction and around 6 per cent in those who have had a previous infarct. If a surgical operation is undertaken within 3 months of a myocordial infarct, the risk of re-infarction is about 30 per cent and, if within 3–6 months, about 15 per cent. Of these, one-third to a half are silent – they present with cardiac failure, hypotension, arrhythmias or on routine investigation. Postoperative infarcts can occur within the first 5 days although most occur within the first 3 days; one-third to a half are fatal. There is some evidence that careful invasive intraoperative monitoring of high risk patients will reduce the incidence of infarction considerably (Wells and Kaplan, 1981). In a large study of non-cardiac operations it was found that of the 25 000 patients who had had coronary angiography in CASS (coronary artery surgery study), myocardial infarction within 6 months of surgery was not a significant risk factor (Foster *et al.*, 1986). It is the degree of left ventricular damage that is important. Thus post-infarction patients at low risk (no severe resting or exercise ischaemia or left ventricular dysfunction) may be candidates for important surgery (i.e. for resectable tumours) after 4–6 weeks (Weitz and Goldman, 1987). Other risk factors for myocardial infarction include age over 70 years, evidence of cardiac failure, a murmur of mitral regurgitation, ventricular extrasystoles on an electrocardiogram (ECG), preoperative hypertension, intraoperative hypotension and in some studies, a prolonged operation time. An abnormal electrocardiogram, with ST-segment and T-base changes, was an important risk factor in the large series.

Risk of cardiac failure

The chief risk is with preoperative evidence of cardiac failure – either severe symptoms, objective signs (third heart sound or raised JVP) or radiological evidence of heart failure. In addition there is a risk with any significant valve disease. Two-thirds of the patients who have postoperative heart failure have none of these features, but are invariably over 60 years.

Arrhythmias

Though difficult to predict there is an increased incidence in patients with previous arrhythmias, cardiac failure or chronic obstructive airway disease.

Hypertension, anticoagulant therapy and antibiotic prophylaxis will be considered later.

Cardiac risk index

A large pool of information has come from Goldman and his colleagues at the Massachusetts

Table 1.1 The Cardiac risk index

Findings	Points
1. History	
(a) Age > 70 years	5
(b) Myocardial infarct in previous 6 months	10
2. Physical examination	
(a) S_3 gallop or raised JVP	11
(b) Significant aortic stenosis	3
3. Electrocardiogram	
(a) Non sinus rhythm or atrial extrasystoles	7
(b) > 5 ventricular extrasystoles any time preoperatively	7
4. Poor general medical condition†	3
5. Operation	
(a) Intraperitoneal, thoracic or aortic	3
(b) Emergency	4

Point total	No or minor complications (%)	Life-threatening‡ complications (%)	Cardiac deaths
0–5	99	0.6	0.2
6–12	96	3	1
13–25	86	11	3
> 26	49	12	39

Key
†K < 3.0 mmol/litre, HCO_3 < 20, urea > 20, creatinine > 260 mmol/litre, PO_2 < 60, pCO_2 > 50 mmHg Abnormal liver (clinical or AST) or bedridden.
‡Myocardial infarct, pulmonary oedema, ventricular tachycardia.

General Hospital. These authors identified the commonest preoperative factors which are associated with life-threatening or fatal cardiac complications after non-cardiac operations. The point scheme is shown in Table 1.1. Weitz and Goldman reviewed this scheme (Weitz and Goldman, 1987) confirming its usefulness, and that recent myocardial infarction can be a lower risk. The risk index has been modified by Detsky *et al.*, (1986) using a nomogram to convert average surgical risk in patients referred for a medical opinion to individual risk. Though stable angina does not appear to be a risk factor in Goldman's index, the modified index adds points for severe and/or constant angina, always accepted by Goldman as likely (he didn't have enough of these patients). Ventricular extrasystoles appear because they are often a marker for more severe heart disease, rather than being important in their own right, so there is no increased risk in the presence of a normal heart. Some of these risk factors are controllable with adequate treatment or delaying surgery well after myocardial infarction.

These risk estimates are useful in directing attention to some important factors, which are often multiple. However they are only approximate and can underestimate the risk; it should be stressed that each patient needs individual clinical assessment.

Ischaemic heart disease

Epidemiology

Ischaemic heart disease, usually manifest by angina pectoris, acute myocardial infarction or sudden death, is probably commoner than generally realized. It is the certified cause of one-third of all male deaths in the UK. The British Regional Heart Study (BRHS) of men aged 40–59, using a questionnaire and electrocardiogram, gave the prevalence of ischaemic heart disease as 25 per cent. In the Whitehall study of civil servants, the prevalence was 17 per cent. The annual heart attack rate (myocardial infarct or sudden death) in the BRHS was 6.2/1000 men/year.

Pathology

Ischaemic heart disease is most commonly caused by atherosclerosis – the degenerative disease causing luminal narrowing of the coronary arteries and other large and medium sized arteries. The atherosclerotic lesions are intimal and contain three cellular elements – smooth muscle, connective tissue and lipid. Complicated lesions contain necrotic debris, haemorrhage and thrombosis. By the time there is symptomatic heart disease there is usually more than 75 per cent narrowing of the luminal area. In addition to the fixed stenosis from the atherosclerotic plaques, there may be sudden progression of the disease from a plaque fissure with intimal and luminal thrombosis and a variable narrowing from coronary spasm. It is this interaction between the fixed lesion and dynamic obstruction mediated by vasoconstriction or thrombosis which explains much of the variable progression and manifestations of ischaemic heart disease.

Pathophysiology

Myocardial ischaemia occurs when there is an imbalance between myocardial oxygen supply and demand. Oxygen demand is determined by heart rate, contractility and left ventricular wall tension (Fig. 1.1). Wall tension is proportional to ventricular systolic pressure and radius and inversely proportional to wall thickness (Laplace's law). Oxygen supply is dependent on coronary blood flow and arterial oxygen availability. Coronary blood flow itself depends on coronary diameter, resistance, the presence of collateral flow, and on the perfusion pressure. Coronary blood flow is autoregulated and is therefore normally relatively independent of coronary perfusion pressure. However, in coronary atherosclerosis, when the

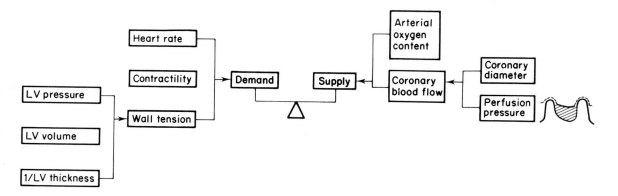

Fig 1.1   The relationship between oxygen demand and supply; imbalance between the two, leads to myocardial ischaemia. Coronary blood flow occurs in diastole – the hatched area between aortic and ventricular diastolic pressures in the small diagram on the right.

vessels become maximally dilated, the flow becomes proportional to the driving pressure. Coronary flow is then related to the difference between the aortic diastolic pressure and left ventricular diastolic pressure and the duration of diastole (*see* Fig. 1.1). The subendocardium of the left ventricle, where the compressive forces are greatest, is at greatest risk of ischaemia.

Anatomy

There are three coronary arteries; the left anterior descending and circumflex arteries which are branches of the left main artery, and the right coronary artery. The left anterior descending coronary artery supplies the anterior wall of the left ventricle and anterior part of the interventricular septum – occlusion of this vessel produces larger myocardial infarcts than occlusion of the other two vessels. The circumflex artery supplies the lateral wall and some of the posterior wall of the left ventricle (this depends on the dominance of the coronary system). The right coronary artery supplies the right ventricle, posterior part of the interventricular septum and some of the posterior wall of the left ventricle. It also supplies the sinoatrial and atroventricular nodes.

Angina pectoris

Angina is a symptom which typically occurs at a certain level of exercise, when the oxygen demand is increased. However, in addition to fixed luminal obstruction from atherosclerosis there can be coronary vasospasm from areas of smooth muscle in the arterial wall. This transient reduction in coronary flow and increased demand with fixed obstruction are equally important causes of myocardial ischaemia. Platelet aggregation may be involved in this reduction in luminal size, either primarily or secondarily to endothelial damage, and may perpetuate coronary spasm by releasing vasoconstrictor substances. These several mechanisms all help to explain the variable symptoms of angina. Although symptoms are broadly related to the severity of the underlying disease, this may not be so in any individual patient.

Angina can also be caused by other coronary diseases (congenital, embolic, vasculitic), valvular disease (especially aortic stenosis), hypertrophic cardiomyopathy, brady- or tachyarrhythmias. It is rarely precipitated by anaemia.

It is important to realize that angina is only one

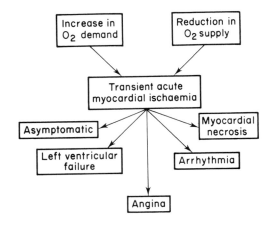

Fig 1.2 Transient myocardial ischaemia causes angina and other clinical effects.

of the manifestations of acute transient myocardial ischaemia. In addition to pain, ischaemia causes abnormal left ventricular function (both decreased systolic contraction and delay in diastolic relaxation) and abnormal metabolism (Fig. 1.2). Ischaemia can also cause pulmonary oedema, without myocardial infarction and arrhythmias. In addition, asymptomatic episodes of myocardial ischaemia recorded by electrocardiography, nuclear or haemodynamic studies may be commoner than symptomatic episodes.

Symptoms

In *stable* angina, symptoms usually occur at a constant level of exercise, with a typical unpleasant, squeezing, tight pressure feeling over the chest, often with dyspnoea. Patients may clench their fist or put the flat of their hand on their chest when describing it and may deny actual pain, when questioned. The symptoms are often worse after meals (hence the tendency to call it 'indigestion'), in the cold, first thing in the morning and with emotion; and if there is spasm the symptoms can vary considerably.

Unstable angina is a term used to describe a group of syndromes intermediate between stable angina and myocardial infarction. It is usually subdivided into new angina, suddenly worsening angina or rest angina. It is this group of patients who have often had sudden worsening of coronary narrowing by atherosclerotic plaque fissuring with the formation of a non-occlusive coronary thrombosis.

Diagnosis

Most patients have no physical signs, although some may have evidence of hyperlipidaemia or a fourth heart sound.

Electrocardiography Electrocardiography which can show virtually any abnormality is the technique most frequently used in the diagnosis of ischaemic heart disease. However ECG readings are normal in at least 50 per cent of patients with angina. If abnormal, there are often non-specific ST-segment and T-wave changes and some patients may have evidence of previous infarction. Typical ST-segment changes are discussed below; T waves may be increased, flattened or inverted (Figs. 1.3, 1.4 and 1.5).

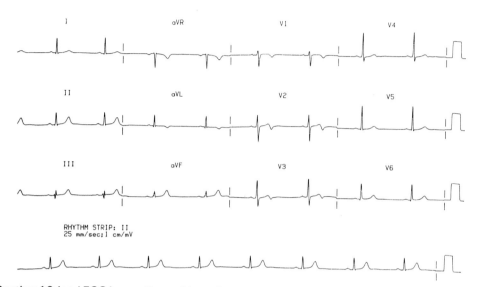

Fig 1.3 Resting 12-lead ECG in a patient with angina caused by severe proximal left coronary disease. The T-waves are biphasic in V2 and V3.

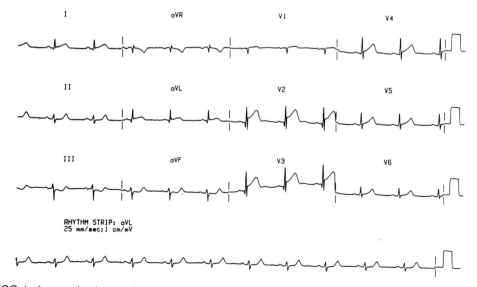

Fig 1.4 ECG during angina in a patient with severe narrowing of the left main coronary artery. There is antero-septal ST-segment elevation.

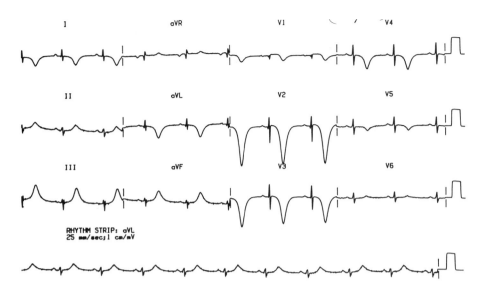

Fig 1.5   Same patient, a few days later, with further angina. There is sharp T-wave inversion. The patient did not have a myocardial infarction, and the ECG returned to normal later.

Exercise testing   Graded maximal exercise testing with a treadmill or bicycle is widely used in the diagnosis of coronary artery disease and in the assessment of its severity. As with all diagnostic tests the usefulness of exercise testing depends on the population being studied. The sensitivity of an exercise test (number of positive tests in those with the disease) is above 75 per cent and the specificity (the number of negative tests in those without the disease) is about 90 per cent. It is therefore not

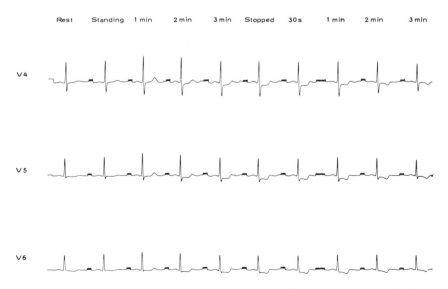

Fig 1.6   Computer processed tracings from leads V4, V5 and V6 before, during and after exercise testing. There is progressively increasing ST-segment depression and T-wave inversion.

helpful in screening asymptomatic patients in whom there is a low incidence of disease.

Many clinical observations are made during exercise testing in an attempt to identify high risk patients: those with triple vessel disease or left main stem disease. In such patients the ST segment depression may occur early, be marked and widespread and may continue for a prolonged time into recovery. There may also be early angina, a fall in systolic blood pressure, a poor heart rate rise and poor exercise duration (Fig. 1.6).

Nuclear imaging Thallium is an isotope taken up by myocardial cells proportional to the blood supply. A 'cold area' is therefore seen after infarction, and when on exercise, decreased perfusion can be detected during myocardial ischaemia. It has a slightly higher sensitivity than exercise testing and is particularly useful when there is an underlying ECG abnormality such as left bundle branch block.

Radionuclide ventriculography is a technique to assess ventricular function. Blood is labelled radioactively and the heart is imaged so that it is in a series of 'gates' in the cardiac cycle. A decrease in contraction, shown by a fall in ejection fraction or abnormal wall motion on exercise has a high sensitivity for coronary artery disease but low specificity.

Treatment

Certain precautions must be taken which are important: smoking must be stopped, weight must be lost, hyperlipidaemia and hypertension treated and anaemia avoided.

Drug treatment

Nitrates These are powerful and useful drugs for the treatment of angina. They relax vascular smooth muscle and produce their effect by two main modes of action. Firstly, venodilatation which causes pooling of blood in the peripheral veins with a consequent reduced venous return. This leads to a reduced left ventricular volume and therefore reduced oxygen demand. They also cause coronary dilatation at both the site of the stenosis and elsewhere and therefore increase oxygen supply. Larger doses cause arteriolar dilatation which can reduce myocardial work. Tolerance develops quickly with sustained use of any preparation. Glyceryl trinitrate sublingually, by tablet or spray, is still the best way of using nitrates (for brief prophylaxis and treatment) though glyceryl

trinitrate tablets deteriorate quickly with moisture and light (less than 8 weeks shelf-life). Various long acting preparations are used by mouth (isosorbide dinitrate or mononitrate) or transdermally but a nitrate-free period is needed to avoid tolerance. Intravenous preparations are widely used in unstable angina and can be used intraoperatively (1–10 mg/hour of isosorbide dinitrate).

Beta-adrenoceptor blocking drugs Beta-blockers are the cornerstone of treatment and because they improve survival after myocardial infarction they are widely used. They work by reducing myocardial oxygen demand on exercise – reducing heart rate, blood pressure and contractility. In patients with predominant coronary spasm they can aggravate the condition because of unopposed alpha-tone. They are contra-indicated in patients with asthma, left ventricular failure, severe bradycardia or peripheral vascular disease and metabolic acidosis. Several preparations are shown in Table 1.2. Cardioselective drugs competitively inhibit beta-1 receptors of the heart but not beta-2 receptors of bronchial or vascular smooth muscle. Drugs with intrinsic sympathomimetic activity (ISA) cause a slightly faster heart rate and may not be quite so effective in patients with angina. A typical dose for angina is propranolol 80 mg b.d., altenolol 100 mg o.d. or metoprolol 100 mg t.d.s.

Table 1.2 Classification of beta-blockers (ISA = intrinsic sympathomimetic activity)

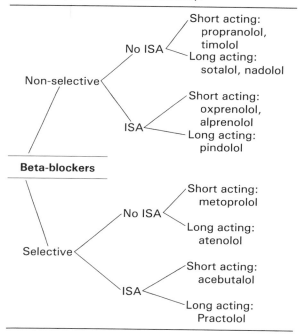

Calcium channel blocking drugs   Calcium ions are essential for the genesis of the cardiac action potential and for myocardial and smooth muscle contraction. Calcium antagonists interfere with the influx of calcium ions into cells in cardiac and smooth muscle and the AV node. In angina they work by reducing myocardial oxygen demand lowering the blood pressure by vasodilation, reducing the heart rate and reducing contractility (they can therefore worsen cardiac failure). They also increase oxygen supply by coronary artery dilatation. However, they can increase demand by two mechanisms and therefore worsen angina; they may cause tachycardia as a reflex sympathetic response to hypotension, and they can reduce oxygen supply by a coronary steal mechanism.

Three drugs are widely used. Verapamil, which has a powerful effect on AV nodal conduction and the SA node. This makes it useful in some arrhythmias and when used as the sole treatment for angina (120 mg t.d.s.). Nifedipine has no effect on the conduction system and is particularly useful in combination with a beta-blocker. The dose in the elderly is 5 mg t.d.s. increasing to 20 mg t.d.s. Diltiazem is in some ways intermediate between the two preceding drugs.

Perioperative drugs   Beta-blockers should be continued, preferably in a long-acting preparation, orally, on the morning of the operation. If the patient is unable to swallow after 24 hours the drug can be given by naso-gastric tube or propranolol or metoprolol given intravenously 6-hourly (for dose *see* acute lowering of blood pressure, p. 33). Nitrates can be continued transdermally or given intravenously.

Coronary angioplasty   Ten to fifteen per cent of patients who have coronary angiography for ischaemic heart disease are suitable for the technique of percutaneous transluminal coronary angioplasty. Discrete atherosclerotic plaques can be compressed and disrupted by the balloon catheter. Complications are inversely related to experience; mortality is about 1 per cent, myocardial infarct rate about 3 per cent and approximately 30 per cent of patients develop re-stenosis in the short term.

Surgery   Coronary artery bypass grafting using saphenous veins or the internal mammary artery has two objectives; to relieve angina and prolong life. For relief of angina it is undoubtedly effective with up to 90 per cent of patients being symptom-free after one year with an operative mortality of 1–3 per cent. Because of such success it should be offered to patients in whom medical treatment has failed and whose lifestyle is limited by angina. Saphenous vein grafts have a fairly high rate of occlusion (2 per cent a year increasing to 5 per cent) so that after 10 years, 30–50 per cent will have angina from graft occlusion or native vessel progression.

The main debate is whether life is prolonged in patients with less severe angina. From large studies the evidence favours surgery in patients with left main stem disease, triple vessel disease, proximal left coronary disease and in certain other subgroups such as those with left ventricular dysfunction (Julian, 1985). Medical treatment is improving all the time and the annual mortality from angina is now 2–3 per cent.

Myocardial infarction

Pathology

Myocardial infarction is caused by prolonged interruption of the blood flow to the myocardium. In two-thirds of patients the infarct is transmural ('Q wave infarct'), usually with total thrombotic occlusion of the related coronary artery. The remainder are subendocardial infarcts ('non-Q wave infarcts') in which there is less myocardial necrosis and a lower incidence of complete occlusion or there may be complete occlusion with a collateral circulation. Both these infarcts are *regional* – involving one segment of the LV; by contrast there may be *diffuse* infarction involving the subendocardial zone of the whole circumference of the left ventricle. This can occur when there is a fall in myocardial perfusion, for example, in cardiogenic shock, postoperatively, after cardiac arrest, or in patients with aortic stenosis.

Symptoms

The chest pain is usually typical although approximately one-third of myocardial infarcts are silent and found only when electrocardiography is carried out later. In fact, half the myocardial infarcts are truly silent, the other half possessing some atypical features which are not always recognized. Other presentations include cardiac failure, angina, embolism or sudden confusion.

Diagnosis

This normally requires a typical history, sequential electrocardiographic change and raised cardiac enzymes. There are no perfect criteria but the definitions proposed by the Nottingham group are helpful (Rowley and Hampton, 1981):

- *Definite myocardial infarction*: typical history, Q waves and/or sequential ST segment and T wave changes plus a rise in cardiac enzymes to more than twice the upper limit of normal (or necropsy evidence).
- *Probable myocardial infarction*: history plus either ECG or enzymes as above.
- *Possible myocardial infarction*: typical history with abnormal electrocardiogram not characteristic of myocardial infarction and a rise in cardiac enzymes less than twice the upper limit of normal.
- *Chest pain query cause*: a useful sub-group of patients admitted with chest pain who have normal ECGs and enzymes and in whom no firm diagnosis is made.

Electrocardiography Some change is always seen in serial electrocardiograms but is dependent not only on the extent and position of the infarction but also its age, the presence of conduction defects, drugs, electrolytes and pericarditis.

The typical sequential change is firstly an increase in the T wave which is peaked or sometimes inverted. During the first 24 hours there is ST segment elevation accompanied by the development of abnormal Q waves or loss of the normal R waves. The ST and T changes can revert to normal over a month (Figs. 1.7–1.10). A Q wave is abnormal in leads 1, 2, AVF if greater than 0.04 seconds, greater than 2 mm and greater than 25 per cent of the following R wave. In the left precordial leads (from V3) a Q wave is abnormal if greater than 0.04 seconds, 2 mm or greater than 15 per cent of the R wave. A Q wave in lead 3 may be normal but is considered to be pathological if it is associated with an abnormal Q wave in lead 2 or AVF. Subendocardial infarction usually produces widespread and persistent ST depression and T-wave abnormalities. However, there can be Q waves in a subendocardial infarct and Q waves may be absent in patients who have transmural infarcts (hence the increasing use of the terms 'Q wave' and 'non-Q wave infarction').

The recognition of a previous infarct is important. Abnormal Q waves can disappear in about one-third of patients after 18 months. There are other causes of anterior Q waves than a previous

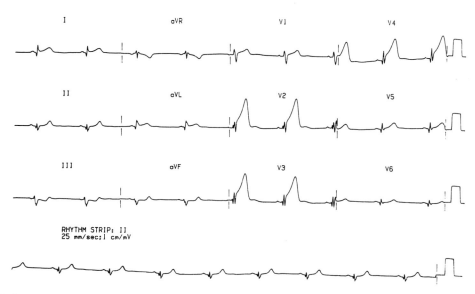

Fig 1.7 Early acute anterior myocardial infarction. There is ST-segment elevation in V2–V4, with increased height of the T-waves. A small Q-wave is seen anteriorly.

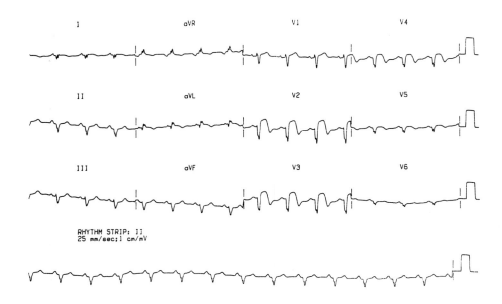

Fig 1.8   Extensive acute anterior infarction – the same patient 2 days later showing sequential changes, and left axis deviation.

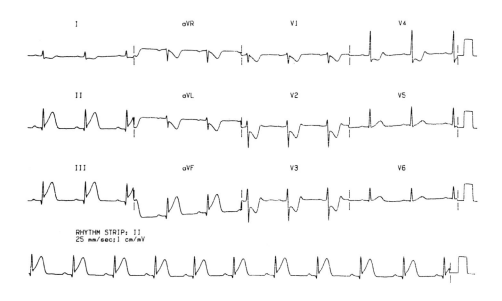

Fig 1.9   Early acute inferior infarction. There is 'reciprocal' ST-segment depression in V2–V4.

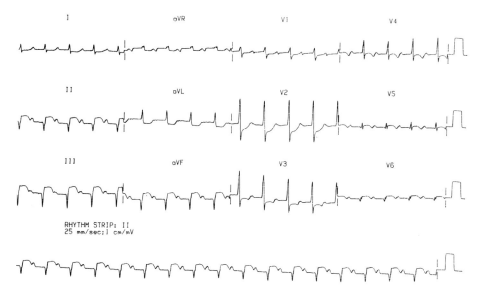

Fig 1.10   Acute infero- postero-lateral infarction. There are classical ECG changes inferiorly and laterally and R > S wave in V1. There is also first degree AV block.

infarct, for example, left ventricular hypertrophy, left bundle branch block, Wolff–Parkinson–White syndrome, and in cardiomyopathies. Poor R-wave progression (failure of the normal rise in R wave voltage across the V leads), may be a sign of an old anterior infarct (Fig. 1.11). However, it may also be due to a normal variant, occurs in cardio-myopathies (Fig. 1.12) or other diffuse muscle disease, left or right ventricular hypertrophy and emphysema.

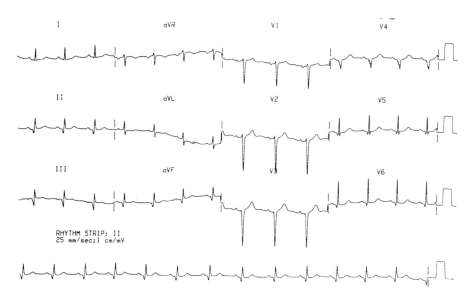

Fig 1.11   12-lead ECG in a 45-year-old man, 2 years after inferior and anterior infarction (with documented occlusion of the right and left coronary arteries). There are abnormal Q-waves in both territories.

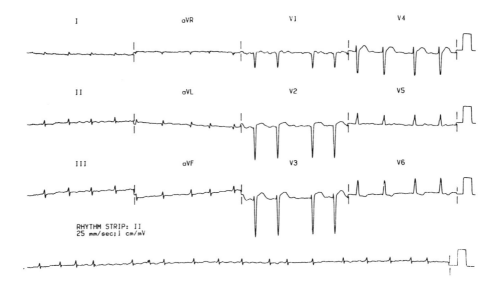

Fig 1.12 ECG in a young patient with severe end-stage dilated cardiomyopathy. There is low limb-lead voltage and poor R-wave progression in the V-leads. Note atrial fibrillation and non-specific ST depression.

Cardiac enzymes Enzymes diffuse through the membranes of damaged cells so that nearly all patients with myocardial infarction have a detectable rise in enzyme activity. The test is therefore very sensitive for myocardial necrosis but there is a lack of specificity leading to false positives in suspected myocardial infarction. There is a lag phase after infarction with a peak proportional to the extent of myocardial necrosis. The time course varies but by 12 hours all cases should have a rise (Fig. 1.13 and Table 1.3).

Table 1.3 Time-course of plasma enzyme-activity after myocardial infarction

Enzyme	Onset of rise (h)	Peak activity (h)	Duration of rise (days)
CK-MB	3–8	16–24	1–4
Total CK	4–8	18–36	3–4
AST	4–8	18–36	3–4
LDH	6–12	48–96	7–14

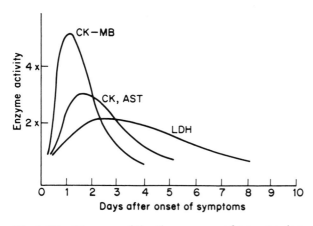

Fig 1.13 Diagram of the time course of enzyme rise after myocardial infarction.

- *Aspartate transferase (AST)* This is present in liver, myocardium, skeletal muscle and kidney. Disease of these organs will all cause a false positive.
- *Lactate dehydrogenase (LDH)* Present in heart, liver, skeletal muscle, kidney, red blood cells and neoplastic tissue, so LDH is raised in disease of many systems – and in haemolyzed blood samples. Isoenzymes are used but are not truly heart-specific.
- *Creatine kinase (CK)* This is present in high concentration in skeletal muscle and in cardiac muscle, brain, thyroid, kidney, gut and other tissues. Many muscle diseases can cause an elevation – intramuscular injections, convulsions, vigorous exercise or alcohol intoxica-

tion. Suxamethonium, especially with halothane, may cause a rise, also cardioversion (a small increase proportional to the energy used and due to skeletal muscle injury), external cardiac massage (may be a large rise in CK) and hypothyroidism. The advantage over AST is that it is normal in heart failure and hepatic disease.

- *Creatine Kinase-MB* This isoenzyme is virtually heart-specific but is more difficult to measure; it is particularly useful post-operatively.

Other specific causes of increased enzyme activity include pulmonary embolism (rise in LDH but only AST if there is cardiac failure) and surgery. In this there is a variable increase in CK, AST and LDH proportional to the skeletal muscle damage. Trauma, coma, drug overdose and hypothermia can all increase enzyme levels.

Treatment

The basis of treatment is careful monitoring and treatment of complications – arrhythmias or cardiac failure. Some of these are considered later. The use of thrombolytic drugs in the early stage is rapidly becoming accepted, with other measures to try and reduce infarct size.

Prognosis

The highest mortality occurs before patients receive medical care – in community studies 25 out of 100 patients with a heart attack (sudden death or myocardial infarct) die without medical attention. The hospital mortality of myocardial infarction is 15–18 per cent, but is about 25 per cent for perioperative infarction. Mortality in patients over 65 years is nearer 30 per cent. After leaving hospital 10–15 per cent of patients will die in the first year, mainly within a few months. The main determinant of survival is the extent of left ventricular damage – more important than the number of diseased coronary arteries. After one year the mortality is about 5 per cent per year.

True left ventricular aneurysms, localized protrusions of the LV walls, are found in about 5 per cent of patients. They may be complicated by cardiac failure, ventricular tachycardia or embolism. When aneurysms are defined on ventriculography as an akinetic (no movement) or dyskinetic (paradoxical movement) segment of LV, they are common.

Sudden death

This is defined as death within 15 minutes of presentation. Most patients have severe, widespread coronary disease and careful studies show an underlying plaque fissure and thrombus. Death is from ventricular fibrillation secondary to myocardial ischaemia.

Valvular heart disease

Valve disease remains a common problem. It is no longer good enough to label a patient with a possible diagnosis; it is usually essential to specify this and assess its severity and importance. Many patients will need a cardiological opinion and this may be followed by echocardiography or Doppler ultrasound for accurate evaluation. With an ageing population aortic stenosis is the commonest and most difficult to assess.

Mitral stenosis

Usually caused by rheumatic fever, the valve progressively narrows and invariably produces breathlessness from the high left atrial pressure and then fatigue from a low cardiac output. It can usually be recognized from the classical physical sign of a rumbling mid-diastolic murmur, with a loud first sound and opening snap in younger patients without valve calcification. The murmur may be inaudible when the cardiac output falls or when the heart rate is fast. Pulmonary oedema can be precipitated by atrial fribillation, pregnancy, infection, exercise or anaesthesia – the latter by fluid overload or perioperative tachycardia. A high left atrial pressure is required to maintain the cardiac output, so patients are more sensitive to overdiuresis. Some patients present with systemic emboli, a reminder of the importance of anticoagulation. The differential diagnosis includes left atrial myxoma and atrial septal defect. The initial treatment is with diuretics but surgery may be needed in patients with moderate symptoms and a small valve area shown by echocardiography or Doppler ultrasound. These non-invasive techniques can accurately quantify the severity, and should be carried out in all patients.

Mitral regurgitation

There are numerous aetiologies, reflecting the relative complexity of the mitral valve apparatus. This has five main components – the annulus, leaflets, chordae tendineae, papillary muscles and ventricular wall. Mitral regurgitation is a common finding in ischaemic heart disease because of papillary muscle necrosis secondary to infarction, rupture of part of a papillary muscle (rupture of the whole papillary muscle is severe and usually fatal) or secondary to dilatation of the left ventricle.

Mitral valve prolapse is a condition in which one or more of the mitral valve leaflets prolapses into the left atrium in systole. It can be primary or secondary. In primary mitral valve prolapse (floppy mitral valve) there is myxomatous transformation of the valve which becomes redundant and the chordae become attenuated. This can occur in Marfan's syndrome and other related connective tissue disorders. Secondary mitral valve prolapse can occur with any disease of the mitral valve apparatus. The normal mitral valve shows mild bulging in systole and this had led to over diagnosis of the condition by echocardiography. Patients with a floppy mitral valve may be asymptomatic or develop paroxysmal tachycardia or atypical chest pain. They are usually of slender build, often with pectus excavatum or a straight back. On auscultation there is a mid-systolic click and late systolic murmur. The condition is usually benign but some patients develop progressively severe mitral regurgitation or chordal rupture and there is a risk of infective endocarditis, embolism and ventricular arrhythmias.

In chronic mitral regurgitation the left atrium becomes huge and thin with increased compliance; it can therefore contain a large volume of regurgitant blood without a rise in pressure and without breathlessness. The left ventricle can tolerate this volume overload for years until it begins to fail. In many patients, symptoms of breathlessness then increase with increasing severity of regurgitation – although breathlessness can be replaced by fatigue. There may be a hyperdynamic apical impulse but the loudness of the pansystolic murmur does not always correlate with the severity of regurgitation. A third heart sound is usually heard with significant mitral regurgitation. In acute mitral regurgitation, occurring from chordal rupture, there can be dramatic pulmonary oedema and only a short systolic murmur.

Aortic stenosis

The commonest cause of aortic stenosis is premature calcification of a congenitally bicuspid aortic valve. Other origins may be rheumatic or from calcification of a normal valve in the elderly but these occur less frequently. There are also several congenital varieties – valvar, supravalvar or subaortic.

As the valve narrows there is progressive concentric left ventricular hypertrophy, increasing LV systolic pressure and maintaining the cardiac output. Symptoms occur late in the course of the disease and include angina, breathlessness, syncope or sudden death. In some aortic stenosis the cardiac output may fail to increase with exercise or surgical stress. Patients are very sensitive to hypovolaemia or vasodilatation. Syncope on exercise is probably due to stimulation of the LV baroreceptors by the high pressure, causing sudden, severe arterial and venous hypotension. The typical signs are a slowly rising pulse and narrow pulse pressure, a heaving or sustained left ventricular impulse and a long harsh systolic murmur in the aortic area. However, it cannot be emphasized enough that these are all difficult to assess, especially in older patients. The pulse characteristic invariably overlaps the normal, the murmur may be quieter in the aortic area than the mitral area where it may mimic mitral regurgitation and as cardiac failure develops the murmur becomes quieter. Even experienced clinicians can have difficulty separating aortic stenosis from mitral regurgitation by the character of the murmur alone.

The electrocardiogram usually shows left ventricular hypertrophy with ST and T changes – although it may be normal in significant aortic stenosis. The chest radiograph shows a normal heart size, often with a left ventricular contour, and there is usually poststenotic dilatation of the ascending aorta. Over the age of 55 years the valve is calcified in all patients with significant aortic stenosis, and this can usually be seen on a lateral film.

Patients with suspected aortic stenosis need careful assessment – perhaps more so than with any other valve disease. The severity is so often underestimated by physicians that patients presenting with 'terminal' cardiac failure are not uncommon. Echocardiography and Doppler ultrasound should be used with a low threshold and have dramatically improved the objective assessment of severity, so that cardiac catheterization is not often needed. The prognosis is usually less than 3 years in patients with symptoms.

Aortic regurgitation

The commonest cause is aortic root dilatation (or annulo-aortic ectasia) in which the histological abnormality is similar to that of Marfan's syndrome. In this condition there is progressive dilatation of the ascending aorta sometimes dramatically altered by dissection. Other causes are bicuspid aortic valve (often associated with some aortic root dilatation), rheumatic heart disease, 'floppy' aortic valve, trauma and inflammatory aortic root disease (syphilis, ankylosing spondylitis and Reiter's syndrome). The combination of aortic stenosis with aortic regurgitation is usually rheumatic and less often calcific.

Moderate aortic regurgitation may be tolerated for years so patients are usually asymptomatic until there is left ventricular failure – which may arise late. The patients then have breathlessness or chest pain may occur. Signs of chronic aortic regurgitation are fairly classical; a wide pulse pressure, hyperdynamic left ventricular impulse, long blowing early diastolic murmur and a systolic flow murmur from the increased stroke volume in all patients with significant regurgitation. There is left ventricular hypertrophy on the ECG and a large heart on chest radiography. In acute aortic regurgitation – commonly from endocarditis – there are none of these signs. The patients may present severely ill with cardiac failure or a shock-like state with a low cardiac output and a quiet diastolic murmur. The treatment is emergency valve replacement.

Prosthetic valve

These are, with examples:

Biological:	homograft	(cadaver aortic valve)
	heterograft	(porcine, e.g. Carpentier–Edwards)
		(pericardial, e.g. Ionescu–Shiley)
Mechanical:	ball-and-cage	(Starr–Edwards)
	tilting disc	(Bjork–Shiley)
	bileaflet	(St Jude)

Prosthetic valves have different properties which suit patients of particular ages. The smaller ones are all relatively stenotic, mechanical valves have a distinct risk of thromboembolism (5/100 patient years) and biological valves may fail after a period of 10 years. All patients with mechanical valves need long-term anticoagulation. If a patient with a prosthetic valve develops cardiac symptoms then it is useful to remember that the valve itself is a likely source of the problem – mechanical failure, thrombosis or endocarditis.

Congenital heart disease

The incidence is 8/1000 live births, and eight lesions account for 80 per cent of the abnormalities. The approximate incidence for infants and children is:

Ventricular septal defect (VSD)	20 %
Patent duct arteriosus (PDA)	15 %
Atrial septal defect (ASD)	10 %
Pulmonary stenosis (PS)	10 %
Tetralogy of Fallot	10 %
Coarctation of the aorta	5 %
Aortic stenosis	5 %
Transposition of the great arteries	5 %

Other abnormalities such as truncus arteriosus, tricuspid atresia, total anomalous pulmonary venous drainage and Ebstein's anomaly are rare. The commonest congenital heart disease is the bicuspid aortic valve which may affect up to 2 per cent of the population. It is only included when it causes aortic stenosis because it usually functions normally until late adult life.

It is not possible to review congenital heart disease in any detail here. Most patients will be under the care of paediatricians or cardiologists. It is important to know that each individual lesion may be of any severity and can improve or deteriorate with time, that is the lesions are variable and dynamic. Three specific neonatal problems are those of cardiac failure (caused, for example, by hypoplastic left heart or coarctation), cyanosis (e.g. transposition or severe Fallot) and patent ductus of prematurity. In the latter, the ductus can be closed pharmacologically with indomethacin (an inhibitor of prostaglandin synthesis) or surgically. Conversely in cyanotic neonates, whose pulmonary flow is dependent on a patent ductus, the ductus can be temporarily kept open with a prostaglandin.

Adult congenital heart disease

The commonest lesions seen in adulthood are ASD, VSD, PDA, PS and coarctation. ASD may present late because the auscultatory findings of a quiet systolic murmur are thought to be insignificant and the fixed splitting of the second sound is missed. The ECG shows partial right bundle branch block and the chest X-ray may show cardiomegaly and pulmonary plethora (often misreported as left ventricular failure or obstructive airways disease). A number of patients will present in middle age with symptoms of heart failure or arrhythmias. There is no risk of endocarditis from an atrial septal defect unless it is associated with mitral regurgitation. Small VSDs have a loud murmur and the only risk is from endocarditis. Large defects may cause heart failure in childhood and may cause pulmonary hypertension. Coarctation of the aorta sometimes presents in adults at a routine examination, or with hypertension, associated aortic valve disease or endocarditis. The blood pressure is usually raised, the femoral arterial pulses delayed or absent, there is a systolic murmur, palpable collaterals and chest radiograph shows an abnormal aorta and rib notching.

Cyanotic heart disease can be classified on the basis of the pulmonary blood flow – increased or not, and on the presence or absence of pulmonary hypertension. Certain features are also usually recognizable clinically.

Diminished pulmonary blood flow without pulmonary hypertension is most often caused by the tetralogy of Fallot (including pulmonary atresia). More rarely there may be obstruction at the tricuspid level in which case the electrocardiogram shows the unusual appearance of left ventricular hypertrophy. Diminished pulmonary blood flow with pulmonary hypertension is the finding in Eisenmenger syndrome in which, there is reversal of a previous left to right shunt (at any level) from severe pulmonary hypertension. Some aspects of pulmonary hypertension are considered later.

Patients with increased pulmonary blood flow have a form of anatomical or functional common chamber (such as transposition or a single ventricle). These patients do have specific surgical risks. Patients with secondary polycythaemia are at risk of postoperative haemorrhage or thrombosis and need venesection with volume replacement if the haemoglobin is over 20 g/dl. Fluid replacement is important during surgery because of the risk of deterioration in renal function. There are risks of endocarditis and paradoxical emboli (including air) and patients with right ventricular outflow obstruction (e.g. tetralogy) will become worse when there is systemic hypotension because this increases the right to left shunting. Stressful situations may also increase the degree of pulmonary stenosis which is often muscular. Severe hypoxic spells in children with a tetralogy are treated with oxygen, morphine, propranolol and sodium bicarbonate.

After total correction or palliative surgery many patients will have abnormal signs and present a new type of disease. Residual mitral regurgitation and paroxysmal atrial arrhythmias are common in older patients after atrial septal defect repair, and hypertension is common after coarctation resection. Residual aortic stenosis is common after aortic valvotomy as is pulmonary stenosis (and trivial pulmonary regurgitation) after pulmonary valvotomy. After correction of tetralogy of Fallot patients may have a residual ventricular septal defect or pulmonary stenosis. There are specific problems with certain operations; after a Mustard operation (intra-atrial baffle) for transposition, patients may develop right ventricular failure, caval obstruction or arrhythmias.

Pregnancy and heart disease

The haemodynamic effects of pregnancy can be dangerous in patients with heart disease. The cardiac output increases by 30–45 per cent until after delivery, with higher peaks during labour. There is a risk of pulmonary oedema in patients with mitral stenosis, and also aortic stenosis. Patients with Marfan's syndrome are at increased risk of aortic dissection. The Eisenmenger syndrome and primary pulmonary hypertension are contraindications to pregnancy. In these the normal fall in peripheral vascular resistance during pregnancy can reduce the preload, the right ventricle can no longer maintain an output, and there is postural hypotension, right ventricular failure and cardiogenic shock.

Patients with mechanical prosthetic valves need to be anticoagulated; warfarin is teratogenic and can be replaced with subcutaneous heparin in the first trimester, and in the last month. On admission heparin is given by intravenous infusion. The favoured method of delivery is vaginal with forceps in the second stage under epidural analgesia. The heparin infusion is stopped and the epidural commenced when the whole blood clotting time and the activated partial thromboplastin time has returned to normal. However, the fall in vascular resistance from an epidural may be harmful in pulmonary hypertension, hypertrophic cardiomyopathy and aortic stenosis.

Infective endocarditis

Infective endocarditis is an illness caused by a microbial infection of a damaged or abnormal cardiac valve or endocardium. The terms 'acute' and 'subacute' are less often used because of their overlap.

Aetiology

The illness requires an abnormal or damaged valve, a platelet–fibrin thrombus, bacteraemia and the presence of agglutinating antibodies. In acute endocarditis, normal valves may be damaged by invasive organisms. In most patients the portal of entry is dental and less often the gastrointestinal or genitourinary tracts.

Clinical aspects

The disease occurs more commonly in men. There is no obvious source of infection in more than 50 per cent of cases and 50 per cent of patients have previously unrecognized heart disease. *Streptococcus viridans* is the commonest infective organism (approximately 50 per cent) and in about 20 per cent it is the *Staphylococcus*. The commonest underlying condition is a congenitally bicuspid aortic valve.

Patients present with manifestations of infection, embolic complications – including neurological, evidence of valve involvement and evidence of an immunological disorder – giving the peripheral stigmata of endocarditis. In right heart endocarditis, usually in illicit drug users, patients may have evidence of infection and an unusual pneumonia (which is embolic in origin). The diagnosis requires at least three sets of blood cultures within 24 hours and treatment requires collaboration between cardiologists and microbiologists.

Prophylaxis of endocarditis

Antimicrobial drugs must be administered to susceptible patients when they are undergoing any procedure which may cause bacteraemia. Recommendations have been put forward by a working party of the British Society for Antimicrobial chemotherapy (BSAC) (Table 1.4).

Table 1.4 The BSAC recommendations for dental procedures

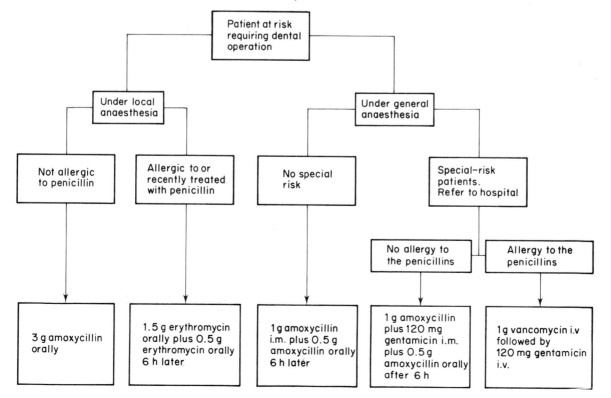

Intramuscular and intravenous antibiotics are given just before induction of anaesthesia; 1.0 g amoxycillin is given in 2.5 ml of 1 % lignocaine hydrochloride; vancomycin, for penicillin allergy, is infused over 60 minutes. For children under 10 years half the dose of amoxycillin and vancomycin is given and those under 5 years of age are given a quarter of the dose.

Special risk patients are:

- Those needing a general anaesthetic who have received penicillin more than twice in the previous month, have a prosthetic valve or who are allergic to penicillin.
- All patients with previous endocarditis.

The recommendations for other procedures are shown in Table 1.5.

Table 1.5   BSAC recommendations for other procedures

Procedure	Valve	Regimen (as in diagram)
Genito-urinary instrumentation	**Native** damaged or prosthetic	i.m. amoxycillin + gentamicin
Obstetric and gynaecological procedures (including IUCD insertion)	Prosthetic only	"
GI endoscopy, barium enema	Prosthetic only	"
Tonsillectomy/ adenoidectomy	**Native** damaged Prosthetic	i.m. amoxycillin two doses i.m. amoxycillin + gentamicin

It is difficult to cover all possibilities. Other procedures which may cause bacteraemia include surgical procedures on any infected tissue and sometimes with bronchoscopy and nasal intubation. Patients with prosthetic valves should certainly be taken very seriously because prosthetic endocarditis has a mortality of about 50 per cent.

Heart muscle disease

This is usually subdivided into those diseases of unknown aetiology – the cardiomyopathies (a pathophysiological classification) and certain specific heart muscle diseases (an aetiological classification).

Specific heart muscle disease

There are many diseases which affect heart muscle:

- Infection (viral, bacterial, protozoal).
- Metabolic/endocrine (thyroid, diabetic, nutritional deficiency, hypokalaemia).
- Connective tissue disease.
- Neuromuscular (muscular dystrophy, Friedreich's ataxia).
- Muscle toxins (ethanol, radiotherapy, antineoplastic drugs).
- Systemic disease (amyloid, sarcoid, haemochromatosis).

Most of these conditions are rare, but acute myocarditis may be common. It is usually caused by a viral infection and by the immune response to this infection. The clinical consequences are determined by the severity of the myocardial injury and therefore vary from being clinically asymptomatic to fulminating cardiac failure. Typically, patients with febrile illnesses have an inappropriate tachycardia, ST/T changes on the electrocardiogram, arrhythmias and a variable degree of cardiac failure. Most patients recover completely but some, an unknown number, progress to a dilated cardiomyopathy.

Cardiomyopathies

These are subdivided into three groups as shown in Fig. 1.14; hypertrophic, dilated and restrictive/obliterative.

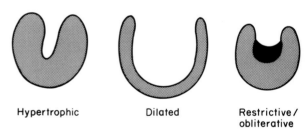

Hypertrophic   Dilated   Restrictive/ obliterative

Fig 1.14   The three pathophysiological types of cardiomyopathy.

Hypertrophic cardiomyopathy

This is an inherited disorder of unknown cause with usually gross hypertrophy of the left ventricle. This is either asymmetric – involving the septum – or concentric. It involves males more than females and half the patients have evidence of autosomal dominant inheritance.

Pathophysiologically there is good systolic function but the left ventricle is stiff and this leads to difficulty in filling in diastole (reduced compliance). Some groups have emphasized the importance of left ventricular outflow obstruction in systole but others think that this obstruction is mythical and unimportant. Patients need a high filling pressure and consequently hypovolaemia or vasodilation should be avoided.

The typical presentation is a young man with breathlessness (from the high left atrial pressure, secondary to the stiff left ventricle) angina (inadequate coronary flow from left ventricular hypertrophy), syncope (from ventricular tachycardia or low cardiac output) and palpitations. However the clinical symptoms can be quite variable. The main physical signs are of a late systolic murmur at the left sternal edge, a jerky pulse and a palpable presystolic left ventricular impulse. The electrocardiogram will show left ventricular hypertrophy and ST/T changes. The echocardiogram is diagnostic showing the hypertrophy with other features of the abnormal pathophysiology. It is important to maintain high index of suspicion of this disease which is potentially very serious. The differential diagnosis is usually from aortic stenosis, mitral regurgitation or a VSD (or sometimes just an athletic heart).

The prognosis is variable and though many patients remain unchanged after a long period of time about 25 per cent develop progressively severe symptoms. Death is often sudden. The symptoms can be relieved with beta-blockers and ventricular tachycardia may be treated with amiodarone, but thorough cardiological assessment is required.

Dilated cardiomyopathy

In this condition, previously known as congestive cardiomyopathy, there is dilatation of the ventricles, and impaired systolic function. It is not rare and usually presents in middle age. Although by definition it is of unknown cause it is probably the end result of muscle damage from a variety of causes. For example about 20 per cent of patients have a history of excess alcohol consumption and 20 per cent have had a severe flu-like illness (with probable myocarditis).

Initially the disease is asymptomatic and patients may be detected because of a gallop rhythm, cardiomegaly or an abnormal electrocardiogram. However patients later develop manifestations of systolic pump failure: they become breathless, fatigued and have fluid retention. They may have arrhythmias, emboli or atypical chest pain.

The diagnosis is basically one of exclusion, that is, of ischaemic or hypertensive heart disease, valve disease especially aortic stenosis and other heart muscle or pericardial conditions. The prognosis is poor, and about 75 per cent of the patients will die within 2 years of presentation. Treatment is for heart failure and some patients will need cardiac transplantation.

Restrictive cardiomyopathy

This is a rare subgroup in which there is restriction to diastolic filling by endocardial or myocardial disease. Systolic function is normal. Later in the disease the ventricular cavities become obliterated by organic material. The usual cause is endomyocardial fibrosis subdivided into a tropical group, with little eosinophilia, and a temperate variety with considerable eosinophilia. These two conditions may really be the same (Loeffler's myocardial disease). The disease may also occur with eosinophilia from other causes.

Patients usually present with progressive right ventricular failure with little cardiac enlargement and a low voltage electrocardiogram. In this way they mimic amyloid disease or constrictive pericarditis.

Pericardial heart disease

Pericardial disease is often underdiagnosed and often asymptomatic.

Anatomically the pericardium is a flask-shaped sac enclosing the heart and roots of the great vessels. There are two sacs – an outer fibrous and inner serous, which has visceral and parietal layers. The visceral layer is the epicardium which covers the heart and vessels and is reflected back to line the outer fibrous layer as the parietal pericardium. The pericardial cavity is between these serous layers.

Acute pericarditis

This is a condition of inflammation of the pericardium from many causes:

- Idiopathic.

- Infective (viral, bacterial including tuberculosis and other).
- Myocardial infarction.
- Neoplastic (metastatic from breast, lung, lymphoma or leukaemia).
- Physical injury (radiation, trauma).
- Connective tissue disease (rheumatic fever, rheumatoid arthritis, systemic lupus, systemic sclerosis).
- Others.

A typical patient has sudden anterior chest pain, worse with inspiration and lying down and often associated with a characteristic creaking pericardial rub. The electrocardiogram shows widespread ST segment elevation.

Treatment is of the underlying disease; if there is associated myocarditis patients need bed rest. There is rarely pericardial tamponade. The natural history is usually self-limiting.

Pericardial effusion

This may occur with any cause of pericardial inflammation. Rapid accumulation of relatively small volumes (250 ml) can cause severe tamponade, but there may be slow accumulation of large volumes without a rise in pressure – dependent on the shape of the pericardial pressure–volume curve.

There may be no symptoms, or symptoms from compression of neighbouring organs or from tamponade.

Pericardial tamponade

In this condition the heart is compressed by excess fluid in the pericardial space. It may be acute or chronic, and is one of the most important, life threatening medical emergencies. It must be recognized clinically.

Acute tamponade characteristically causes an acute illness with progressively falling blood pressure and rising venous pressure, increase in heart rate and breathlessness. It may be necessary to sit patients up to see the high venous pressure. There is usually pulsus paradoxus and the heart sounds are quiet. The usual causes are neoplasm, trauma, idiopathic pericarditis, dissection of the aorta, infective pericarditis or uraemia. The differential diagnosis is that of cardiogenic shock. It may mimic pulmonary embolism, right ventricular myocardial infarction or even obstructive pulmonary disease.

Chronic tamponade may present with breathlessness, ascites and a high venous pressure.

Observation of the jugular venous pressure and arterial blood pressure is important. In tamponade the JVP is elevated; the y descent gradually disappears but inspiration is always associated with an increase in venous return and therefore a fall in venous pressure. Kussmaul's sign (*see* p. 21) is not seen.

Pulsus paradoxus is the exaggeration of the normal inspiratory decline in left ventricular stroke volume and system arterial pressure. It is present when there is a greater than 10 mmHg fall in systolic blood pressure with inspiration, as

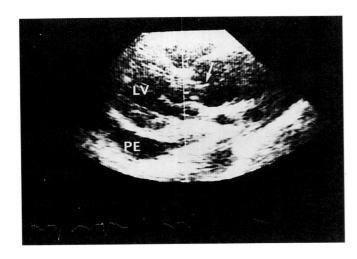

Fig 1.15 Two-dimensional echocardiogram showing a pericardial effusion (PE). (LV = left ventricle). The arrow points to an intimal flap inside an enlarged aortic root – the patients had an aortic dissection (*see* Fig. 1.17).

measured with a sphygmomanometer. During inspiration there is an increase in venous return with an expansion of the right ventricular stroke volume. This, with its associated increase in intra-pericardial pressure, shifts the interventricular septum toward the left ventricle, decreasing left ventricular stroke volume (which is already low). There are probably other factors involved in the pathophysiology of pulsus paradoxus. Paradoxus can also be seen in some patients with massive pulmonary embolus or hypovolaemic shock. In asthma there is an expiratory increase in blood pressure not a fall in pulse pressure.

The treatment of tamponade is pericardio-centesis, usually after confirmation of pericardial fluid by echocardiography (Fig. 1.15). The safest approach is sub-xiphoid.

Pericardiocentesis

Normally performed by cardiologists, it may be needed as an emergency. Haemodynamic support by volume replacement or inotropic drugs can be useful in the short-term. Many sites have been used but the simplest is the sub-xiphoid route which is extrapleural and avoids the coronary and internal mammary arteries. A 5–10 cm, 16–18 gauge needle and cannula is used (short needles for thin patients and long needles for fat patients). The thorax is elevated 25–45 degrees and using aseptic techniques the tissues are infiltrated with lignocaine. The needle, with syringe, is introduced in the angle between the xiphisternum and left ribs, pointed posterior to the rib cage and then advanced at about 45 degrees to the transverse plane aiming at the left shoulder (it is better to inadvertently punc-ture the left ventricle than the thin walled right atrium or right ventricle).

Constrictive pericarditis

In this condition cardiac filling is restricted by a fibrotic or calcified pericardium. It is usually idio-pathic but sometimes follows acute pericarditis or tuberculosis. Cardiac filling only occurs in early diastole and there is no increase in venous return. Hence Kussmaul's sign (an inspiratory increase in venous pressure) can occur but is difficult to detect clinically. The cardiac output is maintained by the high filling pressure (and tachycardia), so that diuretics, or other means of lowering this, such as anaesthesia, are dangerous.

Patients usually present with oedema, ascites and later have pulmonary congestion. There is a low voltage electrocardiogram and pericardial cal-cification may be seen radiologically.

The condition mimics restrictive cardiomyo-pathy although clinically it may be confused with SVC obstruction, liver disease, nephrotic syn-drome, abdominal neoplasm or right heart failure.

Diseases of the aorta

The ageing aorta

The normal aorta increases in length and width with age producing the characteristic 'unfolded' appearance on chest radiographs. The histology is similar to that in more severe forms of aortic dis-ease with elastic fragmentation, fibrosis and cystic medial necrosis.

Aortic aneurysms

Seventy five per cent of aortic aneurysms occur in the abdominal aorta below the renal arteries. They are a consequence of arteriosclerosis which leads to weakening of the aortic wall and they usually co-exist with widespread arteriosclerotic disease.

Thoracic aneurysms may be arteriosclerotic but more often show elastic fragmentation and cystic medial necrosis; 20 per cent of patients with thoracic aneurysms have Marfan's syndrome. They usually occur in the arch or descending aorta while ascending aneurysms may be syphilitic in origin. They present with pain or pressure on local structures, or they may be discovered on a chest radiograph. CT scanning or aortography are the best diagnostic techniques and surgery is con-sidered in patients with symptoms or enlarging aneurysms.

Aortic dissection

Aortic dissection is an acute condition with penetration of a column of blood through an inti-mal tear into the aortic wall. It is caused by a com-bination of hypertension and an abnormally weak aortic wall. Histologically there is cystic medial necrosis but this is not particularly widespread except in patients with Marfan's syndrome. At least 75 per cent of the patients have hypertension, many have extensive atheromatous disease and in a small group of patients there may be a bicuspid aortic valve, coincidental pregnancy or some traumatic procedure.

Classification

The DeBakey classification is shown in Fig. 1.16. In type I the dissection begins in the ascending aorta and extends beyond the arch, in type II it is confined to the arch and in type III it begins in the descending aorta, below the left subclavian artery, and extends distally and very rarely, retrogradely. In practical terms it is easier to classify dissections as either proximal or distal, these occuring in a ratio of 2:1.

Signs and symptoms

A typical patient is a 60-year-old man presenting with sudden, very severe chest pain which migrates or is also felt in the back of abdomen. There are vaso-vagal manifestations and patients may have cardiac failure from aortic regurgitation, syncope from pericardial rupture or profound neurological disturbance from occlusion of an aortic branch vessel. A useful feature is that the patient appears to be shocked but has a normal or high blood pressure.

Once the diagnosis has been thought of, a diagnostic technique is urgently required. Two-dimensional echocardiography can show proximal dissec-

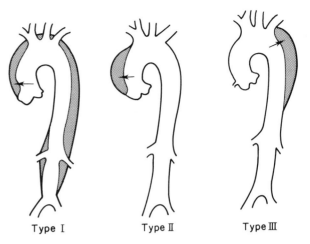

Type I   Type II   Type III

Fig 1.16   The three types of aortic dissection.

tions (*see* Fig. 1.15), computerized tomography (CT) is more accurate in demonstration (Fig. 1.17) and aortography may be needed to define the full extent and evaluate aortic regurgitation.

Urgent treatment is needed to lower the systolic blood pressure to 100–120 mmHg – usually with a combination of sodium nitroprusside and intravenous beta-blockade. The treatment is surgery for proximal dissection and medical for distal dissection unless there are complications.

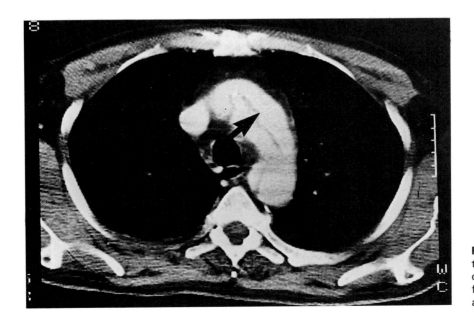

Fig 1.17   CT scan (contrast-enhanced) in aortic dissection. The intimal flap is seen in the aortic arch (arrow).

Thromboembolic disease

Pulmonary emboli break off from thrombi in veins of the pelvis, thighs or calf. They are common, often undiagnosed, potentially preventable and often fatal. The incidence is unknown but they are thought to occur in 1 in 20 of hospital in-patients. Ten per cent of patients with a pulmonary embolus will die.

Deep venous thrombosis (DVT)

The risk factors of DVT are age over 40, a previous DVT, malignancy, obesity, prolonged immobility, cardiac failure, varicose veins, the oral contraceptive, and certain forms of surgery. For example, after hip surgery under general anaesthesia the incidence is 50–80 per cent and after abdominal or thoracic surgery it is 20–30 per cent.

The physical signs are unreliable but include fever, local pain, swelling or oedema. However, 50 per cent have no signs and 50 per cent of patients who are thought to have a clinical DVT do not. Diagnosis is by I^{125} fibrinogen scanning, venous Doppler, plethysmography or venography 'the gold standard'. Treatment is with anticoagulation.

The evidence favours more widespread prophylaxis of DVT in high risk situations. Subcutaneous heparin is administered in 5000 units every 8 or 12 hours for 7–10 days. A higher dose may be needed in orthopaedic surgery – a dose large enough to keep the activated partial thromboplastin time (PTT) in the high–normal range.

Pulmonary embolism

It cannot be stressed enough that the clinical diagnosis of pulmonary embolism is very poor. In many patients it is found unexpectedly at post-mortem; on the other hand, pulmonary embolus may be clinically over diagnosed. In some large series up to 40 per cent of patients who have had a pulmonary angiogram for suspected pulmonary embolism do not have any evidence of this.

Typically there are three clinical syndromes:

• Pulmonary infarction.
• Acute breathlessness.
• Massive pulmonary embolus.

The so-called classic triad of pleural pain, breathlessness and haemoptysis occurs in less than 1 in 5 patients. However, the combination of breathlessness and tachypnoea is highly sensitive. A DVT is clinically diagnosed in less than half the patients and a small proportion have a pleural rub or wheeze.

Massive pulmonary embolus

The clinical features are collapse or syncope with chest pain, respiratory distress, hypotension, tachycardia and peripheral vasoconstriction and anxiety. There is often a right ventricular gallop, raised venous pressure and loud pulmonary second sound although these are difficult signs to detect. Patients may only be hypotensive when they sit or stand. ECG abnormalities are proportional to the severity of the embolus which produces its effect by mechanical obstruction and pulmonary vasoconstriction. Most patients with massive embolism will have some ECG change but with a sub-massive embolus only about 75 per cent will. The commonest findings are non-specific ST/T changes. About 25 per cent will have the classic findings of right axis deviation, right bundle branch block or an $S_1Q_3T_3$ pattern. The chest radiograph in massive pulmonary embolus may show oligaemia (or be remarkably normal in an ill, breathless patient). With smaller pulmonary emboli there may be lower lobe infiltrates, pleural effusions or a raised diaphragm.

Diagnosis

Ventilation–perfusion (V/Q) lung scanning is the most widely used technique. Perfusion scanning is carried out after intravenous injection of isotopically labelled macro-aggregated albumin particles and ventilation scanning after the inhalation of the gas krypton or xenon (Fig. 1.18). A normal perfusion scan rules out the diagnosis of pulmonary embolus but an abnormal scan is common in lung disease. Probability estimates rather than definite diagnoses must be made; multiple, segmental or lobar V/Q mismatches have a high probability of pulmonary emboli whereas small sub-segmental mismatches have a low probability of emboli. Pulmonary angiography is the 'gold standard' for diagnosis, but it needs experience in a catheter laboratory and in interpretation.

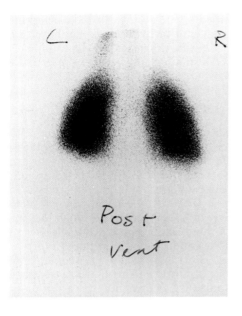 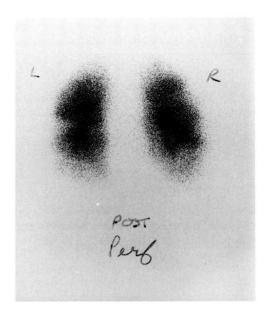

Fig 1.18   Lung scan in a patient with pulmonary emboli: showing (a) ventilation (normal) and (b) perfusion (multiple segmental defects).

Treatment

Patients with DVT and pulmonary embolus are anticoagulated. Patients with a massive embolus need emergency resuscitation often with cardiac massage. If the venous pressure is low then intravenous dextran can help, and intravenous inotropic drugs may be needed to support the acutely failing right ventricle. Fifteen thousand units of heparin are given intravenously and emergency pulmonary embolectomy considered for patients with a systolic blood pressure less than 90 mmHg, urine output less than 20 ml/hour and PO_2 less than 60 mmHg after one hour of maximal treatment.

Thrombolytic therapy with streptokinase, urokinase or tissue plasminogen activator have been used to lyse thrombi in the deep venous system and emboli in the pulmonary circulation. Although there is clinical improvement with these drugs they are expensive, have side-effects and have not been widely used.

Anticoagulant therapy

Heparin

Heparin combines with antithrombin III, a natural inhibitor of the clotting system. The complex inactivates thrombin and other clotting factors and prevents the conversion of fibrinogen to fibrin. Only a small dose of heparin is needed to prevent the initiation of thrombosis because of the amplification of the clotting cascade. A larger dose is needed to prevent clot extension or propagation. Heparin also reduces the effect of thrombin on platelets in pulmonary emboli therefore reducing vasoconstrictor and bronchoconstrictor substances. It has an immediate anticoagulant effect and a short half-life (90 minutes) but can be reversed with protamine.

To anticoagulate patients, 5000 units of heparin are given as an intravenous bolus then 40 000 units in 24 hours with a pump. The PTT can be monitored and maintained at 1.5 to 2.5 times the prepheparin control, mainly to make sure that enough heparin is given. The dose can then be adjusted in steps of 2500–5000 units/day if necessary.

Warfarin

Warfarin is an inhibitor of vitamin K which is required for the hepatic synthesis of a number of clotting factors. It reduces factor VII quickly, prolonging the prothrombin time (PT) before it has a significant anticoagulant effect. Because of this and an early reduction in protein C (a naturally occurring substance which limits thrombosis and initiates fibrinolysis), it is important to overlap treatment with warfarin and heparin for at least 5 days. The usual dose of warfarin is 10 mg/day for 3 days then 3–5 mg/day depending on the PT. This should be maintained at a ratio of 2.0–3.0, or 3.0–4.5 for recurrent emboli, arterial grafts or prosthetic valves. Treatment is usually continued for 3–6 months. The antidote to warfarin is fresh frozen plasma or vitamin K_1 (which acts more slowly and leads to refractoriness in re-anticoagulating). There is a long list of important drug interactions with warfarin antagonized by barbiturates or cholestyramine and potentiated by cimetidine, amiodarone, metronidazole or liver disease, for example.

Anticoagulants and surgery

Patients on long-term anticoagulants, in particular those with prosthetic valves, need careful management. A simple procedure is to stop warfarin 3 days before surgery and allow the PT to fall within 20 per cent of normal. The warfarin is restarted 2 days later. For patients at high risk of thromboembolism i.e., with mechanical valves in the mitral position, heparin (intermittent subcutaneous or intravenously) is used until 6 hours before operation and resumed 12 hours later.

Pulmonary hypertension

Pulmonary hypertension is defined as a pulmonary artery pressure greater than 30/15 mmHg or a mean of 20 mmHg (measured from mid chest).

The normal pulmonary circulation has a low resistance with a large reserve for high flow with little increase in pressure. There must therefore be a considerable reduction in the size of the vascular bed before significant pulmonary hypertension

develops. The pulmonary circulation is responsive to many factors and in particular vasoconstriction occurs with hypoxia, potentiated by acidosis and alpha-adrenergic agonists. Vasodilation may occur with beta-adrenergic agonists and prostacyclin. The thin-walled right ventricle behaves differently to the left ventricle. There is a sharp decrease in right ventricular stroke volume with only a small increase in pulmonary artery pressure. Also an increase in filling pressure has less effect on the right ventricle than the left.

Causes of pulmonary hypertension

Increased resistance to pulmonary venous drainage

This may be at three levels: the left ventricle, left atrium or pulmonary veins. The common causes are left ventricular failure and mitral valve disease but include constrictive pericarditis and the rare pulmonary veno-occlusive disease. In these conditions there is initially a passive increase in pulmonary artery pressure but later, especially in mitral stenosis, there may be reactive pulmonary vasoconstriction.

Increased resistance to flow through the pulmonary vascular bed in diseases with hypoxia

There are two important groups: disease of the lung parenchyma and airways (chronic obstructive airways disease or fibrosing diseases) and hypoventilation (neuromuscular, chest wall disease or

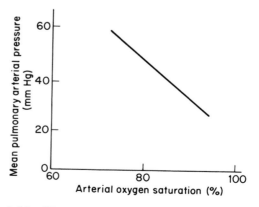

Fig 1.19 Diagram of the relation between the mean pulmonary artery pressure and arterial oxygen saturation in a patient with chronic obstructive pulmonary disease.

diseases with decreased ventilatory drive). In these pulmonary conditions the main factor causing pulmonary hypertension is hypoxic pulmonary vaso-constriction (Fig. 1.19). There are contributing factors from polycythaemia with increased viscosity, and from reduction in the size of the vascular bed – pulmonary hypertension becomes inevitable when more than half the vascular bed is destroyed.

Obstruction of the pulmonary vascular bed

The commonest cause is pulmonary thrombo-embolism; other diseases include parasitic disease, neoplasm and peripheral pulmonary stenosis.

Primary pulmonary hypertension (see below)

Increased pulmonary blood flow

When pulmonary blood flow from a large left-to-right shunt exceeds the reserve capacity, there will be a passive increase in pulmonary artery pressure. However there may be an additional increase in pulmonary resistance, either functional from vaso-constriction or fixed, with a similar histology to that of primary pulmonary hypertension. The latter may be partly a persistence of the normal fetal pattern of high resistance. Typically patients with large atrial septal defects develop pulmonary hypertension during their life while patients with ventricular septal defects have pulmonary hypertension from a young age.

Miscellaneous group

These include high-altitude exposure, intravenous drug abuse, haemoglobinopathies, drugs.

Primary pulmonary hypertension

In this condition there is no obvious cause; it is thought that the pulmonary arteries and arterioles are initially hyper-reactive to constrictive stimuli. There may be occult venous thrombosis with pulmonary emboli or *in situ* thrombosis, congenitally abnormal vessels or arteritis. The characteristic pathology is onion skin intimal thickening of the small vessels, thickening of the wall and plexiform lesions (proliferation of cells in dilated sacs).

The disease is commonest in women aged 20–30 years who present with exertional dyspnoea, syncope, chest pain or fatigue. The physical signs are usually more obvious than in other causes of pulmonary hypertension. There may be peripheral cyanosis, a prominent 'a' wave in the jugular venous pulse and characteristic auscultatory

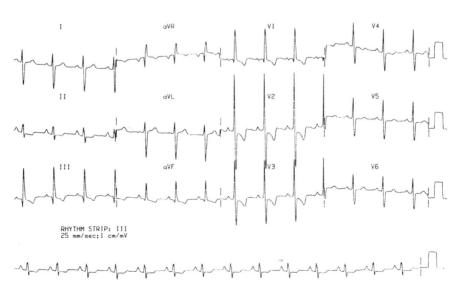

Fig 1.20   Electrocardiogram of a patient with primary pulmonary hypertension showing severe right ventricular hypertrophy.

findings (a fourth heart sound, ejection click, tricuspid regurgitation and loud pulmonary second sound). The ECG may show right atrial and right ventricular hypertrophy (Fig. 1.20) and the chest X-ray shows a large main pulmonary artery with pruning of the peripheral vessels. Differential diagnosis is from all other causes of pulmonary hypertension, especially mitral stenosis and multiple pulmonary emboli.

Some patients respond to vasodilator drugs (such as nifedipine or prostacyclin) but without heart/lung transplantation the average death occurs within 3 years of presentation. Patients may collapse suddenly for example during induction of anaesthesia or angiographic procedures. The mechanism for this collapse is not clear but it may be from further constriction of the pulmonary vascular bed with worsening right heart failure or arrhythmias, or sometimes from peripheral vasodilatation with a reduction in venous filling. All patients are anticoagulated because it is never possible to exclude thromboembolic disease.

Cor pulmonale (pulmonary heart disease)

This is defined as right heart disease (hypertrophy or dilatation), secondary to pulmonary hypertension caused by parenchymal lung or pulmonary vascular disease. Thus the causes are those of precapillary hypertension (not the first group above).

In most patients the respiratory symptoms outweigh those from the heart. Patients may develop oedema, ascites or a raised venous pressure. The most useful diagnostic findings arise from electrocardiography. There may be right atrial or right ventricular hypertrophy, right axis deviation, partial right bundle branch block and inverted T waves over the right praecordial leads.

Cardiac failure

Cardiac failure is traditionally defined as a state in which the heart fails to maintain an adequate cardiac output for the needs of the body, despite normal filling pressures. The term is generally used for a collection of symptoms and signs which may complicate any form of heart disease. The commonest cause is hypertensive heart disease, followed by coronary heart disease (or a combination of both). Less common causes are valve disease, cardiomyopathy, pericardial disease, arrhythmias and drugs (beta-blockers, calcium antagonists).

Pathophysiology

The cardiac output is the product of the heart rate and the stroke volume and the three determinants of stroke volume are the preload, afterload and contractility. In order to understand these relationships and how they may be altered in disease or by treatment, it is of considerable practical use to have a clear visual understanding of the basic framework of the mechanics of the pressure-volume loop of the ventricle.

In the normal cardiac cycle, when the mitral valve opens the left ventricle fills along the diastolic pressure–volume curve (Fig. 1.21(a) line 1). At the onset of systole, contraction begins; this is initially isovolumic (a rise in pressure but no change in volume, line 2) until the aortic valve opens. Blood is then ejected into the aorta (line 3) until the aortic valve closes. This is followed by isovolumic relaxation (line 4). The stroke volume is the horizontal distance of this loop, from end-diastole to end-systole.

If the preload is increased – that is the end-diastolic volume (which is mainly governed by the venous return and the blood volume with a contribution from atrial contraction), then the loop will enlarge to the right (Fig. 1.21b). If the ventricle

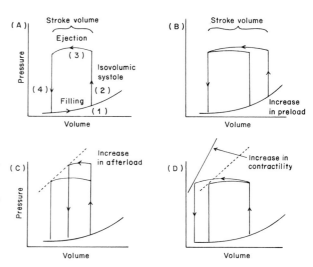

Fig 1.21   Four diagrams of pressure-volume loops of the left ventricle. (a) shows the four normal phases of the cardiac cycle, (b) shows the effect of an increase in preload, (c) an increase in afterload and (d) an increase in contractility (*see* text). The dotted line in (c) and (d) and the arrowed line in (d) is the isovolumic pressure line.

contracts to the same aortic pressure then the stroke volume will increase. This is the Frank–Starling law of the heart which states that 'the mechanical energy of contraction is dependent on the length of the muscle fibres'. It is limited by the steep slope which eventually leads to a high end-diastolic pressure transmitted back to the lungs; the critical pressure for pulmonary oedema is 24 mmHg. When the left ventricle is diseased it is stiffer (less compliant), and the slope is steeper. When there is a fall in preload (i.e. in fluid depletion) there is a fall in stroke volume.

If the afterload is increased then the stroke volume falls (Fig. 1.21c). Afterload, defined as the stress (force per unit area) in the ventricular wall during ejection, is largely determined by the arterial pressure and also by the size of the left ventricle (from Laplace's law). This effect is of greatest importance when there is reduced contractility and is the explanation for the beneficial effect of afterload reduction in the treatment of cardiac failure.

The third determinant of stroke volume is contractility, that is cardiac performance which is independent of preload or afterload. It is represented by the isovolumic pressure line seen in Fig. 1.21(d). This is the linear relationship of the maximum pressure that the ventricle can generate at any given end-diastolic volume and is a good measure of contractility. If the contractility is increased, the line is shifted up and to the left so that at any given end-diastolic volume and arterial pressure, stroke volume will increase.

Another widely used format which is based on the Frank–Starling mechanism, is the 'ventricular function curve'. This relates cardiac index (or some other measurement of cardiac performance such as stroke volume) to the preload which is most easily measured as the left ventricular end-diastolic pressure (Fig. 1.22). With increased contractility (i.e. with sympathomimetic drugs) the curve is shifted up to the left and in heart failure the curve moves to the right and becomes flatter.

When the cardiac output falls in disease two powerful neurohumeral mechanisms swing into action to try and maintain cardiac output and arterial pressure. The sympathetic nervous system is stimulated (from baroreceptors in the carotid sinus and aortic arch) and this causes tachycardia, increased contractility, venoconstriction, peripheral arterial vasoconstriction, renal sodium retention and stimulation of the renin–angiotensin system. The renin–angiotensin system is also stimulated directly and this causes fluid retention,

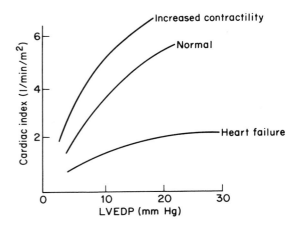

Fig 1.22 Left ventricular function curves – the relationship between cardiac index and preload (LVEDP, left ventricular end diastolic pressure).

peripheral vasoconstriction, stimulates ADH release and aldosterone production.

The fluid retention, partly a result of the body's attempt to increase the preload of the heart, eventually leads to peripheral oedema and then pulmonary oedema. The body's need to maintain arterial pressure for perfusion of vital organs can become harmful by the profound vasoconstriction.

These are acute changes seen in acute left ventricular failure or in shock states; the chronic response of the heart is to enlarge (and therefore increase the end-diastolic volume) and to hypertrophy (which reduces afterload).

The syndrome of congestive heart failure

The clinical manifestations of cardiac failure depend on the degree of pulmonary oedema, low cardiac output, fluid retention or ventricular dysfunction. If there is sudden onset, then there may be the shock-like state of massive myocardial infarction, pericardial tamponade or the slower development of classical congestive heart failure.

The first symptom is usually breathlessness on exercise (partly from the high end-diastolic pressure but also related to metabolic factors) and later orthopnoea, cough and paroxysmal nocturnal dyspnoea. If the cardiac output is low, patients will complain of fatigue, and in acute failure they are anxious or restless. There may be a gallop rhythm, raised venous pressure, evidence of a large left ventricle, oedema (which occurs after at least 4 litres of fluid have been retained), fine inspiratory crackles and later hepatomegaly and cardiac cachexia.

It cannot be stressed enough that a patient's symptoms of breathlessness or fatigue correlate poorly with the severity of left ventricular dysfunction, measured by echocardiography or nuclear methods. The careful elucidation of physical signs, study of electrocardiograms and chest radiographs may be needed to detect relatively asymptomatic patients with severe disease.

Treatment of heart failure

- Treat the cause – such as valve disease or hypertension.
- Treat the precipitating cause – such as infection, arrhythmia, anaemia or pulmonary emboli.
- Treat the overt manifestations of cardiac failure.

Diuretics

These reduce excess preload by a direct venodilating effect and by reducing the fluid overload through natriuresis and diuresis. The LVEDP is lowered below the level which causes pulmonary congestion (Fig. 1.23); because of the steep diastolic pressure–volume curve (*see* Fig. 1.21), a reduction in LV volume causes a greater reduction in pressure.

Thiazides are given for mild symptoms (*see* hypertension) and loop diuretics for more severe symptoms (frusemide 40–80 mg, rarely much

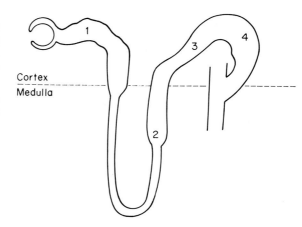

Fig 1.24 Sites of diuretic action in the kidney. 1 the proximal tubule (mannitol), 2 the ascending loop of Henle (frusemide), 3 the cortical diluting segment thiazides) and 4 the distal tubule (spironolactone, amiloride).

higher; bumetanide 1–2 mg (Fig. 1.24). The loop diuretics can be given intravenously for acute pulmonary oedema. Potassium-sparing diuretics can be useful (spironolactone 50–200 mg, amiloride 5–20 mg). Although diuretics reduce fluid retention and relieve breathlessness, they lower the stroke volume and too high a dose can severely reduce the cardiac output. Prolonged use may cause hypokalaemia or hyperuricaemia.

Vasodilators

Vasodilators are now well established in the treatment of moderate to severe heart failure. Nitrates reduce the preload as do diuretics, and there is an increasing earlier use in acute left ventricular failure. Drugs which reduce the afterload (such as hydralazine) will increase the cardiac output. Some drugs, such as angiotensin converting enzyme (ACE) inhibitors (*see* hypertension) have a combined effect on preload and afterload. This group of drugs produce a sustained haemodynamic and clinical improvement, producing vasodilatation by reducing angiotensin II dependent vasoconstriction. They also reduce angiotensin II stimulated thirst, ADH production and aldosterone fluid retention.

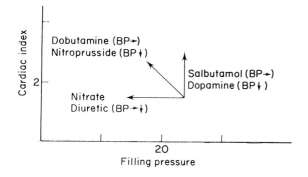

Fig 1.23 Diagram of the expected general effect of cardioactive drugs in heart failure (large arrows), based on studies in acute myocardial infarction. The small arrows in brackets give the likely directional change in sytemic arterial pressure.

Positive inotropic drugs

Digoxin Digoxin has a narrow therapeutic ratio (the relation between its clinical and toxic effects).

Its main use is to control atrial fibrillation. Although it does have an inotropic effect this is small and may not be worthwhile. Digoxin toxicity causes anorexia, fatigue, visual disturbance and confusion in the elderly. It may cause sinus bradycardia or atrioventricular block, ventricular extrasystoles or many other arrhythmias including atrial tachycardia with variable block. Toxicity is more likely in the presence of hypokalaemia or cardiac failure and digoxin levels may be increased by a number of drugs such as amiodarone or verapamil. Digoxin blood levels, measured 6 hours after a dose, can be helpful: if less than 1 ng/ml patients are not toxic but if greater than 3 ng/ml they are more likely to be.

Other inotropic drugs

These can be useful for short-term use in some acute situations to try and reverse the vicious circle of hypotension and poor coronary flow. However, they can increase myocardial ischaemia and cause cell damage and arrhythmias. They lose their effec-

Table 1.6 Classification of adrenergic receptors

Adrenergic receptor	Site	Action
Beta$_1$	Myocardium	Increased contractility
	SA node	Increased heart rate
	AV conduction	Enhanced conduction
Beta$_2$	Arterioles	Vasodilatation
	Lungs	Bronchodilation
Alpha	Peripheral arterioles	Vasoconstriction

receptors and more than 15 stimulates alpha receptors and can cause potentially harmful peripheral vasoconstriction.

Dobutamine Dobutamine is a synthetic beta$_1$ agonist with slight beta$_2$ properties. The latter vasodilator properties make it useful in patients with severe low output heart failure (*see* Fig. 1.23).

Table 1.7 Sympathomimetic drugs

Agent	Site			Dose	Indications
	α	B$_1$	B$_2$		
Adrenaline	+ +	+ +	+	0.5–1.0 mg	Cardiac arrest
Noradrenaline	+ +	+ +	0	1–20 μg/min	Need for vasoconstriction Superceded by dopamine
Isoprenaline	0	+ +	+ +	1–10 μg/min	AV block
Dopamine	+ +	+ +	*	0.5–5.0 μg/kg/min	Oliguric shock
Dobutamine	+	+ +	+	2.5–10.0 μg/kg/min	Cardiogenic shock

*specific vasodilator receptors

tiveness with continued administration by desensitizing the myocardial beta-adrenergic receptors; this has been found to occur in 'failing' hearts. The largest groups are sympathomimetic drugs which stimulate adrenergic receptors (Tables 1.6 and 1.7), but there are newer non-glycoside, non-sympathomimetic drugs being investigated.

Dopamine Dopamine is an endogenous precursor of noradrenaline which stimulates alpha, beta$_1$ and specific dopamine receptors in the renal arteries. The response is related to the dose; 2–5 μg/kg/hour mainly stimulates specific dopamine receptors. More than 5 μg/kg/hour stimulate beta$_1$

Salbutamol Salbutamol, a beta$_2$ stimulant, has its main effect by peripheral vasodilatation.

Hypertension

There is no clear separation between a normal and raised blood pressure so definitions of hypertension vary. Definitions include the level of blood pressure which is greater than the epidemiological normal or one at which detection and treatment does more good than harm. A blood pressure of less than 140/90 mmHg is normal in adults and greater than or equal to 160/95 is raised. Between these readings is 'borderline' hypertension. Some authors choose a slightly higher level and for patients over the age of 60 years would restrict the term hypertension to pressures greater than 175/100 mmHg. Therapeutic studies use the term mild hypertension for diastolic blood pressures of 90–104, moderate hypertension for 104–114 and severe hypertension for greater or equal to 115.

Haemodynamically the mean arterial pressure is determined by the product of flow (cardiac output) and resistance (total peripheral resistance) – a mechanical Ohm's law. From Poisseuille's formula, resistance is inversely proportional to the fourth power of the radius, hence the great importance of the radius. So hypertension basically is an abnormality of vascular resistance. An increase in cardiac output (from increased contractility or increased blood volume) can contribute to hypertension and may be found in borderline or mild hypertension but this would not be relevant without an increase in peripheral resistance. The latter might occur from neural mechanisms (the autonomic nervous system), local mechanisms (some abnormality of vascular smooth muscle contractility) or humoral factors (such as the renin–angiotensin–aldosterone system).

Hypertension is the most important cause of cardiovascular mortality and this mortality is related to the level of blood pressure (and to the systolic more than the diastolic). It is common; 10–20 per cent of the adult population at some time have a diastolic pressure greater than 100 mmHg.

Blood pressure is variable – at all levels. The variability is partly due to the technique of measuring it but there is also a natural variability. Considerable circadian variation occurs and also variation from day to day. There is also an alarm reaction when the blood pressure is measured by a doctor (less so when measured by a nurse) – this may often be a rise of 10–15 mmHg.

Causes of hypertension

- *Essential* (95 per cent) There are genetic, racial and environmental factors; the latter include salt and alcohol consumption, obesity and social status.
- *Renal* (5 per cent) This occurs with renal artery stenosis, acute and chronic glomerulonephritis, chronic pyelonephritis, polycystic kidneys, hydronephrosis, collagen vascular disease and trauma.

- *Endocrine* (1 per cent) Phaeochromocytoma, primary aldosteronism, Cushing's syndrome, hyperparathyroidism and renin secreting tumours.
- *Other rare causes* Coarctation of the aorta, polycythaemia and the contraceptive pill.

Measurement of blood pressure

The patient should be relaxed, comfortable, resting and the position noted. The cuff should be the correct size (13–15 cm but larger in the obese) and the arm should be horizontal and at heart level. A cuff which is too small will over estimate the blood pressure and the arm dangling down will add an effect from hydrostatic pressure. Korotkoff phase 5 is used to measure the diastolic pressure.

Assessment of severity

Apart from the measurement of the blood pressure itself the severity is assessed by looking for evidence of target organ damage; fundi, kidney, heart or brain. The grade 1 and 2 changes of hypertension in the fundi are changes of arteriosclerosis and seen as part of the ageing process. Grade 3 fundi are those with haemorrhages and exudates; however, if patients have flame-shaped haemorrhages and a high blood pressure then they have accelerated (or malignant) hypertension, a term originally restricted to those with grade 4 fundi (papilloedema).

All patients need measurement of full blood count, electrolytes, urea, creatinine, urine testing, an electrocardiogram, chest radiograph and measurement of urinary vanilmandelic acid (VMA) excretion. A smaller number need specific investigations for endocrine or renal disease.

Phaeochromocytoma

Although rare (0.1 per cent of hypertension), it is important because hypertensive crises can be precipitated by drugs, anaesthesia, parturition or surgery. These tumours arise from chromaffin cells in the sympathetic nervous system. Most patients describe headache, palpitations, anxiety or sweating, and in 50 per cent of patients the symptoms and hypertension are paroxysmal. There may be orthostatic hypotension. Urinary VMA excretion is measured but there are occasional false negative results and some false positive results when there is sympathetic overactivity (extreme anxiety, cardiac failure or the use of vasodilators). To lower the blood pressure patients need initial treatment with an alpha-blocker (phenoxybenzamine) followed by a beta-blocker (propranolol).

Treatment of hypertension

Treatment may be started if the diastolic pressure is greater than 100 mmHg on three occasions (perhaps higher in a woman). There is a case to treat patients with levels of diastolic blood pressure of 90–99 mmHg if there is evidence of target organ damage. Treatment would normally be started without delay for a diastolic blood pressure greater than 120 mmHg.

Surgical operations should be deferred if the diastolic blood pressure is greater than 110 mmHg. If 90–110 mgHg, patients may need treatment later but they will need careful monitoring of blood pressure during and after surgery. Drugs should not be stopped before anaesthesia.

- *Non-drug treatment* of hypertension includes weight reduction in the overweight, reduction of salt intake and alcohol consumption, stopping the contraceptive pill or nonsteroidal anti-inflammatory drugs, stopping smoking (a potent risk factor for cardiovascular disease). Other factors such as increasing exercise, reducing dietary fat and relaxation may be useful.
- *Drug treatment.* Patients are usually started on a beta-blocker or thiazide diuretic and then a combination of both. If this fails then a vasodilator is added. There is increasing tendency to use calcium antagonists or angiotensin converting enzyme inhibitors earlier in treatment.

Examples of drugs (Fig. 1.25)

- *Thiazide diuretics.* These include bendrofluazide 5 mg, cyclopenthiaxide 0.5 mg
- *Beta-blockers* (*see* p. 7). These have their effect

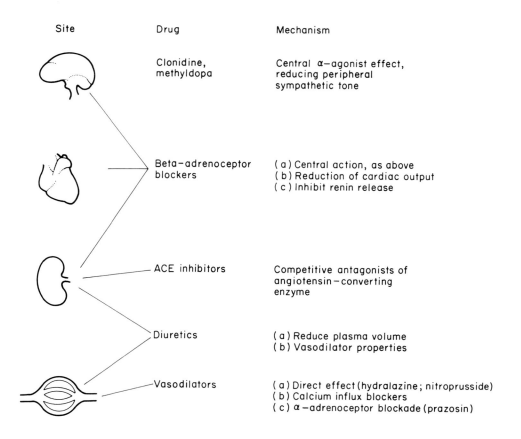

Site	Drug	Mechanism
	Clonidine, methyldopa	Central α–agonist effect, reducing peripheral sympathetic tone
	Beta–adrenoceptor blockers	(a) Central action, as above (b) Reduction of cardiac output (c) Inhibit renin release
	ACE inhibitors	Competitive antagonists of angiotensin–converting enzyme
	Diuretics	(a) Reduce plasma volume (b) Vasodilator properties
	Vasodilators	(a) Direct effect (hydralazine; nitroprusside) (b) Calcium influx blockers (c) α–adrenoceptor blockade (prazosin)

Fig 1.25 Classification and mechanisms of hypotensive drugs, based on their main site of actions.

by inhibiting the renin–angiotensin system, reducing cardiac output, reducing sympathetic outflow and may have a central effect on alpha adrenergic receptors.

- *Vasodilators.* These have a direct effect on smooth muscle. Hydralazine (75–150 mg) and calcium antagonists (dose as for angina) are often used; minoxidil and diazoxide are for refractory hypertension, and sodium nitro-prusside for emergency treatment. When used alone they usually cause reflex tachycardia.
- *Angiotensin converting enzyme inhibitors.* These drugs prevent the formation of angio-tensin II and hence lower the blood pressure through reduced peripheral vascular resistance. The most tried is captopril (25–150 mg), or enalapril (10–40 mg).
- *Centrally acting drugs.* Methyldopa (500–1500 mg) has a central alpha agonist effect reducing sympathetic outflow. Clonidine has limited use because of the rebound hypotension which can occur when it is suddenly stopped.

Emergency treatment of hypertension

Acute lowering of blood pressure is rarely required; there are four main indications.

- Dissection of the aorta with raised blood pressure.
- Hypertensive encephalopathy (a very high press-ure with fluctuating neurological signs or fits).
- Eclamptic toxaemia.
- Phaeochromocytoma.

Drugs used acutely by injection: sodium nitro-prusside, a precise drug but not easy to set up (0.5–1.5 μg/kg/minute), or hydralazine (5–25 mg i.m. or i.v. bolus, repeated hourly). These drugs tend to produce a reflex tachycardia. Intravenous labetalol is preferred in some units (1 mg/kg), and other drugs such as sublingual nifedipine, may find more use in the future. During surgery intravenous beta-blockade (0.5 mg propranolol every 2 minutes up to 5 mg, or metoprolol 1–2 mg/min up to 10 mg) can be used when there is also a tachycardia.

Urgent oral treatment is required for accelerated hypertension or hypertension with left ventricular failure.

Systolic hypertension

Systolic blood pressure increases progressively in the elderly because of decreased distensibility of the aorta and major vessels by arteriosclerosis. Treat-ment of this has been advocated because of the associated increased risk of stroke and heart failure but there is no evidence of benefit.

Cerebral autoregulation

This is the mechanism which maintains a constant cerebral blood flow during changes in systemic arterial pressure. It is achieved by constriction of arterioles as the blood pressure rises and dilatation as the blood pressure falls. The lower limit of brain autoregulation in a normotensive patient is a mean arterial pressure of 60–70 mmHg (Fig. 1.26). The lower limit in a hypertensive patient is about 120 mmHg. Below this the brain compensates by increasing oxygen extraction until symptoms of brain hypoxia develop – discomfort, dizziness, sleepiness, nausea then loss of consciousness. It is important to be aware of the correlation between the lower limit of autoregulation and the usual blood pressure because of the need to lower blood pressure gradually.

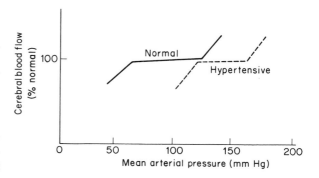

Fig 1.26 Diagram of autoregulation of the cerebral blood flow with change in arterial pressure in normal and hypertensive subjects (from Strandgaard).

Arrhythmias

An arrhythmia is any cardiac rhythm other than normal sinus rhythm. There is much to gain from a careful history. Patients who describe episodes of fast irregular palpitation probably have atrial fibrillation, and rarely multiple extrasystoles. The sudden onset of rapid palpitations is likely to be a true paroxysmal tachycardia. Patients with a slightly increased rate or a more forceful or vague heavy beating may be describing a normal heart rate. Patients who have syncope or near syncope may be describing symptoms from either a bradycardia or tachycardia.

Mechanisms of arrhythmias

There are three basic mechanisms – re-entry, abnormal automaticity and triggered activity.

Re-entry (circus movement)

This is the probable mechanism of the majority of supraventricular tachycardias and some ventricular tachycardias. It requires the presence of a dual circuit which may be large, such as the accessory pathway in Wolff–Parkinson–White syndrome, or tiny in distal Purkinje tissue or ischaemic myocardium. The typical onset is with a premature

ectopic impulse which approaches the dual circuit and finds one limb still refractory (unidirectional block); the impulse can then travel back slowly through this pathway (retrograde conduction) (Fig. 1.27A). This can then reactivate the previous circuit causing a single re-entry beat or a re-entry (or circus movement) tachycardia.

Abnormal automaticity

There is an increased rate of spontaneous depolarization of cells in latent or ectopic pacemakers or in myocardial cells (Fig. 1.27B). This is a less common mechanism than previously thought. Beta adrenergic stimulation, hypokalaemia and hypoxia can all stimulate automaticity.

Triggered automaticity

Under certain circumstances an action potential may be followed by unexpected oscillations or after depolarizations (Fig. 1.27C, arrow), which may produce one or more premature action potentials or a tachycardia. Digoxin can cause after depolarizations, which have also been found in mitral valve tissue and coronary sinus fibres.

Investigation

A 12-lead electrocardiogram may reveal an accessory pathway (see Fig. 1.46), QT prolongation, arrhythmia or evidence of underlying heart disease. Ambulatory electrocardiography with portable ECG tape recorders has an important role in the diagnosis of arrhythmias and assessment of treatment, but symptoms must be correlated with any arrhythmia. Transtelephonic ECG monitoring is used for patients with less frequent arrhythmias. Small portable recorders can be taken home for many weeks; when the patient has symptoms the recorder is applied to the chest and a short period of ECG is recorded on tape so this can be replayed over a telephone. Invasive electrophysiology is the use of intracardiac electrodes to record and stimulate the heart in the analysis of brady- and tachycardias. It is an important investigation in intractable or potentially lethal arrhythmias and enables better antiarrhythmic therapy to be found and assessment for pacemaker treatment or surgery.

(A)

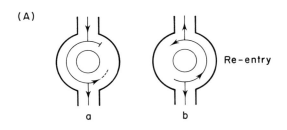

Re-entry

a   b

(B)

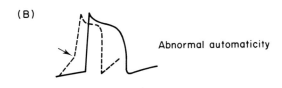

Abnormal automaticity

(C)

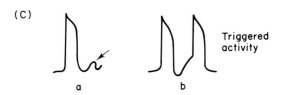

Triggered activity

a   b

Fig 1.27 The three basic mechanisms of arrhythmias (see text). A: diagram of initiation of re-entry (a and b). B: an action potential with increased automaticity (dotted line). C: an afterdepolarisation (arrow) may cause a triggered action potential.

Normal rhythms

In normal sinus rhythm the rate is 60–100/minute. Sinus arrhythmia is slightly irregular either with respiration or not. Some patients may have a wandering atrial pacemaker in which there are various P wave morphologies with a slightly varying heart rate. This is usually a normal finding but many occur in the sick sinus syndrome (*see* below).

Bradycardias and disturbances of conduction

Sinus bradycardia

The sinus rate is less than 60/minute. It occurs in healthy, fit adults, during sleep and with carotid sinus pressure. It may occur with raised intracranial pressure, obstructive jaundice, hypothyroidism and drugs such as digoxin and beta-blockers.

Sinus disease

This is the usual cause of a slow sinus rate other than in athletes.

Sinus node dysfunction   This typically occurs in acute inferior myocardial infarction either from direct ischaemia or excess vagal tone). If there is haemodynamic deterioration, patients may respond to atropine or isoprenaline.

Sick sinus syndrome   This is fairly common in the elderly; it is idiopathic and rarely caused by coronary or congenital heart disease. The sinus node becomes fibrosed or atrophic and there is some degree of degenerative change in the atria and conducting system. Patients may present with syncope, or near syncope. ECG findings include sinus bradycardia, sinoatrial block in which there is intermittent absence of the P wave, usually followed by junctional or ventricular escape, or complete sino-atrial block (or sino-atrial arrest) in which there is permanent absence of the P waves (Fig. 1.28). There may be paroxysmal atrial fibrillation (the so-called bradycardia–tachycardia syndrome, Fig. 1.29). Indeed, sino-atrial disease may be the underlying cause of lone atrial fibrillation – hence the potential danger of cardioversion in this condition. The prognosis is good but symptoms are relieved with a pacemaker.

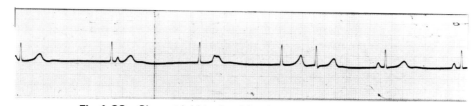

Fig 1.28   Sino-atrial block with a junctional escape rhythm.

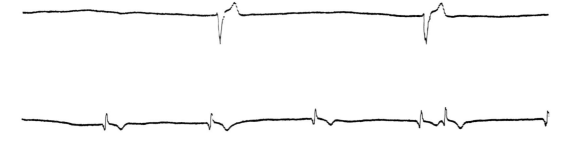

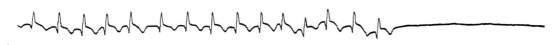

Fig 1.29   Sino-atrial arrest with ventricular and then junctional escape, a run of supraventricular tachycardia, then SA arrest (the three strips are continuous).

Atrioventricular block

In this there is delay or block of conduction of the cardiac impulse between the atrium and the ventricles. It may be pathological or physiological during a supraventricular tachycardia. The most important factor is the site of block in the conducting system. If the block is high, in the AV node, there is a stable junctional escape pacemaker; if the block is low, below the AV node, there is an unstable pacemaker in the Purkinje cells.

First degree AV block   Each impulse is conducted but there is delay so the PR interval is longer than 0.20 seconds. It is usually caused by disease in the AV node but it can be lower in the conducting system (*see* Fig. 1.10). It is seen in inferior myo-

progressive prolongation of the PR interval followed by a dropped beat. It is invariably caused by disease of the AV node and is therefore usually benign (Fig. 1.30).
- In Mobitz type 2 block there is intermittent block without progressive PR prolongation. This is always infranodal and therefore potentially serious. It occurs with anterior myocardial infarction, bundle branch fibrosis and cardiomyopathies and usually requires treatment with a pacemaker (Fig. 1.31).
- 2:1 AV block. When the ratio between the P waves and the QRS complex is 2:1 it is not possible to classify the block into Type 1 or 2, although the QRS complex is usually wide in Type 2 block.

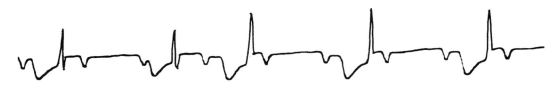

Fig 1.30   Second degree AV block. This is initially 2:1, then there is an episode of Mobitz type 1 (Wenckebach) block.

cardial infarction, myocarditis including rheumatic fever and with certain drugs (such as digoxin, beta-blockers, verapamil). It may occur in the presence of increased vagal tone or hypoxia. No treatment is required.

Second degree AV block   Some impulses are con-

- High grade block. Two or more atrial impulses are blocked without being complete.

Third degree or complete AV block   All the impulses are blocked and there is a subsidiary escape pacemaker. In AV nodal block there will be

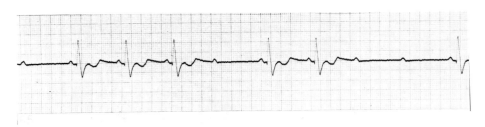

Fig 1.31   Type 2 second degree AV block.

ducted and some blocked. Two distinct types occur.
- In Mobitz type 1 (Wenckebach) block there is

narrow complexes and a rate of 40–50 which increases with exercise or sympathetic stimulation. In infranodal block the QRS complexes are wide

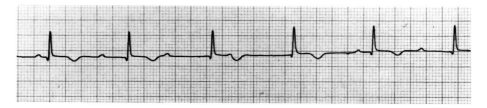

Fig 1.32   Complete AV block.

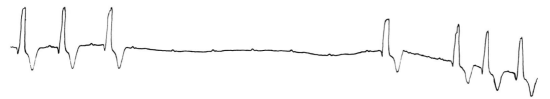

Fig 1.33   Ventricular asystole.

and the rate 20–40 (Fig. 1.32). The usual cause is age related idiopathic bundle branch fibrosis – a degenerative process not caused by coronary disease.

• Ventricular asystole is usually the end result of type 2 second degree block or occurs in infra-nodal complete block (Fig. 1.33). It can occur with a vagal storm – for example profuse vomiting.

• AV dissociation is the independent beating of the atria and ventricles; it is not a primary arrhythmia, but the result of another disorder. It should not be used to describe AV block and can be seen when there is no AV block (usually with a sinus bradycardia and an accelerated junctional

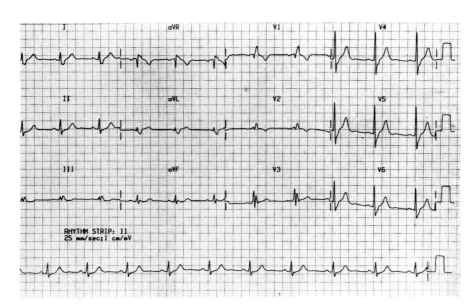

Fig 1.34   Isolated right bundle branch block in a patient with an otherwise normal heart.

rhythm, *see* Fig. 1.28). When the atria and ventricles are at the same rate it has been called isorhythmic, but this is one of many unnecessary terms. Usually no treatment is needed.

Intraventricular block

- Right bundle branch block, (described in the section on ECGs), is often found in healthy hearts – 0.3 per cent of the population over the age of 40 years in the Framingham Survey (Fig. 1.34). It may also be found in ischaemic

1.8) and in left posterior block there is abnormal right axis deviation. Bifascicular block is block in two fascicles, most commonly a combination of right bundle branch block and left anterior fascicular block. This may be seen in acute myocardial infarction but is usually caused by idiopathic fibrosis (Fig. 1.36). The risk of developing complete heart block is only about 1 per cent per year and prophylactic pacing is not required except in some symptomatic patients.

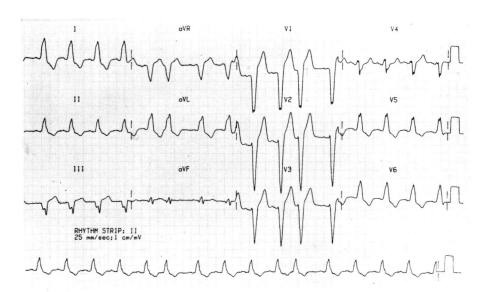

Fig 1.35   Left bundle branch block (and atrial ectopics).

heart disease, cardiomyopathies, bundle branch fibrosis, atrial septal defect and pulmonary emboli.
- Left bundle branch block is more rarely a normal variant (Fig. 1.35). It may occur in ischaemic or hypertensive heart diseases, calcific aortic valve disease, cardiomyopathies, or bundle branch fibrosis. It is rarely rate dependent – either with an increased heart rate, or more rarely bradycardia dependent.
- Fascicular block (hemiblock) is a block in one of the three main fascicles or bundles of the conducting system. In left anterior fascicular block there is abnormal left axis deviation (*see* Fig.

Supraventricular arrhythmias

Atrial extrasystoles   An extrasystole is the premature discharge of an ectopic impulse. There is therefore a premature, abnormally shaped P wave which may not be conducted to the ventricles (Fig. 1.37) or be followed by a normal or aberrant QRS complex (Fig. 1.38). Aberrant ventricular conduction is an important concept. It is a common occurrence when a premature beat arrives when one of the bundle branches (usually the right) is still refractory. It is particularly important in the diagnosis of tachycardias and is considered in more detail below. Atrial extrasystoles are usually normal but

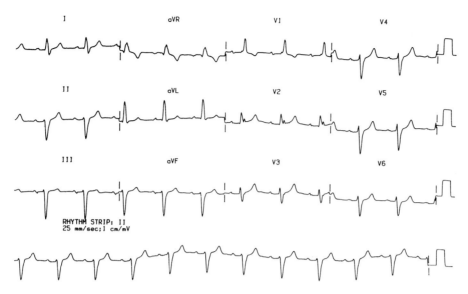

Fig 1.36   Bifascicular block (right bundle branch block and left anterior fascicular block). There is also first-degree AV block (this combination is sometimes called trifascicular block).

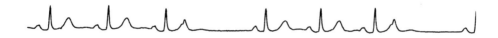

Fig 1.37   Nonconducted atrial extrasystoles (on the T-wave of the third ORS complex).

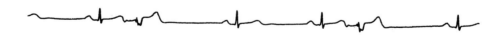

Fig 1.38   Atrial extrasystoles with aberrant conduction.

they increase with stress, alcohol, caffeine, tobacco and some antiarrhythmic drugs. They also increase with atrial distension. They only rarely require treatment when their frequency leads to a fall in cardiac output.

Supraventricular tachycardias (Table 1.8)

Sinus tachycardia   Sinus tachycardia is usually a normal response to certain illnesses. There are rare

Table 1.8   Narrow QRS tachycardias

Sinus tachycardia
Automatic (ectopic) atrial tachycardia
Atrial flutter
Atrial fibrillation
Re-entry (circus movement) tachycardia:
   1. atrioventricular nodal;
   2. accessory pathway (WPW);
   3. concealed accessory pathway.

pathological sinus tachycardias some of which may be produced by a sinoatrial re-entry mechanism.

Ectopic atrial tachycardia   This occurs particularly with organic heart disease such as myocardial infarction, chronic lung disease, infections, excess alcohol consumption, digoxin toxicity and neoplastic invasion of the heart. Each complex is preceded by an abnormal P wave. In multifocal atrial tachycardia, the heart rate is greater than 100 with at least three different P wave forms (Fig. 1.39). These arrhythmias can be difficult to treat and are often resistant to cardioversion. Drugs which inhibit AV nodal conduction such as digoxin, beta-blockers or verapamil usually slow the heart rate and verapamil may have a more specific effect in multifocal tachycardia. Drugs which reduce automaticity – such as disopyramide – may be effective. In patients with obstructive airways disease the arrhythmias may be related to theophylline administration.

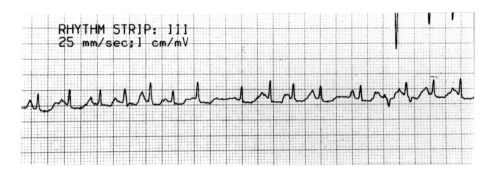

Fig 1.39   Multifocal atrial tachycardia.

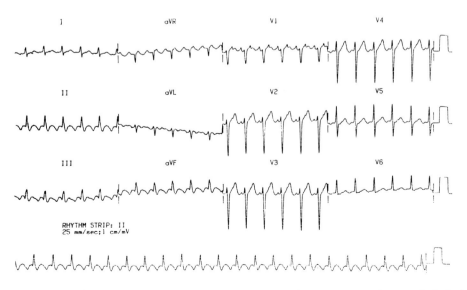

Fig 1.40   Atrial flutter with 2:1 AV block (the saw-tooth waves are only seen inferiorly).

Atrial flutter   This is probably caused by an intra-atrial re-entry mechanism. Electrocardiographically there are saw tooth waves inferiorly and variable atrioventricular block (Fig. 1.40). The ventricular rate may be slowed with drugs which inhibit AV nodal conduction e.g. (as above); if persistent and especially if symptomatic, the best treatment is cardioversion (patients invariably respond to a low energy of 25–50 watt seconds).

Atrial fibrillation   This is the commonest tachyarrhythmia (in the Framingham study the incidence was 1.7 per cent of the population, increasing with age). Commonest associated diseases are hypertension, cardiac failure and rheumatic heart dis-

ease. Some patients may have thyrotoxicosis but one-third of patients have no overt heart disease – 'lone' atrial fibrillation. On the ECG there are no P waves but irregular, fast 'f' waves (Figs. 1.41 and 1.42). The ventricular rate is fast and can be slowed with digoxin or verapamil. Patients with underlying mitral valve disease, dilated cardiomyopathy, thyrotoxicosis and associated sinoatrial disease should be anticoagulated.

Re-entry supraventricular tachycardias   Most patients with a regular narrow complex tachycardia fall into this group which is subdivided into those with re-entry in the AV node and those involving an accessory pathway. The accessory pathway may be

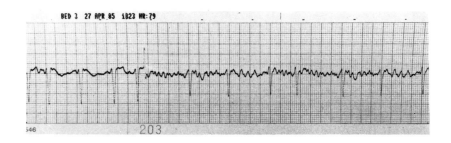

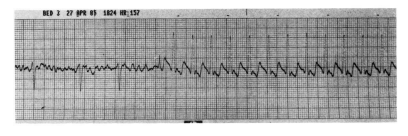

Fig 1.41   Onset of atrial fibrillation which spontaneously changes to atrial flutter in the lower strip (strip continuous).

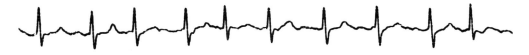

Fig 1.42   Atrial fibrillation (with barely visible 'f' waves).

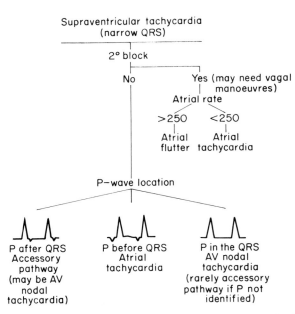

Fig 1.43 Diagram for recognition of narrow QRS tachycardias. The presence or absence of AV block and the position of the P-wave usually allows classification of the arrhythmia (from Bär, 1984).

overt, as in the Wolff–Parkinson–White (WPW) syndrome, or concealed (that is, it only conducts in the retrograde direction). The ventricular rate during tachycardia is usually between 120–230 beats/minute with a mean of 170. Patients with accessory pathways tend to be younger with faster rates and more often developing aberrant conduction. A simple flow chart giving an approach to diagnosis of supraventricular tachycardia is shown in Fig. 1.43. In AV nodal re-entry there is retrograde conduction to the atrium simultaneously with anterograde conduction to the ventricles, so the P wave is not seen. With accessory pathways retrograde conduction is later, and the P is after QRS complex (Fig. 1.44). Supraventricular tachycardia with aberrant conduction (RBBB) at onset is illustrated in Fig. 1.45.

It is important to recognize the WPW syndrome on the resting electrocardiogram because it mimics many other ECG abnormalities (Fig. 1.46). The prevalance is about 1.5/1000 patients and at least 10 per cent of these patients have arrhythmias. The usual pathway of a tachycardia is anterogradely over the AV node and retrogradely through the accessory pathway. Sometimes there is anterograde

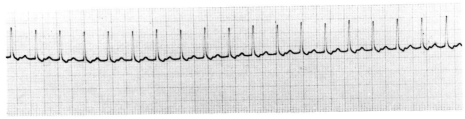

Fig 1.44 Supraventricular tachycardia (SVT) using an accessory pathway (retrograde P waves).

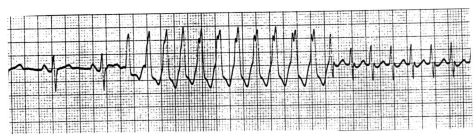

Fig 1.45 Supraventricular tachycardia with aberrant conduction (RBBB) at onset.

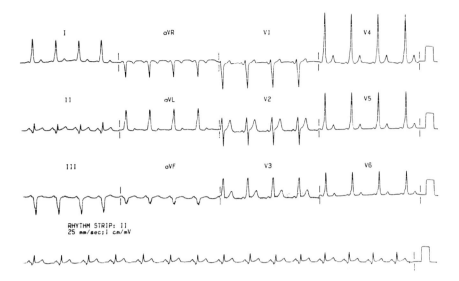

Fig 1.46 Wolff–Parkinson–White syndrome. Note that P-R and delta waves (the apparent inferior Q-waves mimics myocardial infarction).

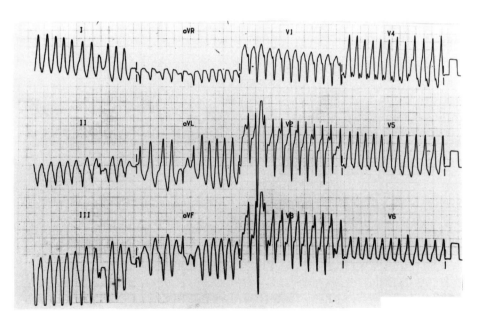

Fig 1.47 Wide complex tachycardia seen during SVT in Wolff–Parkinson–White (WPW) syndrome.

conduction over the accessory pathway – producing a wide complex tachycardia (Fig. 1.47). Digoxin should be avoided in WPW syndrome because it shortens the refractory period of the accessory pathway and increases the tachycardia rate (which can be lethal in atrial fibrillation).

Treatment for SVTs is required in prolonged or symptomatic episodes. Autonomic manoeuvres, which stimulate the parasympathetic nervous system and impair AV nodal conduction, may stop the attacks (carotid sinus pressure, Valsalva manoeuvre, dive reflex, retching, drugs to elevate the blood pressure). Intravenous verapamil is the drug of choice. Other antiarrhythmic drugs can be used and synchronized cardioversion is safe and effective. Attacks may be prevented by drugs which inhibit AV nodal conduction or which have an effect on other parts of the re-entry circuit or the initiating ectopics. For intractable arrhythmias other techniques are rarely used – surgery, catheter ablation or antitachycardia pacemakers.

Junctional rhythm or nodal rhythm This is usually secondary to failure of the sinus node – in sino-atrial disease, myocardial infarction, digoxin toxicity, atrio-ventricular block and in some normal people – especially during the night in children and in athletes. The usual rate is 40–60 and the P wave may be before, during or after the QRS complex (Fig. 1.48). Its position is dependent on the difference between anterograde and retrograde conduction, not the origin of the impulse. Accelerated junctional rhythm (rate 60–100) is often seen

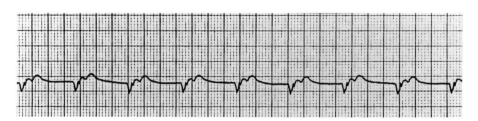

Fig 1.48   Junctional rhythm (P between the QRS and T wave).

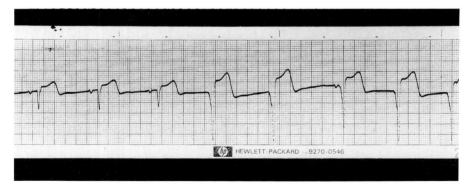

Fig 1.49   Onset of idioventricular rhythm.

in inferior myocardial infarction and digoxin toxicity and there will usually be AV dissociation.

Ventricular arrhythmia

Accelerated idioventricular rhythm is a benign 'escape' arrhythmia seen commonly with sinus bradycardia in inferior myocardial infarction (Fig. 1.49). The rate is 50–100/mm.

Ventricular extrasystoles are common in normal people, increasing with age. Even frequent and complex extrasystoles can occur in normal people. Asymptomatic patients with no evidence of cardiac disease do not need treatment. Ambulatory electrocardiography has revealed their incidence – uniform ventricular extrasystoles in 50 per cent of young people and multiform in 10 per cent of normal people. They may be precipated by caffeine, alcohol, sympathomimetic drugs and stress. Ventricular extrasystoles are also common in cardiac disease, especially coronary disease, cardiomyopathies, mitral valve prolapse and with bradycardias. When secondary to cardiac disease they are more likely to be frequent or complex, that is multiform (different shapes), repetitive such as couplets or triplets, or R-on-T extrasystoles (Fig. 1.50). In patients with coronary disease, especially after a myocardial infarction they are associated with lower ejection fractions and an increased risk of sudden death but it has never been shown that their treatment is beneficial. If there is haemodynamic disturbance from their frequency, class 1 antiarrhythmia drugs can be used, intravenous lignocaine being the most commonly used drug.

Ventricular tachycardia

Ventricular tachycardia is usually a serious arrhythmia, occurring with coronary disease or with a cardiomyopathy, sometimes in other forms

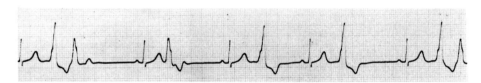

Fig 1.50 Coupled ventricular extrasystoles with two forms and couplets (two consecutive VEs at beginning and end of strip).

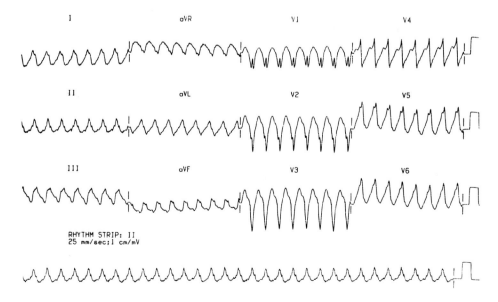

Fig 1.51 Ventricular tachycardia.

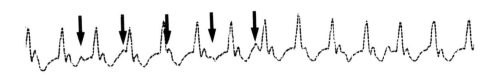

Fig 1.52   Ventricular tachycardia. The arrows point to the dissociated P-waves. The end of each triphasic QRS complex superficially mimics a P-wave.

of cardiac disease and sometimes with a totally normal heart when it may be benign (Fig. 1.51). However, this latter occurrence is very rare.

Difficulty in ECG diagnosis often occurs because the appearance may be mimicked by a supraventricular tachycardia with aberrant conduction (Table 1.9). Atrioventricular dissociation occurs in about half the patients and this may be evident clinically (cannon waves, changing intensity of first sound, changing systolic blood pressure) or on the electrocardiogram. The independent P waves may be seen (Fig. 1.52) or there may be fusion or capture beats – at a certain critical timing a sinus impulse may capture the ventricles producing a normal complex or may fuse with the ventricular complex producing an intermediate shape. In the remainder of the patients

Table 1.9   Wide QRS tachycardias

Ventricular tachycardia
Supraventricular tachycardia with:
1. aberrant conduction;
2. pre-existing bundle branch block;
3. anterograde conduction over accessory pathway;
4. drugs which widen the QRS.

there is retrograde conduction to the atria which may be in a 1:1 ratio producing regular P waves or there may be varying retrograde block. Other ECG guides to ventricular tachycardia, rather than supraventricular with aberrant conduction, include a QRS duration greater than 0.14 seconds, QRS axis less than $-30°$, a concordant praecordial pattern (all complexes in the same direction) and certain QRS configurations (Fig. 1.53).

Patients with ventricular tachycardia may be surprisingly uncompromized but if it is sustained they require treatment. Intravenous lignocaine is the drug of choice but cardioversion is needed if there is hypotension or cardiac failure.

Atypical ventricular tachycardia (torsades de pointes) is a polymorphous ventricular tachycardia with the ECG pattern showing alternating QRS polarity in an undulating pattern (twisting of the points) (Fig. 1.54). It is usually associated with underlying prolongation of the QT interval which may be congenital or acquired from potassium or magnesium deficiency, antiarrhythmic or psychotropic drugs, bradycardias or underlying myocardial disease, rarely ischaemic. This arrhythmia is dangerous and a precursor of ventricular fibrillation; patients respond to beta-blockers, phenytoin or overdrive pacing.

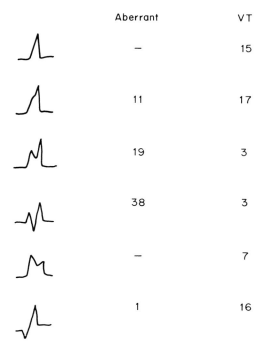

	Aberrant	VT
	–	15
	11	17
	19	3
	38	3
	–	7
	1	16

Fig 1.53 Appearance of QRS morphology in lead V1 during wide complex tachycardias with RBBB pattern. The numbers of patients with SVT with aberrant conduction or VT are given. Thus a triphasic complex is invariably SVT and a monophasic complex is VT (from Wellens, 1982).

Table 1.10 Vaughan Williams' classification of anti-arrhythmic drugs

	Class 1	Class 2	Class 3	Class 4
a	Quinidine Procainamide Disopyramide	Propranolol (etc) Bretylium	Amiodarone (Disopyramide) (Sotalol)	Verapamil Diltiazem
b	Lignocaine Mexilitine Tocainide			
c	Flecainide Encainide			

Ventricular fibrillation, recognized by the absence of normal complexes (Fig. 1.55), causes cardiac arrest, and should be treated with immediate cardioversion.

Antiarrhythmic drugs

The Vaughan Williams classification of anti-arrhythmic drugs is widely used; it is based on the drugs' electrophysiological effect on the action potential (AP) in tissue models (Table 1.10). The classification is theoretically useful but of poor clinical value, and there is no place allowed for digoxin. In practical terms it is more useful to divide up drugs into their main site of action (Table 1.11). For doses, *see* Table 1.12.

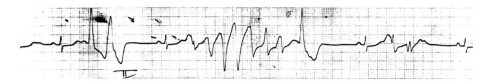

Fig 1.54 An episode of Torsades de Pointes in a patient with QT prolongation.

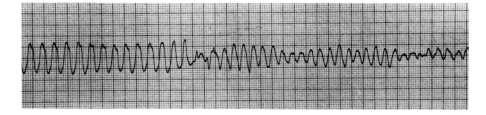

Fig 1.55 VT degenerating into ventricular fibrillation.

Table 1.11   Classification of antiarrhythmic drugs based on their main site of action

Atrium	Accessory pathway	AV node	Ventricle
Quinidine	Quinidine	Digoxin	All class 1 drugs
Procainamide	Procainamide	Beta-blockers	Amiodarone
Disopyramide	Disopyramide	Verapamil	
Amiodarone	Amiodarone		
	Flecainide		

Class 1 drugs slow the rate of rise of the AP by decreasing the fast inward sodium current, and slow the rate of diastolic depolarization. 1a drugs lengthen the AP duration, 1b shorten its duration and 1c have no effect. Class 2 drugs block the effect of catecholamines on the AP and class 3 prolong the AP duration. Class 4 drugs impair calcium transport into the cell (the main current in the SA and AV nodes).

Cardiac pacing

Temporary pacemakers

Temporary pacemakers are used for prophylaxis in patients at high risk of complete heart block or bradycardia and for urgent treatment in patients with sino-atrial or AV conduction disease. Before surgery, prophylactic pacing is required in untreated complete heart block, type 2 second degree AV block, symptomatic sino-atrial disease (i.e. sinus bradycardia with syncope) and symptomatic bifascicular block. If patients are candidates for permanent pacemakers, they should, if possible, be inserted preoperatively. Patients with chronic bifascicular block do not need prophylactic pacing in the absence of syncope or higher grade block.

Permanent pacemakers

Permanent pacemakers are implanted for symptomatic complete heart block or sino-atrial disease and sometimes in symptomatic second-degree block. The implantation rate in the United Kingdom is 150/million population (in the United States it is three times higher), and many patients are aged over 80 years.

The classification of types of pacemakers has been simplified by a generic code of five letters (Fig. 1.56). The first letter is the chamber-paced (V – ventricular, A – atrium, D – dual), the second is the chamber-sensed (V, A, D or 0 for none), the third is the way the pacemaker responds (T – triggered, I – inhibited, D – dual or O – none). The fourth letter describes the programmability and the fifth antiarrhythmic functions. Programmable pacemakers can have their electrical characteristics altered externally (the rate, output, sensitivity, mode of function etc.). Dual chamber or physiological pacemakers are increasingly used to maintain the normal atrio-ventricular sequence – stroke volume may then be increased by up to 30 per cent. Other pacemakers are rate-responsive and increase their rate with exercise.

Pacemaker problems

The two main problems with pacemakers are the pacemaker syndrome and interference. In the former there is a symptomatic fall in cardiac output secondary to ventriculo-atrial conduction. Interference may be caused by myopotentials from skeletal muscle contraction, from domestic appliances, weapon detectors and NMR. There are small risks of severe interference from diathermy. For safety the indifferent diathermy plate should be kept as far from the pacemaker and heart as possible and the active, cutting diathermy not used near the pacemaker or its electrode. Short bursts of diathermy should be used and the ECG monitored. This may show that the pacemaker changes to a fixed rate unit. This also happens when a magnet is put over the pacemaker and is a common method of routine testing. There should be particular care with complex, programmable pacemakers.

Halothane and related gases raise the threshold for capture, and should not be used.

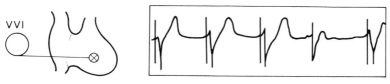

Fixed rate ventricular pacing, now rarely used. There is a risk of ventricular arrhythmias (pacing on the T wave, 4th complex).

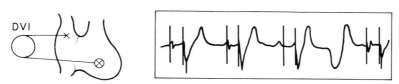

Ventricular demand pacing, the commonest mode. Pacing is inhibited by a sensed ventricular impulse (the 4th QRS above)

AV sequential pacing; after sensing the ventricle, both chambers are paced. This mode ignores spontaneous P waves (3rd complex).

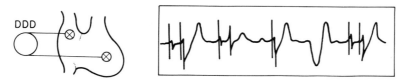

The optimal sequential unit which senses and paces both chambers. The first complex is paced AV sequential, the second is a normal QRS after atrial pacing, the third is ventricular pacing triggered by sensed, normal atrial activity.

Fig 1.56   Classification of pacemakers. The generic code is explained in the text. The commonest is a ventricular demand (VVI).

Electrocardiography

Knowledge of electrocardiography is essential in medicine. Three particular difficulties seem to arise. Firstly, lack of theoretical knowledge of the basic ECG pattern in different leads, secondly lack of knowledge of the wide variety of normal patterns and thirdly lack of awareness of the non-specificity of many abnormal findings.

Theoretical basis

The electrocardiogram is a graphic record of the electrical potentials produced by the heart. By convention when a current flows towards an

Table 1.12   Antiarrhythmic drugs

	Intravenous dose loading	maintenance	Oral dose loading	maintenance	Common side-effects	Comments
Procainamide	50–100 mg in 2 mins. up to 500 mg-IG	2–6 mg/min		1–1.5g 8 hrly (durules)	Myocardial depression SLE Vasodilatation	Caution with severe heart failure, shock heart block.
Disopyramide	2 mg/kg in 10 mins	0.4 mg/kg/hr	400 mg	1–200 mg 6 hrly or 250–375 mg 12 hrly (retard)	Myocardial depression Anticholinergic	Caution as above, and with prostatic symptoms.
Lignocaine	75–100 mg in 1–2 mins. then 10 mg/min for 20 mins	1–2 mg/min (up to 4 mg) (25 mg bolus for break-through VT)			Confusion Fits	Half dose if CF, shock, liver disease, > 70 yrs. More effective with normal/high K.
Mexilitene	250 mg in 15 mins	0.5–1.0 mg/min		150–250 mg 8 hrly	c.f. Lignocaine nausea, vomiting	
Flecainide	150 mg in 10–30 mins			100 mg bd, increasing by 50 mg to 300 mg bd	Dizziness, blurred vision, pro-arrhythmic, modest myocardial depression, prolongs conduction.	Caution with CF, sinus node disease and AV block
Amiodarone	2–5 mg/kg in 2 hrs (centrally)		200 mg tds (600 mg tds if urgent/week)	200 mg od	Corneal microdeposits photosensitivity, thyroid dysfunction, alveolitis etc.	Caution with S.A. disease & Dig/Warfann effect
Verapamil	5–10 mg bolus in 1 min. repeat at 30 mins			40–120 mg tds	Bradycardia, hypotension, AV blocks	Not with B-blocker (reverse hypotension with i/v Ca gluconate)
Propranolol	0.5 mg every 2 mins. up to 5 mg					
Metoprolol	1–2 mg/min up to 10 mg					

Table 1.12 (*cont.*)   Antiarrhythmic drugs

	Intravenous dose loading	maintenance	Oral dose loading	maintenance	Common side-effects	Comments
Phenytoin	250–500 mg at < 50 mg/min					For Digoxin-induced arrhythm
Bretylium	5 mg/kg	5 mg/kg 6–8 for 48 hrs			Hypotension	For resistant V.F.
Digoxin	0.5 mg in 30 mins repeat 3–6 hrly		1 mg or 0.25 mg bd (for slow effect)	0.25 mg o/bd		

Key
CF = cardiac failure
SA = sinoatrial
SLE = systemic lupus erythematosis

electrode it is represented by an upright deflection, and away by a negative deflection. The amplitude of the deflection is maximal when the direction of the electrical activity is towards a lead and least when it is perpendicular to the lead.

It is easiest to understand the derivation of the QRS complex in the chest leads in the horizontal plane. The interventricular septum is depolarized from the left to the right side causing a small positive deflection in V1 and small negative in V6 (Fig. 1.57). When the bulk of the ventricles are depolarized there is a larger force from the left ventricle downwards and to the left.

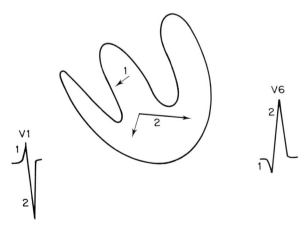

Fig 1.57 Diagram of the basis of the derivation of the QRS complex in the chest leads. The initial septal depolarization (1) is followed by a ventricular depolarization (2).

The limb leads are in a frontal plane and they are best explained from the hexaxial reference system. It is assumed that the heart is in the centre of an equilateral triangle, the apices of which are the right arm, left arm and left leg (Einthoven's triangle hypothesis, Fig. 1.58). Lead 1 records the potential difference between the left arm and right arm (and so on with the other leads) and the unipolar leads, which have to be augmented, record from their respective limbs. It is easier to draw the triangle with the axis of the leads through zero. The electrical forces produced by the heart are represented by a vector – an arrow with direction and magnitude. All the limb lead patterns can then be derived in this frontal plane in the same way as Fig. 1.57.

Normal electrocardiogram

Electrocardiograms should always be read systematically, starting with the calibration, looking for artifacts, measuring the rate, rhythm and the axis. The calibration mark must show 10 mm for 1 millivolt. At the normal paper speed of 25 mm/second each very small square has a width of 0.04 seconds; the rate is 1500 divided by the number of small squares (HR = 60, *see* Fig. 1.32; HR = 214, *see* Fig. 1.45). The axis is the main direction of electrical forces. All parts of the electrocardiogram (P, QRS, T) have an axis at different times and usually we are only concerned with the mean, frontal plane QRS axis. It is determined by finding the frontal plane lead with the most equiphasic

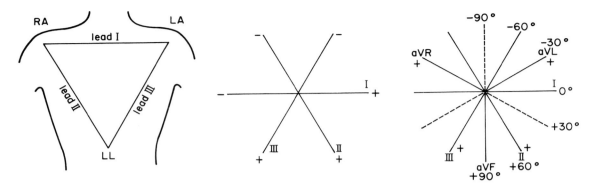

Fig 1.58 Diagram of the derivation of the hexaxial reference system. Einthoven triangle on the left is drawn through zero in the centre and completed on the right.

deflection; the mean frontal plane QRS axis is at right angles to this lead. Look at the lead at right angles and see if the direction is positive or negative, and this gives the axis to the nearest 30°. It can be adjusted to 15° depending on whether the most equiphasic deflection is slightly positive or negative. The normal mean QRS axis is from −30° to +90°; more negative is left axis deviation (−75°, *see* Fig. 1.36) and to the right is right axis deviation (+120°, *see* Fig. 1.20). Only by consciously measuring the axis in ECGs can fascicular block be recognized.

The P wave represents depolarization of the atrium; the amplitude is normally less than 2.5 mm and the duration less than 0.12 seconds. The PR interval is the time for the impulse to travel from the SA node to the ventricles and is measured from the beginning of the P to the beginning of the QRS complex in a limb lead. It is normally 0.12–0.20 seconds. The QRS complex represents depolarization of the ventricles. A Q wave is an initial downward deflection, the R wave is the first upward deflection (with or without a preceding Q) and the S wave is a downward deflection after the R wave.

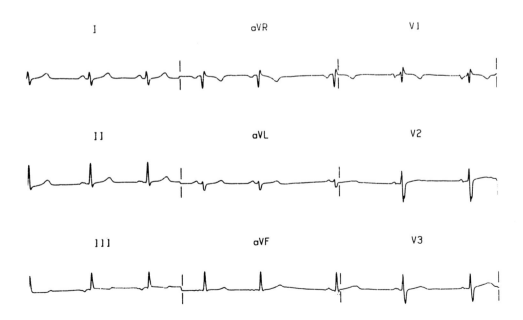

Fig 1.59 Left atrial hypertrophy in a patient with mitral stenosis.

R' is a second upward deflection and QS is a single negative deflection. The R wave height in the chest leads is normally progressively larger from V1 to V6. The T wave represents ventricular repolarization and the axis is normally in the same direction as the QRS complex – that is the angle between the mean QRS vector and the mean T wave vector can be up to 45° in the frontal plane.

Abnormal electrocardiograms

Atrial hypertrophy

In left atrial hypertrophy the P wave duration exceeds 0.10 seconds, it is notched in lead 2 and the terminal component of the P wave has an axis shifted to the left and posteriorly. This is recognized by a negative terminal deflection in lead 3 and a diphasic P wave in V1 with a wide and deep terminal component (Fig. 1.59). It is an important finding in the left atrial hypertrophy of mitral valve disease but also it is a common sign of left ventricular disease, including hypertension, when the left atrium is contracting against a stiff left ventricle.

Ventricular hypertrophy

The left ventricular voltage is increased so the height of the R wave in lead V5 or V6 added to the depth of the S wave in V1 or V2 is greater than 35 mm. The R in V5 may be greater or equal to 26 mm and R in V6 greater or equal to 18 mm. In the limb leads the sum of R in lead 1 and S in lead 3 is greater or equal to 25 mm (Fig. 1.60). These criteria require a QRS duration of less than 0.12 seconds and are for adults over 16-years-old. There may be associated left atrial hypertrophy and in more severe left ventricular hypertrophy there may be ST segment and T wave inversion in the leads with the highest voltage. The ECG criteria do not have a high sensitivity. Right ventricular hypertrophy is a rare finding – the R wave is greater than the S wave in V1 and R less than S in V5 and V6. There is usually right axis deviation (see Fig. 1.20).

Low voltage

This is present when the largest QRS deflection in the limb leads is less than 5 mm and the largest in the praecordial leads less than 10 mm. It may be a normal variant or is seen in emphysema, coronary disease, pericardial effusion, myxoedema or obesity.

Bundle branch block

In right bundle branch block there is a delayed activation of the right ventricle (see Figs. 1.34, 1.61).

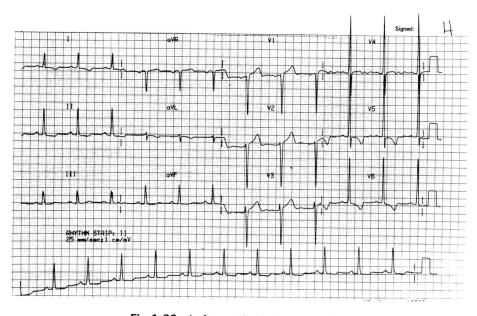

Fig 1.60   Left ventricular hypertrophy.

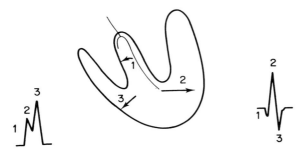

Fig 1.61 Diagram of the ECG appearance in leads V1 and V6 in right bundle branch block (RBBB). The initial depolarization (1) is normal, but right ventricular depolarization (3) is delayed.

So V1 has an 'RSR' complex and repolarization is in an opposite direction. There is a delayed S wave in V6. The QRS duration is 0.12 seconds or more and if it is 0.10–0.12 seconds the pattern is partial right bundle branch block. In left bundle branch block there is reversal of the normal septal depolarization. The right praecordial leads show a QS complex, or an initial R and deep S and the left praecordial leads are broad and notched without the normal septal Q wave. The QRS duration is greater than or equal to 0.12 seconds, and there are secondary ST segment and T wave change (Figs. 1.35, and 1.62).

An RSR complex in V1 with a normal QRS duration may be a normal variant (*see* Fig. 1.59), incomplete right bundle branch block, right ventricular hypertrophy or posterior myocardial infarction. A dominant R in V1 can also be seen in Wolff–Parkinson–White syndrome.

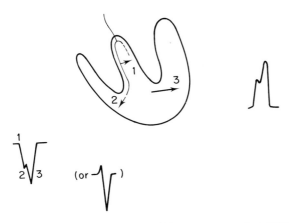

Fig 1.62 Diagram of the ECG appearance in LBBB. Septal depolarization is opposite to normal.

ST/T changes

ST-segment depression may occur with myocardial ischaemia or a sub-endocardial infarct, or it may be reciprocal to a raised ST-segment in myocardial infarction. It is seen in bundle branch block and may be seen in severe left or right ventricular hypertrophy, in patients on digoxin (Fig. 1.12) or with hypokalaemia and in patients after tachycardia. ST segment elevation may be a normal variant if slight, occur in acute or old myocardial infarction or in pericarditis. Minor T wave changes occur in a large number of cardiac diseases, electrolyte and drug abnormalities and in normal people. Non-diagnostic ST segment and T wave changes are the commonest abnormalities seen in electrocardiograms and should be reported as 'non-specific ST/T wave changes', not as 'ischaemic change'.

Potassium effect

In hyperkalaemia the T wave becomes tall and peaked, the R wave voltage falls, the QRS widens and the ECG becomes increasingly bizarre. In hypokalaemia the T wave voltage falls and there is an increased U wave. The ST segment may be depressed in a trough-like manner (Fig. 1.63). Large U wave may be seen in normal patients especially athletic, with a bradycardia or left ventricular hypertrophy.

Echocardiography

Echocardiography is an important non-invasive investigation that utilizes ultrasound to study the dimensions and movements of cardiac structures. An ultrasound transducer on the chest wall produces pulses of ultrasound (frequency 2–3.5 megahertz in adults) which are reflected from interfaces between structures with different acoustic properties.

In M mode echocardiography a single beam passes through parts of the heart. The motion (M for motion) of the aortic valve, mitral valve and the left ventricle are recorded on a strip-chart (Fig. 1.64). The main use of M mode echocardiography is for accurate measurement of left ventricular dimensions (Table 1.13).

In two-dimensional (or cross-sectional) echocardiography multiple beams of ultrasound are used from either a mechanical rotating head or from a phased array system with multiple transducers. A large slice through the heart is imaged in

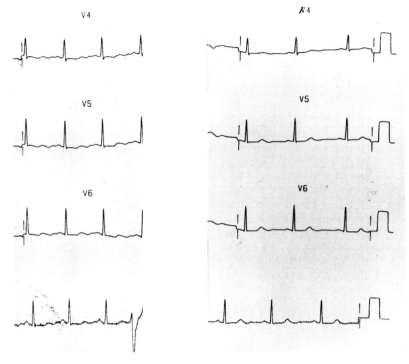

Fig 1.63   Changes of hypokalaemia. (a) Serum potassium 3.2, (b) 4.1 on the right (*see* text).

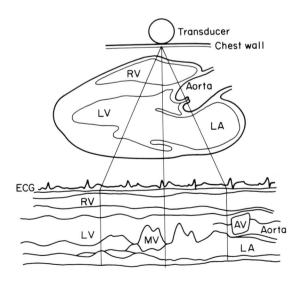

Fig 1.64   Diagram of a 2-D image of the heart (above) and of an M-mode echocardiographic strip (below).

Table 1.13(a)   Normal echocardiographic values

Left ventricular end-diastolic dimension (LVEDD)	3.5–5.6 cm
Left ventricular end-systolic dimension (LVESD)	2.5–4.1 cm
Septal and posterior wall thickness	0.7–1.1 cm
LV fractional shortening: $\dfrac{(LVEDD-LVESD)}{LEVDD}$	0.30–0.40
Aortic root diameter	2.0–3.7 cm
Left atrial dimension	1.5–4.0 cm

Table 1.13(b)   Normal haemodynamic values (mmHg. Zero mid-chest)

Right atrium	mean 0–8 (a = 7, v = 5)
Right ventricle	15–30/0–8
Pulmonary artery	15–30/3–12 mean 9–16
Pulmonary wedge	mean 1–10
Left ventricle	100–140/3–12
Aorta	100–140/60–90
Cardiac index	2.5–4.2 litre/min/m^2
Ejection fraction	50–80 %

different planes, producing detailed anatomical information (Fig. 1.64). This technique has revolutionized many aspects of cardiac diagnosis including complex congenital heart disease. Measurements of left ventricular size and performance can be made from the two-dimensional images.

Common uses for echocardiography include the assessment of the severity of valve disease, quantitive assessment of left ventricular function in overt or suspected cardiac failure and in pericardial disease, endocarditis or disease of the ascending aorta.

Doppler echocardiography provides information about the velocity of blood flow in the heart and is usually performed in conjunction with cross-sectional echocardiography. The Doppler effect is the change in frequency of sound caused by the motion of the source or observer. In the heart a frequency shift occurs when a sound wave strikes moving red blood cells. The velocity of blood flow can be related to the frequency shift, and the Doppler shift is then analyzed spectrally to provide a graphic display of blood flow velocity.

It is a rapidly developing technique which has considerably increased the ability to assess certain cardiac conditions, such as the severity of stenotic valves. Cardiac output can be measured from the aortic systolic velocity curve. Colour Doppler allows real time, two-dimensional blood flow imaging.

These non-invasive diagnostic techniques provide enough informative in the assessment of the severity of valve disease to avoid cardiac catheterization. The main reason to catheterize patients now is to determine the severity of coronary artery disease.

Bedside right heart catheterization

In critically ill patients it can be important to know the filling pressure of the heart. This will then establish whether circulatory failure is secondary to heart failure, to hypovolaemia or to inappropriate vasodilation in normovolaemic shock. Observation of the jugular venous pressure or measurement of the central venous pressure is often adequate, but when there is underlying heart disease, and sometimes in severely ill patients, there is a discrepancy between the filling pressures of the right and left heart. In ischaemic heart disease the pressure is likely to be higher on the left but it will be higher on the right in pulmonary embolism or right ventricular infarction.

In the absence of mitral stenosis or pulmonary hypertension the left ventricular filling pressure (LVEDP) is the same as the mean pulmonary artery wedge pressure or the pulmonary artery diastolic pressure (PADP). (The pressure is transmitted retrogradely from the left atrium to the pulmonary arteries – which are end arteries). The wedge pressure is measured by impacting a catheter in a small branch of the pulmonary artery; with a balloon catheter it is measured by occluding a larger branch by blowing up the balloon – the pulmonary arterial occlusive pressure.

Technique

A balloon catheter is introduced through a sheath in a large central vein (subclavian or jugular). It is passed to the SVC, the balloon inflated and the catheter then floats to the right atrium, right ventricle and into the pulmonary artery. In patients with a very low cardiac output radiographic screening is helpful. Although the technique is simple, correct calibration of the pressure transducer and accurate recording of the pressure is more difficult and requires technical knowledge and experience. There are many potential complications – those of the vein puncture, arrhythmias in the right ventricle, damage to the tricuspid or pulmonary valves, rupture of the pulmonary artery or pulmonary infarction and infection.

It is most convenient to use the PADP measured at end-expiration. The cardiac output can be measured at the same time by thermodilution, though the catheters are expensive and the actual value rarely affects management. If the PADP is too low plasma expansion is needed and if too high, vasodilation or diuretic therapy (*see* Table 1.13). The JVP or CVP are normally measured in cm of water and the PA pressure in mmHg (pressure in cm of water = 1.36 × pressure in mmHg).

A typical appropriate use would be in a severely ill, haemodynamically unstable patient who is not responding to what is thought to be the correct therapy. It can also be used to monitor patients during anaesthesia; a rise in pressure may be true left ventricular failure or from a rise in LVEDP from reduced compliance, during episodes of myocardial ischaemia.

References

Bär, F.W., Brugada P., Dassem, W.R.M. and Wellens, H.J.J. (1984). Differential diagnosis of tachycardia with narrow QRS complex (shorter than 0.12 seconds). *American Journal of Cardiology* **54**, 555–60.

BSAC Working Party. (1982). The antibiotic prophylaxis of infective endocarditis. *Lancet* **2**, 1323–6.

Detsky, A.S., Abrams, H.B., Forbath, N., Scott, J.G., Hilliard, J.R. (1986). Cardiac assessment for patients undergoing noncardiac surgery. A multifactorial clinical risk index. *Archives of Internal Medicine* **146**, 2131–4.

Foster, E.D., Davis, K.B., Capenter, J.A., Abele, S. and Fray, D. (1986). Risk of noncardiac operation in patients with defined coronary disease: The Coronary Artery Surgery Study (CASS) registry experience. *Annals of Thoracic Surgery* **41**, 42–9.

Goldman, L. (1983). Cardiac risks and complications of noncardiac surgery. *Annals of Internal Medicine* **98**, 504–13.

Julian, D.G. (1985). The practical implications of the coronary artery surgery trials. *British Heart Journal* **54**, 343–50.

Logue, R.B. (1986). Evaluation and management of patients with heart disease who undergo noncardiac surgery. In: *The Heart*. Edited by Hurst, J.W. McGraw-Hill, New York. 1511–1519.

Rowley, J.M. and Hampton, J.R. (1981). Diagnostic criteria for myocardial infarction. *British Journal Hospital Medicine* September: 253–8.

Strandgaard, S., Olesen, J., Skinhøj, E. and Lassen N.A. (1973). Autoregulation of brain circulation in severe arterial hypertension. *British Medical Journal* **1**, 507–10.

Weitz, H.H. and Goldman, L. (1987). Noncardiac surgery in the patient with heart disease. *Medical Clinics of North America* **3**, 413–32.

Wellens, H.J.J., Bär, F.W.H.M., Vanagt, E.J.D.M. and Brugada, P. (1982). Medical treatment of ventricular tachycardia: considerations in the selection of patients for surgical treatment. *American Journal of Cardiology* **49**, 186–93.

Wells, P.H. and Kaplan J.A. (1981). Optimal management of patients with ischaemic heart disease for non cardiac surgery by complementary anesthesiologist and cardiologist interaction. *American Heart Journal* **102**, 1029–37.

Wolf, M.A. and Braunwald, E. (1984). General anaesthetic and non cardiac surgery in patients with heart disease. In: *Heart Disease*, pp. 1911–22. Edited by Braunwald, E. W.B. Saunders, Philadelphia.

Further reading

Braunwald, E. (Ed). (1988). *Heart Disease*. Third Edition. W.B. Saunders, Philadelphia.

Hurst, J.W. (Ed). (1986). *The Heart*. Sixth Edition. McGraw-Hill, New York.

Marriott, H.J.L. (1983). *Practical Electrocardiography*. Seventh Edition. Williams and Wilkins, Baltimore.

Schamroth, L. (1982). *An Introduction to Electrocardiography*. Sixth Edition. Blackwell Scientific Publications, Oxford.

Weatherall, D.J., Ledingham, J.G.G. and Warrell, D.A. (1987). Cardiovascular disease (Section 13). In: *The Oxford Textbook of Medicine*. Second Edition. Oxford University Press, Oxford.

2
Respiratory Disorders

Martyn Partridge

Introduction

The importance of respiratory disease

Infections of the respiratory tract are one of the major reasons for consultation in general practice. Chronic bronchitis accounts for the loss of 30 million working days a year in the UK. Lung cancer is the commonest cancer in males and in Scotland and some American States it has become commoner than breast cancer in females. The prevalence of asthma has trebled over the last 40 years. It is therefore no surprise that respiratory disorders are a major problem to the anaesthetist. Postoperative pulmonary complications include hypoxaemia, atelectasis, aspiration, embolism, effusion and pneumonia. A history of lung disease is the most important risk factor from a list which includes age, obesity, smoking, acute infections and pre-existing respiratory disease. In this chapter there is a description of the clinical features and investigation of respiratory disease followed by sections on airway narrowing, restrictive lung disorders, infections, respiratory failure and sleep apnoea syndromes.

The lungs

The function of the lungs is to permit rapid passage of oxygen from air to blood and to allow carbon dioxide to pass readily in the reverse direction. This function is achieved using a series of branching airways. From the trachea the major bronchi divide into lobar, segmental and sub-segmental bronchi for 23 generations becoming progressively smaller at each division. The terminal bronchioles have occasional air sacs budding from their walls, but eventually the alveolar ducts are reached which are completely lined with alveoli. Throughout their length the airways are lined with a varying thickness of pseudostratified columnar epithelium which contains a variety of other cells such as goblet cells, ciliated cells, Kulchitsky cells and Clara cells (which may be responsible for secretion of a surfactant like-substance). The proportion of bronchial glands and smooth muscle varies with division of airway and with disease. The airways are accompanied by pulmonary and bronchial arteries and lymphatics. The parasympathetic nervous supply is from the vagus, stimulation of which has a constricting effect on the airways and a secretory effect on the glands in the airway wall. There is a sympathetic supply from the stellate ganglion and the thoracic sympathetic trunk, but the numerous alpha and beta adrenoreceptors in the airway walls probably respond to circulating chemicals and catecholamines rather than to stimulation of the sympathetic nervous system. Alpha receptor stimulation may cause airway narrowing, and beta receptor stimulation, broncho-dilation and reduction in vascular permeability. Disorders of the structure and function of the lungs may give rise to a variety of symptoms.

Symptoms of respiratory disease

Cough

Coughing is one of the major defence mechanisms of the respiratory tract. It is initiated by stimulation of receptors in the bronchial wall which may be caused by foreign bodies, irritant gases or infective agents. After sudden contraction of the expiratory muscles against a closed glottis, the glottis is opened and the obstructed air is rapidly released shearing mucus from the airway walls. If a bout of coughing is prolonged the resulting rise in intra-thoracic pressure may impede venous return to the heart leading to syncope. Coughing may result from almost any disease affecting the lungs and occasionally from heart failure or oesophageal disease. The most threatening pathologies are those of lung cancer or tuberculosis in which the chest radiograph is usually abnormal. Two other common causes of a persistent cough may occur without chest radiographic abnormality; coughing associated with sinus disease and coughing due to asthma.

A cough may not be productive of sputum, but the presence of sputum is always abnormal. Normal subjects produce approximately 150 ml of secretion/day and this is wafted gently mouthwards by ciliary action, collecting airborne particles and humidifying the inspired air. These secretions are then usually swallowed without the individual being aware of their production. In smokers the quantity of mucus is increased and it is more tenacious, and the ciliotoxic effect of smoking leads to the continous gentle movement of secretions being replaced by bulk movement by coughing.

Haemoptysis

Haemoptysis always requires further investigation. Occasional confusion may occur with blood arising in gums, nose or pharynx and occasionally oesophageal bleeding produces fresh blood whose gastrointestinal source is not obvious because it has not been altered by contact with acid. Panendoscopy may then be necessary. Of the causes of 'true' haemoptysis a bronchial carcinoma is the most important, its major characteristic being the persistence of the symptom. Haemoptysis associated with bronchiectasis is usually initially bright red and then darkens and diminishes over the subsequent few days. It is an uncommon, but important symptom of pulmonary infarction and also occurs in patients with pulmonary oedema and mitral stenosis. If the patient with haemoptysis has a normal chest radiograph, has only had one occurrence, and is a life long non-smoker then further action may not be necessary. All other patients require further investigation or follow-up.

Chest pain

Chest pain as a symptom of respiratory disease occurs in patients with pleurisy or pulmonary infarction and may also be a presenting feature of a bronchial carcinoma. In those with severe cough, secondary muscle pains and cough fractures of the ribs may develop. Patients who become very breathless on exertion may also develop a dull exertional chest pain. This is not always due to associated coronary artery disease and the pain usually *follows* the onset of breathlessness and may reflect the work load of the respiratory muscles.

Breathlessness

The origin of the sensation of breathlessness remains unclear. It is usually sensed when the respiratory muscles have to work unduly hard to maintain a normal tidal volume and this occurs when disease has led to increased airway resistance and decreased compliance. It also occurs when respiratory muscle activity is increased because of hyperventilation; this may occur in response to demands, or as a response to change in blood gas tensions produced by alteration in lung mechanics. The correlation between the subjective sensation of breathlessness and objective measurement of functional derangement is not always close. Disparity may reflect rate at which function has declined, with some degree of adaptation occurring with the more slowly progressive pathologies. For these reasons any scoring of subjective sensation may be better replaced by a scale of 'disability' based upon the patient's stated exercise tolerance (Table 2.1).

The list of potential causes of breathlessness is long, and classification may involve separation according to systems, to rate of onset, or whether breathlessness is due to hyperventilation or abnormal lung mechanics. However, clinical features, a chest radiograph and measurement of spirometery will be sufficiently diagnostic in the majority of

Table 2.1   A five grade system suitable for recording patient's stated exercise tolerance

Grade	Exercise tolerance
Grade 1	Normal
Grade 2	Able to walk with normal people of his own age and sex on the level, but unable to keep up on hills and stairs
Grade 3	Unable to keep up with normal people on the level, but the patient can walk long distances at his own pace
Grade 4	Unable to walk more than 900 metres (100 yards) on the level before being stopped by breathlessness
Grade 5	Unable to walk more than a few steps without breathlessness and becomes breathless on washing and dressing

cases. It is the patients who are breathless with normal clinical and chest radiographic findings who cause most confusion. In such cases it is important to exclude a variable cause of breathlessness, such as asthma, to exclude 'silent' pulmonary emboli and to consider very carefully the possibility of a systemic cause such as anaemia, thyrotoxicosis, obesity or respiratory muscle weakness. Breathlessness is usually worse on exertion and deterioration on lying down (orthopnoea) is well recognized as a symptom of cardiac failure. However, in patients with diaphragm weakness, breathlessness may also occur when recumbent because the intra-abdominal contents then elevate the weakened diaphragm restricting pulmonary expansion.

Evaluation and investigation of the respiratory system

Clinical examination

Clinical assessment of the patient with respiratory disease involves general and chest examination.

General examination

Cyanosis

Central cyanosis is assessed by examination of the inside of the lips and the tongue and may be difficult to detect. To produce cyanosis 2–3 g/100 ml of reduced haemoglobin are required. However, it is more evident in patients with polycythaemia than those with anaemia, while some patients, such as those with emphysema, may only desaturate on exercise.

Finger clubbing

Finger clubbing consists of painless bulbous thickening and swelling of the soft tissues at the base of the nail with the result that the angle between nail base and adjacent skin is lost. Palpation reveals the nail to be freely depressable in the soft tissues. If there is doubt examine the index finger for it is usually the more abnormal. The condition may be congenital or acquired, but the pulmonary causes are the most important and frequent and the commonest are bronchial carcinoma, fibrosing alveolitis, asbestosis and cystic fibrosis.

The hands

The hands may also reveal signs of carbon dioxide retention. The peripheral veins may be dilated and if the arms are outstretched and the wrist dorsiflexed with fingers apart a flapping tremor may develop in the presence of significant increases in carbon dioxide tension.

Lymphadenopathy

Examination of the cervical and supraclavicular lymph nodes is essential. Both are common sites of spread from a bronchial carcinoma and may also be involved in cases of sarcoidosis or lymphoma. Axillary lymph nodes are rarely enlarged in respiratory disease, the rare exception being when tumour has invaded the chest wall.

The chest

Inspection

A note is made of whether the patient appears breathless at rest or whether inspiration is limited by pain. Chest wall inspection will reveal significant thoracic cage deformity, such as a kyphoscoliosis, and may provide useful clues as to the presence of longstanding airway disease. In these cases lung hyperinflation leads to an increase in the antero-posterior thoracic diameter giving the so called 'barrel chest'. Severe air flow limitation is likely to be accompanied by indrawing of the intercostal spaces and use of the accessory muscles of respiration, such as sternomastoid.

Percussion

The percussion note is increased over hyperinflated lungs and symmetrically increased over a large bulla or pneumothorax. Dullness to percussion suggests the presence of either consolidation or fluid, but may occur to a lesser extent over large tumours or airless lung.

Auscultation

Auscultatory findings are often described with difficulty because of confused terminology. Clinically useful signs are those of bronchial breathing and whispering pectoriloquy, wheezes and crackles. In patients with consolidation the percussion note is reduced and harsh central airway (bronchial) breath sounds are transmitted through the consolidated lung to the stethoscope on the chest wall.

If there is doubt as to whether the harshness truly represents bronchial breathing, comparision is made with the other lung or the patient is asked to whisper. Whispering pectoriloquy is often a more easily determined, 'all or none' phenomenon. Whispering, being high pitched, is filtered by air filled lung and is normally inaudible. Airless lung conducts these high pitched sounds so that whispered speech becomes intelligible in patients with consolidation. Wheezes are merely due to vibration of the airway wall and whilst helpful as a sign of probable disease it must be stressed that the presence of the sign carries no significance as to diagnosis or potential for reversibility. All that wheezes is not asthma and not all asthma wheezes. Crackles may occur in patients with pulmonary fibrosis, pulmonary oedema, bronchiectasis or airway disease and the timing of crackles in inspiration may be of more diagnostic value than their character. In patients with severe airway narrowing crackles may be wrongly attributed to associated oedema or fibrosis whereas they may be present in early inspiration purely as a result of the airway disease; one explanation is that they are due to the airways reopening after having closed towards the end of the preceeding expiration. Crackles occuring in mid inspiration are found in patients with bronchiectasis, and late inspiratory crackles occur in those with pulmonary oedema. In patients with pulmonary fibrosis (fibrosing alveolitis or asbestosis) the crackles may occur throughout inspiration, but are usually loudest at the end.

Radiographic examination

Proper assessment of the patient with respiratory disease may involve standard chest radiography, isotope lung scanning, ultrasound or computerized tomography.

Chest radiograph

The standard PA chest radiograph remains the single most important investigation performed on patients with respiratory disease. Every opportunity should be taken to look at films to build up an image of normality so that abnormalities can subsequently be quickly recognized. Pulmonary changes may consist of discrete lesions (single or multiple), diffuse changes, or changes involving the pleura or chest wall. Single coin lesions may be due to a bronchial carcinoma, metastatic carcinoma, TB, histoplasmosis, a hamartoma, abscess,

rheumatoid nodule or fungal ball. Multiple coin lesions are most commonly due to metastases from an extrathoracic tumour, but may also be due to abscesses, rheumatoid nodules, infarcts or lymphoma. Cavitating lesions are usually due to a carcinoma or infection, but pulmonary infarction sometimes leads to cavitation especially if it involves the upper lobes. Widespread alveolar shadowing may be due to pulmonary oedema or infection. Other more diffuse shadowing may reveal diagnostic clues by virtue of the zones which are maximally involved. Upper zone shadowing may be infective (e.g. TB and klebsiella), fibrotic (e.g. ankylosing spondylitis, silicosis, burnt out phase of sarcoid) or allergic (e.g. bronchopulmonary aspergillosis, or extrinsic allergic alveolitis). Bilateral lower zone shadowing with loss of volume suggests the possibility of fibrosing alveolitis or asbestosis (for the latter look for corroboratory pleural plaques). Unilateral translucency may be due to soft tissue loss, such as mastectomy or absence of pectoralis major, but may also be due to lung disease, such as McLeod's syndrome, pneumothorax or lobar collapse with compensatory over-inflation of the remaining lung. Homogeneous uniform opacification is usually due to airless lung, fluid, infarction or solid tumour. If a whole hemithorax is involved and opaque and the mediastinum is shifted toward the abnormality it is due to collapse. If away from the opacification the diagnosis is likely to be a large pleural effusion. Lesser quantities of fluid in the pleural space leads to obliteration of the costophrenic angle and with moderate quantities, shadowing with a classical upper border which is curvilinear towards the axilla. Common pitfalls in interpretation of a standard chest radiograph involve a failure to compare the two sides, failure to look behind the heart shadow (for a left lower lobe collapse or hiatus hernia) and a failure to obtain old films for comparison.

Isotope ventilation and perfusion lung scanning

Isotope ventilation and perfusion lung scanning has its major role in the diagnosis of pulmonary thromboembolic disease. If a technetium macroaggregate perfusion scan is normal on four views within four days of onset of suggestive symptoms then a significant pulmonary embolus is extremely unlikely. If the perfusion scan shows inhomogeneity then this may reflect either pulmonary vascular occlusion or hypoxic vasocontriction in areas of diminished ventilation, and a ventilation scan is then essential. Whilst xenon is still sometimes used, it is only the wash-in and wash-out images that are useful, for the equilibration picture represents lung volume rather than ventilation. The ultra short life krypton 81 is to be preferred and matched ventilation and perfusion defects would suggest airway disease and hypoxic pulmonary vasoconstriction, whilst impaired perfusion in a normally ventilated region (an unmatched defect) suggests pulmonary thromboembolic disease.

Ultrasound of the chest

Ultrasound of the chest has a limited, but useful role in elucidating the nature of shadows close to the chest wall. Normal lung tissue conducts sound poorly, but an ultrasound performed with a probe in the intercostal window reveals echoes from the visceral and parietal pleura and then a non echogenic zone. A solid lesion (tumour or consolidation) adjacent to the chest wall reflects masses of echoes and can be distinguished from a pleural effusion where the picture is of chest wall and parietal pleural echoes separated by an echo free zone from the visceral pleura and lung edge. Ultrasound examination may thus be useful in determining the best site for pleural aspiration.

Computerized tomography of the chest

Computerized tomography of the chest is largely replacing conventional linear tomography and playing an increasing role in evaluation of patients with respiratory disease. The current indications for CT scans are:

* Assessment of operability of bronchial carcinoma (see p. 77).
* Assessment of spread and response to chemotherapy in other tumours that have spread to, or arisen in the mediastinum (e.g. germ cell tumours).
* Diagnosis of bronchiectasis.
* Elucidation of unexplained plain chest X-ray shadows, especially in the mediastinum and the paravertebral gutter.

Lung function tests

The function of the lungs is to maintain normal and nearly constant oxygen and carbon dioxide pressures and content in the arterial blood in all phy-

siological circumstances. This is achieved by the efficient transfer of gas between alveolar air and the blood passing through the alveolar capillaries. This involves four processes:

* *Ventilation* – the delivery of inspired air to the alveoli by the bellows action of the lung.
* *Pulmonary capillary blood flow* – delivery of blood to the pulmonary capillaries by the action of the right ventricle.
* *Diffusion* – the passage of gases from blood to air.
* *Adequate control of the above stages.*

Testing of lung function therefore involves either direct measurement of ventilation, pulmonary capillary blood flow and diffusion or measurements which reflect the consequences of their derangement. Standard testing would therefore include measurement of:

* Ventilatory capacity
  1. dynamic lung volumes e.g. $FEV_{1.0}$, FVC, flow volume curves and PEFR;
  2. static lung volumes e.g. TLC.
* Gas transfer
  1. transfer factor for carbon monoxide;
  2. blood gases.

Spirometry

The expiratory spirogram is performed on a low resistance spirometer and the patient inhales maximally then breathes out as hard and as far as possible. Measurement is made of the amount of air expired and at the rate at which it is exhaled. From the spirogram are measured the $FEV_{1.0}$ and the FVC. The forced expiratory volume in 1 second ($FEV_{1.0}$) is the volume of air expelled in the first second of a forced expiration starting from full inspiration. The forced vital capacity (FVC) is the volume of air expelled by a maximal expiration after a maximum inspiration. Normal subjects exhale 70–75 per cent of that volume in the first second of a maximum expiration. The cardinal feature of airway narrowing is prolongation of expiration so that FEV/FVC ratio may fall to 40–45 per cent (Fig. 2.1). In restrictive disorders the $FEV_{1.0}$ and FVC are reduced by the same proportion giving an FEV/VC ratio of greater than 75 per cent.

The peak expiratory flow rate (PEFR) is the greatest flow that can be sustained for 10 milliseconds on forced expiration starting from full inspiration; it is measured in litres/minute with a Wright's peak flow meter or Mini peak flow meter.

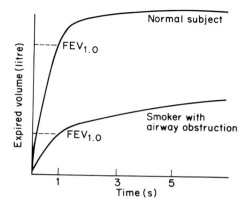

Fig 2.1 Spirogram for a normal subject and a smoker with airway obstruction. Note that the smoker is still exhaling at 7 seconds – prolongation of expiration is one of the cardinal features of airway narrowing.

Flow volume curves

The spirogram plots exhaled volume against time. If we instead plot exhaled volume against flow rate we produce a curve or loop which assumes a differing shape in different situations and in different diseases. The explanation for these differences is complex and in some areas contentious, but in their simplest form these curves provide useful clues as to the cause of airway narrowing in individual cases. The normal expiratory flow volume curve

has a characteristic shape with an early peak which corresponds to the peak expiratory flow rate measured on a Wright's peak flow meter. The flow rate then declines in a roughly linear fashion towards end-expiration. Much of the expiratory curve, especially toward residual volume, is independent of effort and provided a minimal driving pressure is applied the curve is very reproducible. At residual volume the patient breathes in to total lung capacity and a semi circular inspiratory loop is recorded. Figure 2.2 shows some examples of normal and abnormal flow volume curves. These can detect disease at an early stage, can often help determine the likelihood of there being significant emphysema, and are invaluable in cases of upper airway obstruction.

Total lung capacity (TLC)

Total lung capacity is measured either in a body plethysmograph or by a helium dilution method. The latter assumes that inert and insoluble helium is not absorbed and the patient breathes in and out of a bag of known volume containing a known concentration of gas until equilibration has taken place with the gas in the lungs. Due to slow mixing, equilibration may take up to 15 minutes in patients with severe airway narrowing. In the plethysmographic method the patient sits in an air-tight box and pants or inspires against a closed shutter within the mouthpiece. Inspiration causes intrathoracic air to be decompressed, whilst the air in the box is compressed by the increase in chest volume. The

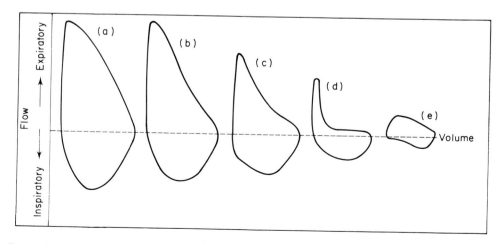

Fig 2.2 Examples of normal and abnormal flow volume curves: (a) Normal. (b) Early airflow limitation (e.g. young smoker). (c) Volume dependent airway obstruction (e.g. asthma). (d) Pressure dependent airway obstruction (e.g. emphysema). (e) Rigid extrathoracic obstruction (e.g. tracheal stenosis).

volume changes must be equal and opposite and the pressure change in the patient's lung is measured in the mouthpiece shutter. Lung volume is calculated by Boyles' law (P1 × V1 = P2 × (V1 + dV)). TLC, however measured, is usually increased in patients with airway disease, with the largest changes occurring in the patient with emphysema and loss of elastic recoil. In patients with parenchymal lung disease such as fibrosis, the lungs are small and stiff. Reduced TLC also occurs in those with reduced respiratory muscle pressures or chest wall deformity.

Carbon monoxide uptake

This test measures the ability of the lungs to transfer gas from alveolar air into pulmonary capillary blood. Carbon monoxide is used because with low concentrations the partial pressure in the pulmonary capillary blood remains low in comparison to that in air, so that the gas is taken up all along the capillaries. The uptake is affected by a membrane component, and by the rate of combination in the red cells. The membrane component is affected by the surface area available for gas exchange, by the correct matching of ventilation and perfusion and also by the thickness of the membrane. The red cell component is affected by haemoglobin and the pulmonary capillary blood volume. Rate of uptake of carbon monoxide (TLCO) is therefore reduced in patients with anaemia, emphysema and interstitial lung disease, but also by reduction in surface area, for example by pneumonectomy. To counteract for such misleading impression of a defect in gas exchange, the rate of transfer of carbon monoxide is usually 'corrected' for effective available alveolar volume (VA). This is done by combining the inspired carbon monoxide with inert helium for a simultaneous measurement of the lung volume available to the test gas. Testing therefore involves the patient taking a vital capacity breath of a known low concentration of carbon monoxide (0.3 per cent) and helium (10 per cent), holding the breath for 10 seconds and exhaling. The first 750 ml are discarded because of dead space contamination, and the next litre analyzed for carbon monoxide and helium concentration. On the assumption that the CO is lost from alveolar gas in propor-

Table 2.2   Typical results of lung function testing in patients with lung disorders

Measurement	Chronic airflow limitation	Chronic airflow limitation with emphysema	Asthma	Restrictive disorders (e.g. pulmonary fibrosis, kyphoscoliosis, respiratory muscle weakness, pleural disease, obesity)
Forced expiratory volume in 1 second ($FEV_{1.0}$)	Reduced	Reduced	Reduced	Reduced
Forced vital capacity (FVC)	Reduced	Reduced	Reduced	Reduced
FEV/VC %	Less than 75 %	Less than 75 %	Less than 75 %	More than 75 %
Residual volume (RV)	Increased	Increased and often markedly increased	Increased	Reduced
Total lung capacity (TLC)	Normal or slightly increased	Increased and often markedly increased	Normal or increased	Reduced
Expiratory flow volume curve (see Fig. 2.2)	Volume dependent airway collapse	Pressure dependent airway collapse	Volume dependent airway collapse	Unhelpful
Transfer factor for carbon monoxide (TLCO)	Reduced	Markedly reduced	Normal or reduced	Normal or reduced
Transfer factor for carbon monoxide per unit lung volume (KCo)	Normal	Markedly reduced	Normal	Normal or reduced

tion to the P_{CO} during breath holding, the TLCO is calculated as the amount of carbon monoxide transferred/minute corrected for the concentration gradient of carbon monoxide across the alveolar capillary membrane (mMol/min/kPa). The KCO is TLCO/VA (mMol/min/kPA/litre) where VA is the alveolar volume obtained by simultaneous inspiration of helium. (KCO is the TLCO/unit volume, or is the amount of CO transferred/minute corrected for the concentration gradient of carbon monoxide across the alveolar capillary membrane per unit volume.) Because the uptake of carbon monoxide is dependent upon haemoglobin concentration the TLCO and KCO may be high if extra haemoglobin is available for uptake because of either polycythaemia or because of intra-alveolar haemorrhage. In the latter case the carbon monoxide uptake is increased for the first 24 hours or so after intrapulmonary bleeding. The haemoglobin is later denatured and the KCO rapidly returns to base line. The measurement has proved useful in elucidating the cause of unexpected radiographic shadowing and in monitoring the response to treatment in patients with diseases such as Goodpasture's syndrome or idiopathic pulmonary haemosiderosis which are associated with intra-alveolar haemorrhage.

Table 2.2 summarizes typical patterns of abnormality of lung function tests in some of the commoner respiratory disorders.

Blood gas estimation

The ultimate measurement of lung function is the measurement of blood gases, abnormalities of which reflect severe derangement of one or more of the four components of lung function. There are four causes of hypoxaemia at normal altitude:

- hypoventilation
- diffusion impairment
- shunt
- ventilation and perfusion mismatching,

and two causes of increased arterial CO_2

- hypoventilation
- ventilation and perfusion mismatching.

Hypoventilation is commonly the result of non pulmonary disorders and CO_2 retention and hypoxaemia always coexist. The hypoxaemia can be easily abolished by increasing the inspired oxygen concentration, but P_{CO_2} will only be normalized by increasing ventilation. Hypoventilation may be due

to disorders of the respiratory centre (e.g. drug overdose), disorders of the medulla (e.g. encephalitis), cervical cord (trauma), anterior horn cell (e.g. poliomyelitis), motor nerve (e.g. Guillain-Barré), neuromuscular junction (e.g. myasthenia gravis), respiratory muscles (muscular dystrophy), thoracic cage trauma or upper airway obstruction (see sleep apnoea).

Diffusion limitation as a cause of hypoxaemia is uncommon. Whilst it may theoretically occur in fibrosing alveolitis, alveolar cell carcinoma or asbestosis, the concept of 'alveolar capillary block' seems unlikely; massive membrane thickening would be needed to explain the blood gas disturbance. It is more likely that the hypoxaemia in these diseases reflects secondary ventilation/perfusion imbalance.

Ventilation perfusion mismatching is the commonest cause of both hypoxaemia and CO_2 retention. In the normal lung, pulmonary vasoconstriction in response to hypoxia (and to a lesser extent bronchodilation in response to hypercapnoea), continually match local ventilation and perfusion, in spite of large variations in both variables between top and bottom of the lung. The major cause of ventilation and perfusion imbalance in disease is intra-regional inhomogeneity of ventilation so that perfusion exceeds ventilation and blood passes through without gas exchange occurring; arterial oxygen levels fall and carbon dioxide levels rise. Such inequality of ventilation occurs in airway disease, emphysema and fibrotic conditions. Primary abnormalities of distribution of perfusion also occur, for example in patients with pulmonary thromboembolism and in those with raised left atrial pressure.

Hypoxaemia may also result from shunts. These may occur because of a cardiac septal defect, a patent ductus arteriosus or because of an intrapulmonary arteriovenous malformation. The term shunt is also applied to what is really an extreme form of ventilation/perfusion inequality when blood passes through a completely unventilated consolidated lobar pneumonia. With shunts pure oxygen will not improve the PaO_2 to normal levels.

Indications for lung function tests Simple tests performed frequently are often of more value than detailed tests made only occasionally. Formal lung function tests may be needed for one of several reasons:

- Diagnosis – only asthma is defined in terms of an abnormality in function and therefore only asthma can be diagnosed by these tests. However, other diagnoses may be suggested by certain patterns of functional abnormality. For example severe airway narrowing, large lungs, reduced CO uptake and pressure dependent collapse on the flow volume curve would be suggestive of the presence of emphysema (see Table 2.2).
- Assessment of severity and monitoring of progression of disease or response to therapy. This applies most often to patients with pulmonary fibrosis e.g. fibrosing alveolitis or sarcoidosis.
- Determination of relative contribution of cardiac, respiratory or extrathoracic disease to the sensation of breathlessness.
- Detection of upper airway obstruction by measurement of flow volume curves (see Fig. 2.2).
- Monitoring intra-alveolar haemorrhage.
- Assessment of fitness for surgery. For extrathoracic surgery, spirometery ± blood gas estimation alone may be sufficient. For planned cardiac, oesophageal or pulmonary surgery, more detailed testing is often necessary (see p. 77 for 'assessment of operability').

Bronchoscopy

Fibreoptic bronchoscopy has now been available for 20 years and is an important tool in the management of patients with respiratory disease. It has largely superseded rigid bronchoscopy although the latter still has a role in children, for the removal of foreign bodies, for photography and more recently for laser resection of major airway tumours where it is used in conjunction with the fibrescope. The major advantages of the fibreoptic bronchoscope are that more of the bronchial tree can be visualized particularly in the upper lobes. It can be performed safely and comfortably under topical anaesthesia on an out-patient basis. The major indication is diagnostic, but the technique may be useful therapeutically in patients with sputum retention, especially in the critically ill patient being mechanically ventilated. Further intensive care indications are to assess the patency and position of the endotracheal tube and also with intubation, especially in those with severe maxillo-facial injuries. The major indication for diagnostic bronchoscopy is in patients with suspected bronchial carcinoma where bronchial mucosal samples may be taken for histological examination and brush biopsies and washings taken for cytology. In suspected tuberculosis and in immunosupressed patients with opportunist infections, the procedure is helpful in obtaining samples for microbiological examination.

Lung biopsy

The lung may be biopsied via the bronchoscope, through the chest wall or by means of a thoracotomy. Selection of the appropriate approach depends on whether the lesion is discrete or diffuse, its position, and the likely diagnosis. With localized lesions beyond the range of the bronchoscope, either fine needle aspiration biopsy or cutting needle biopsy (Trucut) would be performed under radiological screening. The former procedure produces samples suitable for cytological examination, but trucut biopsy produces a core of tissue which can be processed histologically. With diffuse lung disease, transbronchial lung biopsy via the fibreoptic bronchoscope is usually the most appropriate technique. The bronchoscope is passed in the normal way to a segmental bronchus and the forceps advanced into the abnormal area under screening. At the end of a deep inspiration the forceps are opened, the patient fully exhales and the forceps are closed, trapping bronchial mucosa, a subcarina, and lung tissue. Such biopsies provide a high diagnostic yield in sarcoidosis, tuberculosis, diffuse malignancy or lymphoma, and in patients with opportunist infections especially with pneumocystis carinii. It is a much less useful procedure in fibrosing alveolitis where the small samples make it difficult to determine whether there is any excess of fibrous tissue or alveolar inflammation.

Broncho-alveolar lavage

This simple technique presupposes that cells washed from the lung may bear some relationship to the pathological processes taking place in the surrounding tissue. The technique is under evaluation, but some aspects are of value. During routine bronchoscopy the tip of the instrument is wedged in a radiographically abnormal segment and 50–100 ml aliquots of buffered normal saline are passed into the lung during inspiration and then aspirated. Twenty to eighty per cent of the instilled fluid is recovered some of which is sent for bacteriological culture and may be useful in diagnosing TB.

Cytological examination of the fluid may be helpful in pneumocystis infections and also in recovering asbestos bodies. A negative culture is essential if the rest of the lavage fluid is to be examined. Most recent interest has been in the interpretation of the differential cell count in the lavaged fluid. In normal subjects macrophages account for 91–93 per cent of the recovered cells with 1 per cent polymorphs and 5–7 per cent lymphocytes. In cases of unexplained diffuse pulmonary shadowing a lymphocyte count of over 30 per cent is suggestive of active sarcoidosis. Neutrophilia, in the absence of infection, is suggestive of a significant degree of pulmonary fibrosis. These findings may have importance in the selection of patients with diffuse lung disease for steroid therapy.

Pleural biopsy

Pleural effusions may arise as a result of a number of diseases, but the two commonest reasons for large unilateral effusions are malignancy and tuberculosis. Simple aspiration and cytological and bacteriological examination may be helpful, but a general rule should be never to aspirate an undiagnosed effusion without also performing a biopsy, because the yield with that technique is so much greater. Under local anaesthesia an Abrams' needle is inserted and multiple biopsies taken with the cutting surface at each hour of the clock face other than 12. The latter is omitted because a biopsy performed with the cutting edge pointing upwards runs the risk of damage to the intercostal vein, artery and nerve lying in the groove on the inferior surface of the rib above. In both TB and malignancy, biopsy produces a diagnosis in 60–80 per cent of cases.

Diseases of the respiratory system

Diseases of the airways

Diseases of the airways involve changes in the lumen, the airway wall or changes outside the bronchial wall. Most will result in some airway narrowing and limitation to air flow. Such obstruction may be localized (in the larger airways), or more generalized with narrowing of all of the medium and small airways.

Table 2.3 lists the commonest causes of generalized airway narrowing and Table 2.4 gives some causes of localized obstruction. It will be apparent

Table 2.3 Causes of generalized airway obstruction

Asthma
Chronic bronchitis
Emphysema
Bronchiectasis
Cystic fibrosis
Fungal hypersensitivity
Obliterative bronchiolitis
?Fibrotic disease

Table 2.4 Causes of localized obstruction

Vocal cord paresis	Post-tracheostomy
Laryngeal carcinoma	stenosis
Tracheal carcinoma	Laryngomalacia
Bronchial carcinoma	Relapsing polychondritis
Foreign bodies	Extrinsic compression
Obstructive sleep	Fungal hypersensitivity
apnoea	

that asthma, chronic bronchitis, emphysema and chronic airflow limitation are the commonest causes of generalized airway narrowing and prior to a detailed description of each we must think clearly about classification and terminology.

Clinicians talk of a chronic bronchitic to convey an image of a breathless patient and yet the epidemiologist's definition mentions only a chronic productive cough. Others talk of a patient as having emphysema and yet this is strictly a pathological diagnosis characterized by destruction and distortion of alveolar sacs. The definition of asthma is more widely accepted and yet the magnitude of reversibility needed to fulfill the diagnosis has never been clarified. Terminologically the problem can be solved, for the basic problem is of airway obstruction which limits airflow. The purist will realize that air flow may also be limited by a reduced driving pressure (such as fibrotic disease or muscle weakness), and so airway narrowing or obstructive airway disease are the terms to be preferred. Where we must not permit confusion is in the classification of these diseases. Whilst overlap does occur there are many reasons why we should take a 'constituent disease' approach to the problem of generalized airway narrowing. The Venn diagram in Figure 2.3 shows one possible classification and shows the separation of generalized airway narrowing into two main disease groups. The diagram shows that some patients may have a persistent cough and sputum production for more

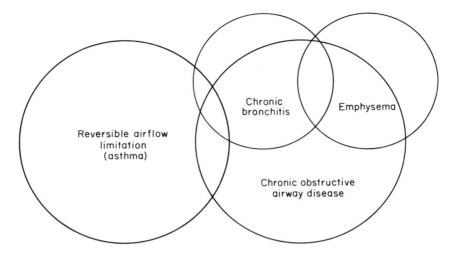

Fig 2.3   A Venn diagram showing the division of generalized airway diseases into asthma on the left hand side of the diagram, and predominantly irreversible disease on the right hand side of the diagram.

than 3 months of each year for 3 consecutive years (chronic bronchitis) and that this may or may not coexist with chronic airway obstruction. It also exemplifies the overlap in that some patients with asthma develop a fixed component to their airway narrowing and some with irreversible airway disease have some response to bronchodilators. However, the main feature of the diagram is that it demonstrates that the majority of patients with generalized airway narrowing fall into one of two groups; those with smoking induced predominantly irreversible airway obstruction (alias chronic bronchitis, emphysema, chronic airflow limitation, etc.,) and those with predominantly reversible airway narrowing which is called asthma. The diagnostic label attached to a patient determines treatment and each patient should be carefully positioned to the left or to the right of the Venn diagram. Only in this way will we avoid dangerous under-treatment of asthma, and avoid inappropriate treatments such as steroids and theophyllines being given to those with predominantly irreversible disease (from smoking).

Asthma

The most widely accepted definition of asthma is that it is a disease characterized by airway narrowing which varies in severity over short periods of time either spontaneously or as a result of treatment. Whilst traditionally classified as extrinsic or

intrinsic this offers no particular merit for our treatment or further understanding of the disease. The major clinical features are of cough, breathlessness and wheeze of varying severity. It may be associated with a personal history of the related conditions of hay fever or nasal polypi, or with a family history of these disorders.

Epidemiology

Studies of prevalence vary according to whether we discuss the number suffering from asthma at one point in time (current prevalence) or whether, with a variable disease, we include all who have ever had the disease (cumulative prevalence). In the UK various studies have shown current prevalence rates in children of 2–4 per cent and cumulative rates of 3–7 per cent. Current prevalence rates in adults range from 1–5 per cent of the population. Prevalence varies from one country to another and within the UK there is evidence of the disease becoming commoner in the last 40 years, although this may in part reflect changes in diagnostic practice. The death rate peaked in the early 1960s as a probable result of patients delaying seeking medical advice because of the introduction of self help with high dose isoprenaline inhalers. The mortality then remained constant for a decade, but recent evidence suggests a further UK increase involving all age groups although the biggest increase in deaths have occurred in the 5–34 age group. Boys are twice as likely to have asthma as girls whilst in adults both sexes are equally affected. Fifty per cent of patients will have developed asthma by the age of 10 years, but 50 per cent of children will be symptom free by the age of 20 years.

Pathogenesis

A cardinal feature of asthma is that the patients exhibit bronchial hyper-reactivity or bronchial hyper-responsiveness to inhaled substances. Appreciation of this basic excessive irritability is central to our current understanding of asthma. The manifestations of the disease arise when these irritable airways come into contact with a trigger factor. Thus:

Asthma = Bronchial hyper-responsiveness + Trigger

The list of trigger factors is enormous ranging from inhaled allergens such as pollen and house dust mite, through to exercise, infections, laughter and menstruation, to occupational factors, food and alcohol. Most patients with asthma have multiple triggers and the majority cannot be identified. Management of the disease has correctly moved away from 'trigger factor management' to treatment of the underlying hyper-reactivity and inflammation. Whilst the hyper-reactivity is a central feature the mechanism of its production is not clear and its relationship to chemical mediator release poorly understood. Current interest involves the substance platelet activating factor which seems to be capable of producing prolonged bronchial hyper-reactivity even in normal subjects. Irrespective of whether a trigger factor is physical such as exercise or an IgE mediated antigen/antibody reaction, the result is a release of chemical mediators from mast cells. Sometimes there may be a neurogenic interplay and with a minority of triggers, stimulation of vagal receptors in the bronchial mucosa may stimulate bronchoconstriction independently of mediator release. The pathological features of asthma include infiltration of the bronchial walls with inflammatory cells (neutrophils and eosinophils), mucosal oedema, mucus plugging and bronchial smooth muscle hypertrophy and contraction. All these factors can be produced by the mediators contained in, or produced by, mast cells. Some are preformed and contained in granules within the mast cell and these include histamine and eosinophil and neutrophil chemotactic factors which attract neutrophils and

eosinophils to the site of mast cell degranulation. In addition to the release of preformed inflammatory chemicals mast cell degranulation is associated with a release of arachidonic acid. This serves as a substrate for cyclo-oxygenase and lipoxygenase enzymes which synthesize prostaglandins and a variety of leukotrienes, differing types being capable of causing the smooth muscle constriction, mucosal oedema, mucus secretion and bronchial epithelial damage which is characteristic of asthma. This bronchial epithelial damage seems to correlate well with the degree of bronchial hyper-reactivity and such damage has been seen in mucosal biopsy samples taken from patients who are relatively symptom free from their asthma at the time of biopsy. This demonstration of damage and irritability even when patients are well is now changing the emphasis of asthma therapy away from first aid relieving bronchodilator treatment towards much more aggressive regular anti-inflammatory regimes.

Diagnosis

A clear history of variable breathlessness and wheezing, variable PEFRs, and a response to bronchodilators is diagnostic. The problem arises with children where symptoms may be confused with infection and in adults where the variability of the disease may not be apparent. Children should never be given antibiotics for respiratory symptoms without a consideration of the diagnosis of asthma and the question 'has the child ever wheezed?' should always be asked. If doubt persists a simple exercise test can be performed; 6 minutes free running with PEFR measurement before and for 12 minutes afterwards will produce a post exercise fall in PEFR of more than 15 per cent in the asthmatic child. In adults every symptomatic patient with severe airway narrowing should at some time have a formal 10-day diagnostic trial of prednisolone 40 mg daily, monitored by 3 times daily PEFRs. This will ensure that a label of 'chronic bronchitis' is never mistakenly applied to the potentially more treatable condition of asthma.

Treatment

For the patient with very occasional symptoms a beta agonist bronchodilator such as inhaled salbutamol or terbutaline is required, and the patient given careful instruction in the correct use of either a metered dose inhaler, a dry powder rotahaler or a spacer inhaler. With more frequent symptoms the need is not for more broncho-dilators, whether beta agonist or theophylline, but for specific preventative anti-inflammatory measures; a damping down of the underlying bronchial irritability. In a child the first choice may be cromoglycate which is safe and effective, but has the disadvantage of a minimum three times daily regime. For other children and for adults, inhaled steroids (beclomethasone or budesonide) are necessary. These need to be taken regularly from the same range of inhalational devices as are available for bronchodilators. Inhaled steroids have the advantage that they are effective, remarkably free of side-effects and are delivered direct to the site of action. They need only be taken twice daily to achieve effect. For patients who are still inad-equately controlled on standard doses of inhaled steroids, or for those who need frequent courses of oral steroids, the introduction of higher dose beclomethasone (up to 2000 μg/day) has improved control. Although clinical problems are unlikely, patients on these latter doses should be considered to have a minor degree of hypothalamo-pituitary-adrenal suppression and operations and periods of stress should be covered as for those on oral steroids. The treatment of asthma is summarized in Fig. 2.4.

The anaesthetist's involvement with asthmatic patients pertains to the perioperative care of the asthmatic having elective or emergency surgery, and the intensive care of the patient with acute severe asthma.

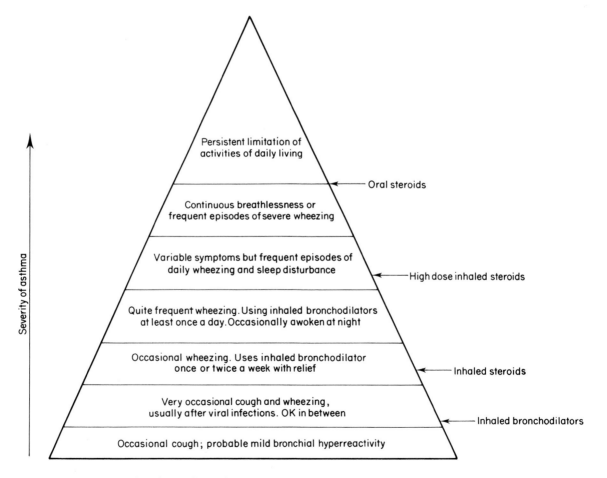

Fig 2.4 A treatment plan for asthma. Note that inhaled bronchodilators are always preferable to tablets. Night-time wheezing reflects poorly controlled asthma. Improving treatment usually abolishes nocturnal waking. If persistent symptoms occur, a bed-time dose of theophylline may be indicated.

Management of asthmatic patients having elective surgery

Patients with asthma should be treated in the weeks prior to surgery so that their disease is well controlled by the time of admission. Knowledge of the epithelial damage and bronchial hyper-responsiveness that can be present even in the mild asthmatic (mentioned earlier) emphasizes the need for a low threshold for intervention with inhaled steroids. If there is any doubt about the control of the patient's airways they should undergo a period of domiciliary peak flow monitoring. If readings are reduced, and especially if there is diurnal variability then a regular inhaled steroid should be introduced. Perioperatively the patient may require oral or parenteral steroid cover and nebulized bronchodilators should be available, but the aim should be good preoperative control of disease rather than perioperative first aid with high dose bronchodilators. If this policy is adopted the risk of further airway narrowing in response to endotracheal intubation, coughing or drugs will be reduced.

Drugs which release histamine or cause bronchoconstriction should be avoided, e.g. morphine, tubocurarine and neostigmine.

Emergency surgery

With non elective surgery the anaesthetist will be faced with the patient whose asthma may or may not be well controlled. Historical evidence of night time wheezing or early morning waking would certainly suggest uncontrolled disease. The lesser degrees of uncontrolled hyper-reactivity may not be apparent. Clinical and spirometric assessment is essential and if there are doubts about pre-existing control, or if the patient was on oral or high dose inhaled steroids, then parenteral hydrocortisone should be given with the premedication. Intraoperative worsening of airway narrowing may indicate the need for hydrocortisone, aminophylline or salbutamol. The latter should be used with caution in the presence of halothane and dosage of aminophylline should be calculated carefully and adjusted if the patient was on previous oral theophylline therapy. It should be given by slow infusion over 20 minutes. Postoperatively, nebulized beta agonists should be available in a dose of salbutamol 2.5 mg q.d.s. Aminophylline suppositories are associated with variable and unpredictable absorption and have been superseded by the availability of nebulized bronchodilators.

Acute severe asthma

Patients and doctors frequently underestimate the severity of asthma. The only safe way to manage patients admitted to hospital with acute severe asthma is to make an initial objective assessment with recording of peak expiratory flow rate and arterial blood gas tensions, and to repeat these measurements frequently until one is sure that the patient is responding to treatment. Listening to wheezes is a notoriously unreliable guide to the severity of asthma! Assessment is clinical, spirometric and by blood gas estimation. A chest radiograph is always performed to exclude a complicating infection or pneumothorax. All patients with acute severe asthma need to be taken seriously and treated energetically, but if any of the following features are present the situation is imminently life-threatening and the patient requires intensive care and probably mechanical ventilation:

- Exhaustion.
- Disturbance of consciousness.
- Inability to talk because of breathlessness.
- Tachycardia greater than 120/minute.
- Pulsus paradoxus.
- Central cyanosis.
- Pneumothorax or pneumo mediastinum.
- Pa_{O_2} less than 60 mmHg (8 kPa).
- Pa_{CO_2} greater than 45 mmHg (6 kPa).
- ECG evidence of right heart strain.

Treatment of acute severe asthma

All patients are distressed and require reassurance, rehydration and oxygen. The excessive minute ventilation plus inadequate oral intake of fluid leads to dehydration. Oxygen is given in concentrations of 28–35 per cent, or higher as necessary, via a venti-mask. Although respiratory efforts are initially well preserved, if the patient is exhausted uncontrolled oxygen may give rise to CO_2 retention. Sedation is never given and specific therapy with steroids and bronchodilators is introduced as quickly as possible. Oral prednisolone (40 mg daily) may be sufficient for the minor to moderately severe attack with i.v. hydrocortisone being reserved for those with incipient ventilatory failure. The hydrocortisone hemisuccinate salt should always be used and not the phosphate salt which gives anogenital pruritus. Hydrocortisone is not totally innocuous and when given intravenously can cause urticaria and increased bronchospasm – this is more likely in aspirin sensitive asthmatics. If it is indicated, the initial bolus is given in a dose of 4 mg/kg body weight followed by 3 mg/kg body weight/6 hours.

Nebulized salbutamol is given to adults in a dose of 2.5–5.0 mg, 4-hourly. A lower dose should be given in patients with coronary artery disease and the patient should be questioned as to the presence of chest pain after the first dose. The nebulized anticholinergic agent ipratropium bromide has little advantage over salbutamol, but if the patient has a poor response to the first dose of beta agonist 250–500 micrograms of ipratropium may be given. Even when diluted with normal saline, paradoxical bronchoconstriction may occur with this product. Aminophylline is not necessary for most patients with asthma, but may be indicated for those with severe disease. A loading dose of 5 mg/kg body weight is given intravenously by slow infusion over 20–30 minutes. If the patient was previously on an oral theophylline preparation, plasma theophylline levels should be measured and i.v. aminophylline dosage adjusted accordingly. If an emergency theophylline assay is not available, the loading dose should be halved if the patient had never previously had a theophylline blood level measurement, or omitted if the patient's previous theophylline therapy had been laboratory titrated (the assumption being that the plasma theophylline level is then in the normal range). Maintenance therapy with aminophylline is given in a dose of 0.5 mg/kg body weight/hour. If the patient has heart failure or liver disease the dose should be reduced by a third, or preferably plasma levels should be estimated. Aminophylline may be cumulative if continued for more than 24 hours and prescribers should be aware that concomitant prescription of erythromycin and cimetidine reduces theophylline clearance.

The commonest indication for artificial ventilation of patients with severe asthma is exhaustion. If the $PaCO_2$ is raised on admission and does not fall within the first 3–4 hours, or if it rises, mechanical ventilation is indicated. Intubation and artificial ventilation of severe asthmatics require considerable skill and continued observation for the development of a pneumothorax. If the patient fails to improve with conventional treatment and mechanical ventilation, some workers have reported benefit from ether. Halothane has bronchodilator activity and probably relaxes smooth muscle and antagonizes the bronchoconstrictor effects of histamine and acetylcholine. However, its usage may be limited in these patients by its negative inotropic effect and predisposition to catecholamine induced cardiac arrhythmias which may be aggravated by hypoxia. Ether has similarly been known to be a bronchodilator for over 70 years and if problems arise with halothane or if there is no success with steroids, bronchodilators and halothane anaesthesia, then ether may have a role in a life-threatening situation.

Recovery

Peak flow rates should show some response pretty promptly, but PaO_2 remains low for 10–14 days. As the patient improves, night time dipping of peak flow rate often becomes apparent and the third and fourth nights in hospital may be particular periods of danger. Steroids should be continued for a minimum 14-day course and metered dose inhaled bronchodilator therapy should always be re-instituted at least 24 hours before the patient is discharged from hospital, to ensure that no deterioration occurs when the nebulizer is stopped. These patients should be reviewed within one week of discharge, for 'asthma deaths' frequently involve patients recently discharged from hospital. Every admission of a patient with acute severe asthma is a reflection of the failure of their previous therapy:

- Was the patient using the inhaler satisfactory?
- Was the patient on adequate preventative therapy with inhaled steroids?
- Did the patient act appropriately to the worsening asthma and appreciate the severity? If not, further advice should be given and the patient issued with a peak flow meter for home monitoring.

Drugs to avoid in asthma

Aspirin has been known to be capable of inducing asthma for 50 years and such attacks may be fatal. Typically an acute attack develops within 2 minutes to 2 hours after taking aspirin and the patient is likely to have taken the drug before with impunity. About 2 per cent of British asthmatics are aspirin sensitive and the mechanism results from an imbalance between bronchodilator and bronchoconstricting prostaglandins. Other prostaglandin inhibitors such as non steroidal anti-inflammatory agents may cause similar, but less severe problems. Aspirin sensitive asthmatics may also react adversely to intravenous hydrocortisone and to the yellow colouring agent tartrazine. Paracetamol is likely to be a safer mild analgesic or anti pyretic for patients with asthma.

Beta blockers are well recognized to have an adverse effect when given orally or intravenously to patients with asthma. Less well known is the adverse affect of the ocular beta blocker (Timolol) which is an effective treatment for glaucoma. Just one or two eyedrops may be sufficient to provoke asthma and should be avoided in patients with asthma.

Chronic obstructive airway disease (chronic bronchitis and emphysema)

Chronic obstructive airway disease is the 'English disease' and causes the loss of 30 million working days/year in the UK and 25 000 deaths. There is evidence of a decline in the number of men suffering from the disease, but as with lung cancer it is becoming more common amongst women. Whilst occasional non smoking patients are still seen, in whom some occupational or environmental factor has initiated the disease, the majority of patients are suffering from the effects of cigarette smoke inhalation. However, not all smokers develop the disease and this has led to a search for a susceptibility factor which is possibly inherited. One such factor that is known is alpha$_1$ anti-trypsin deficiency which is inherited in an autosomal recessive fashion. Alpha$_1$ anti-trypsin is a serum protein which can inhibit proteolytic enzymes and in its absence neutrophil elastase, cathepsin and other proteases which are released in response to infections and smoking, have an unhindered field in which to break down elastin, collagen and basement membranes producing emphysema at young ages. This condition is rare and does not explain the susceptibility of the majority of cases although a similar unproven imbalance between proteases and inhibitors may be responsible. Dutch workers have suggested that there may be an aetiological overlap between asthma and the susceptible smokers and pointed out that IgE and eosinophil levels in these patients may be raised and that they may have some degree of bronchial hyper-responsiveness. However, the apparent eosinophilia probably represents the increased total white cell count found in smokers, and the bronchial hyper-reactivity is more likely to be an acquired effect than a predisposing cause.

Pathology

The major feature of this group of diseases is airway obstruction. This is due to factors within the lumen, within the airway wall and outside the airway wall. The effect of smoke is to cause mucus gland hyperplasia. In normal subjects the glandular layer represents only 20–35 per cent of the thickness of the airway wall, but in smokers it may increase to 70 per cent with the thickening impinging upon the airway lumen. This overgrowth of glands is associated with an outpouring of larger than normal quantities of mucus, and the mucus itself is abnormally tenacious. It is ineffectively cleared from the airway because of the stunting and paralyzing effect that smoke has upon the airway cilia, with the result that secretions obstruct the lumen, further reducing airway calibre. If destruction and distortion of airsacs is present (i.e. emphysema), there is further airway narrowing. This occurs because normally elastic lung tissue exerts a spring like or guy-rope like radial traction on the airway maintaining patency. If this spring is over stretched as in emphysema, radial traction is reduced.

Most of these pathological changes are irreversible. Stopping smoking leads to a diminution in mucus production and a diminution in chest infections, but airway narrowing is unchanged. Once the damage is done spirometry or PEFR do not improve, but the subsequent rate of decline reverts to that of age alone and is in parallel with that of the non smoker. By the time FEV$_1$ has fallen below 1 litre, 5-year mortality rates are approximately 40–50 per cent.

Diagnosis and clinical features

The major clinical features relate to airway narrowing and breathlessness and this may or may not be accompanied by the chronic sputum production of chronic bronchitis. Clinical examination, spirometry and chest radiograph may all be helpful in diagnosis and in assessment of severity, but the major point of differentiation is to separate this disease from the more treatable condition of asthma. There may be historical clues in the form of a family history of atopic disease or a clear history of variability, but in the 5th and 6th decades these clues are often absent even in those subsequently shown to be asthmatic. All breathless patients are worse on waking, but a history of premature waking especially around 4 am would be more suggestive of asthma than smoking induced airway obstruction. Wherever there is doubt, a properly controlled trial of oral steroids is required, with prednisolone 40 mg/day being given for 10 days. Response is monitored by the patient making peak flow rate recordings 3 times daily throughout the 10 day period. Those with a significant improvement in flow rate have, by definition, asthma whilst the others have (smoking induced) chronic obstructive airway disease.

Clinical features and pathophysiology

The main symptom suffered by these patients is breathlessness and a productive cough may be present. The more severe cases tend to separate into two clinical syndromes, pink puffers and blue bloaters, although no division is ever absolute and there is considerable overlap of features. The terms are a convenient shorthand method of describing two types of patients with chronic airway disease.

Pink puffers Pink and puffing patients work hard at breathing, hyperventilate the better ventilated parts of the lung and manage to maintain relatively normal oxygen and carbon dioxide levels at rest. Once demands are increased by exercise they desaturate and their sensation of breathlessness increases. These patients are usually very underweight. This is probably because of the increased energy cost of breathing in conjunction with the simple difficulty of using the upper air passages for eating and breathing at the same time. Chewing is especially unpleasant for breathless patients and high calorie liquids or semi-solid feeds are to be preferred. These patients have an increased total lung capacity, reduced carbon monoxide uptake and pressure dependent airway collapse on the flow volume curves. They rarely develop oedema or cardiorespiratory failure until late in the course of the disease. Pathologically it is likely that these patients have more emphysema than the blue bloaters.

Blue bloaters As the name implies the blue bloater is characterized by cyanosis and fluid overload. For a similar degree of air flow limitation these patients are often not consciously short of breath (although exercise tolerance is usually similarly limited). Polycythaemia is common and may be considerable if the patient continues to smoke whereby the hypoxic stimulus to red cell production is joined by the stimulus of increased carboxy haemoglobin levels. These patients fail to attempt the hyperventilation undertaken by the pink puffer and become relatively insensitive to a rise in carbon dioxide levels. Hypoxaemia then becomes the stimulus to respiration and leads to constriction of muscles in the walls of the pulmonary arteries which with time becomes fixed. The low pressure pulmonary circuit becomes a higher pressure system in which even atheroma may develop. Pulmonary hypertension increases the work of the right side of the heart leading to right ventricular failure. Hypoxaemia also leads to changes in the renin-angiotensin-aldosterone system giving rise to intra and extracellular fluid shifts which contribute to the oedema of right heart failure.

Treatment for obstructive airway disease

These patients require firm, repeated and unequivocal advice to stop smoking. Most will experience some subjective benefit from the use of a beta agonist inhaler such as salbutamol or terbutaline, and there may be a small objective improvement. Synergism is occasionally demonstrated by the addition of an anti-cholinergic agent such as ipratropium bromide. No benefit is achieved by use of theophyllines or steroids. Exercise should be encouraged for although this may produce breathlessness, regular activity has been shown to increase subjective comfort and exercise tolerance. For very breathless pink puffers judicious use of supplemental oxygen during exertion can be helpful. Placing a cylinder near to the bed with a long lead of tubing and soft nasal cannulae permits the patient to breathe oxygen during simple activities of daily living such as dressing and shaving. For patients with previous episodes of right heart failure longer term oxygen breathing for a minimum of 15 hours/day has been shown to prolong survival. Such quantities cannot be provided by cylinders and oxygen concentrators are therefore prescribed.

Acute exacerbations of breathlessness may be experienced by both pink puffers and blue bloaters. The cause is often unclear. Detailed studies have shown that an infective cause may only be discovered in about half of the cases (20 per cent viral, 30 per cent bacterial). Rhinoviruses are the commonest viral aetiology and *Haemophilus influenzae* and *Streptococcus pneumoniae* the commonest bacteria.

Respiratory failure is defined rather arbitrarily as a blood oxygen tension below 60 mmHg (8 kPa) with or without a $P\text{CO}_2$ above 49 mmHg (6.5 kPa). It is most likely to occur in those with the more severe air flow limitation ($FEV_{1.0}$ below 1 litre) and more in the blue bloater. It may be acute, occurring temporarily during an infective exacerbation of the chronic condition or as a result of sedation – some people live in symbiosis for long periods with appalling blood gas tensions. This group of patients will present special problems to the anaesthetist, on the intensive care unit during severe exacerbations of disease and more commonly will require care and assessment perioperatively. The problems encountered relate to sputum, fixed airway narrowing, loss of responsiveness to CO_2, difficulties of ventilation, and problems associated with provision of adequate analgesia.

Elective surgery

If the patient is still smoking they require clear advice to stop at least 6 weeks before their operation. This time is needed to permit some reduction in sputum production and to allow for some recovery in tracheobronchial clearance. A similar time is needed for improvement in immunoregulatory T cell activity, alveolar macrophage function and natural killer cell activity. Abstinence from smoking for this period may also reduce the rate of thromboembolic phenomena, probably by reducing platelet adhesiveness. If clinical, spirometric and radiographic assessments suggest that the patient is a borderline candidate for general anaesthesia, assessment at 6–8 weeks before operation also leaves time for adequate trials of bronchodilators, weight reduction and instruction in postoperative breathing techniques by the physiotherapist.

Emergency surgery

Smoking cessation remains vital and if surgery can be delayed for 12–24 hours then there may be benefit to the borderline patient. This length of time leads to rapid decline in carboxyhaemoglobin and nicotine levels, reducing their deleterious effect on cardiovascular function. Carboxyhaemoglobin reduces tissue oxygenation by reducing the amount of haemoglobin available for oxygen carriage, and also has a weak negative inotropic effect on the heart. This reduced oxygen supply is compounded by the increased myocardial oxygen demands which nicotine produces by increasing heart rate and blood pressure. Whilst objective benefit may be slight, the patient with seriously impaired airway function should be given nebulized beta agonists (salbutamol or terbutaline) and probably an anticholineric agent (ipratropium bromide). For those with secretions, physiotherapy is required pre-

operatively and the importance of postoperative cooperation is stressed to the patient in advance. The level of preoperative PaO_2 is less predictive for postoperative complications than is the PCO_2, and blue bloaters and others with a raised PCO_2 are likely to require postoperative ventilatory support. With the pink puffer the need is to try and avoid high airway pressures and baro trauma to the emphysematous lung and the anaesthetist needs to be constantly aware of the possibility of development of a pneumothorax. Postoperative opiates should be avoided wherever possible in CO_2 retaining blue bloaters, or given in very low intravenous doses in conjunction with extra dural local anaesthetics. In the pink puffer, analgesia must be sufficient to allow the patient to maintain his accustomed hyperventilation.

Other generalized airway diseases

Bronchiectasis

Bronchiectasis is a disease characterized by permanent dilatation of the bronchi accompanied by destructive changes in the bronchial wall. It may occur as a complication of childhood pneumonia, whooping cough or tuberculosis or as a result of bronchopulmonary aspergillosis or cystic fibrosis. It is commoner in patients with rheumatoid arthritis and may also present in adult life as a result of acquired hypogamma globulinaemia. It is occasionally asymptomatic and occasionally intermittently symptomatic, but for many it is a disease associated with a daily cough, productive of large quantities of sputum with frequent infective exacerbations. Despite the descriptive dilatation of airways there is often coexisting generalized airway narrowing and breathlessness. About 50 per cent of patients with bronchiectasis have haemoptysis at some time. The clinical features are usually suggestive of the diagnosis. The plain chest radiograph may show a non specific increase in bronchovascular markings or more suggestive tram lining or double line shadows due to thickening and swelling of bronchial walls. Bronchography is a useful diagnostic procedure, but modern CT scanning permits excellent visualization of saccular and cylindrical dilatation of bronchi. Intermittent courses of high dose antibiotics (e.g. amoxycillin 3 g twice daily) are necessary to control exacerbations of bronchial sepsis. There is no place for long term antibiotic therapy. Clearance of sputum is essential and postural drainage is valuable. It is however time consuming and a better compromise is the use of forced expiratory techniques. The patient adopts a procedure similar to that for measuring peak expiratory flow rate and a prolonged expiration is followed by a bout of coughing and expectoration. This can be repeated several times and if done 3–4 times daily is probably more effective than postural drainage performed only once.

Operations performed on patients with bronchiectasis require skilful anaesthesia. Bronchodilators, antibiotics and physiotherapy are given preoperatively. Frequent rigorous endobronchial suction is needed during the operation. Oxygenation and ventilation are not usually a problem in those with bronchiectasis but adequate pain relief is essential to ensure adequate coughing and to permit postural drainage and forced expiratory techniques.

Obliterative bronchiolitis

Obliterative bronchiolitis is a rare condition characterized by generalized narrowing and damage to the smaller airways. It may occur after certain childhood viral infections and also occurs as a manifestation of rejection in patients who have had heart and lung transplants. It has been reported in association with rheumatoid arthritis and may be commoner in those with that condition who have been treated with penicillamine. It is managed in the same way as chronic obstructive airway disease and the narrowing is not usually reversible.

Localized airway disorders

Bronchial carcinoma

The commonest carcinoma in males and the second commonest in females, bronchial carcinoma is predominantly a smoking induced disease. Histological types include squamous cell carcinoma (50 per cent), adenocarcinoma (15 per cent), large cell undifferentiated (15 per cent) and small cell carcinoma, including oat cell (20 per cent). Alveolar cell carcinoma may be a separate entity or may merely represent an alveolar pattern of spread of an adenocarcinoma. It constitutes less than 1 per cent of the total.

Clinical features

These patients may present with symptoms from the primary tumour such as increased cough, breathlessness or haemoptysis, or as a result of local or distant spread. They may thus develop pleural effusions or chest wall pain from spread outwards, or oesophageal compression, vena caval obstruction or nerve palsy (recurrent laryngeal, phrenic, sympathetic) from mediastinal invasion. Distant spread is commonly to brain, bone, liver, adrenal or skin. Symptoms may first arise from such secondaries.

A number of non metastatic manifestations of bronchial carcinoma can be considered under the headings of endocrine, neuromuscular and skeletal, and renal.

Endocrine complications

The commonest endocrine complication is hypercalcaemia which is usually due to the tumour producing parathormone fragments rather than being due to bone secondaries. Significant elevation of serum calcium causes nausea, vomiting, bowel and urinary disturbances, confusion and coma. The complication is a sign of advanced disease and if the tumour itself cannot be treated the hypercalcaemia is treated with minimal success by intravenous fluids and steroids, or more competently by the use of mithramycin or calcitonin. The syndrome of inappropriate ADH secretion is the second commonest endocrine complication and is characterized by dilutional hyponatraemia with low plasma sodium and urea and reduced plasma osmolality and increased urine osmolality. Very low sodium levels may be associated with confusion, fitting and fatal cerebral oedema. First aid treatment is by strict fluid restriction (500 ml intake/24 hours) or with life-threatening hyponatraemia by a combination of a loop diuretic, hypertonic saline and anti-epileptic therapy, given in an intensive care setting. If the primary tumour can be treated by chemotherapy or other means the syndrome resolves. If more time is needed pending these measures demeclocycline is given. This blocks the effect of inappropriate antidiuretic hormone on the kidney, but takes approximately 8 days to take effect. ACTH production produces unexpected hypokalaemia or hyperglycaemia in a patient with a bronchial carcinoma. The patients rarely survive long enough for the ACTH produced by the tumour to cause a true Cushing's syndrome. Whilst cranial diabetes insipidus occasionally occurs, modern methods of investigation suggest that it is probably due to secondary spread of tumour rather than being a non metastatic manifestation.

Neuromuscular and skeletal complications

Peripheral neuropathies, mononeuritis, cerebellar degeneration, the myasthenic syndrome and proximal myopathies may all occur as a non metastatic complication of a bronchial carcinoma. Hypertrophic pulmonary osteo-arthropathy also occurs and is characterized by vascular overgrowth and periosteal new bone formation at the ends of long bones. This produces painful swelling of wrists and ankles and the patient usually also has finger clubbing. It never occurs in patients with oat-cell carcinoma. The aetiology is unknown, but it involves an afferent vagal pathway and efferent hormonal pathway. The symptoms resolve dramatically following either treatment of the tumour or vagotomy.

Renal complications are uncommon, but a particularly resistant nephrotic syndrome may develop in association with bronchial carcinoma probably related to immune complex deposition in the kidney. Treatment is of the primary lung tumour and neither steroids, azathioprine or cyclophosphamide have much effect on urinary protein loss.

Diagnosis of bronchial carcinoma

Diagnosis of bronchial carcinoma may involve chest radiography, cytological examination of the sputum, bronchoscopic biopsy, percutaneous needle biopsy or less commonly biopsy of a distant lymph node or metastasis.

Treatment

Sadly, the disease remains a major killer and the options for treatment depend on histological type. Small cell (oat-cell) carcinoma have nearly always metastasized at presentation (whether apparent or otherwise) and these cases have median survival of approximately 3 months from diagnosis. The only possible treatment is combination chemotherapy, with various regimes producing similar results; overall median survival increasing to approximately 12 months with treatment. Adenocarcinomas and squamous cell carcinomas are best treated surgically and whilst older text books mentioned 25 per cent of patients being suitable for operation and 25 per cent of these being alive at 5 years these figures are overoptimistic. With better

selection of patients for surgery and avoidance of unnecessary thoracotomies, only 10–12 per cent of patients are operable and better selection will hopefully lead to increased 5-year survival rates.

Assessment for operability involves consideration of age, possibility of metastases and pulmonary function. There is no definite upper age limit for pulmonary resection, but above the age of 73 or 74 such major surgery often dates even the biologically youthful. If there are no clinical or biochemical features to suggest extrathoracic metastases staging for operation involves CT scanning of the thorax. Whilst tumours do occasionally spread to bone, liver or brain without associated mediastinal involvement this is uncommon. If the CT scan shows no evidence of chest wall involvement and no mediastinal extension or lymphadenopathy then pulmonary surgery may proceed. If lymph node enlargement is visualized this should not be regarded as a contra indication to surgery but rather mediastinal exploration should be planned, for the lymph nodes may be enlarged for benign reasons (e.g. draining an area of pneumonia, sarcoid reaction, etc). The false negative rate for mediastinal CT scanning may be highest with adenocarcinomas which seem to have a propensity for involving lymph nodes without necessarily causing their enlargement.

Lung function Arbitrary values of spirometry below which pulmonary resection is hazardous are often quoted (e.g. FEV< 1.4 litre precludes pneumonectomy). However, these values bear no relationship to the patient's sex or size nor consideration of the lung to be resected. A previous generation of thoracic surgeons used as reassurance the fact that patients could walk a flight of stairs without undue distress and this proved a not unreasonable predictor of postoperative status. It should always be assumed that a pneumonectomy may be necessary for a tumour may be more extensive than envisaged, or mobilization may lead to distant damage necessitating more extensive resection. The lung to be removed may or may not be contributing to overall pulmonary function and this should be borne in mind. If the FEV1 is 1.4 litres for example, but the whole of the lung has collapsed beyond a main bronchial tumour, the patient's lung function is probably good and will be no worse following resection of the collapsed lung. Assessment for operability should therefore involve mediastinal CT scanning and other imaging techniques or mediastinal biopsy as appropriate, and an assessment of likely postoperative pulmonary function based upon formal preoperative lung function tests, assessment of exercise tolerance and assessment of preoperative contribution to function of the tissue to be resected. In borderline cases this contribution may need to be assessed further by radioactive isotope studies. However the greatest advances in lung cancer will only occur if the incidence of smoking decreases.

Other causes of localized airway narrowing

Foreign bodies may produce localized airway obstruction and the trachea may be obstructed by extrinsic compression due to thyroid enlargement. Tracheal obstruction may also result from post tracheostomy stenosis, tracheal tumours or subglottic laryngeal carcinomas and these may sometimes mimic more widespread airway obstruction and bronchitis. In such cases of extrathoracic airway obstruction, measurement of flow volume curves (see Fig. 2.2) may prove very useful.

Mediastinal glands may cause compression of the bronchi and the superior vena cava. The effects may only become apparent when the patient is lying flat. General anaesthesia of these patients can be hazardous.

Restrictive disorders

Whilst the airway disorders of asthma, obstructive airway disease and lung cancer are numerically the commonest, restrictive disorders include a range of disease processes of considerable importance. Restriction implies small lungs but it is essential to emphasize that the lungs may be small because of lung disease, pleural disease, chest wall disease, neuromuscular disease or intra-abdominal disorder.

Restrictive lung disorders

The three most common parenchymal lung disorders in this category are sarcoidosis, fibrosing alveolitis and asbestosis. All provide a similar problem to the anaesthetist with ventilation/perfusion mismatching leading to hypoxaemia. CO_2 retention and right heart failure are only late complications. Artificial ventilation can be difficult because of poor lung compliance, and because lung volumes are reduced coughing is often ineffective postoperatively.

Sarcoidosis

Sarcoidosis is a granulomatous disorder of unknown aetiology which can affect any part of the body. Irrespective of presentation or organ of maximum involvement there is an intrathoracic disorder in nearly 90 per cent of cases. Respiratory changes may be asymptomatic or associated with a cough or breathlessness. Whilst 50 per cent of the chest X-ray abnormalities consist of bilateral hilar lymph node enlargement, and 30 per cent pulmonary infiltration, 10 per cent of patients have irreversible fibrosis at presentation. Diagnosis is confirmed histologically by biopsy of bronchial mucosa, lung, liver, lymph node or Kveim test. The highest positive yields are for bronchial biopsy (positive in 70 per cent of cases shown subsequently to have active sarcoidosis) and transbronchial lung biopsy (80 per cent positive). Chest radiographs reveal shadows and apparent structural changes may not correlate with degree of functional impairment. Detailed lung function testing is essential in the assessment of these patients. As in fibrosing alveolitis the commonest abnormality is for there to be restrictive spirometry (both $FEV_{1.0}$ and FVC reduced), a reduction in total lung capacity, and a variable reduction in TLCO and KCO. Prognosis in most patients with untreated pulmonary sarcoidosis is excellent; most resolve without therapy. However some, especially negroes, develop severe widespread pulmonary damage and disability. Broncho alveolar lavage may be helpful in distinguishing those with an active lymphocytic alveolitis from those with irreversible fibrotic disease. Whilst steroids can cause regression of some of the pulmonary changes, it has not been proven that their use alters long term outlook. Extrathoracic manifestations of sarcoidosis include erythema nodosum, skin infiltration, polyarthralgia, bone destruction, cardiac involvement, uveitis, lymphadenopathy, hepatosplenomegaly, intracranial and meningeal deposits and hypercalcaemia and hypercalcuria. Some manifestations of sarcoidosis are known to be associated with certain HLA types, for example sarcoid arthritis and erythema nodosum are more likely to occur in females who are HLA-B8, A1, CW7 and DR3.

Fibrosing alveolitis

Cryptogenic fibrosing alveolitis, as the name implies, is of unknown aetiology. In a minority it develops against a background of one of the connective tissue disorders such as rheumatoid arthritis, SLE, systemic sclerosis and Sjogrens' syndrome. Small lungs co-exist with diminished CO uptake, and progress to cause hypoxaemia and terminally, CO_2 retention. With prolonged or profound hypoxaemia, pulmonary hypertension and right heart failure develop. The major symptoms are of cough and breathlessness and 40 per cent of cases have finger clubbing. Nearly all have showers of late inspiratory crackles. The chest radiograph shows shrunken lungs with predominantly lower zone fibrosis. Diagnosis involves exclusion of alternative diagnoses by transbronchial lung biopsy or a positive diagnosis of fibrosing alveolitis by percutaneous drill biopsy or thoracotomy. The disease is commoner in females in the sixth and seventh decades of life, but all ages and both sexes can be affected. Response to treatment is unpredictable. A minority respond to large doses of oral steroids. Other immunosuppressive agents such as cyclosporin are not of proven value although azathioprine has a steroid sparing effect. About 10 per cent of patients with cryptogenic fibrosing alveolitis develop a complicating lung cancer. In the younger patient heart and lung transplantation may be considered, but for the older breathless patient who does not respond to steroids, palliative oxygen therapy is the best that can be offered.

Asbestosis

Asbestos exposure can give rise to benign pleural plaques and calcification, to malignant tumours of the pleura (mesothelioma) or to pulmonary fibrosis (asbestosis). The fibrosis mainly involves the lower lobes and is suffered by those exposed to the mineral fibres in their occupation either by involvement in its production or use (e.g. insulating workers, gas mask assemblers, naval dock yard personnel, etc). Patients with asbestosis usually have finger clubbing and basal crackles and they develop progressive shortness of breath and eventually cardiorespiratory failure. If they still smoke they have a $90 \times$ normal risk of developing lung cancer.

Other restrictive lung disorders

Other restrictive lung disorders are less common, but include other occupational diseases such as, silicosis and coal-workers pneumoconiosis. A rarer group of pulmonary fibrotic conditions occur in association with chronic active hepatitis and Crohn's disease and ulcerative colitis. The latter is sometimes also associated with bronchiectasis.

Diseases of the pleura

A pleural effusion is an accumulation of excess fluid within the pleural space. They are traditionally classified according to their protein content as either a transudate (less than 3 g of protein/litre) or exudates (more than 3 g of protein/litre). Possible causes are listed in Table 2.5 but it should be recalled that there are also other types of fluid that may accumulate within the pleural space. An empyema is a collection of pus: a haemothorax may occur following trauma or in association with a pneumothorax, and chylothorax is due to accumulation of lymph in the pleural space. Such chylothoraces may occur as a result of damage to the thoracic duct by carcinomatous or lymphomatous infiltration and also as a complication of surgery or central line insertion into the *left* internal jugular vein.

True pleural effusions usually present with shortness of breath or with symptoms of the underlying cause. Before a radiograpic abnormality is obvious 300 ml of fluid is required in the pleural space; the appearance as described on p. 61. In undiagnosed cases aspiration *and* pleural biopsy is essential (p. 67). It is useful to consider the aetiology within the context of the overall condition of the patient and to know of the commoner causes amongst those listed in Table 2.5. Small to moderate sized bilateral effusions are usually due to cardiac failure. If there are corroboratory signs of cardiac dysfunction diuretics are instituted or increased, and aspiration or further investigation only indicated if the effusion

Table 2.5 Causes of pleural effusions

Transudates	Cardiac failure, hypoproteinaemia (renal disease, liver disease, mal digestion, and mal absorption, constrictive pericarditis)
Exudates Infective	Pneumonia, tuberculosis, associated with subphrenic abscess and pancreatitis, and infectious mononucleosis
Inflammatory	Following myocardial infarction, rheumatoid arthritis, systemic lupus erythematosus, rheumatic fever and sarcoidosis
Malignant	Primary (mesothelioma) and secondary bronchial, prostatic, ovarian, bowel etc
Traumatic	Associated with spontaneous pneumothorax
Vascular	Pulmonary Infarction

fails to resolve. Large unilateral effusions are usually due to malignancy although in those aged under 40 and in Asian immigrants the possibility of tuberculosis should be considered. In young ladies presenting with pleuritic pain and pleural shadowing consider the possibility of SLE and in men with unexplained bilateral disease consider rheumatoid disease. The pleural manifestations may pre-date the arthritis. In both sexes at any age, pleural involvement without obvious cause should always raise the possibility of pulmonary thrombo-embolism and infarction.

Aspiration of pleural fluid produces rapid improvement in symptoms and in cases awaiting anaesthesia such aspiration should be performed at least 24 hours preoperatively. Recurrent effusions associated with malignant disease may require repeated aspiration, tube drainage and chemical pleurodesis, talc pleurodesis or pleurectomy. The choice of technique depends upon rate of recurrence, cell type and expected survival.

Chest wall deformity

A mild restrictive defect with diminution of all lung volumes may occur with kyphosis, but in general the effects on the heart and lung are negligible with deformities such as kyphosis, pectus excavatum and pectus carinatum. Scoliosis however, may be associated with marked cardiorespiratory dysfunction. Eighty per cent of cases are idiopathic and this is commonest in girls and usually convex to the right. Many neuromyopathic processes may also lead to scoliosis, for example Friedrich's ataxia, muscular dystrophy and neurofibromatosis. The amount by which the lung volumes are reduced in scoliosis depends on the severity of the deformity and clinical problems are common if the angle of the scoliosis is greater than 90°. Lung volumes are reduced; CO uptake is usually normal, and in most scoliotics the only abnormality in blood gases is usually slight reduction in PO_2. However respiratory failure may occur and this is usually initially only present at night. Hypoxia causes vasoconstriction and this increases pulmonary vascular resistance, but these patients also develop pulmonary hypertension because the pulmonary vascular bed is too small to accommodate the whole cardiac output especially on exertion. Eventually right heart failure and respiratory failure progress.

Respiratory muscle weakness

The diaphragm is the major inspiratory muscle augmented during time of increased ventilatory demands by inspiratory rib-cage muscles and sterno mastoids. These are voluntarily and involuntarily controlled muscles whose function can be impaired with over inflation of the lung, by thoracic cage deformity and by fatigue which may occur secondary to blood gas disturbances. These in turn occur because of mechanical derangement. They may also under-perform because of impairment of cerebral function or drug overdose and also because of damage to spinal cord, myoneural junction (e.g. myasthenia gravis) or peripheral nerve (e.g. Guillain-Barré). This latter disorder is a not uncommon reason for a patient's admission to an intensive care unit. Weakness and paralysis develop in the extremities and ascend proximally. Fifty per cent of cases follow a viral infection and the main danger of the disease is the often unrecognized onset of respiratory muscle weakness and failure. Very frequent measurements of vital capacity need to be made and failure is often precipitated by retained secretions and inability to cough. The patients may also develop autonomic imbalance and cardiac arrhythmias. If mechanical ventilation is needed, this may need to be prolonged, but with support a moderate to complete recovery is made in the majority of cases. Neither steroid therapy nor plasmaphoresis have been shown to produce definite benefit.

Obesity

This subject is logically considered under the heading of restrictive disorders. Obesity is a major risk factor for anaesthesia and even in those without any demonstrable pulmonary pathology, hypoxaemia is common. The mechanism for this is not entirely certain, but radio-isotope studies have shown diminished basal ventilation and the deranged blood gases probably reflect airway closure during tidal breathing. Splinting of the diaphragm and lower chest wall by abdominal adiposity and decreased basal ventilation are associated with diminished coughing and clearance of secretions. Postoperative atelectasis is therefore common. Some of these patients also suffer ventilatory abnormalities during sleep (*see* p. 84).

Pneumothorax

Pneumothorax means literally air within the pleural cavity. It may occur spontaneously as a result of rupture of a pleural bleb; something which is more likely in tall young males. It also occurs frequently in association with asthma, obstructive airway disease, fibrotic lung disease and cystic fibrosis. Corticosteroid therapy frequently delays healing of a pneumothorax but may also be associated with an increased incidence of the condition. Iatrogenic pneumothoraces also result from needle biopsy of the lung, transbronchial lung biopsy and as a complication of cannulating the subclavian vein. Mechanical ventilation with high inflation pressures in a patient with underlying lung disease is associated with a significant increased risk of the disease. A large pneumothorax, however produced, results in smaller than normal lungs and there is an immediate fall in arterial oxygenation. However, hypoxic vasoconstriction causes a reduction in perfusion of the affected lung returning arterial oxygen content to normal within a few hours. Interestingly the symptom of breathlessness often diminishes over the same time course. If the patient is being ventilated the pleural defect is likely to remain open. Unless the lung is fixed to the chest wall by adhesions, it will collapse and as pleural pressure rises a tension pneumothorax results with mediastinal displacement compromising cardiac filling. At operation a tension pneumothorax readily ensues as nitrous oxide rapidly diffuses into the pneumothorax. The percussion note becomes hyper-resonant over the appropriate hemithorax, breath sounds become diminished or absent, and eventually trachea and apex beat are displaced to the opposite side. Blood pressure falls, there is a reflex tachycardia, and relief of the positive intra-pleural pressure is then required. This may be performed by formal drainage or in an emergency with any large bore needle. Firm guide-lines about who requires intercostal intubation are difficult. Whilst the ventilated patient and the patient with a completely collapsed lung and an abnormal remaining lung clearly require intercostal tube drainage, it is probable that we are over invasive with many other patients. For those with underlying lung disease the degree of subjective distress may be a better guide than the actual degree of pulmonary collapse. For those with normal underlying lung, observation alone is often sufficient, but if there is more than a 50 per cent reduction in radiographic lung volume simple aspiration of air is a reasonable initial step with tube drainage being performed only if there is a failure of re-expansion. Twenty per cent of pneumothoraces recur in the first year and for these surgical pleurectomy is the only therapy guaranteed to be successful. For the patient unable to undergo such a procedure talc pleurodesis may be attempted.

Infections of the respiratory system

Community acquired pneumonia

Community acquired pneumonia remains a common condition and can be a life-threatening event even in previously healthy young adults. These patients frequently require admission to intensive care units and there is evidence that the mortality has not been reduced over the last 25 years despite more effective antibiotics. Clinical features include cough, fever, pleuritic chest pain and breathlessness, with examination findings of bronchial breathing and whispering pectoriloquy. The chest radiograph may show either lobar or more widespread pneumonic shadowing. The patient frequently develops severe hypoxaemia due to a combination of shunt of blood through unventilated lung, and due to ventilation/perfusion mismatching secondary to airway secretions. In addition to general support and oxygen therapy prompt administration of an appropriate antibiotic is essential. Its choice depends on an understanding of the organisms likely to be responsible. Several surveys have given conflicting results usually because they involve a large proportion of cases where the organism was not isolated because of pre-treatment with antibiotics. Counter current immunoelectrophoretic studies on urine or sputum permit detection of the capsular antigen of most types of pneumococcal (*Streptococcus pneumoniae*) infection for 24–48 hours after starting antibiotics. Studies of pneumonia which have utilized this technique have identified the cause of the pneumonia in most cases and have shown that 80–90 per cent of patients are suffering from pneumococcal (*Str. pneumoniae*) infection which is by far the commonest cause of community acquired pneumonia. This requires treatment with high doses of benzylpenicillin (although amoxycillin would be an acceptable alternative); it should be recalled that a bacteraemia is very common with pneumoccal infection and a meningitis or an endocarditis may also develop. The second commonest cause of community acquired pneumonia is infection with mycoplasma and although this usually takes a milder course it is not always benign and protracted illness and death can occur. Infection with *Legionella pneumophila* is the next commonest and both this and mycoplasma have systemic effects on liver function and gastro-intestinal disturbance. Both respond to early treatment with erythromycin. *Haemophilus influenzae*, Q-fever and influenzal pneumonia are much less common. *Staphylococcus aureus* infection is unusual other than in the context of an influenza epidemic, cystic fibrosis or in intravenous drug abusers.

Hospital acquired pneumonia

The same organisms causing community acquired pneumonia may affect the patient in hospital, but different pathogens are likely if the patient has pre-existing lung disease or if they have recently had surgery or been pre-treated with other antibiotics. Pneumonia complicating chronic bronchitis is often due to *H. influenzae* or *Str. pneumoniae*. It responds to amoxycillin. Fifty per cent of all pneumonias developing in hospital patients are due to Gram-negative organisms. These reach the lung by aspiration from the upper airway, via infected inhalational equipment, or by bacteraemic spread from an extrathoracic source. Because the organisms may usually be found in the upper airways, incriminatory proof of them as a cause for a lower respiratory infection may be difficult. The commoner organisms are *Klebsiella pneumonia, Pseudomonas aeruginosa* and *Escherichia* coli. *E. coli* can exist in the stomach when antacids are administered prior to surgery. If there is subsequent inhalation of gastric contents an *E. coli* pneumonia may occur. Each hospital should have an antibiotic policy for dealing with these bacteria, probably involving use of aminoglycosides. Anaerobic bacteria may also be aspirated and these have a tendency to cause tissue necrosis and abscesses. Many respond to penicillin, but combination with metronidazole is safer. Hospital acquired staphylococcal infections may occur post-operatively as a result of aspiration, but may also result from colonization of intravenous lines. In the latter case multiple septic pulmonary infarcts may develop. Flucloxacillin is the initial choice, but alternative agents such as fusidic acid or gentamicin may be used according to local antibiotic policies and resistance patterns.

HIV related pulmonary disease and other opportunist infections

Patients may be immunocompromized by virtue of their underlying disease or by its treatment such as steroids given after transplantation. They may have a predisposition to 'normal' bacterial infections or tuberculosis or they may develop infection with unusual organisms such as *Pneumocystis carinii*, CMV, and *Nocardia*. Much current concern involves patients with human immunodeficiency virus infection and the acquired immunodeficiency syndrome. The anaesthetist may encounter these patients in their normal work or as a result of an intensive care commitment. Patients with acquired immunodeficiency due to HIV infection may suffer from normal bacterial respiratory infections, opportunist pulmonary infection, lymphoid interstitial pneumonitis or Kaposis sarcoma of the lung. Experience from the USA and in this country suggests that the commonest opportunist infection is with *Pneumocystis carinii*. The major clinical features of this are fever (90 per cent of cases), dyspnoea on exertion (75 per cent), hypoxaemia (80 per cent), diffuse interstitial shadowing (80 per cent) and sputum production (30 per cent). Tuberculosis is also common, but it manifests itself in an unusual fashion with mid and lower zone shadowing, usually without cavitation. Non pulmonary manifestations of tuberculosis are common. Legionella infection is less frequent than originally reported. On admission of a patient with HIV infection and radiographic pulmonary shadowing numerous tests are needed. Routine blood and sputum cultures are obtained and the patient is then started on appropriate antibiotics for community acquired pneumonia e.g. amoxycillin and erythromycin. This avoids the risk of patients dying of pneumococcal pneumonia or mycoplasma infection pending a search for opportunist disease. Sputum is sent for fungal culture and in the USA induction of sputum by means of nebulized saline produces samples for cytological examination which have proved diagnostic of pneumocystis in 80 per cent of cases. These figures have not been matched in the UK. Management therefore involves either empirical therapy with high dose trimethoprim/sulphamethoxazole, or preferably fibre optic bronchoscopy, bronchoalveolar lavage and transbronchial lung biopsy. This permits a firm diagnosis which makes future management and estimation of prognosis easier. Infection with pneumocystis foretells a poor prognosis. If respiratory failure intervenes during the first attack of this infection, the survival rate is less than 14 per cent.

Adult respiratory distress syndrome (ARDS)

Adult respiratory distress syndrome is an acute respiratory failure occurring in patients with previously normal lungs and left ventricles who develop a low pressure pulmonary interstitial oedema and subsequent thickening of the air blood interface. It occurs after infections, trauma, aspiration, inhalational injury or overdose. An inflammatory response is triggered which is mediated by compliment activation, macrophage activity and influx of polymorphs into the alveolar septa. These changes are accompanied by further release or production of inflammatory mediators which cause endothelial cell damage, increased pulmonary capillary permeability and pulmonary capillary hypertension. The result is an increase in lung water, a progressive increase in alveolar arterial oxygen tension difference, reducing PaO_2 and increased intrapulmonary shunt. The chest radiograph shows increased intra-alveolar and interstitial shadowing and eventually hypoxaemia worsens despite all therapy and CO_2 retention follows. Respiratory infection, whether a precipitant of adult respiratory distress syndrome or a result, seems to be an important predictor of outcome. In patients at risk from ARDS or who are developing it, every effort should be made to avoid additional infection and subsequent tissue destruction. Good medical and nursing hygiene is essential and selective decontamination of the oropharynx and gastro-intestinal tract may reduce the risk of patients infecting themselves. Maintenance of oxygenation whether by intermittent positive pressure ventilation, PEEP or CPAP or with high frequency ventilation or membrane oxygenation have all been attempted. Despite this and greater understanding of the condition, the mortality remains unchanged at about 45 per cent.

Respiratory failure

Respiratory failure (defined on p. 74) may occur in patients suffering from any of the airway or restrictive disorders already discussed and their treatment has been considered earlier. It may also occur after drug overdosage or as a consequence of sleep apnoea syndromes.

Type 1 respiratory failure is said to be present when PaO_2 is decreased with a normal or low $PaCO_2$. Type 2 respiratory failure, also known as ventilatory failure, is present when the low PaO_2 is accompanied by a raised PCO_2. It will be recalled from the section on lung function that hypoxaemia may occur as a result of hypoventilation, shunt, ventilation/perfusion mismatch or diffusion impairment, but the commonest causes are ventilation/perfusion mismatching and hypoventilation, and these are the two causes of rising CO_2 tension. Therapy must be directed at the underlying pathology with antibiotics, bronchodilators and physiotherapy designed to reduce the degree of VQ mismatching or shunting and supplemental oxygen provided. If doubt exists about the ventilatory responsiveness to CO_2, inspired oxygen concentrations are incremental with PaO_2 being checked to ensure effectiveness of the increase, and $PaCO_2$ being checked to ensure identification of unexpected rises. If hypercapnia is present, clearance of secretions is essential; formal or mini tracheostomy may be indicated for this reason alone. A progressive rise in $PaCO_2$ in spite of these measures merits consideration of elective mechanical ventilation. This would be the logical next step in a patient with pneumonia, chest trauma or drug overdose. However, if the patient has a long standing neuromuscular disorder, scoliosis or severe chronic obstructive airway disease, very careful consideration is required. If the patient previously had a very poor exercise tolerance, was breathless at rest and rarely left the house mechanical ventilation is not usually justified. Whilst it may correct the gas tension abnormalities it is often impossible for the patient to be subsequently weaned from the machine. No firm guide-lines can be given and these decisions remain some of the most difficult in medicine. In the non ventilated patients, CO_2 retention can give rise to confusion and drowsiness and this may make even low dose continuous oxygen therapy difficult. Respiratory stimulants such as Doxapram may be useful in correcting raised CO_2 levels following injudicious or uncontrolled oxygen therapy; it has no other role and efforts are better directed at clearing airway secretions and maximizing bronchodilator therapy.

Fat embolism

Some degree of marrow fat embolization of the lungs and pulmonary insufficiency follow almost universally after trauma and long bone fracture. It is usually mild or even asymptomatic but may cause severe and fatal illness. The severity may reflect associated stress factors such as haemorrhage or shock and unnecessary handling or delayed immobilization of the limb increases the risk. Major clinical features are of respiratory insufficiency, cerebral involvement and a petechial rash, but unexplained fever, tachycardia, jaundice and renal dysfunction are part of the clinical picture.

Anaemia, thrombocytopenia and fat macro-globulinaemia may be noted but the respiratory features predominate in the majority of cases. Whilst a number of treatments have been attempted including steroids, alcohol, heparin and aprotinin, the major need in the severe case is for supplementary oxygen and ventilatory support.

Sleep apnoea syndrome

Ventilatory abnormalities during sleep are common and disturbances of gas exchange which are present during wakefulness are likely to worsen at night as a result of hypoventilation, diminished mucociliary clearance and recumbency. Recent attention has involved the subject of abnormal apnoea during sleep. All subjects have some spells of sleep apnoea and periodic apnoea occurs for example as a normal phenomena during the transition from wakefulness to sleep. The diagnosis of pathological sleep apnoea syndrome is fulfilled by subjects having apnoeas lasting more than 10 seconds during sleep and occurring more than 30 times during a 7 hour sleep. The syndrome may be divided into:

- Obstructive sleep apnoea, where air flow ceases despite continuation of abdominal and thoracic inspiratory movements.
- Central apnoea: where cessation of air flow is accompanied by cessation of respiratory efforts.
- Mixed obstructive and central apnoeas.

Central apnoeas have been studied for a long time and can occur in patients with encephalitis, brain stem disease, Ondine's curse, myxoedema or supratentorial space occupying lesions.

Periodic obstructive sleep apnoea has attracted most recent attention. It occurs usually in subjects with a predisposing structural abnormality who develop an additional functional upper airway obstruction during sleep. Such functional hypo-tonicity of lateral pharyngeal wall and genioglossus is maximal during REM sleep and the tongue and lateral pharyngeal walls cause obstruction so that air flow at the nose and mouth ceases despite respiratory efforts. The short thick fat neck of the obese patient is one structural predisposition and others include miocrognathia, macroglossia and tonsillar and adenoid hypertrophy. Nasal obstruction (whether due to colds, deviated septa or post-operative nasal packing), by reducing negative

intrapharyngeal pressures, will enhance the chance of suction collapse of the upper airways during sleep. Alcohol and some other drugs also increase the frequency of apnoeas.

Clinical features which should suggest the possibility of the obstructive sleep apnoea syndrome are severe snoring and nocturnal thrashing associated with significant daytime sleepiness and intellectual deterioration. The obese patient forms the single largest group of affected subjects, but unexplained pulmonary hypertension and right ventricular hypertrophy have been reported in children on ENT waiting lists for tonsillar and adenoid surgery. The periodic apnoeas during sleep may last up to 45 seconds each and may recur 30 to 50 times per hour so that the patient may spend a considerable part of each night apnoeic. This leads to hypoxaemia, CO_2 retention, polycythaemia, pulmonary hypertension, systemic hypertension and fluid retention and eventually these abnormalities become severe and persist during wakefulness. There is a significant associated risk of cardiac arrhythmia and sudden death.

Treatment is of the underlying condition wherever possible e.g. tonsillar and adenoid surgery, weight reduction and nasal reconstruction, and also avoidance of alcohol and nocturnal sedation. In resistant cases of obstructive sleep apnoea tracheostomy has been performed, but positive nasal airway pressure systems used during sleep are now attracting attention.

Conclusion

Postoperative pulmonary problems involve the risk of hypoxaemia, atelectasis, aspiration, effusion and pneumonia. Age, smoking, obesity and previous lung disease are major factors in the development of these complications. A clear understanding of respiratory disorders is essential for the skilful anaesthesia of these patients. Postoperative analgesia is necessary to aid cooperation and to aid basal ventilation, cough and expectoration, but it may contribute to problems by virtue of hypoventilation and by inducing both central and obstructive apnoea. This chapter has covered these subjects along with some aspects of respiratory management that may be encountered in the intensive care unit. Further information may be found in the reading list below.

Further reading

Editorial. (1986). Adult respiratory distress syndrome: a clinical view. *The Lancet* **ii**, 439.

Jones, R.M. (1985). Smoking before surgery; a case for stopping. *British Medical Journal* **290**, 1763–4.

Partridge, M.R. (1984). Sleep apnoea syndromes. In: *Anaesthesia Review 2*, pp. 2–20. Edited by Kaufman, L. Churchill Livingstone, London.

Prys–Roberts, C. (1986). Anaesthesia and severe pulmonary disease. *British Journal of Hospital Medicine* 43–5.

Robertson, C.E., Stedman, D., Sinclair, C.J., Brown, D. and Malcolm–Smith, N. (1985). Use of ether in life threatening acute severe asthma. *The Lancet* **i**, 187–9.

3
Interpretation of X-Rays

David Grant

Introduction

The aims of this chapter are to provide a frame-work for evaluation of the chest X-ray and to emphasize the importance of an organized approach to film viewing. The radiological appearances of disease are presented in association with relevant pathology and examples have been chosen of problems in everyday clinical practice.

Assessment

The majority of errors in radiological assessment are due to failure of observation rather than incorrect interpretation. The frontal chest X-ray is the most useful projection used in the routine assessment of the chest. A large number of abnormalities are readily apparent, but a systematic approach is necessary to detect the more subtle presentations of serious disease. It may also reveal additional lesions not obvious on cursory examination.

The image seen on a frontal chest X-ray is a summation of densities between the anterior and posterior chest walls and represents the condensation of the thoracic contents into a 2-D image. Individual structures are perceived as a result of differences in density between soft tissue, air and bone. Where these differences are large, abnormalities are readily apparent and the sensitivity of the technique is high. Conversely contiguous structures of a similar density may be difficult to see. It is possible however to infer their presence either by displacement of or loss of outline of normal structures. The disappearance of the outline of normal structures is known as the 'Silhouette Sign' and is extremely important for localization of lesions (Felson, 1973). This is particularly relevant to the emergency situation where the frontal projection is often the only view possible. A table of localization by loss of outline is shown in Table 3.1.

A number of factors influence detection of disease on the radiograph. It is useful to consider them in terms of the intrinsic properties of the lesion, the radiography, and the observer. The nature of the lesion is obviously important in the detection of disease. Large objects of high density are easy to visualize. Small objects of similar density to the surrounding soft tissue or those located in areas partially obscured by overlying structures, such as the retrocardiac area are more difficult to see. Similarly the sensitivity of the technique is markedly increased if the objects are of high density or of a non-anatomical shape. Thus linear structures or structures with sharp angles become readily apparent, whereas those which present with ill-defined margins or curve contours are more easily missed. A high standard of radiography is essential for the early detection of disease. In particular, penetration of the film and accurate positioning of the patient are factors that reflect the quality of the radiography and should form part of the assessment of the radiograph. Finally, one should consider the experience of the observer, the level of observer fatigue, and the lighting conditions in which the X-rays are reviewed as these are significant factors influencing the ability to detect disease.

Table 3.1 Localization by loss of outline

Ascending aorta	Right upper lobe
Right heart border	Right middle lobe
Right hemi-diaphragm	Right lower lobe
Aortic knuckle	Left upper lobe
Descending aorta	Posterior chest
Left heart border	Lingula (segment of left upper lobe)
Left-hemi-diaphragm	Left lower lobe

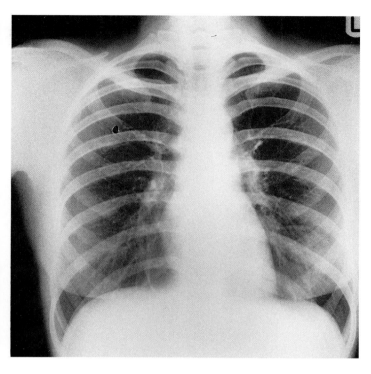

Fig 3.1 Normal frontal chest radiograph. PA projection.

The following method of film viewing is submitted as a guide-line. Like the physical examination of the patient, the clinician will develop his own particular routine. The exact order of the investigation or assessment is irrelevant so long as a repeatable system of viewing is used. The radiographic factors to be checked on each patient include the name of the patient, date of examination and presence or absence of any appropriate side marker. These may seem trivial points but can save a great deal of confusion at a later date. As previously mentioned, the centering of the film and the degree of penetration should be noted. An acceptable level of penetration is one in which the outlines of the vertebral bodies can just be discerned behind the cardiac silhouette. The degree of inspiratory diaphragmatic excursion should be such that, in the postero–anterior (PA), seven anterior ribs or ten posterior ribs are visible. This ideal situation is not always possible and frequently the depth of inspiration is poor e.g. the postoperative period. It should be appreciated however, that in these cases basal lesions may be missed. The trachea, mediastinum, heart and aorta are the midline structures and they should be assessed in terms of position, contour, size and in the case of the trachea, calibre. The normal appearance is shown in Fig. 3.1. From superiorly to inferiorly, the mediastinal margin is formed by the brachiocephalic vessels, the ascending aorta and the superior vena cava. The right cardiac border consists of the right atrium. The right ventricle is an anterior structure and in the normal situation does not form part of the right heart border. The left mediastinal margin is formed by the aortic knuckle, immediately below which is the pulmonary trunk and the left pulmonary artery. There is a small bulge inferior to this in the cardiac outline due to the left atrial appendage. The remainder of the left heart border is formed by the left ventricle. The left atrium does not form either of the lateral borders in the normal situation, but in cases of pathological enlargement, this posterior structure may be seen as a double density behind the cardiac silhouette with a lateral margin extending behind the right heart border (Fig. 3.2). In cases of gross left atrial enlargement, the left main bronchus becomes elevated and more horizontal in its position as the abnormal cardiac chamber expands. The pulmonary hila should be evaluated for their relative position, and the left hilum is usually between 1 and 1.5 cm higher than the right. The densities should be equal and the

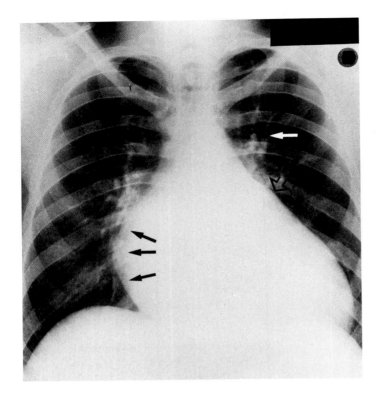

Fig 3.2 Cardiomegaly secondary to mitral valve disease.

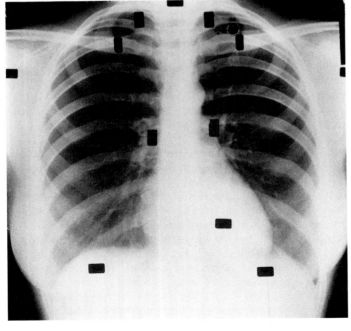

Fig 3.3 Frontal radiograph illustrating 'review areas'.

Key
Solid black arrows − enlarged left atrium.
Open black arrow − enlarged left atrial appendage.
White arrow − upper lobe venous blood diversion.

shape and size must be noted. The hilar shadows are almost exclusively formed by the pulmonary arteries and veins. The normal bronchial walls are normally so thin that they cannot be detected at this distance from the tracheal bifurcation and thefore do not form part of the normal hilum. The lateral margin of the hilum is usually concave, rarely straight and almost never convex. Indeed convexity should be regarded as a sign of disease until proven otherwise. The angle formed between the superior pulmonary vein as it crosses the descending branch of the pulmonary artery is always concave in the normal situation. Lung fields should be of equal trans-radiancy with equality of retrocardiac densities and of lung markings. The horizontal fissure which separates the right upper from the right middle lobe is usually the only fissure frequently seen in the frontal projection. It extends from the lateral pleural surface, approximately in the line of the fourth intercostal space towards the mediastinum. It is rarely complete in its medial portion. Its significance is that its relative position may be altered by volume loss in either of the adjacent lobes. Preservation and symmetry of the costophrenic and cardiophrenic angles should be observed. The cardiophrenic angle is frequently a little indistinct due to the presence of a fat pad but in the normal situation the cardiac silhouette may be traced to its intersection with the diaphragm without any additional alteration in contour. Normal fat pads may be quite large, in which case further evaluation to exclude a mediastinal mass may be required. Diaphragmatic contour and relative position should be studied. The right hemi-diaphragm is frequently slightly higher than the left, although the situation may be reversed in the presence of gross gastric or colonic distention. Diaphragmatic calcification is an important observation, especially in the context of industrial (asbestos) exposure. Evaluation of the diaphragmatic contour in relationship to chest disease includes the area beneath the hemi-diaphragm. Bone texture, density and integrity should be included on the check list as well as the symmetry of the overlying skinfolds. Although clinically apparent, superficial skin nodules may cause confusing shadows on the chest X-ray and the knowledge of any superficial lesions should be matched with radiological appearances. Nipple shadows are frequently seen in the frontal projection in the 5th intercostal space. They appear as round soft tissue densities which are usually symmetrical. Round soft tissue densities which are not symmetrical and which are in a slightly abnormal situation may be differentiated from nipple shadows by taking a frontal X-ray with nipple markers. Finally the assessment for foreign bodies forms an integral part of film viewing of particular relevance are the positions of endotracheal and naso-gastric tubes. The position of central venous lines and catheters should also be scrupulously observed.

The above comments are relevant both to the PA and the AP frontal projections. Accurate assessment of cardiac size is only possible in the PA projection as this projection minimizes any magnification effects produced as the result of geometrical enlargement. A number of systems have been devised for assessment of cardiac size but the two most useful and frequently employed methods are the transverse cardiac diameter and the cardiothoracic ratio. The transverse cardiac diameter refers to the maximum diameter of the heart in the frontal projection. The upper limit of normal for the adult male is regarded as 15.5 cm, and for the adult female 14.5 cm. The cardiothoracic ratio refers to the ratio of the maximum transverse diameter of the heart as compared to the maximum diameter of the thoracic cage as measured from the internal aspect of the ribs. A figure of 50 per cent is accepted as the upper limit of normal. The latter measurement should be interpreted with some caution in people with a small heart, as a considerable degree of cardiac enlargement would have to occur before the ratio becomes abnormal. A more useful index is the serial measurement of transverse cardiac diameter. A difference of 1.5 cm is generally regarded as significant enlargement.

Cardiac size and contour in hypertension

Cardiac enlargement and in particular left ventricular hypertrophy is a recognized feature of hypertension. However it should be noted that a considerable degree of ventricular hypertrophy may be present without any pathological increase in cardiac size. The most striking changes in cardiac chamber size occur in those situations in which there is volume overload or in which there is evidence of cardiac failure. Left ventricular enlargement classically produces an apex which occupies a more lateral and inferior position to that normally expected. However selective cardiac chamber

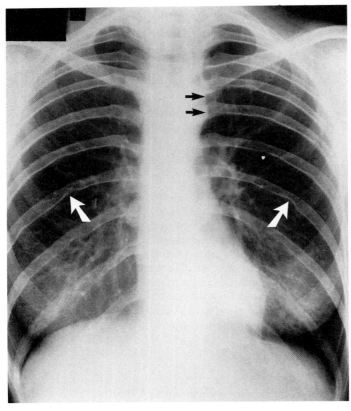

Fig 3.4   Coarctation of the aorta.

Key
Black arrows – flattened aortic knuckle.
White arrows – rib notching.

enlargement is difficult to diagnose accurately on the plain film and may indeed be misleading.

The chest X-ray may reveal signs suggestive of underlying aortic coarctation as a cause for hypertension. The radiological abnormalities include possible increasing size, abnormal configuration to the aortic knuckle and rib notching (Fig. 3.4). Cardiac size in coarctation is dependent upon the degree of pressure overload and the extent of any associated aortic valve disease resulting in regurgitation. In the latter, there will be associated left ventricular enlargement. The aortic configuration is classically described as the double aortic knuckle or '3' sign. This is formed by the combination of proximal bulging of the left subclavian artery or aortic arch, together with a distal post-stenotic dilatation of the descending aorta. It should be noted that the aortic knuckle may be in an abnormally high or low position or relatively incon-

spicuous, and thus the double knuckle sign, although useful if present, does not exclude the diagnosis if absent. Bilateral rib notching is a sign of severe coarctation and affects the inferior aspects of the 4th to 8th ribs. Coarctation is the commonest cause of rib notching, but it is not pathognomonic of coarctation and occurs in obstruction of the superior vena cava, neurofibromatosis and systemic to pulmonary arterial shunts. The Blalock operation anastomosing the subclavian and pulmonary arteries is an example of this and is a cause of unilateral notching. In coarctation, the notching is produced by hypertrophy of the posterior intercostal arteries. The first two ribs are not affected as the intercostal arteries in this region arise from the superior intercostal branch of the costocervical trunk of the subclavian artery and not directly from the aorta. Definitive diagnosis is by aortography. The clinical association with Turner and Klippel–Feil syndromes should be remembered.

Review areas

Despite careful evaluation of the X-ray film, errors in observation may still occur, particularly at those sites at which there are overlapping structures. The following review areas should be scrutinized before declaring a film to be normal (*see* Fig. 3.3). They include:

- lung apices
- retrocardiac density
- pulmonary hila
- diaphragm
- sub-diaphragmatic space
- rib convexities
- posterior rib angles
- clavicles and acromioclavicular joints
- humeral heads

The latter are included in the review areas as they are often visualized on a routine frontal chest X-ray and may reveal evidence of systemic disease, such as metastasis or erosive arthropathy.

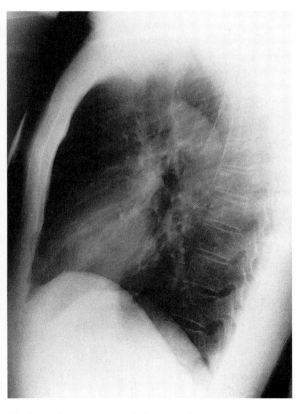

Fig 3.5 Normal lateral chest radiograph.

The lateral chest X-ray

The interpretation of the lateral chest X-ray can be difficult (Fig. 3.5). In the majority of cases an additional lateral projection seldom results in any alteration in patient management. It is rare to be able to perform a useful lateral X-ray in the emergency situation. This emphasizes the need for accurate interpretation of the frontal projection and the importance of the ability to localize an abnormality by the loss of its normal outline (Silhouette Sing). The film is probably best assessed by artificially dividing the contents of the thoracic cavity into those areas that normally appear dark on the lateral film, the central area of relative soft tissue density (white), and the bony margins and diaphragm of the thoracic cavity.

Three regions are classically described as radiolucent (dark) (*see* Fig. 3.6 overleaf). The anterior or retrosternal triangle is an area situated between the chest wall anteriorly, the cardiac shadow posteriorly and the margin of the brachiocephalic vessels superiorly. This area normally maintains a radiolucent appearance and its abolition provides a clue to the presence of an anterior mediastinal structure. The relative size of the retrosternal space will diminish in cases of right ventricular enlargement as this chamber extends up the anterior chest wall. The second area of darkness on the film is the retrotracheal space. This is a quadrilateral shaped bounded anteriorly by the posterior wall of the trachea and the collapsed wall of the oesophagus. Together their combined wall thicknesses should not exceed 5 mm. The floor is the apex of the aortic arch and the posterior margin is formed by the vertebral bodies. The third and probably most significant of all is the retrocardiac lucency. This posterior area displays a caudally progressive increase in the degree of radiolucency, such that the posterior lung bases are considerably darker than the regions at the level of the aortic arch. In simple terms this means that as the observer scans the film from its superior to inferior aspects, the vertebral bodies become more distinct. Loss of definition of the vertebral bodies in this site, or loss of the radiolucency is an important marker of lower lobe pathology.

Within the lung fields, the fissures are best appreciated on the lateral view. The horizontal fissure extends from the hilum to the anterior chest wall. The oblique fissure passes in a diagonal course from approximately the level of the body of T5, through the hilum and the mid portion of the

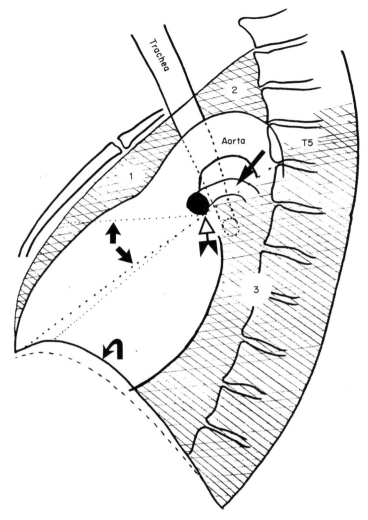

Key
Short black arrows – horizontal and oblique fissures.
Long black arrow – left pulmonary artery.
Curved black arrow – diaphragm.
Open tailed arrow – right pulmonary artery.
1 – retrosternal radiolucency.
2 – retrotracheal radiolucency.
3 – retrocardiac radiolucency.

Fig 3.6   Diagram to illustrate areas of radiolucency in the lateral projection.

cardiac silhouette, terminating 5 cm posterior to the anterior chest wall at the lung base. Displacement of the fissures from these normal positions is again a marker of pathology.

The central soft tissue densities consists of the cardiac silhouette inferiorly and the arch of the aorta superiorly. Immediately inferior to this

parallel to the aortic arch is the left pulmonary artery as it extends superiorly and postero-laterally towards the left lung. At its origin there is an approximately circular area of increased density which is due to the right pulmonary artery seen end-on. The soft tissue density of the cardiac silhouette should be uniform as any abnormal or wedge shape

Table 3.2   Patterns of pulmonary collapse in the frontal and lateral projections

Region	Frontal view	Lateral view
Right upper lobe	Region of increased density in right upper zone.	Obliteration of the horizontal fissure pivoting at the hilum.
	Elevation of the horizontal fissure pivoting upward from the hilum.	Anterior displacement of the oblique fissure.
	Oblique fissure visualized with a concave upward margin as a result of the volume loss.	Increased density in the right upper zone.
	Ipsilateral hilum is elevated.	
	Trachea displaced to the right.	
	Compensatory over inflation of the right middle and right lower lobes.	
	Diaphragmatic position relatively unaffected.	
Left upper lobe	Poorly defined area increased shadowing in the left upper zone resulting in a blurred appearance.	Wedge shaped area of increased density in upper zone.
	Possible associated ill-defined opacity in the upper and mid zones.	NB. If collapse is total then the left upper lobe may be effaced with the mediastinum and no significant opacity demonstrated.
	Loss of outline of the aortic knuckle and left hilum.	
	Possible associated loss of outline of the cardiac silhouette.	Anterior displacement of the oblique fissure.
	Displacement of the trachea to the left.	
Right middle lobe (Fig. 3.7)	Region of increased shadowing in the right mid zone with associated blurring and loss of outline of the right heart border.	Increase in the opacity of the cardiac silhouette.
	Possible depression of the lateral aspect of the horizontal fissure.	Approximation of the horizontal and inferior portion of the oblique fissure.
	NB. If collapse is total then visualization may be very difficult.	
Lingula	Loss of outline and blurring of the left heart border.	Increased opacity of the cardiac silhouette.
Right lower and left lower lobes (Fig. 3.8)	Wedge shaped region of increased density at the lung base with the apex at the hilum and the base of the wedge toward the diaphragm. Collapse occurs postero medially.	Displacement of the oblique fissure inferiorly and posteriorly.
	Visualization of the oblique fissure.	Loss of definition of the posterior border of the hemi-diaphragm.
	Elevation of the ipsilateral hemi-diaphragm.	Increase in ratio opacity posteriorly with loss of the normal retrocardiac lucency.
	Variable mediastinum shift.	Loss of definition of vertebral bodies due to overlying parenchymal shadowing.

increase in density may reflect disease in either the middle or lingula lobes. As in the frontal projection the outlines of the hemi-diaphragms should be clearly seen with sharply defined posterior diaphragmatic recesses. The right hemi-diaphragm may be traced in its entirety from the posterior recess to the anterior chest wall, but the left hemi-diaphragm has an incomplete anterior margin at its junction with the heart. A further though slightly less reliable way of differentiating the left and right hemi-diaphragms is that the gastric air bubble is projected under the left side.

Finally the skeletal anatomy should be assessed, and in the lateral view the sternum is seen to its best advantage. The vertebral bodies should be evaluated for evidence of bone destruction, collapse or anterior erosion which may be the only sign of a posterior mediastinal mass.

Consolidation and collapse

Both consolidation and collapse produce an increase in the degree of radiopacity on the X-ray film. There are differences in the patterns produced, but the end result is often a mixture of the two pathologies. It is beyond the scope of this chapter to deal in detail with the subtle differences in type of parenchymal consolidation or interstitial shadowing. However, it is useful to consider the lung as composed of tubular structures, i.e. the bronchi, lymphatic and blood vessels together with the actual organs of gas transfer, i.e. the lung parenchyma, airspaces and interstitial tissue.

Consolidation

The manifestations of consolidation effect either the airspaces or the interstitial tissues or both. It is rare to have pathology purely restricted to one of these subdivisions and in terms of the overall appearance a number of generalized statements can be made. Acinar shadows are classically poorly defined fluffy shadows with a tendency to confluence. There may be an associated air bronchogram; usually there is little if any associated collapse and the overall distribution is non-segmental. The hallmark of consolidation is the air

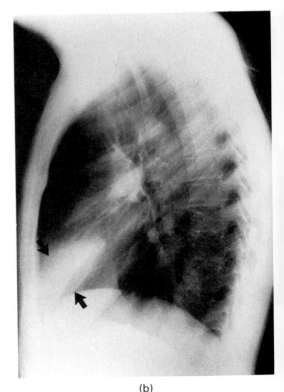

(a)

Key
(a) Long black arrow – right middle lobe collapse.
(b) Short black arrows – increased cardiac opacity secondary to middle lobe collapse.

(b)

Fig 3.7 Right middle lobe collapse – (a) frontal and (b) lateral (c) projections.

bronchogram. This is the result of airless parenchyma surrounding patent bronchi. Radiologically it appears as a region of increased density within the lung fields within which one can see branching radiolucent structures, the bronchi. The significance of the air bronchogram lies in the fact that it indicates parenchymal disease and implies that the air conduction pathways of the lung are patent. The commonest causes of an air bronchogram are pneumonia, radiation pneumonitis and alveolar cell carcinoma.

Collapse (atelectasis)

The radiological appearance of collapse may be divided into those directly attributable to volume loss and those secondary to it. The direct sign of volume loss is displacement of the adjacent interlobar fissures. Indirect signs are all ipsilateral. They include a generalized or localized increase in radiographic density over the appropriate lung field, elevation of the hemi-diaphragm and displacement of the adjacent hilum and mediastinum. If the degree of collapse is severe, there may be associated rib crowding as a result of the relatively

decreased expansion of the chest wall on that side (Grainger and Allison, 1986). The exact pattern of collapse and the degree to which the indirect signs are manifest depends upon which segment of the lung is affected and this is considered in Table 3.2. The appearance in both the frontal and lateral views are described, though in practise the lateral view rarely provides additional information.

Foreign bodies

One of the commonest causes of localized collapse is inhalation of a foreign body. Those at risk are anaesthetized patients and children. Radiology aims to visualize and to localize the inhaled object (Fig. 3.9). It should be stressed however, that although radiology provides a valuable contribution, the next line of investigation of suspected inhaled foreign body is bronchoscopy.

Radiological signs

- Atelectasis.
- Obstructive emphysema.
- Pneumonia.

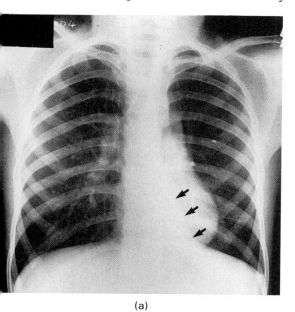

(a)

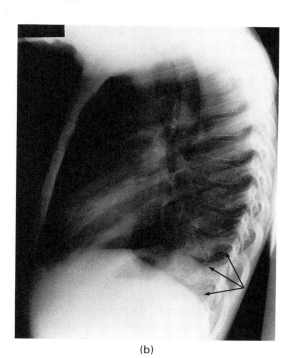

(b)

Fig 3.8   Left lower lobe collapse – (a) frontal and (b) lateral projections.

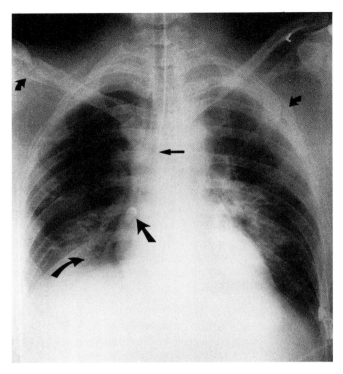

Key
Short curved arrows – fractures.
Horizontal arrow – E/T tube malpositioned in right main bronchus.
Oblique arrow – inhaled tooth.
Curved arrow – partial right lower lobe collapse.

Fig 3.9 Inhaled foreign body.

The X-ray in cases of suspected obstructive emphysema should be evaluated on the frontal view in both inspiration and expiration. The purpose of the expiratory film is to confirm the presence of air trapping which is the hallmark of obstructive emphysema. The appearances in inspiration are those of an increased trans-radiancy of the abnormal lung field with decrease in the vascular markings within the abnormal region. The lung volume and the mediastinal position may be normal. On the expiratory film, the lung volume and trans-radiancy of the abnormal side remain unaltered in contrast to the normal smaller lung which decreases its lung volume. The ipsilateral hemi-diaphragm remains splinted and unchanged from its inspiratory position. There may be associated shift of the mediastinum to the contra-lateral (normal) side. It should be noted that the angula-tion of the right main bronchus favours inhalation into the right lung.

Pneumothorax, pneumomediastinum and pneumopericardium

Pneumothorax

Pneumothorax may be encountered in anaesthetic practice. Although it is most frequently spontaneous, it may be iatrogenic and the result of insertion of central venous lines or consequent upon positive pressure ventilation. It manifests a spectrum of severity from the relatively uncom-

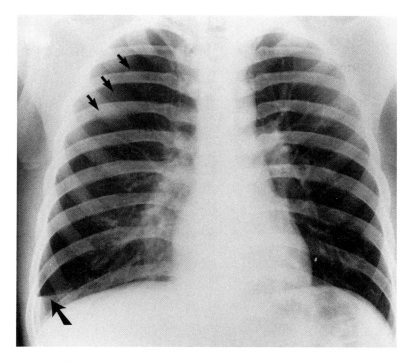

Key
Short arrows – lung edge.
Large arrow – small pleural effusion (haemothorax).

Fig 3.10   Simple pneumothorax.

plicated closed pneumothorax to the potentially life-threatening tension state. It should be noted that significant tension states may be present with radiologically small pneumothoraces. The term simple pneumothorax refers to air within the pleural space at atmospheric pressure. The radiological signs are all ipsilateral and include increased trans-radiancy of the lung field, visualization of a lung edge, failure of vascular markings to extend to the edge of the lung field, absence of vascular markings within the pneumothorax and a small associated haemothorax evident as blunting of the ipsilateral costophrenic angle (Fig. 3.10). Atelectasis and incomplete re-expansion are frequent complications. Failure to re-expand a pneumothorax with a chest drain *in situ* suggests the possibility of a broncho-pleural fistula. The position of the free intra-pleural air depends upon the position of the patient. The commonly described apical pneumothorax is demonstrated when the patient is in the erect position, but medially located pneumothoraces are common in children and with the patient in the supine position. The term tension pneumothorax refers to air within the pleural space at a greater than atmospheric pressure with consequent impairment of venous return and compression of the contralateral lung. Penetrating chest trauma may produce a check valve effect at the site of the pleural defect leading to an increase in intra-pleural pressure with each successive respiratory excursion. Barotrauma, the result of positive pressure ventilation, may also produce a significant tension state. The key radiological signs are contralateral mediastinal shift and contralateral tracheal displacement. The ipsilateral hemi-diaphragm is depressed (Fig. 3.11). Clinical suspicion of a tension pneumothorax should be excluded by insertion of an 18-gauge needle irrespective of the radiographic appearance.

Pneumomediastinum

Air within the mediastinum may be the result of spontaneous or traumatic introduction. Interstitial

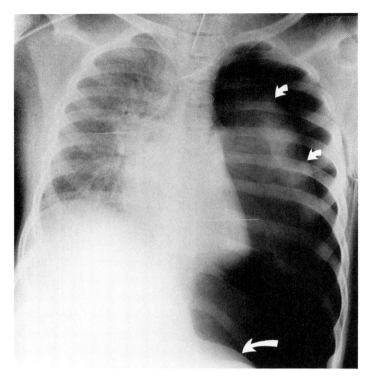

Key
Short arrows – lung edge.

Fig 3.11   Tension pneumothorax.

pulmonary emphysema as a complication of asthma or positive pressure ventilation, is a recognized cause of pneumomediastinum. Radiological signs of air within the mediastinum include streaky lucency outlining the aortic knuckle, pulmonary trunk and/or the cardiac border (Fig. 3.12). The mediastinal pleura may be displaced and the diaphragm separated from the cardiac silhouette as a result of air extending under the pericardium. There may be an associated pneumothorax or subcutaneous emphysema. Unlike pneumothorax, the distribution of air is unaffected by the alteration of the patient's position.

Pneumopericardium

Air within the pericardial cavity is unusual and generally consequent upon penetrating trauma. The radiological signs suggest that the gas is confined to the pericardial cavity and does not extend beyond the aortic root. The distribution of intra pericardial air is positionally dependent and may be associated with a blood/air fluid level.

Pulmonary interstitial emphysema (PIE)

Extra alveolar dissection of air into the interstitium of the lung is a rare complication of asthma but it is more frequently seen in babies receiving positive pressure ventilation (Fig. 3.13). Respiratory embarrassment is due to splinting of the interstitium of the lung which effectively compromises both respiration and venous return. Radiological signs may be unilateral or bilateral and consist of linear/streaky lucencies extending into the lung fields from the pulmonary hila producing a characteristic branching pattern. Small cyst-like collections of gas within the lung or in a subpleural location may be seen (Rohlfing et al., 1976).

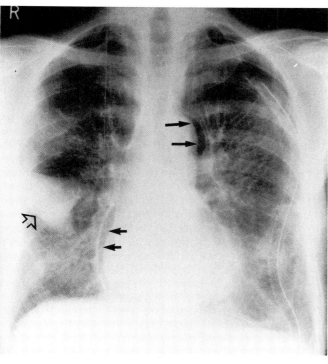

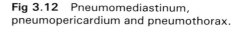

Fig 3.12 Pneumomediastinum, pneumopericardium and pneumothorax.

Key
Short arrows – pneumopericardium.
Long arrows – pneumomediastinum.
Open arrow – loculated fluid.

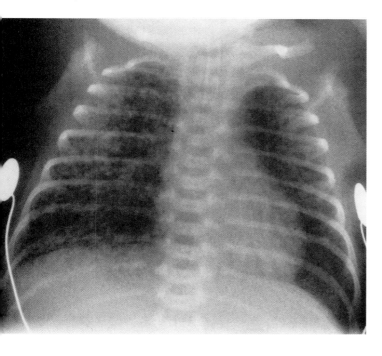

Fig 3.13 Pulmonary interstitial emphysema.

Pneumothorax is a recognized complication of cyst rupture and may be of the tension type.

Rib fractures

The role of the chest X-ray in suspected rib fracture is to identify complications of the fracture such as pneumothorax or pulmonary contusion, rather than the individual fracture sites themselves. Demonstration of the exact site of fracture is of secondary importance and rarely alters patient management and it is for this reason that additional views are rarely warranted. The frontal projection is adequate for the majority of cases, although it should be remembered that approximately 15 per cent of rib fractures will be missed in this projection. The majority of fractures occur in the mid axillary line and affect the 5th to the 9th ribs. However, fractures of the upper three ribs are markers of severe trauma and may be associated with mediastinal injury. In particular injury may be sustained to the brachiocephalic trunk and the aorta. Associated vascular injury may be as high as 10 per cent and the patient should be evaluated with a view to possible CT and formal angiography if clinically indicated. A flail chest, the result of multiple consecutive rib fractures, may compromise ventilation. Underlying pulmonary collapse is common

and the patient often requires positive pressure ventilation with its attendant risks of pneumothorax and pneumomediastinum, etc. Fractures of the lower three ribs may be associated with damage to the liver, spleen or kidneys and injury to these organs is most easily excluded by ultra-sound. Pulmonary contusion, haematoma and tracheo bronchial trauma are all associated with chest trauma. Pulmonary contusion, or bruised lung, manifests radiologically patchy areas of consolidation which do not conform to any anatomical distribution. A contrecoup abnormality may be present and complications are very rare. Pulmonary haematoma is a more severe injury in which there are focal areas of loculated blood within the pulmonary parenchyma. These may be single or multiple and they are often of water density. Subsequent cavitation may occur within the lesions and may be associated with air/fluid level. Frequently these are situated toward the lung edge in a subpleural location. A small haemorrhagic pleural effusion is often present. Complications include infection and pulmonary abscess.

Tracheobronchial trauma implies that very severe force has been sustained. The radiological signs include pneumothorax if the injury is distal to

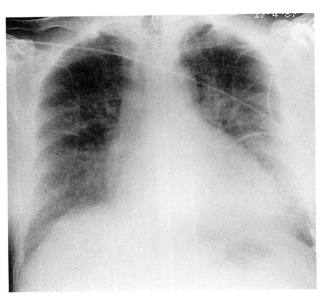
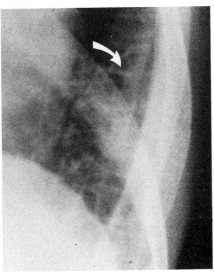

Fig 3.14   Pulmonary oedema, Inset; septal lines.

Key
White arrow – septal (Kerley B) line.

which is often medial in position, associated with an appearance described as 'falling lung' in which the lung has become detached from the lung root and has dropped to the bottom of the chest when viewed in the erect position (Greenbaum, 1982).

Pulmonary oedema

Pulmonary oedema reflects an accumulation of fluid within the interstitium of the lung which eventually progresses to involve the airspaces (Fig. 3.14). The chest X-ray is both more sensitive and more specific than clinical examination and it plays a key monitoring role. Pulmonary oedema is a non-specific response to a variety of pulmonary insults. The commonest cause is secondary to left heart failure.

Radiological signs

The earliest radiological sign of cardiogenic pulmonary oedema is upper lobe vascular redistribution. The calibre of the upper lobe veins becomes equal or greater than those of the lower lobe when the radiograph is taken with the patient in the erect position. Other radiological signs are described, which are present irrespective of the aetiology of the pulmonary oedema. They may be divided in terms of interstitial and airspace oedema. Signs of interstitial oedema include loss of vascular sharpness, peribronchial thickening and ill defined haziness in the lower zones. As the interstitial oedema accumulates, fluid becomes visible in the interlobular septa (Kerley B-lines), and subsequently in the subpleural spaces i.e. effusions. Airspace shadowing is visible as patchy areas of poorly defined shadows of increasing density predominantly in lower zones which coalesce and may produce an air bronchogram. Extension of the shadowing to the subpleural zones produces the classical bat-wing appearance. Resolution of the signs of oedema occurs in reverse order.

Cardiac size

Normal cardiac size has previously been discussed. Cardiac enlargement is common in cardiogenic pulmonary oedema, but may not always occur. Its appearance depends upon the speed of onset of the oedema. If the latter is very rapid, there may be insufficient time for cardiac enlargement to have occurred. There is an important subgroup of causes of pulmonary oedema in which the cardiac size is normal. This group includes cerebral trauma or cerebral infection, narcotic overdose, aspirin overdose, inhalation of noxious gases, adult respiratory distress syndrome and fat embolism. The complications of pulmonary oedema are usually overshadowed by the underlying cause. Infection is the most frequent complication and occurs in the soggy lung tissue. Differentiation between pulmonary oedema and superadded infection can be extremely difficult, particularly if the judgement has to be made on a single film. Serial films are very helpful in this regard e.g. unilateral shadowing which gradually increases in the context of previously resolving pulmonary oedema would favour the diagnosis of infection.

Adult respiratory distress syndrome (ARDS)

The clinical and radiological features of this syndrome tend to be similar regardless of the aetiology. The principle radiological abnormality is airspace consolidation (Greene, 1987). There is a spectrum of radiological severity and the disease tends to evolve over the course of approximately 1 week. Appearances may be considered as early, intermediate and late. The initial chest X-ray may be normal, despite the clinical onset of respiratory failure. The intermediate group is characterized by patchy bilateral areas of poorly defined consolidation which progress to larger areas of confluent consolidation. Air bronchograms are a prominent feature. The later phase demonstrates some decrease in the confluent consolidation, but an increase in the streaky interstitial shadowing, producing a mixed interstitial and airspace picture. The appearances of adult respiratory distress syndrome have been confused with pulmonary oedema, but it should be noted that upper lobe vascular redistribution, cardiac enlargement and pleural effusion are characteristically absent. The major complications of ARDS is infection. Subsequent complications are usually the result of treatment and predominantly those of positive pressure ventilation i.e. pneumothorax, pneumomediastinum, and interstitial emphysema (Goodman and Putman, 1983).

Pleural effusion

Abnormal collections of pleural fluid may be transudate, exudate, blood, pus or chyle but on conventional radiology they all appear similar. The radiological signs of pleural fluid are dependent upon the position of the patient and major differences occur between the erect and supine positions.

Frontal radiograph – erect position

The most characteristic and earliest sign of pleural fluid is loss or blunting of the ipsilateral costophrenic angle. With further increases in the extent of pleural fluid, the outline of the hemi-diaphragm becomes blurred and there may be a fluid meniscus adjacent to the lateral chest wall, in which the meniscus is concave superiorly. A further increase in the amount of fluid causes the lower chest to become homogeneously opacified and gradually the ipsilateral lung field become opaque. Contra-lateral mediastinal shift may be present with very large effusions.

Frontal radiograph – supine position

In the supine position fluid is distributed more uniformly along the posterior chest wall. There is an increased radio-opacity of the ipsilateral lung field and a homogeneous opacification tracing the contour of the lung separating it from the chest wall and producing an apical pleural cap. As in the erect position, contra-lateral mediastinal shift may be present with very large collections of fluid.

Pleural fluid may accumulate in unusual positions or manifest unusual radiological signs. Loculated pleural fluid is frequently observed in cases of resolving left heart failure. The radiological sign is a homogeneous fluid density, intimately related to a pulmonary fissure or the chest wall (Fig. 3.15). It has a sharply defined margin, usually biconvex if within the fissure, or convex toward the lung if adjacent to the chest wall. The opacity disappears as the cardiac failure resolves and reappears as it

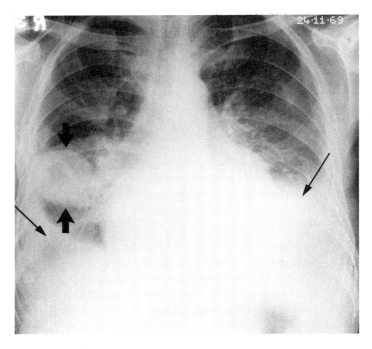

Key
Short arrows – encysted pleural fluid.
Long arrows – pleural effusions.

Fig 3.15   Loculated pleural effusion.

deteriorates. It can be confused with a broncho-genic carcinoma, but the clinical history, relationship to the fissure and disappearance with resolution of cardiac failure mitigate against this.

Pleural fluid may track up the lateral chest wall as a lamellar effusion. This is frequently observed in children and in cases of resolving cardiac failure. The effusion extends superiorly from the lung base and parallel to the lateral chest wall.

Sub-pulmonary collections of fluid may produce an apparent elevation of the diaphragm. In the erect frontal view, there is an increased radio-opacity of the ipsilateral diaphragm with the apex of the diaphragm displaced laterally. The lateral diaphragmatic contour has a relatively vertical slope and is associated with an unusually straight medial portion. If the effusion is left-sided, there may be wide separation of the gastric air bubble from the overlying apparent diaphragm. When present on the right side the diagnosis may be a little more confusing, in which case the lateral decubitus position may be of value. This projection demonstrates mobile fluid as it moves from sub pulmonary location to parallel the contour of the dependent lateral chest wall.

Thromboembolic disease

The radiological diagnosis of thromboembolic disease is based on multiple investigations and this reflects the lack of a single effective screening test (Windebank, 1987). There are large variations in sensitivity and specificity of the various imaging techniques. The chest X-ray is performed as the initial investigation in nearly all patients. It is abnormal in an extremely high percentage of cases (approximately 90 per cent), but unfortunately the appearances are almost invariably non-specific. In broad terms, pulmonary infarction correlates with a generalized increase in radiographic density, whereas pulmonary embolism correlates with areas of hypoperfusion and consequent decreased radiographic density. Radiological signs of consolidation and parenchymal volume loss associated with displacement of the hemi-diaphragm and pleural effusions are all described in cases of pulmonary infarction, but are non-specific findings. It should be noted that a normal chest X-ray does not exclude the diagnosis of pulmonary embolism. Radiological investigation progresses from the least invasive and least specific chest X-ray to the most invasive and most diagnostic pulmonary arteriogram.

Between these two extremes, radioisotope scanning using either isolated perfusion studies or a combination of ventilation and perfusion studies can yield very useful information and obviate the need for further investigation. Results of isotope studies are expressed in terms of probability, but in clinical practice a negative perfusion study effectively excludes pulmonary embolic disease and this is unquestionably the most useful result.

Ascending leg venography is frequently used in the assessment of suspected deep vein thrombosis and pulmonary embolic disease. A positive venographic study will obviate the need for pulmonary angiography since the medical treatment is identical. However, it should be noted that approximately one-third of patients with pulmonary embolism have negative venograms.

Pulmonary arteriography is the definitive test in the diagnosis of embolic disease. It is also the most invasive diagnostic test with an attendant mortality (0.5 per cent) and therefore it should be used selectively. Angiographic assessment is most beneficial in those patients at high risk from anti-coagulation, in whom long term anti-coagulation is proposed, and in whom pre-existing parenchyma lung disease renders interpretation of the isotope scan difficult.

In summary, a normal chest X-ray does not exclude the diagnosis of pulmonary embolism, but a negative isotope perfusion study does. Pulmonary arteriography is the most accurate diagnostic test in the investigation of pulmonary embolic disease.

Aneurysm, rupture, and dissection of the thoracic aorta

Plain film radiology is still useful in the investigation of aortic disease. Its limitations should be appreciated, however, and further investigation by computed tomography or angiography should almost certainly follow. Computed tomography provides far greater diagnostic and localizing information than the plain film (Mirvis, 1987).

Radiological signs of aneurysm on the conventional chest X-ray (frontal view)

Plain film radiology demonstrates a widening of the mediastinum with a distortion or loss of the normal aortic contour (Fig. 3.16). There may be associated calcification within the wall of the aorta,

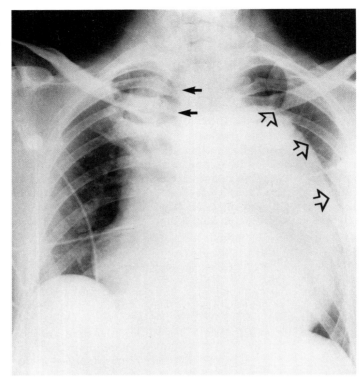

Key
Open arrows − margin of aneurysm.
Solid arrows − tracheal displacement.

Fig 3.16 Aortic aneurysm.

and if this is confined to the ascending aorta then a diagnosis of syphilitic aortitis should be considered. Hypertension and artheroma are much more common and may produce the same appearance. On the lateral view, there may be evidence of pressure erosion of the adjacent bone i.e. the sternum in the case of the ascending aorta or the anterior margins of the vertebral bodies in the descending thoracic aorta.

Aortic dissection and rupture

Accurate localization and the extent of the diseased aortic segment have implications for treatment. However, as previously mentioned to obtain this information computed tomography or angiography are required (Fig. 3.17). Computed tomography has the advantage that it is safe, accurate, non-invasive and provides additional information of the extent of any mediastinal or pericardial haemorrhage.

Radiological signs indicative of aortic dissection or tear may be described in terms of the likelihood of underlying aortic pathology. The most suspicious radiological sign is visualization of the right paraspinous and pleural reflection line, or shift of the trachea and oesophagus to the right. In the correct clinical context, these radiological signs suggest the probability of aortic tear is over 90 per cent. Individual displacement of either the oesophagus (or nasogastric tube) or the trachea to the right is associated with the probability of aortic tear in 70 per cent of cases. Fractures of the first and second ribs carry an association of 10 per cent. Other non-specific radiological signs include pleural effusion, left apical extrapleural haematoma, loss of visualization of the aortic knuckle and displacement of mural calcification away from the lateral aortic margin (Marnocha and Maglinte, 1985).

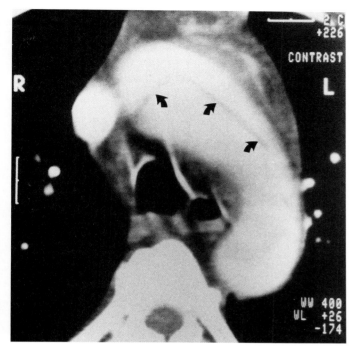

Fig 3.17 CT scan demonstrating dissection of the thoracic aorta.

Key
Arrows – aortic dissection flap.

Acute diaphragmatic rupture/hernia

Diaphragmatic hernia may remain relatively asymptomatic until strangulation occurs and it is frequently missed at the time of the original injury. Radiological signs include loss of clarity of the diaphragmatic outline, elevation of the diaphragm, associated pleural effusion and abnormally positioned loops of gas filled bowel. The latter is the most useful and easily appreciated radiological sign. Both ultra-sound and computed tomography may be required to determine diaphragmatic integrity.

Oesophageal rupture

Unlike diaphragmatic herniation, oesophageal perforation is almost never asymptomatic. The earliest radiological sign is pneumomediastinum. The classically described left-sided pleural effusion is a late sign and its absence should not exclude the diagnosis. Widening of the mediastinum and associated hydro or hydro-pneumothorax may be present if the mediastinal pleura is disrupted. The combination of pneumomediastinum and left pleural effusion is highly suggestive of oesophageal rupture. Complications are mediastinitis and infection.

Pneumonia

Pneumonia is often divided into lobar, broncho and interstitial types. This classification can provide some insight into the causative organism, but its usefulness is limited by the inconsistent patterns of shadowing displayed. Lobar pneumonia is an example of infection which is primarily sited in the peripheral airspaces of the lung parenchyma e.g. TB, klebsiella, and streptococcus (Fig. 3.18). Bronchopneumonia has a different primary site of inflammation, in that the conducting airways and proximal lung parenchyma are predominately

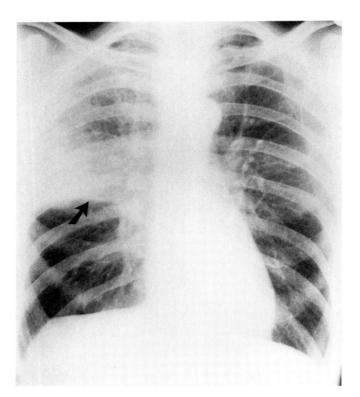

Key
Arrow – horizontal fissure.

Fig 3.18   Lobar pneumonia.

affected e.g. haemophilus and staphylococcus. Interstitial pneumonia is primarily located within the connective tissue of the pulmonary parenchyma and this type of infection is typified by mycoplasma or pneumocystis. Radiological signs are usually non-specific and the appearances depend upon the causative agent and level of immunocompetence of the host. The appearances include patchy or diffuse areas of consolidation with a tendency to confluent shadowing as the infection progresses. Other radiological signs include air bronchogram, pleural effusion, patchy atelectasis, cavitation and lymphadenopathy. The latter is unusual in bacterial pneumonia with the exception of TB. The above changes tend to evolve over a period of 24–48 hours. In cases of dramatic radiographic change over several hours, the following differential diagnosis should be considered: pulmonary oedema, atelectasis, aspiration and pulmonary haemorrhage.

Aspiration pneumonia

The pulmonary response to aspiration is a combination of infective and inflammatory changes depending upon the nature of the material aspirated. The distribution of abnormalities on the chest X-ray may suggest the diagnosis with the right side more frequently involved than the left and with preferential involvement of the posterior segments of the upper and lower lobes. Nevertheless any zone may be affected and the appearances may mimic pneumonia with the signs previously described. Complications include atelectasis, pulmonary abscess, pulmonary oedema.

Although the general features of pneumonia have been described, some radiographic appearances may narrow down the differential diagnosis and provide an insight into the likely causative organism. As previously mentioned, hilar lymphadenopathy is relatively unusual in simple bacterial pneumonia. However, in primary TB, unilateral lymphadenopathy involving the pulmonary hilum is present in approximately 80 per cent of cases. In viral and fungal pneumonia there is often bilateral nodal enlargement. Cavitating pneumonia suggests infection with staphylococcus, klebsiella or TB. Staphylococcal pneumonia frequently cavitates in childhood. Bulging of the inter lobar fissures suggests klebsiella as a possible underlying organism, or the development of a pulmonary abscess. The radiological manifestation of active tuberculosis differ, depending upon whether the infection is primary or secondary. Primary infection involves a previously unexposed host. The features are those of consolidation in any zone, hilar lymphadenopathy (almost always unilateral or at the very least asymmetrical), pleural and/or pericardial effusion and possible miliary spread. The appearances of secondary infection include consolidation (principally at the lung apex or in the apical segments of the lower lobes), cavitation (predominately at the lung apex), pleural effusion and possible miliary spread. Complications include pleural effusion, empyema, pulmonary abscess and pneumothorax secondary to pneumatocele rupture.

Pneumonia in the immuno-suppressed or the immuno-compromised patient

Depression of the immune system extends the range of pathogens capable of invading the pulmonary parenchyma. The radiographic appearances of the more commonly encountered infections may be atypical due to the lack of/or the unusual nature of the patient's response. Frequent radiological monitoring is essential in this group. Simultaneous infection with multiple organisms and reactivation of previously inactive TB is common. One of the most frequent pathogens encountered in the immuno-compromised patient is *Pneumocystis carinii*. The radiological signs of pneumocystis infection are those of a diffuse interstitial lung infiltration with multiple linear shadows, initially distributed around the perihilar regions. The periphery of the lung fields are relatively spared in the early stages, but the distinction is obliterated as the disease progresses and a more ground-glass appearance is seen. The latter is due to airspace shadowing with consequent air bronchograms as the alveoli fill with exudate. Late development of air or air/fluid filled cysts occurs throughout the

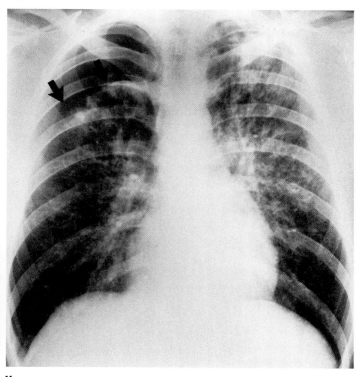

Fig 3.19   Pneumocystis pneumonia.

Key
Arrows – pneumothorax, lung edge.

lung fields with no particular preference of localization. Pneumothorax and/or pneumo-mediastinum are recognized complications (Gamsu *et al.*, 1982).

Acquired immune deficiency syndrome (AIDS)

The pulmonary manifestations of AIDS may be divided into infective and malignant disease. Pneumocystis is one of the commonest infections and radiologically a ground-glass or diffuse veiling of the lung field may suggest the diagnosis (Fig. 3.19). Pulmonary nodules are very unusual in pneumocystis and much more suggestive of TB or fungal infection. In the malignant category Kaposi's sarcoma should be considered. Hilar lymphadenopathy is a feature of TB or malignant disease and again it is very unusual in pneumocystis (Suster *et al.*, 1986).

Legionnaires' disease

Legionella pneumophila is a cause of a potentially fatal lobar pneumonia and is most clinically severe in the elderly, chronically sick or immuno-suppressed.

The principle radiological feature is that of air space shadowing. There is no characteristic appearance, but early findings often include poorly defined round areas of consolidation which coalesce and spread throughout the lung. The lower lobes are the most frequently involved site and 30 per cent of cases are unilateral. Small pleural effusions are common, but large effusions suggest associated cardiac failure. Radiological resolution is typically very slow, may be incomplete and does not correlate with clinical improvement (Evans *et al.*, 1981).

Neonatal respiratory distress

It is beyond the scope of this chapter to provide a detailed consideration of respiratory distress in the neonate (Alford and Kattwinkel, 1983). However, the radiographic appearances of five causes of neonatal respiratory distress which may require management on the intensive care unit are described.

Hyaline membrane disease

The radiological signs in hyaline membrane disease are principally those of under-aeration due to progressive atelectasis. The appearances on the frontal

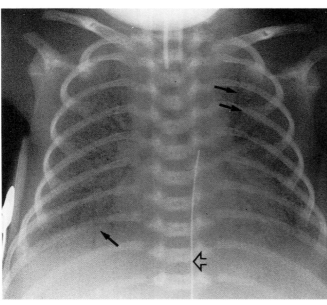

Fig 3.20   Hyaline membrane disease.

Key
Solid arrows – air bronchograms.
Open arrow – umbilical arterial catheter.

chest X-ray are those of bilateral small volume lungs, with faint diffuse granularity throughout the lung fields (Fig. 3.20). As the disease progresses, there is increasing granularity with evidence of air bronchograms and loss of the cardiac and diaphragmatic outlines. Finally this progresses to a total 'white-out' of both lung fields. Complications occur both due to the disease and the treatment. Complications of the disease include pneumonia and left-to-right shunt due to delayed closure or re-opening of the ductus arteriosus secondary to hypoxia. Iatrogenic complications are those secondary to positive pressure ventilation.

Meconium aspiration

In contrast to hyaline membrane disease, the lung volumes are large and the lung fields hyper-expanded. There are patchy areas of airspace shadowing associated with more focal area of hyperinflation (Fig. 3.21). Pleural effusion is present in approximately one-quarter of cases. Complications include pneumothorax, pneumo-mediastinum and infection.

Congenital diaphragmatic hernia

The radiological signs depend upon whether or not the intrathoracic loops of bowel contain gas. In cases of gas filled bowel, there are multiple thin walled radiolucent structures projected within the lung fields. The mediastinum may be displaced to the contralateral side. In the absence of gas filled bowel, the diagnosis is difficult, but may be clarified by introducing a little air into the GI tract and then repeating the frontal radiograph. Alternatively ultrasonic detection of the diaphragmatic defect may prove diagnostic. Congenital diaphragmatic hernia is almost invariably left-sided. Complications include acute respiratory distress, strangulation of herniated abdominal contents and ipsilateral pulmonary hypoplasia.

Congenital lobar emphysema

The key radiographic feature is unilateral hyperinflation with increased volume of the affected lobe and depression of the ipsilateral hemi-diaphragm. The mediastinum may be displaced to the contralateral side. Vascular markings are present, though widely separated and this differentiates this appearance from pneumothorax. Air trapping with ipsilateral hyperinflation persists on an expiratory film. There is a 50 per cent incidence of associated congenital heart disease.

Tracheo-oesophageal fistula (TOF)

Radiological appearances of TOF are those of over expanded large volume lungs with possible patchy areas of airspace shadowing due to aspiration.

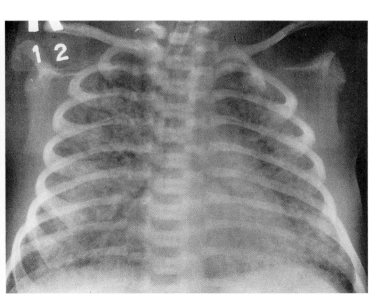

Fig 3.21   Meconium aspiration.

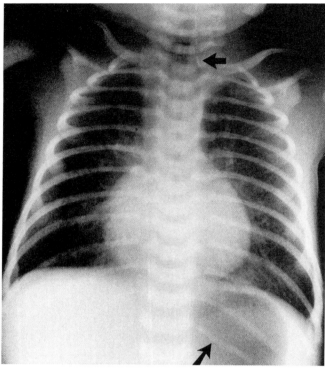

Fig 3.22   Oesophageal atresia.

Key
Horizontal arrow – oesophageal catheter.
Oblique arrow – 13th rib.

There is frequently gaseous oesophageal distension proximal to the level of an almost invariably associated atresia and the trachea may be compressed by the gas filled oesophagus. Abdominal gaseous distension is also frequently apparent and often included within the chest X-ray in an infant. As part of the underlying dysplasia, there may be 13 pairs of ribs. The major complication is aspiration pneumonia, and with this in mind, the diagnosis should be confirmed by insertion of a radio-opaque oesophageal tube which will also establish the level of atresia (Fig. 3.22). Radiological contrast agents are unnecessary for the diagnosis and may induce further aspiration. As part of the general dysplasia, there is an association between oesophageal atresia and vertebral, vascular, renal, radial and ano-rectal anomalies.

Conclusion

The lung fields tend to be symmetrically reduced in size in cases of hyaline membrane disease, and increased in size in meconium aspiration. Unilateral hyperinflation is suggestive of congenital lobar emphysema. Congenital diaphragmatic hernia is almost invariably left-sided. Oesophageal atresia is associated with tracheo-oesophageal fistula in 90 per cent of cases and radiological contrast agents are not necessary to establish the diagnosis of atresia. The use of the contrast medium gastrografin is absolutely contra-indicated in cases in which pulmonary aspiration is a possibility. The hyperosmolar nature of the contrast medium may induce pulmonary oedema.

References

Alford, B.A. and Kattwinkel, J. (1983). Neonatal respiratory distress. In: *Critical Problems in Diagnostic Radiology*, pp. 63–99. Edited by Armstrong, P. Lippincott, Philadelphia.

Evans, A.F., Oakley, R.H. and Whitehouse, G.H. (1981). Analysis of the chest radiograph in Legionnaires disease. *Clinical Radiology* **32**, 361–5.

Felson, B. (1973). *Chest Roentgenology*. W.B. Saunders, Philadelphia.

Gamsu, G., Hecht, S.T., Birnberg, F.A., Coleman, D.L. and Golden, I.A. (1982). Pneumocystis carinii pneumonia in homosexual men. *Americal Journal of Roentgenology* **139**, 647–51.

Goodman, L.R. and Putman, C.E. (1983). *Intensive Care Radiology: Imaging of the Critically Ill*, 2nd Edition. W.B. Saunders, Philadelphia.

Grainger, R.G. and Allison, D.J. (1986). *Diagnostic Radiology*, Vol 1, pp. 113–365, Churchill Livingstone Edinburgh.

Greenbaum, E.I. (1982). *Radiology of the Emergency Patient: An Atlas Approach*, pp. 183–282. John Wiley & Sons, Chichester.

Greene, R. (1987). Adult respiratory distress syndrome: acute alveolar damage. *Radiology* **163**, 57–66.

Marnocha, K.E. and Maglinte, D.D.T. (1985). Plain-film criteria for excluding aortic rupture in blunt chest trauma. *American Journal of Roentgenology* **144**, 19–21.

Mirvis, S.E., Kostrubiak, I., Whitley, N.O. *et al.* (1987). Role of CT in excluding major arterial injury after blunt thoracic trauma. *American Journal of Roentgenology* **149**, 601–605.

Rohlfing, B.M., Webb, W.R. and Schlobohm, R.M. (1976). Ventilator-related extra-alveolar air in adults. *Radiology* **121**, 25–31.

Suster, B., Akerman, M., Orenstein, M. and Wax, M.R. (1986). Pulmonary manifestations of AIDS: review of 106 episodes. *Radiology* **161**, 87–93.

Windebank, W.J. (1987). Diagnosing pulmonary thromboembolism. *British Medical Journal* **294**, 1369–70.

Acknowledgements

I would like to express my sincere thanks to the Department of Radiology, University College Hospital, London from which the majority of radiographs were obtained. This collection of X-rays was acquired during my former attachment to the Department as a Senior Registrar.

In particular I wish to express my appreciation to Dr K.M. Walmsley, Consultant Radiologist, Royal Free and University College Hospital and Dr W.P. Whitear, Senior Registrar, University College Hospital for Figures 3.4 and 3.22 respectively.

4

Endocrinology

Mark Vella and John Betteridge

Diabetes mellitus

Diabetes mellitus comprises a heterogenous group of disorders characterized by chronic hyperglycaemia and a propensity to develop multisystem complications. It is a common condition, affecting 1–2 per cent of Caucasian populations, though its prevalence increases with age and it is seen in all ethnic groups. Indeed studies on Asian communities around the world have consistently shown a higher diabetes prevalence than in other local groups. In the UK, the age-adjusted prevalence of diabetes is approximately four times higher in Asian than in European residents.

Table 4.1 Clinical features of insulin dependent and non-insulin dependent diabetes

	IDD 'juvenile-onset' (Type 1)	NIDD 'maturity-onset' (Type 2)
Age	Usually < 30 years	Usually middle-aged and over
Sex	M ⩾ F	F > M
Onset	Abrupt	Gradual
Weight loss	Marked	Often obese
Ketosis	Common	Absent
Plasma insulin/ C-peptide	Absent or reduced	Normal or raised
Treatment	Insulin and diet	Diet ± oral hypogly-caemics (insulin on occasion)
HLA associations	(B8, B15) DR3, DR4	None

Table 4.2 Diabetes-related disorders

- Associated with other endocrine disorders (Cushing's syndrome, acromegaly, phaeochromocytoma)
- Gestational diabetes
- Pancreatic disease (carcinoma of the pancreas, chronic pancreatitis)
- Drug-induced   e.g. Corticosteroids
  - Thiazide diuretics
  - Diazoxide
  - Streptozocin
- Genetic syndromes
  1. Familial   e.g. Acanthosis nigricans
     - Haemochromatosis
     - Laurence–Moon–Biedl syndrome
     - Myotonic dystrophy
     - DIDMOAD
     - Prader-Willi syndrome
  2. Chromosomal   e.g. Down's syndrome
     - Klinefelter's syndrome
     - Turner's syndrome
- Tropical diabetes ('J-type', 'Z-type')

Primary diabetes is classified into insulin-dependent (IDD) and non-insulin dependent diabetes (NIDD) but this division, is by no means clear-cut (Table 4.1). Secondary causes of diabetes are shown in Table 4.2.

The diagnosis of diabetes mellitus has recently been reconsidered by the World Health Organisation with an intermediate category of glucose intolerance short of diabetes entitled 'impaired glucose tolerance' as seen in Table 4.3.

Aetiology

Insulin dependent (or Type 1 or IDDM) diabetes is aetiologically distinct from the commoner non-insulin dependent (or Type 2) diabetes, though both are still poorly understood. Interactions

Table 4.3 Diagnostic blood glucose levels following 75 g oral glucose tolerance test (OGTT)

Diabetes mellitus (DM)	
Fasting	$\geq$ 6.7 mmol/litre
and/or	
2 hours after glucose load	$\geq$ 10.0 mmol/litre
Impaired glucose tolerance (IGT)	
Fasting	5.6–6.7 mmol/litre
and	
2 hours after glucose load	6.7–10 mmol/litre

These figures refer to the concentration of glucose in venous whole blood.

between genetic, environmental and immunological factors lead to destruction of the β-cells of the pancreatic islets and thus insulinopaenia with consequent IDDM. The most popular working hypothesis suggests that genetic susceptibility is conferred by genes in linkage disequilibrium with HLA DR3 and DR4 on the short arm of chromosome 6. Approximately 95 per cent of IDDM patients are positive for either or both antigens compared to 60 per cent of the control population. There are strong, but less powerful, associations with HLA B8 and B15.

The agent that initiates and sustains B-cell damage is as yet unknown though there are two main contenders. The viral theory is supported by evidence of increased frequency of IDDM in autumn and winter together with numerous anecdotal reports of the disease developing days or months after a viral infection. Increased Coxsackie virus IgM antibody titres at diagnosis also suggest a causal role for this virus.

The second contender is autoimmunity. Patients with newly diagnosed Type 1 diabetes show various immunological abnormalities including complement fixing antibodies to islet cells (CF-ICA), lymphocytic infiltration of the islets, abnormal leucocyte migration inhibition and raised K-cell levels. There is evidence that these phenomena may damage pancreatic β-cells with loss of insulin secretory capacity. The level of CF-ICA at the time of diagnosis is 70–80 per cent compared to 0.1–1 per cent in the general population and as they have been detected several years before presentation in some subjects their presence is considered, by some, to be the most specific immune marker.

It has been postulated that the combination of the inherited HLA DR3 and 4 and an exogenous antigen such as a virus are presented to the immune system and this triggers the formation of B lymphocytes and K-cells which cross react with the pancreatic B-cell, resulting in insulin insufficiency.

Non-insulin dependent diabetes (Type 2 diabetes, NIDDM) has a strong hereditary component, though the mode of inheritance is as yet unknown. In studies of identical twins 90 per cent are concordant for NIDDM compared to 50 per cent concordance for IDD. A multiple gene inheritance is suggested by studies that show that about 20 per cent of patients with NIDDM have siblings with this form of diabetes compared to 2 per cent who have siblings with IDDM.

The insulin gene has been directly analyzed by recombinant DNA technology in an attempt to identify genetic markers of NIDDM. There is a highly polymorphic region of DNA near the 5^1 end of the insulin gene on chromosome 11. This region has been broadly divided into short or large 'insertions' depending on its length. Preliminary evidence suggests that NIDDM is associated with the large DNA insertion.

Recent attention has also focused on the role of insulin resistance in the causation of NIDDM. Insulin, like most polypeptide hormones, interacts with highly specific glycoprotein receptors on cells which sets off a chain of intracellular events. NIDDM patients have been shown to have both insulin receptor and post-receptor defects. The nature of these defects remains unclear but may be responsible for the deterioration of glucose tolerance with age. The relative contribution of insulin resistance and impaired β-cell function in the development of NIDDM remains the subject of much debate. Whereas IDDM patients have a subacute or acute presentation with the development of severe symptoms over days, NIDDM patients have a more insidious onset and the condition is often diagnosed on routine urine testing.

A rare form of diabetes referred to as non-insulin dependent diabetes of the young (or NIDDY) cannot be classified under either group. This condition appears to be inherited as a simple autosomal dominant trait. It usually presents below the age of 30 years and is characterized by the absence of ketonuria and the gradual onset of symptoms. Common symptoms of diabetes mellitus include polyuria, polydipsia, weight loss, recurrent infections, weakness and paraesthesiae. Difficulties in classification have already been mentioned.

Management of diabetes

The aim of treating diabetes is primarily to save life and alleviate symptoms. However with the realization over the past decade that poor control increases the risk of specific diabetic complications modern management aims to achieve near normal glycaemic control over the years to prevent or delay the development of complications.

Urine testing for glucose has largely been superceded by the far more useful and accurate blood glucose monitoring with glucose-oxidase reagent strips (e.g. BM strips, Glucostix) or with hand-held digital read-out meters. But perhaps the most clinically significant impact has been in the use of glycosylated haemoglobin (HbA1) and frugosamine measurements. Glucose has the ability to fix to free amino groups of proteins to form a reversible compound known as a Schiff's base. A stable ketoamine compound may then be formed by the Amadori reaction. The ketoamine linkage between glucose and haemoglobin takes place at the valine residue at the terminal end of one or both β-chains of haemoglobin. Measurement of HbA1 provides a fairly accurate assessment of overall glycaemic control, during the preceding 4–6 weeks. The fructosamine assay is an index of the degree of non-enzymatic glycosylation of serum proteins and provides an overall assessment of glycaemic control over the preceding two weeks. In the modern approach to diabetic management, patients, particularly those with IDDM, are encouraged to measure and record their own blood glucose measurements at home (home blood glucose monitoring) and on clinic visits overall glycaemic control is assessed with glycosylated haemoglobin or fructosamine assays.

Diet

Dietary measures are employed in the management of diabetic patients to optimize blood glucose control, to lessen hypoglycaemic risk and to achieve weight loss in the obese. The British Diabetic Association has recently reviewed its dietary recommendations. In brief, fat intake should be reduced to 35 per cent at the expense of foods rich in saturated fatty acids (i.e. spreading and cooking animal fats, dairy products and meat products wtih a high fat content). Secondly, carbohydrate intake could be increased to meet the energy needs, particularly those foods with a high fibre content.

Oral hypoglycaemic drugs

Sulphonylureas These drugs are used when dietary manipulation fails in the NIDDM patient. Their mechanism of action is not fully understood but in the short term plasma insulin concentrations rise because of stimulation of first phase insulin release (release of preformed insulin from the beta cell). In the longer term, insulin levels return to pretreatment levels but blood glucose levels remain reduced and there is evidence to suggest that sulphonylureas increase insulin receptor numbers in peripheral tissues, thus enhancing the action of insulin.

The sulphonylureas are, in general, rapidly absorbed from the gastrointestinal tract and are tightly protein bound in the plasma to albumin. There are significant differences in the plasma half-life of the various sulphonylurea drugs (Table 4.4) ranging from gliquidone with a half-life of 1.4 hours to chlorpropamide with a half-life of 36 hours. The shorter-acting preparations are usually given two or three times daily and the longer-acting drugs once daily. Discrepancies exist between the plasma half-life of the drugs and the duration of effective hypoglycaemic action and sulphonylureas with intermediate plasma half-lives are often effective in once-a-day dosage. The usual dosage requirements are shown in Table 4.4. No therapeutic advantage is achieved by exceeding the maximum dose but the risk of side-effects is increased.

The sulphonylureas differ in their metabolism as might be expected from their different duration of action. Gliquidone is excreted almost entirely as inactive metabolites in the bile whereas acetohexamide is reduced rapidly in the liver to a

Table 4.4   Sulphonylureas

	Dosage (mg)	Plasma half-life (hours)
First generation		
tolbutamide	500–2000	4–5
chlorpropamide	100–500	36
tolazamide	100–1000	7
acetohexamide	250–1500	6–8
Second generation		
glibenclamide	2.5–20	5
glibornuride	12.5–75	8
glipizide	2.5–40	3½
gliclazide	40–320	10–12
gliquidone	45–180	1½

metabolite that has more hypoglycaemic action than the parent drug which is excreted in the urine. Tolbutamide is rapidly carboxylated in the liver to the metabolically inert carboxytolbutamide which is excreted in the urine while chlorpropamide is excreted very slowly in the urine as an unchanged drug and as hydroxylated or hydrolyzed metabolites.

Side-effects with sulphonylureas are rare (< 1 per cent in large series) and generally confined to mild gastrointestinal upsets and allergic dermatitis. Blood dyscrasias and hepatic toxicity are exceedingly rare. However certain specific side-effects should be emphasized. Chlorpropamide may occasionally precipitate water intoxication by sensitizing the distal renal tubule to antidiuretic hormone and this sulphonylurea is the one most frequently associated with a disulfiram-like reaction (flush, tachycardia and headache) following alcohol. Compounds which interfere with the urinary excretion of the sulphonylureas or their protein binding such as salicylates, probenecid, coumarin anticoagulants and phenylbutazone may potentiate the hypoglycaemic action. In addition, inhibition of hepatic enzyme activity by drugs such as chloramphenicol, phenylbutazone and coumarin anticoagulants may have similar effects. Certain drugs may exacerbate diabetes and lead to loss of diabetic control with sulphonylureas. These include thiazide and other diuretics, corticosteroids, oestrogens, phenothiazines, phenytoin, nicotinic acid, isoniazid, calcium channel blockers and sympathomimetics.

Hypoglycaemic reactions although rare in comparison to those caused by insulin are an important problem in the use of sulphonylureas. These reactions are more likely to occur in the elderly and if hepatic or renal impairment is present. Irregular food intake and excess alcohol intake which inhibits hepatic gluconeogenesis, are also important contributory factors. More rarely other endocrine deficiency states particularly of the pituitary, adrenal and thyroid may exacerbate hypoglycaemia and drugs such as beta-blockers and MAOI inhibitors may mask the symptoms of hypoglycaemia and interfere with normal recovery mechanisms. Serious sulphonylurea-induced hypoglycaemia needs treatment with constant intravenous glucose infusion often for prolonged periods. These drugs augment the insulin response to exogenous glucose and so may produce further hypoglycaemia following bolus administration of glucose.

Biguanides Only one of these guanidine derivatives, metformin, remains available in the UK. The mechanism of action of metformin is not fully elucidated but its major effects include inhibition of hepatic gluconeogenesis, enhanced peripheral glucose utilization and reduced glucose absorption from the gut. These effects appear to be independent of insulin. A possible mechanism to explain these diverse effects is the binding of the drug to mitochondrial membranes with alteration of the surface potential. Metformin is rapidly excreted unchanged through the kidneys with a short plasma half-life.

Gastrointestinal side-effects, particularly nausea and diarrhoea are relatively common with metformin. Appetite is decreased which can be an advantage in the obese patient. Skin rashes, a metallic taste in the mouth and myalgia are rare. A potential major side-effect of the biguanides is lactic acidosis due to increased anaerobic glycolysis. Phenformin has been withdrawn in the U.K., and many other countries as it was the major cause of lactic acidosis. The risk is much less with metformin especially with careful selection of patients.

Guar fibre The galactomannan, guar gum, obtained from the Indian cluster bean is the most effective of the non-absorbable carbohydrates in lowering post-prandial glucose levels. There are several palatable preparations of guar on the market but gastrointestinal side-effects limit their use in many patients. There may be advantages in mixing guar with food rather than taking it in water prior to a meal.

Use of oral hypoglycaemic agents

For practical purposes the use of sulphonylurea and biguanide drugs is confined to the patient with NIDDM. However drug therapy is only introduced if dietary measures alone fail to restore normoglycaemia (> 50 per cent patients). Metformin is a useful agent in the obese patient and weight gain is less of a problem than with sulphonylureas. This drug is best avoided in the presence of renal, hepatic or cardiac impairment and chronic alcholism because of the increased risk of lactic acidosis. The usual starting dose is 850 mg after the evening meal and the dose is increased to a maximum of 3 g/day in divided doses although many physicians would not use more than 1.5 g/day. Initial gastrointestinal side-effects often

Table 4.5   Contraindications to oral hypoglycaemic agents

Biguanides
Insulin-dependent diabetes mellitus
Diabetic ketoacidosis, hyperosmolar nonketotic
   coma
Major surgery, severe infection, trauma
Renal and hepatic impairment
Pregnancy
Cardiac failure and ischaemic heart disease
Alcoholism
Sulphonylureas
Insulin-dependent diabetes mellitus
Diabetic ketoacidosis, hyperosmolar nonketotic
   coma
Major surgery, severe infection, trauma
Hypersensitivity
Pregnancy
Severe renal or hepatic impairment

disappear with time and hypoglycaemia does not occur.

A sulphonylurea is usually the treatment of choice in the non-obese patient and choosing from the many available is difficult. There are no overwhelming advantages with the newer second generation drugs. It is best to become familiar with two or three agents and tailor the appropriate drug to the appropriate patient based on the patient's age and the presence of renal or hepatic impairment. The short-acting compounds (e.g. tolbutamide) have advantages in the elderly as the risk of accumulation is less. In younger patients a compound effective on a once-daily dosage aids compliance. In renal impairment compounds excreted in the urine should be avoided. In this situation gliclazide and gliquidone are useful in that they are principally metabolized and excreted by the liver. However these drugs would be best avoided in hepatic insufficiency.

As sulphonylureas and biguanides have different modes of action a synergistic effect can be obtained by using a combination of these drugs. However it is probably better to proceed to insulin therapy. Contraindications to oral hypoglycaemics are shown in Table 4.5. Glymidine is a hypoglycaemic agent related to the sulphonylureas without cross allergy with the other sulphonylureas and can be used in patients with a history of allergy to these compounds.

Insulin

The aim of insulin treatment is to improve diabetic control without producing disabling hypo-

Table 4.6(a)   Classification of insulins by duration of action

Duration of action	Formulation
Short-acting	• Neutral soluble
	• Acid soluble
Intermediate-acting	• Isophane
	• Lente
Long-acting	• Ultralente
	• Protamine zinc insulin

Table 4.6(b)   Some insulin preparations available in the UK

Type	Manufacturer	Species	Approximate duration of action (hours)
• *Short-acting*			
Soluble	Wellcome	Beef	6–8
Hypurin Neutral	CP Pharm.	Beef	6–8
Actrapid MC	Novo	Pig	6–8
Humulin S	Eli Lilly	Human (CRB)	6–8
Velosulin	Nordisk	Pig	6–8
• *Intermediate*			
Neuphane	Wellcome	Beef	12–18
Insulatard	Nordisk	Pig	12–18
Humulin 'I'	Eli Lilly	Human (CRB)	12–16
Monotard	Novo		
• *Long-acting*			
Humulin Zn	Eli Lilly	Human (CRB)	16+
Ultratard HM	Novo	Human (EMP)	24+
Lentard	Novo	Pig and beef	18–24

glycaemic attacks. Insulin is indicated for the young ketosis-prone IDDM and for the NIDDM patient in whom diet and maximal oral agents have proved unsuccessful. Insulin is classified according to formulation or duration of action (Tables 4.6(a) and (b)).

Short-acting insulins   Short-acting insulins are true acidic solutions of 'soluble' insulins, whose pH is restored to 7.0 after buffering with acetate or phosphate. It is preferable to use a neutral insulin if this is to be mixed in a syringe because the extended action insulins themselves are of neutral pH.

Intermediate-acting insulins   Intermediate-acting insulins are based on the complexing of insulin molecules to protamine, a large protein derived from salmon sperm. These 'isophane' insulins are produced in highly purified beef, pork or human varieties. The prolonged effect of insulin zinc suspensions (Lente insulin) is based on the fact that neutral insulin can be precipitated by an excess of zinc.

Long-acting insulins   Long-acting insulins are produced by using both protamine and zinc as complexing agents to further extend the insulin's duration of action. Insulin zinc suspensions are pure crystals of zinc insulin which are useful in providing basal insulins upon which may be superimposed multiple injections of soluble insulin during the day before meals.

Insulin types are further subdivided according to their animal source (beef, pork, human) (Table 4.7). The amino acid sequence of human insulin differs from porcine insulin by one residue at the C terminal position on the B-chain. Human insulin varies from beef insulin by three amino acids at position A8, A10 and B30. Pork and human insulins appear to behave in a similar fashion though bovine insulins may be of slower onset – this may be due to reversible binding with insulin antibodies. Species difference is only one of the variables concerned in immunogenicity.

Table 4.7   Amino acid changes in beef, pig and human insulin

	B30	A8	A10
Human	Threonine	Threonine	Isoleucine
Pork	Alanine	Thronine	Isoleucine
Beef	Alanine	Alanine	Valine

Indeed, antibody formation is provoked by impurities such as proinsulin, insulin derivatives and breakdown products such as desamido insulin and insulin ethyl esters. The clinical significance of these antibodies remains to be fully explained but they are associated with insulin resistance seen in some diabetics taking beef insulin particularly; they may also prolong the half-life of some injected insulins thus delaying recovery from hypoglycaemia. There have also been suggestions that they cross the placenta to cause neonatal hypoglycaemia and that they may have a role in the causation of autonomic neuropathy by cross-reacting with nerve growth factor.

Indications for human insulins which provoke fewer antibodies, are few. These include insulin allergy, patients with fat atrophy and those requiring high doses, and when insulin is required only temporarily, e.g. in pregnancy or perioperatively. However, some companies are withdrawing their pork insulins as they move to the production of human insulin by genetic engineering techniques.

Use of insulin

It is difficult to mimic normal pancreatic insulin release with injected insulins but this is the basis of insulin therapy. IDDM patients inject themselves subcutaneously with insulin one or more times a day.

Endogenous insulin production may still be present in some patients and one injection of a depot insulin prior to breakfast may provide reasonable control. Soluble insulin can be added if post-breakfast hyperglycaemia is a problem. However most IDDM patients are better controlled on multiple daily insulin injections. A commonly used regime consists of twice daily injections (30–40 minutes before breakfast and 30–40 minutes before the evening meal). A combination of a short-acting and an intermediate-acting insulin is given at each injection.

Some patients prefer to split the evening injection and give the soluble insulin prior to the evening meal and the intermediate-acting insulin at bedtime. This approach gives more flexibility in the timing of the evening meal and also reduces hypoglycaemic reactions in the early hours of the morning if this is a problem. A further useful regime is to take a long-acting insulin at bedtime to provide a basal level of insulin together with preprandial soluble insulin before the main meals. This regime has become more popular since the introduction of pen-injection devices such as 'Novopen' which make insulin injections much more convenient.

A relatively recent introduction to insulin therapy has been miniature portable insulin pumps which can be programmed to provide different rates of basal insulin subcutaneously with bolus insulin to cover meals. Good glycaemic control can be achieved with this technique of constant subcutaneous insulin infusion (CSii) but it has not proved as popular in the UK as in the USA partly due to the cost of the pumps. Patients also need to be well-motivated and meticulous in the use of CSii if problems are to be avoided. Much research is currently underway in the miniaturisation of pumps and the development of glucose sensors. Implantable pumps are also being studied.

In the future isolated pancreatic beta-cell transplantation may provide a means of 'curing' IDDM and early treatment of IDDM patients with immunosuppressive therapy may prevent further immune-mediated beta cell damage.

Subcutaneous injection of insulin needs to be balanced against a regular carbohydrate intake if hypoglycaemia is to be avoided. The carbohydrate should preferably be high in fibre and refined sugars should be avoided. An exchange system is used where the patient learns the amount of various carbohydrate foodstuffs which contain 10 g of carbohydrate. The exchange system enables the patient to consume roughly the same amount of carbohydrate at each meal but to vary the type. A typical patient may take 50 g of carbohydrate or five carbohydrate exchanges for each of three main meals with 10–20 g carbohydrate as mid-meal or bedtime snacks. Additional carbohydrate is necessary to cover the additional energy expenditure of sporting activities.

The dose of insulin is adjusted on the basis of blood glucose measurements with reagent strips. Blood samples are easily obtained with automatic finger-pricking devices (Autolet, Autoclix, Autolance) which are painless and quick. Preprandial glucose levels of 5–7 mmol/litre are optimal.

Intercurrent illness in the diabetic on insulin demands special care. The secretion of 'stress' hormones (cortisol, growth hormone, catecholamines) which are insulin antagonists leads to increased insulin requirements. Frequent blood glucose measurements are necessary and make insulin adjustments easier. An unfortunate mistake (still made too often) is for the patient to reduce or stop insulin during an infection which reduces the appetite or produces vomiting leading to failure to take the normal carboyhdrate intake. This can lead to rapid development of ketoacidosis. On the contrary insulin injections should be maintained and often increased. If necessary the carbohydrate intake can be maintained in liquid form such as leucozade. If vomiting persists hospital admission and intravenous fluid therapy is required.

Hypoglycaemia

The symptoms and signs of hypoglycaemia are shown in Table 4.8. Most hypoglycaemic attacks occur in patients on insulin but it is important to remember that this can be a serious problem in patients on sulphonylurea therapy.

Table 4.8　Symptoms and Signs of hypoglycaemia

Sweating Nervousness Palpitations Trembling Paraesthesiae Numbness Intense hunger Pallor	Due to catecholamine release
Restlessness Agitation Irritability Loss of memory Drowsiness Slurred speech Confusion Headache Unsteadiness Blurring of vision Convulsions Coma Diplopia Hyperreflexia Extensor plantar reflexes Paraplegia Hemiplegia Monoplegia	Due to neuroglycopenia

Hypoglycaemia is very distressing to the patient, relatives and friends and steps are taken in the education and management of the patient to avoid this, yet maintain as near as possible normoglycaemia.

Hypoglycaemic symptoms develop when blood glucose levels fall to 2.5 mmol/litre. In the short term the brain is solely dependent on glucose for fuel and neuroglycopenia together with sympathetic activation associated with hypoglycaemia produce the symptoms (see Table 4.8). If diabetics constantly have high blood glucose levels they may develop hypoglycaemic symptoms at a higher level of glucose.

Hypoglycaemic reactions are more common at certain times depending on the type of insulin regime. For instance, hypoglycaemia will occur mid-morning if the dose of the soluble insulin injected prior to breakfast is too high. If the dose of intermediate-acting insulin taken at this time is too high then hypoglycaemia will occur in the afternoon.

In patients taking a large single dose of intermediate or long-acting insulin once a day before breakfast hypoglycaemia may be particularly troublesome in the late afternoon or at night. Patients are particularly prone to hypoglycaemia prior to meals and timing of meals is therefore very important and they should not be taken late. Mid-meal snacks are also important to buffer the insulin action at the time of maximum activity.

Physical exercise may also be an important cause of hypoglycaemia if appropriate additional carbohydrate is not taken. Heavy alcohol intake may cause profound hypoglycaemia through inhibition of the enzymes of gluconeogenesis in the liver.

Diabetic patients carry glucose tablets at all times and identification cards giving instructions for first aid in the event of hypoglycaemia. If in doubt a blood glucose test may be performed. Some patients do not have warning symptoms of hypoglycaemia particularly those with autonomic neuropathy. Occasionally difficulties arise as the mental confusion and disorderly and aggressive behaviour due to neuroglycopenia make the patient reluctant to accept treatment.

Treatment of hypoglycaemia

If the patient is able to swallow, a useful first aid measure is to give glucose dissolved in milk. A glucose solution administered by a syringe into the side of the mouth is useful in bypassing clenched teeth. If the patient is stuperose and unable to swallow, glucose is administered intravenously, e.g. 25–50 ml of a 50% glucose solution. This may have to be repeated and a continuous infusion set up if overdosage is suspected or a long-acting sulphonylurea is the cause. An alternative is to give glucagon (1 mg) intramuscularly. Glucagon raises the blood glucose by mobilizing liver glycogen. The injection may be repeated if necessary after 10 minutes. The patient should be given glucose orally as soon as this is possible. Glucagon may be ineffective if stores of liver glycogen are low and alternative measures are necessary if there is no response after 15 minutes.

Diabetic ketoacidosis

As a cause of death, diabetic ketoacidosis (DKA) has become less important since the advent of insulin therapy. The mortality associated with this medical emergency is still in the region of 5 per cent because it is often precipitated by severe illness such as myocardial infarction or pancreatitis.

DKA is the most serious of the metabolic abnormalities of insulin deficiency and is characterized by the accumulation of organic acids (acetoacetate and β-hydrobutyrate) and acetone in the blood (up to 15 mM). These abnormalities are a direct result of insulin deficiency. Hepatic glucose output is increased three-fold and this together with decreased tissue utilization of glucose produces marked hyperglycaemia. The major precursors for hepatic gluconeogenesis are amino acids which lead to a negative nitrogen balance. Adipose tissue lipolysis is uninhibited leading to release of free fatty acids (FFA) and increased flux to the liver. Mitochondrial β-oxidation of FFA produces excess acetyl CoA which cannot enter the Krebs cycle and condenses to form ketones. In addition to this massively increased production of ketones the ability of tissues, particularly muscle, to utilize ketones as fuel is impaired in insulin deficiency. The accumulation of ketones leads to severe metabolic acidosis. The hyperketonaemia together with marked hyperglycaemia produces a massive osmotic diuresis and resultant water and electrolyte loss. This loss is often exacerbated by fluid losses related to vomiting.

Clinical features of diabetic ketoacidosis

Nausea, vomiting and drowsiness (sometimes coma) are common. Respiration is characteristically deep and sighing (Kussmaul's breathing) due to the severe acidosis. Acetone may be detected on the breath. It is important to remember the gastro-intestinal symptoms that can accompany DKA, particularly severe abdominal pain which may mimic an intra-abdominal catastrophe. Marked signs of dehydration are present with tachycardia and hypotension. Signs of an underlying precipitating cause such as myocardial infarct, sepsis or pancreatitis may be present.

Laboratory findings show very high blood glucose, the bicarbonate is very low and arterial pH may be below 7. Blood and urine ketones are high. Leucocytosis may be present in the absence of infection perhaps related to the hypertonic plasma. A raised serum amylase is not uncommon and does not necessarily indicate pancreatitis.

Treatment

The key initial management of DKA is the replacement of the fluid deficit (often approximately 6 litres). Physiological saline (0.9%) should be administered rapidly, 1 litre over 30 minutes followed by a further litre over the next hour. In the absence of shock and hypotension some physicians advocate the administration of 0.45% saline as the deficit of water is relatively greater than that of sodium. After the initial rapid infusion, fluid should be given at a rate of 1 litre over 2 hours. Fluid therapy is changed to 5% dextrose when the glucose level falls below 10 mmol/litre. If severe metabolic acidosis (pH < 7.0) is present most physicians would give 50–100 mmol over 30–60 minutes and then repeat until the pH rises above 7.0. Bicarbonate is reserved for the severe cases only, as the metabolism of ketones produces bicarbonate when insulin administration is started and too rapid an increase in pH may be associated with a rapid fall in CSF pH. In addition red cell 2,3-diphosphoglycerate is reduced and the shift in oxygen dissociation curve by bicarbonate administration may further impair tissue oxygen delivery.

The initial plasma potassium may be normal or even slightly elevated but total body potassium levels are markedly depleted (up to 10 mEq/kg). With treatment of DKA, potassium rapidly passes intracellularly and plasma levels may fall precipitously. For this reason potassium replacement (40 mEq/litre of fluid administered) is started at the outset.

In general fluid management is more easily regulated if central venous pressure is monitored.

Urine output needs to be carefully assessed and a urinary catheter is passed if necessary. A nasogastric tube is passed in the unconscious patient and when gastric stasis occurs.

Intravenous insulin therapy is commenced as soon as possible. After a bolus dose of 10 units of soluble insulin a continuous insulin infusion is given. Insulin resistance is quite marked and when acidosis is severe 10–12 units/hour may be required. This is monitored by frequent blood glucose measurements and the infusion rate is gradually reduced depending on the response. There is no doubt that continuous insulin infusion produces less hypoglycaemia and less hypokalaemia compared to the older regime of bolus high dose insulin. As the patient recovers subcutaneous insulin is recommenced.

Frequent biochemical monitoring is required for the successful management of DKA and it is best to keep a progress chart and detail the response of important parameters. Blood glucose should be measured every 30 minutes in the early stages. This can be done at the bedside with the glucose oxidase testing strips. Potassium measurments are required every 2 hours and replacement is adjusted accordingly. Continuous ECG monitoring with T-wave assessment is useful as a measure of plasma potassium. Arterial blood pH and bicarbonate is repeated after 2 hours and further bicarbonate may be required if the pH is slow to correct. The treatment of DKA may be complicated by the precipitating event, usually sepsis, myocardial infarction or pancreatitis. However shock, cerebral oedema, disseminated intravascular coagulation and adult respiratory distress syndrome can occur with DKA alone.

Lactic acidosis

The incidence of lactic acidosis in the diabetic population has been reduced since the removal of the biguanide drug phenformin from the market. However accumulation of lactate and metabolic acidosis still occurs. It may be seen in association with DKA, hyperosmolar non-ketotic coma, various causes of shock and occasionally occurs spontaneously. The pathogenesis of lactic acidosis, particularly its spontaneous development in the diabetic is not understood. However, increased muscle lactate production and failure of hepatic uptake of lactate may be important in the other causes.

Clinical features include depression of consciousness, deep sighing respiration, dehydration and abdominal pain. Arterial pH is low with a reduction in plasma bicarbonate and an increased anion gap without ketonaemia. Plasma lactate levels are greater than 5 mmol/l. Other causes of acidosis have to be excluded. Treatment involves correction of the acidosis which often requires large amounts of bicarbonate.

Hyperosmolar non-ketotic coma

This condition is generally seen in a newly presenting NIDDM patient or develops in a patient with known NIDDM. It is characterized by severe hyperglycaemia, hyperosmolality and dehydration. By definition this occurs in the absence of ketonaemia. The pathogenesis is uncertain but it has been suggested that there is sufficient insulin to inhibit lipolysis but not hyperglycaemia.

Impaired consciousness is common and focal neurological signs may be present or generalized seizures may develop. In some cases the condition appears to have been precipitated by administration of some drugs – diuretics and corticosteroids in particular.

Typical biochemical findings show marked hyperglycaemia, a high plasma osmolality (> 310 mOsm) and a raised urea. The plasma sodium is often normal because of the redistribution of intracellular and extracellular fluids secondary to the hyperglycaemia.

Hyperglycaemic hyperosmolar coma is treated with fluids and insulin. Hypotonic saline is sometimes necessary. Small amounts of insulin only are required. The thrombotic tendency is increased markedly and most physicians anticoagulate these patients with heparin.

Complications of diabetes

Diabetic neuropathy

Several patterns of diabetic neuropathy are well recognized (Table 4.9), affecting approximately 13 per cent of all diabetics. The commonest is symmetrical sensory polyneuropathy affecting all modalities of sensation resulting in numbness, tingling and parasthesiae, usually in the feet, with reduction in knee and ankle jerks and vibration sense. Neuropathy is responsible for serious foot problems. Ulcers result from unnoticed mechanical or thermal injuries. Loss of the normal arches of

Table 4.9   Types of diabetic neuropathy

Symmetrical sensory neuropathy
Monoeuritis simplex or multiplex
Diabetic amyotrophy
Autonomic neuropathy

the foot lead to excess callus formation on the plantar surface of the metatarsal heads. The circulation is actually increased in these patients and oedema is not uncommon, probably due to abnormal vasomotor function and arterio-venous shunting. The neuropathic ulcer or callus may become infected and in severe cases leads to osteomyelitis, thrombotic arterial occlusion and gangrene; amputation of the digit is then essential. Because of these potentially disastrous consequences diabetic patients with peripheral neuropathy are carefully educated in foot care and have regular chiropody.

Neuroarthropathy or Charcot's joints results from loss of pain sensation and bone rarefaction. The usual precipitating event is minor trauma and osteolysis; subluxation and joint disorganization rapidly develop leading to gross deformity of the joint. Diabetes is the commonest cause of neuroarthropathy affecting the feet.

A second type of diabetic neuropathy consists of multiple or isolated involvement of peripheral or cranial nerves. The third and sixth nerves are the commonest cranial nerves involved, the onset tending to be rapid and painless. Mononeuritis of the ulnar, radial, medial, femoral, popliteal and other nerves is occasionally seen. These lesions almost always recover.

Diabetic amyotrophy is an asymmetrical motor neuropathy presenting as a painful, progressive weakness and wasting of the proximal muscles of the lower limbs. It usually occurs in patients over 60 years of age and carries a good prognosis if glycaemic control is improved. The currently held view is that the anterior (motor) spinal nerve roots bear the brunt of the damage.

Neuropathic damage in the diabetic may also affect the autonomic nervous system. Clinical features are listed in Table 4.10. Cardiopulmonary arrest has been reported, particularly during and after surgery, and absence of the normal respiratory responses to hypoxia and hypercapnia has been incriminated as the aetiological factor. Cardiac parasympathetic damage must be detected in diabetics suspected of having autonomic

Table 4.10 Clinical features of autonomic neuropathy

Oesopahgeal atony
Gastroparesis
Nocturnal diarrhoea
Postural hypotension
Absent sinus arrhythmia
Gustatory sweating
Absent sweating in feet
Impotence
Retrograde ejaculation
Bladder dysfunction
Cardiorespiratory arrest
Increased pupil size and resistance to mydriatics
Loss of awareness of hypoglycaemia

neuropathy before they are subjected to an anaesthetic. Five standard cardiovascular autonomic function tests based on measurements of variations in heart rate are commonly used (Table 4.11).

A particularly distressing form of neuropathy is painful neuropathy which in severe cases is accompanied by anorexia, weight loss and marked depression. Occasionally patients with this condition have committed suicide. The pain which is usually in the legs has a peculiar burning quality and is unremitting. Sleep is disturbed and patients cannot bear the touch of the bedclothes. Sometimes the pain is described as being like a tight band round the leg. Objective physical signs of neuropathy may be few. Occasionally the distribution of the pain involves the abdomen and intra-abdominal pathology may be suspected.

Table 4.11 Values of cardiovascular autonomic function

	R/R interval ratio on ECG	
	Normal	Abnormal
Para-sympathetic tests		
Valsalva manoeuvre	> 1.21	< 1.10
Deep breathing response	> 15 beats min	< 10 beats min
Standing up (30:15 ratio)	> 1.04	< 1.0
Sympathetic tests	*mmHg*	
Blood pressure response to standing (mmHg fall in systolic)	< 10	> 30
BP response to sustained handgrip (mmHg rise in diastolic)	> 16	< 10

Neuropathic pain eventually improves after many months. Sometimes intensified diabetic control may help and there are reports of help from antidepressants and/or phenothiazines. Phenytoin and carbamazepine have also been used with some success. In addition to painful neuropathy, the entrapment neuropathies, e.g. carpal tunnel syndrome are more common in diabetic patients.

The aetiology of neuropathy is unclear. There is evidence for small vessel disease (thickening of the capillary basement membrane leading to capillary occlusion) in peripheral nerves, but its relation to blood glucose levels is unknown. Possible biochemical causes of diabetic neuropathy include protein glycosylation, decreased myo-inositol levels which normally play a critical role in phospholipid synthesis to form myelin, and thirdly an increase in sorbitol (through the activity of the enzyme, aldose reductase) which accompanies high glucose levels. No therapeutic agent has been convincingly shown to be beneficial in diabetic neuropathy, though aldose-reductase inhibitors (currently under clinical evaluation) by diminishing levels of sorbitol, have led to an improvement in nerve conduction in some studies but not in others.

Diabetic nephropathy

Renal failure is a major cause of death in diabetics under the age of 30. The incidence of diabetic nephropathy is related to the duration of diabetes with two peaks being observed, the first at 15 years and a smaller peak occurring 30 years after diagnosis.

The earliest functional change in kidneys of diabetic patients is a raised glomerular filtration rate (GFR). This is followed by renal hypertrophy and this stage is accompanied by intermittent microalbuminuria. This amount of albumin is not detected by conventional 'Albustix' testing and requires radioimmunoassay for its detection. However recently dip-stick tests have been developed. Both this and the raised GFR can be reversed by strict glycaemic control. Once 'Albustix'-positive albuminuria develops, improved glycaemic control does not delay deterioration.

The characteristic lesion is nodular glomerular sclerosis first described by Kimmelstiel and Wilson. Electron micrographs show increased deposition of hyaline material which progresses to nodule formation. Diffuse glomerular sclerosis is a second but less specific finding and is due to generalized basement membrane thickening. Subintimal hyaline thickening of the arterioles is widespread in the diabetic kidney and often involves the efferent as well as the afferent arterioles.

Testing of urine samples for proteinuria and in the future, microalbuminuria, should be routine clinical practice. Furthermore, blood pressure must be regularly checked since it has been shown that high BP enhances the development of diabetic nephropathy and that early aggressive antihypertensive treatment reduces the rate of decline in GFR. There is current interest in dietary protein restriction which, in diabetics with elevated urinary albumin excretion, has resulted in both a reduction in GFR and in microalbuminaria. In addition there is particular interest in the role of angiotensin-converting enzyme inhibitors in the treatment of the diabetic hypertensive. Once creatinine values have reached levels of 700–800 mmol/litre, long-term continuous ambulatory peritoneal dialysis, haemodialysis or renal transplantation becomes necessary.

Diabetic retinopathy

Diabetic retinopathy is the commonest long-term complication of diabetes and the commonest cause of blindness in adults between the ages of 30 and 65 years of age in the UK. Table 4.12 lists the retinal abnormalities characteristic of diabetic retinopathy.

The duration of diabetes and suboptimum glycaemic control are the two main risk factors associated with the development of retinopathy and therefore every effort is made to ensure normoglycaemia in the diabetic. Background retinopathy is not associated with any visual impairment and no specific treatment is indicated.

Table 4.12 Classification of diabetic retinopathy

'Background'	Retinal vein dilation
	Microaneurysms
	Haemorrhages ('dot', 'blot')
	Hard exudates
Maculopathy	Circinate maculopathy
	Macular oedema
Preproliferative retinopathy	Venous beading
	Venous reduplication
	Soft exudates ('cottonwool spots')
Proliferative retinopathy	New vessel formation
	Fibrous proliferation
	Vitreous haemorrhage

The reversibility of early diabetic retinopathy with tightened diabetic control has been the subject of recent controversy. Various anecdotal reports have described the disappearance of retinal abnormalities with improved control but three major controlled studies utilizing CSii have disappointingly shown transient deterioration with the development of cottonwool spots in the initial phase of therapy. In the longer run however CSii leads to slower deterioration of retinopathy. It is thought that impaired retinal perfusion secondary to diminished nutrient substrate during improved control may be responsible for transient deterioration. It has been suggested that 're-entry' to normoglycaemia should be a gradual process.

Maculopathy, preproliferative and proliferative retinopathy can be successfully managed with retinal photocoagulation (xenon arc or argon laser) which destroys areas of retinal ischaemia, reduces oedema and obliterates new vessels directly. The rationale for this ablation therapy is the reduction of growth factor production by the ischaemic retina which has angiogenic properties. Diabetic retinopathy is symptomless until well-advanced and therefore all diabetics must have regular visual acuity checks, and ophthalmosocopic examination (using a mydriatic). IDDs should be checked every 5 years for the first 10 years, then yearly thereafter, whereas NIDDs are best checked yearly. If new vessels, preproliferative changes or macular oedema are visualized, prompt referral to the ophthalmologist is mandatory.

Diabetes and atherosclerosis

Diabetes mellitus is a risk factor for both an excess incidence of and mortality from coronary, cerebrovascular and peripheral vascular disease. Thus, a diabetic has twice the risk of myocardial infarction than a non-diabetic. The atheroma itself is not distinct from that of the non-diabetic but is more extensive and develops at an earlier age.

Possible explanations for the increased risk of atheroma include hypertension, abnormal lipid and lipoprotein metabolism, abnormal blood rheology and coagulation. Hypertriglyceridaemia is particularly common in diabetics and high density lipoproteins are generally low in NIDDM but normal or raised in IDDM. Red cell deformability is diminished in diabetics whereas platelet aggregability, mean platelet volume nad platelet diameter are increased. Furthermore various coagulation factors are higher and fibrolytic factors lower in diabetes. All these observations are consistent with the hypothesis that they might play a role in the pathogenesis of the vascular complications in diabetes.

Diabetes and pregnancy

The last decade has seen an overall downward trend in obstetric mortality and morbidity associated with diabetes with perinatal mortality figures in the better centres approaching those found in the general population. The complications (Table 4.13) associated with diabetic pregnancy are related to poor glycaemic control and therefore emphasis has been placed on maintaining normoglycaemia both before conception and during pregnancy. Fasting plasma glucose concentrations should be kept between 3.3 and 5.5. mmol/litre with postprandial levels below 8 mmol/litre throughout the pregnancy. Strict antenatal care is required preferably in a joint diabetic/obstetric clinic together with at least twice daily injections of short and medium acting insulins. Hospitalization in the late third trimester is no longer mandatory with adequate home monitoring of blood glucose levels. In most centres, unless obstetric considerations dictate otherwise, pregnant diabetic women are allowed to go to term and hopefully normal spontaneous vaginal delivery.

Strict diabetic control, with hourly checks on maternal blood glucose is important in *labour*. A 5 % dextrose infusion is recommended at a rate of 500 ml 4-hourly. Insulin can be administered intravenously by a motorized syringe pump at a variable rate starting at 1 unit hourly; alternatively 4 units of soluble/neutral insulin can be placed in a bag of dextrose. After the first hour the following strategy is then recommended:

- If blood glucose is less than 5.0 mmol/litre reduce insulin to 2 units/500 ml by changing the bag.
- If blood glucose is between 5–10 mmol/litre continue same regimen.
- If blood glucose is greater than 10 mmol/litre increase insulin to 8 units/500 ml by changing the bag.

Using these methods, it is easy to prevent starvation ketosis whilst maintaining an empty stomach so that general anaesthesia can be given should an emergency Caesarian section be necessary. After delivery, maternal insulin requirements drop dramatically and the insulin dose should be reduced appropriately.

Diabetes may be diagnosed for the first time during pregnancy, but if it remits after delivery, then it may be called gestational diabetes. It is usually asymptomatic and therefore detected by routine screening for glycosuria usually between 28 and 32 weeks of gestation. The diagnosis needs to be confirmed on oral glucose tolerance testing as the renal threshold for glucose absorption falls in pregnancy especially in the third trimester. In obstetric clinics in the USA, the overall incidence varies between 1.5 and 2.5 per cent. Gestational diabetes causes fetal problems similar to those seen in insulin-dependent diabetics. Fetal macrosomia and neonatal hypoglycaemia are the most significant but can be prevented by appropriate management which may involve insulin treatment to keep preprandial blood glucose values below 5.5 mmol/litre.

Care of the diabetic patient undergoing surgery

The risks of surgical procedures are greater for diabetics than non-diabetics. Of equal importance to preoperative metabolic control are the effects of diabetic complications. The increased incidence of atheroma increases the risk of coronary thrombosis during surgery but perhaps more important is the potentially dangerous but often asymptomatic autonomic neuropathy which has been associated with cardiorespiratory arrest and cardiac arrhythmias. Postoperatively there is also a substantial morbidity because of sepsis secondary to impaired neutrophil function and poor wound

Table 4.13 Complications of diabetic pregnancy

Fetal	Maternal
Large for dates	Hydramnios
Macrosomy	Hypoglycaemia
Congenital malformation	(especially 1st
(sacral dysgenesis)	trimester)
CNS/Cardiovascular	Ketoacidosis (especially
abnormalities	2nd trimester)
Intrauterine thrombosis	Pre-eclampsia
Hyperinsulinaemia	Premature labour
Neonatal	Increased placental size
– hypoglycaemia	
– respiratory distress	
– hypocalcaemia	
– hypomagnesaemia	
– jaundice	

healing due to vascular diseases, neuropathy and impaired protein synthesis.

The metabolic changes associated with surgery are due to a combination of stress and starvation. High concentrations of the anti-insulin hormones (cortisol, catecholamines, glucagon and growth hormone) are found and, together with partial insulin resistance during surgery, result in hyperglycaemia, negative nitrogen balance and an increased metabolic rate. Furthermore, lactate and pyruvate levels, as well as ketone bodies increase, though less so than in starvation. The extent of these changes depend on the length of the operation, and the presence or absence of sepsis or shock.

In order to achieve as near normal metabolic control as possible planning is necessary. The most important point to consider is whether the diabetic has any of the potentially hazardous complications. Besides a full clinical history and examination, the following should also be available in every longstanding diabetic going to theatre.

Urinalysis for protein.
Blood urea, electrolytes and creatinine estimation.
ECG (with continuous recording to about 40 beats after standing to calculate the 30:15 ratio, i.e. the R-R interval at the 30th and 15th beat after standing).

A ratio of less than 1.03 indicates borderline or definite autonomic neuropathy and thus not only is monitoring of the cardiovascular parameters essential during surgery, but their display or recording should be carefully scrutinized.

Guidelines to management

Non-insulin dependent diabetics

Diet controlled

if blood glucose is less than 10 mmol/litre, manage as non-diabetic

if blood glucose is more than 10 mmol/litre, add insulin as discussed below

Tablet controlled

stop all tablets on day of operation

if blood glucose less than 4 mmol/litre, give i.v. 500 ml 5 % dextrose over 4 hours

if blood glucose 4–10 mmol/litre, treat as non-diabetic

if blood glucose more than 10 mmol/litre for

lengthy operations, add insulin as discussed below

start i.v. glucose if oral feeding is likely to be delayed for more than 6 hours

Insulin-dependent diabetes

- Admit patient 1–2 days before surgery and substitute long-acting insulin with 2 or 3 times daily short and medium-acting insulin.
- Reduce evening preoperative intermediate-acting insulin by 20–30 per cent.
- Day of operation

Minor surgery Set up 5 % dextrose drip 500 ml to run in over 4 hours. If blood glucose is more than 10 mmol/litre, add 8 units of neutral/soluble insulin to the *bag*. If blood glucose is less than 10 mmol/litre add 4 units of insulin (no insulin if less than 4.0 mmol/litre). If surgery is later in the day, give patient normal dose of short acting insulin and a light breakfast. Monitor blood glucose 2 hourly and set up dextrose drip as above before the operation. In both cases, the dextrose infusion is continued until normal eating is resumed.

Major surgery Various regimens have been described. A common technique is to add insulin to a 5 or 10 % dextrose solution but disadvantages include adsorption of insulin to the plastic material and the inability to allow finer adjustments. Alternatively insulin is infused separately with the aid of a syringe pump or paediatric burette which is attached by a small volume-connecting tube to the same cannula used for the dextrose infusion. This technique allows precise and immediate changes and adsorption loss is clinically insignificant. A constant rate infusion device (e.g. IVAC drip monitor) is necessary however and requires constant supervision. The initial insulin infusion rate is usually 2 units hourly (using soluble

Table 4.14 Suggested rates of insulin infusion (with simultaneous 10 % dextrose/KCl infusion)

	B Sugar (mmol/litre)	Insulin dose rate (units/hr)
Initially	–	2
After 2 hours	< 5	1
	5–10	2
	10–20	3
	> 20	4

insulin) and the infusion fluid should be 500 ml of 10 % dextrose with 10–20 ml potassium chloride run in over 6 hours. Subsequently, blood glucose levels are checked 2 hourly and insulin infusion rates and blood glucose levels plotted against time. The insulin dose rate is adjusted as suggested in the Table 4.14. Blood glucose should be kept between 6.0 and 10.0 mmol/litre. The infusion is continued until oral feeding resumes.

The following points should also be borne in mind for all diabetics:

- Blood glucose can be monitored using BM or Glucostix test strips, or preferably, with a reflectance meter.
- If possible, put diabetic patients first on the morning list.
- The physician normally caring for diabetics should always be informed and their care shared.
- If there is sepsis, or corticosteroids are being administered insulin requirements are markedly increased.

Emergency surgery

Management in situations requiring emergency surgery is virtually identical to that discussed above though severe hyperglycaemia and/or severe keto-acidosis (pH < 7.1, plasma HCO_3 < 12 mmol/litre) should be treated first because mortality is high. In older patients, adequate hydration preoperatively is also essential.

An important potential trap is the 'acute abdomen' that often accompanies diabetic ketoacidosis, or the high leucocyte count (often exceeding 20×10^9/litre) seen with moderate or severe acidosis which is of no diagnostic value, and like the abdominal pain soon resolves with appropriate medical treatment.

The pituitary and hypothalamus

The pituitary gland (weight $\approx$ 0.5–1.0 g) lies in a bony fossa in the sphenoid bone called the sella turcica (the pituitary fossa). The gland has two parts which have different embryological origins and different functions. The anterior pituitary or adenohypophysis is formed from an upgrowth of the primitive pharynx known as Rathke's pouch whereas the posterior pituitary or neurohypophysis is of neural origin. Important anatomical relations of the pituitary which may be affected by an enlarging gland include the optic chiasma which lies above and in front, the hypothalamus and third ventricle above and the cavernous sinuses which lie above and laterally.

The adenohypophysis

The adenohypophysis synthesizes and secretes hormones which act on other target endocrine glands, follicle stimulating hormone (FSH), luteinizing hormone (LH), thyroid stimulating hormone (TSH), adrenocorticotrophic hormone (ACTH) and hormones which act on target tissues, growth hormone (GH) and prolactin. Pituitary hormone secretion is in turn controlled by hypothalamic hormones (either stimulatory or inhibitory) reaching the pituitary through the connecting portal blood system. The hypothalamus itself is responsive to a wide variety of humoral, metabolic, physical and nervous stimuli. *Adrenocorticotrophic hormone* (ACTH) Adrenocorticotrophic hormone is a polypeptide hormone consisting of a single chain of 39 amino acid residues. It is the N terminal part of the molecule (18 amino acids) which is responsible for biological activity. ACTH is produced, together with a related peptide, β-lipotrophin by enzymatic cleavage of a precursor carbohydrate containing molecule, the prohormone pro-opiocortin. Further enzymatic cleavage of ACTH may occur producing corticotrophin-like peptide (CLIP) and a melanocyte stimulating hormone (αMSH). The biological relevance of these substances remains to be determined. β-lipotrophin contains the amino acid sequences of the endorphins and encephalins These opioid peptides (they are also found in brain and are synthesized in neurones) comprise a distinct peptidergic system related to the perception of pain – the endogenous morphine-like agents.

The synthesis and release of ACTH from the anterior pituitary is stimulated by the hypothalamic hormone corticotrophin-releasing factor (CRF). This determines the striking circadian rhythm of ACTH being highest around 8 a.m. and lowest at midnight. This rhythm may be overcome by 'stress' such as fever, hypoglycaemia and trauma. ACTH binds to receptors on adrenocortical cells of the zona reticularis and zona fasicularis and stimulates glucocorticoid and androgen production. ACTH secretion is under negative feedback control by cortisol principally at the hypothalamus.

Thyroid stimulating hormone (TSH)

Thyroid stimulating hormone, a glycopeptide hormone, is the main regulator of thyroid hormone production in the thyroid gland. Its secretion is stimulated by the tripeptide thyrotrophin-releasing hormone (TRH) from the hypothalamus.

TSH is under negative feedback control by the thyroid hormones thyroxine and tri-iodothyronine. TSH binds to a specific receptor on the cell membrane of thyroid cells leading to activation of the adenylate cyclase system and increased levels of cyclic AMP. This then mediates the effects of TSH by interaction with protein kinases which phosphorylate key enzymes in thyroid hormone synthesis.

Prolactin

Prolactin is a peptide hormone comprising 198 amino acid residues (MW $\approx$ 26 000) which is principally involved with the development of the mammary duct system and lactation. Its secretion is under a dominant inhibitory control by dopamine which is synthesized in the hypothalamus and secreted into the hypothalamo pituitary portal system. Secretion is highest at night after the onset of sleep while levels fall during the morning. In pregnancy there is a slow increase in prolactin levels and postpartum the most powerful stimulus to secretion is stimulation of the breast and nipple. Prolactin is increased by stress as well as physical exercise, hypoglycaemia and coitus. Prolactin secretion is stimulated by the injection of TRH although it is unlikely that TRH plays a physiological role in prolactin secretion.

Growth hormone

Growth hormone is a polypeptide hormone with two disulphide bridges of 191 amino acid residues (MW $\approx$ 22 000). It is of interest that there is considerable structural hormology between growth hormone and prolactin. The hormone is secreted in short bursts especially in the first half of the night and during the day levels are low. The regulation of its secretion is complex but is probably modulated by a growth hormone release inhibiting hormone (somatostatin) and more importantly the recently discovered growth hormone releasing factor. In addition growth hormone release is enhanced by dopamine in normal man and α-noradrenergic

pathways via noradrenaline also enhance release in response to hypoglycaemia, glucagon and arginine vasopressin. Growth hormone has a wide spectrum of metabolic effects related to growth. These effects may be direct or indirect through large molecular weight polypeptide mediators called somatomedins or insulin-like growth factors. Somatomedins are produced in the liver in response to the action of growth hormone and have an anabolic action on muscle and fat and promote growth by enhancing cell multiplication.

Gonadotrophins

The gonadotrophins, luteinizing hormone (LH) and follicle-stimulating hormone (FSH) are produced from the same cells of the adenohypophysis. They are glycopeptides with two chains, α and β. In males LH acts on the Leydig cells of the testes stimulating testosterone secretion and FSH stimulates the development of seminiferous tubules as the major inducer of spermatogenesis. In women ovulation is stimulated by LH, the ovarian synthesis of oestrogen and progesterone is increased and the corpus luteum maintained. FSH as its name suggests stimulates follicular development in the ovary.

Gonadotrophin synthesis and secretion is stimulated by the hormone gonadotrophin releasing hormone (LHRH) a decapeptide synthesized in the hypothalamus. Feedback control of gonadotrophin secretion by gonadal hormones is complex and in women there is both positive and negative feedback by oestradiol. In men there is a negative feedback of testosterone on gonadotrophin secretion and in addition further control is exerted by inhibin, a substance produced in the seminiferous tubules.

The neurohypophysis

The neurohypophysis is composed of nerve cells and fibres, the nerve fibres arising from the supraoptic and paraventricular nuclei of the hypothalamus. The hormones vasopressin (antidiuretic hormone) and oxytocin are produced in the cells of these hypothalamic nuclei and reach the neurohypophysis where they are stored and released via connecting nerve fibres of the pituitary stalk.

Vasopressin

This cyclic octapeptide (MW $\approx$ 1000) acts on the renal collecting tubules, increasing permeability to water and so reducing urine volume. The hormone acts through the adenylate cyclase enzyme increasing cyclic AMP levels. It also has an effect on blood vessels and may be involved in the control of hypertension and in the clotting mechanism. It has a very short plasma half-life (approximately 5 minutes) as it exists entirely in free form (unlike most hormones) and is rapidly cleared from the circulation. Vasopressin secretion is controlled by hypothalamic osmoreceptors sensitive to changes in plasma osmolality which is normally tightly controlled (280–290 mosmol/kg). Secretion is also increased by a reduction in plasma volume, emotional factors, stress, pain, exercise and trauma (e.g. surgery). Drugs such as morphine and nicotine also stimulate vasopressin secretion.

Oxytocin

The actions of this hormone which differs from vasopressin by just two amino acids are confined mainly to the breast and uterus during parturition and lactation in animals. The role of this hormone in man remains to be fully determined.

Pituitary tumours

Pituitary tumours account for about 10 per cent of all clinically detectable intracranial neoplasms. They are almost always benign and can either be classified according to their staining characteristics (chromophobe, basophil or acidophil adenomas) or more usefully by their granular content or immunohistochemistry detailing the particular hormone content. Chromophobe adenomas are the most common and tend to be the largest. They can be functionless although hormones are secreted sometimes. Prolactin is the most common hormone secreted whilst growth hormone and ACTH are secreted occasionally. Acidophil adenomas are usually associated with hyperprolactinaemia and with growth hormone excess leading to acromegaly. Basophil tumours are the rarest and usually produce excess ACTH and Cushing's disease. Adenomas producing gonadotrophic hormones or TSH are very rare. Occasionally tumours arise from Rathke's pouch remnants giving rise to a craniopharyngioma. These tumours can be solid or cystic and commonly occur in children.

Clinical features of pituitary tumours

A pituitary tumour may manifest itself by space occupying effects, hypersecretion of a particular hormone or hypopituitarism. In addition it is not uncommon for an enlarged pituitary fossa to be detected incidentally.

Space occupying effects

An enlarging adenoma of the pituitary gland leads to expansion of the pituitary fossa which can be seen on a lateral skull X-ray. Within the fossa, destruction of other secretory cells can occur leading to hypopituitarism. Because of the close vicinity of the optic chiasma (above and in front) visual disturbances are a typical feature of tumours which enlarge and extend upwards out of the fossa (suprasellar extention). Classically upper temporal quadrant field defects occur first because of pressure on the lower fibres of the chiasma. This progresses to bitemporal hemianopia and optic atrophy. More pronounced upward extensions of the tumour may lead to hypothalamic damage with diabetes insipidus, hyperphagia and disturbances of sleep and temperature regulation. Headaches are common and hydrocephalus may occur due to compression of the third ventricle. Sometimes the tumour extends laterally into the cavernous sinus producing paralysis of the cranial nerves supplying the external ocular muscles. With further extension temporal lobe epilepsy may occur. Extension of the tumour downwards into the sphenoid may cause CSF rhinorrhoea.

Hypopituitarism

This is the clinical condition resulting from partial or total pituitary hormone deficiency by an enlarging pituitary tumour. Other pituitary and parasellar lesions may also cause hypopituitarism, e.g. craniopharyngioma and sphenoidal-ridge meningiomas (Table 4.15). Hypotension following postpartum haemorrhage can cause hypopituitarism with failure of lactation (Sheehan's syndrome). With an expanding pituitary tumour there tends to be a progressive loss of function with growth hormone and LH secretion being the first to be affected. Later the secretion of FSH, ACTH and TSH are affected. Prolactin deficiency (except in Sheehan's syndrome) and diabetes insipidus due to either posterior pituitary involvement or damage to the hypothalamus or connecting neurones are uncommon.

The clinical presentation will depend on the pattern of hormone loss. Loss of normal ACTH secretion results in secondary hypoadrenalism with similar symptoms to patients with Addison's

Table 4.15 Causes of hypopituitarism

Tumours	Pituitary adenomas
	Craniopharyngiomas
	Secondary deposits
	Parasellar tumours
	meningioma
	Optic nerve glioma
Ischaemia	Sheehan's syndrome
	(postpartum necrosis)
	Pituitary apoplexy
	Arteritis
	Sickle cell disease
	Diabetes mellitus
	Aneurysm of internal carotid
	artery
Iatrogenic	Posthypophysectomy
	Radiotherapy
Infectious disease	Meningitis/encephalitis
	Malaria
	Tuberculosis
	Syphilis
Granuloma	Sarcoidosis
	Histiocytosis
Hypothalamic disease	Tumours
	Trauma
	Idiopathic (isolated releasing
	factor deficiencies)
	Malnutrition (gonadotrophin
	deficiency)
	Histiocytosis
	Granulomatous disease

disease (*see* p. 147). However because ACTH levels are low (instead of high as in primary adrenal failure) skin pallor is a feature rather than hyperpigmentation. Gonadotrophin deficiency produces secondary gonadal failure with amenorrhoea, genital atrophy, reduced body hair, decreased breast mass and loss of libido in women. Men also show loss of body hair together with impotence, loss of libido, azoospermia and decreased testicular size. Typical skin changes are seen in both sexes with fine wrinkling especially around the eyes.

TSH deficiency leads to secondary hypothyroidism with symptoms similar to those of primary hypothyroidism (*see* p. 136). Growth hormone deficiency is not a problem in adults but leads to short stature in children.

Isolated hypothalamic/pituitary hormone deficiency

Isolated deficiencies of secretion of various anterior pituitary hormones can occur secondary to absence of the appropriate hypothalamic releasing factor. The commonest of these is growth hormone deficiency leading to impairment of linear growth and bone maturation in children. Mental development is normal but the growth rate is abnormally slow (less than 3 cm/year) after the age of 3 years leading to a short child but with normal body proportions. In addition the child is often plump with immature facies, poor muscular development and delayed dentition. The diagnosis is confirmed by growth hormone stimulation tests and it is necessary to exclude other hormonal deficiencies as occasionally these are multiple. Other causes of short stature need to be excluded (Table 4.16). The other endocrine causes of short stature are hypothyroidism, congenital adrenal hypoplasia, Cushing's syndrome, emotional

Table 4.16 Causes of short stature

Familial	
Emotional deprivation	
Endocrine disorders	Hypothyroidism
	Cushing's syndrome
	Pituitary dwarfism
	Congenital adrenal
	hyperplasia
	Sexual precocity
Disease of major	Chronic infections
organs	Heart, pulmonary, renal,
	hepatic and CNS
	disease
	Anaemias
Metabolic diseases	Glycogen storage
	diseases
	Mucopolysaccharidoses
	Galactosaemia
	Fructose intolerance
	Cystinosis
Chromosomal	Trisomy 21
abnormalities	Turner's syndrome
	Gonadal disgenesis
Skeletal diseases	Vitamin D resistant
	rickets
	Achondroplasia
	Hypophosphataemia
	Osteogenesis imperfecta
Malnutrition	Malabsorption states
	Starvation
Low birth weight	Abnormal pregnancy
	Prematurity
	Chromosomal
	abnormalities
	Infections
	Congential abnormalities

deprivation and sexual precocity. However the majority of cases of short stature do not have endocrine causes. Juvenile hypothyroidism leads to retardation of growth with infantile body proportions, immature naso-orbital configuration, delayed bone age and dental development. Neonatal hypothyroidism leads to cretinism and mental retardation. Screening of neonates has been introduced using TSH measurements to detect the condition at an early stage. The high cortisol levels seen in children with Cushing's syndrome affect the release and peripheral action of growth hormone with consequent effects on growth. Congenital adrenal hyperplasia and sexual precocity are associated with initial acceleration of growth but premature fusion of epiphyses occurs with ultimate reduction in height. Emotional deprivation is an important cause of shortness of stature probably secondary to hypothalamic dysfunction.

Absence of the hypothalamic releasing hormone LHRH leads to failure of LH and FSH secretion by the anterior pituitary. These patients with hypogonadotrophic hypogonadism present with delayed puberty. Sometimes this condition is associated with anosmia (Kallman's syndrome) or congenital orofacial abnormalities such as cleft palate, craniofacial asymmetry or hare lip.

Diseases associated with hypersecretion of pituitary hormones

Cushing's disease due to hypersecretion of ACTH from a basophilic-staining adenoma of the pituitary is dealt with on p. 142 in the section on Cushing's syndrome. Pituitary adenomas secreting TSH and gonadotrophins do occur but are rare.

Prolactinoma

This is the commonest of the secretory tumours. However hyperprolactinaemia of lesser degree may be seen in association with other tumours if they interfere with the prolactin inhibiting factor dopamine reaching prolactin secretory cells. A prolactin-secreting adenoma also has to be differentiated from other causes of hyperprolactinaemia (Table 4.17). The clinical features (Table 4.18) are related to the enlarging adenoma and the effects of prolactin excess. In women the condition generally presents at an early stage because of amenorrhoea and commonly the adenoma is confined to the pituitary fossa (a microadenoma). Men tend to present late, often with signs of an expanding pituitary tumour.

Diagnosis of prolactinoma is made by the demonstration of hyperprolactinaemia together with the appropriate imaging techniques. The latest generation of CT scanning machines together with contrast enhancement allow good visualization of the pituitary substance and can identify very small tumours. The recently introduced MRI scanning also gives high definition views of the pituitary gland. However in some cases a presumed diagnosis of prolactinoma has to be made where other causes of hyperprolactinaemia have been excluded but even with the latest imaging techniques no lesion is demonstrable in the pituitary. Dynamic function tests have been advocated in this situation where prolactin secretion is stimulated by TRH injection, insulin hypoglycaemia or the dopamine antagonist metoclopramide. Where there is autonomous production of prolactin an impaired prolactin response would be expected. However such testing does not make a clear distinction.

Table 4.17   Causes of hyperprolactinaemia

Physiological	Pregnancy
	Suckling
Stress	
Pituitary prolactinoma	
Pituitary stalk damage	Head injury
	Surgery
	Tumour
Hypothyroidism	
Renal failure	
Drugs	Dopamine antagonists (phenothiazines, metoclopramide, butyrophenones)
	Dopamine depleting agents (reserpine, methyldopa)
	Oestrogens
Polycystic ovarian disease	

Table 4.18   Clinical features of prolactinoma

Infertility
Amenorrhoea
Galactorrhoea
Impotence
Loss of libido
Gynaecomastia
Headaches
Visual disturbance

Prolactinomas are of special interest because not only may the associated hyperprolactinaemia be controlled with medical therapy but in the vast majority of cases there is actual tumour shrinkage with medical therapy. The dopamine-agonist bromocriptine is the treatment of choice. The drug is started at a very low dose (1.25 mg) with food at bedtime to minimize side-effects. The dose is gradually increased over weeks to 2.5 mg t.d.s. with meals. In small adenomas this dose is often sufficient to fully suppress the hyperprolactin-aemia and to restore normal menstrual function and fertility. Even large prolactinomas with suprasellar extension respond to bromocriptine which is tried even in the presence of visual impairment. If in the rare case there is no response then surgical decompression is required which is often possible by the transphenoidal or trans-ethmoidal route with postoperative bromocriptine therapy. Small prolactinomas may be cured with bromocriptine therapy alone, the drug being withdrawn after 2–3 years. With the larger adenomas, bromocriptine is used in the first instance to control symptoms and reduce the size of the tumour such that more definitive therapy such as transphenoidal adenectomy or radiotherapy may be undertaken. An important point to remember is that the tumour shrinkage effect of bromocriptine is related to reduction in individual cell size secondary to a reduction in the cell's protein (i.e. prolactin) synthesizing capacity. If bromocriptine is stopped there may be a rapid re-expansion of the tumour mass. Prolactin secreting tumours may expand during pregnancy and women previously treated with bromocriptine who become pregnant need careful monitoring during the pregnancy. Although there do not appear to be any teratogenic effects secondary to bromocriptine most physicians recommend stopping bromocrip-tine when pregnancy ensues. Side-effects of bro-mocriptine include nausea, vomiting and postural hypotension. Nasal stuffiness may be trouble-some. In some centres the preferred treatment of microadenomas is selective adenectomy with preservation of the normal part of the pituitary gland.

Acromegaly

Acromegaly is the clinical condition that results from excessive growth hormone secretion over many years. If hypersecretion occurs in adolescence before epiphyseal fusion gigantism

Table 4.19 Clinical features of acromegaly

Related to pituitary tumour
  Visual field defects
  Headaches
  Cranial nerve palsies
  Hypopituitarism
Related to excess GH secretion
  Coarse facial features
  Overgrowth of hands and feet
  Prognathism
  Increased interdental separation
  Macroglossia
  Enlarged supra-orbital ridges and zygomatic
    bones
  Increased sweating
  Thickened greasy skin
  Hirsuties
  Deep resonant voice due to cartilaginous
    proliferation of the larynx
  Carpal tunnel syndrome
  Hypertension
  Cardiomyopathy
  Arthritis
  Secondary amenorrhoea
  Impaired glucose tolerance
  Hyperprolactinaemia
  Hypercalciuria
  Goitre

results. The majority of cases of acromegaly are secondary to a pituitary adenoma (usually acidophil staining) but rarely, pulmonary or pancreatic carcinoid tumours secrete growth hormone. It is an uncommon condition affecting both sexes equally and is sometimes part of the multiple endocrine neoplasia syndrome. In a third of patients the adenoma also produces an excess of prolactin.

The clinical features of acromegaly (Table 4.19) are related to local effects of the pituitary tumour or result from the metabolic effects of excess growth hormone. There is considerable morbidity and mortality from cardiovascular disease partly explained by the frequently observed hypertension and diabetes. A specific cardiomyopathy may occur in acromegaly but is very rare.

The diagnosis of acromegaly is usually made on the clinical appearance. However, because of the slow development of the characteristic features the diagnosis tends to be made late. If past photographs of the patient are studied it is not uncommon to detect the first signs as long as 15 years before the actual diagnosis was made. For this reason the pituitary fossa is expanded in about ninety per cent of acromegalics at diagnosis. Growth hormone levels are elevated which are not suppressed during a glucose tolerance test. Somatomedin C levels are more closely correlated with disease activity.

Acromegaly is generally treated with a combination of pituitary surgery and radiotherapy. Bromocriptine is effective in a minority of patients with reduction of growth hormone levels and improvement of glucose tolerance. However, reduction in tumour mass is only observed when there is concomitant prolactin secretion. A recent therapeutic innovation under clinical trial is the use of somatostatin analogues. Currently these have to be given by injection which limits their usefulness. There have been occasional reports of tumour shrinkage with these agents.

The acromegalic due to undergo surgery requires careful assessment. Hypertension and diabetes mellitus need to be adequately controlled. The enlarged tongue and pharynx, soft tissue swelling of the pharynx and thickening of the vocal cords may pose problems with intubation. A long-bladed laryngoscope and a long endotracheal tube may be necessary. Preoperative treatment with the somatostatin analogues has been advocated to reduce the soft tissue overgrowth.

Diabetes insipidus

This condition results from failure of vasopressin (anti-diuretic hormone, ADH) secretion due to hypothalamic or pituitary damage (cranial diabetes insipidus). It may also be caused by resistance of the renal tubules to the hormone (nephrogenic diabetes insipidus) (Table 4.20). Cranial disease is idiopathic in about a third of cases. Diabetes insipidus may be transient if due to trauma of the hypothalamus or pituitary (e.g. after pituitary surgery). In patients with associated anterior pituitary failure and secondary adrenocortical insufficiency the symptoms of diabetes insipidus may be masked until corticosteroid replacement has been commenced as steroids have a permissive effect on water excretion.

The major symptoms are polyuria and polydipsia. The onset and severity vary considerably but severe cases may lead to dehydration, exhaustion and coma. Other causes of polyuria such as diabetes mellitus, chronic renal failure, hypercalcaemia, hypokalaemia and psychogenic polydipsia have to be excluded. The diagnosis is likely if the plasma osmolality is above

Table 4.20 Causes of diabetes insipidus

Deficiency of vasopressin acquired	Head injury
	Idiopathic
	Neurosurgery
	Tumours (craniopharyngioma, pituitary adenoma, glioma, meningioma)
	Metastatic deposits
	Granulomatous deposits (histiocytosis, sarcoidosis)
	Infections (meningitis, encephalitis, syphilis)
	Vascular (Sheehan's, sickle cell anaemia, aneurysms)
Familial (autosomal dominant)	Pyelonephritis
Insensitivity to vasopressin acquired	Polycystic renal disease
	Hypokalaemia
	Hypercalcaemia
	Drugs (lithium, demeclocycline)
	Amyloid
	Post-obstruction
	Sickle cell disease
	Sarcoid
Familial	X-linked recessive

300 mosmol/kg in the presence of an unconcentrated urine (osmolality of less than 279 mosmol/kg). In difficult cases the water deprivation test is a useful diagnostic procedure. Fluids are withheld (for 8 hours) and urine and plasma osmolality checked hourly. In the normal subject plasma osmolality shows little change but the urine osmolality, should rise above 600 mosmol/kg. If the patient fails to concentrate the urine during the test, vasopressin is administered; in cranial diabetes insipidus but not in nephrogenic disease the urine will concentrate. This needs to be very carefully monitored.

The treatment of choice is the long-acting vasopressin analogue – desmopressin (1-desamino-8-D-arginine vasopressin, DDAVP). This is usually administered intranasally in a dose of 10–40 μg daily. Lysine vasopressin is also available but it has a short duration of action. Parenteral DDAVP is available for postoperative patients and diabetes insipidus can be controlled with a dose of 1–2 μg daily given intramuscularly.

Inappropriate antidiuresis

The syndrome of inappropriate antidiuresis with water retention may occur in a variety of medical conditions (Table 4.21) and can be secondary to certain drugs. The pathogenesis of this condition is not fully understood. There may be ectopic ADH secretion or a failure of normal suppression of ADH secretion in response to a reduction in plasma osmolality. Drugs exert their effects by either stimulating ADH secretion (e.g. vincristine, clofibrate) or increasing renal ADH sensitivity (chlorpropamide, carbamazepine). Often the condition is asymptomatic but confusion, irritability and nausea occur as the plasma sodium concentration falls to about 120 mmol/litre and there is a danger of seizures and coma if the concentration falls lower still. Fluid restriction (0.5–1.0 litre/24 hours) together with attention to the underlying cause is generally very effective treatment. If there is severe hyponatraemia it may be necessary to infuse hypertonic saline in the short term. Occasionally demeclocycline (a tetracycline) is given which impairs renal tubular response to ADH.

Table 4.21   Causes of inappropriate antidiuresis

Trauma	
Tumours	Carcinoma (bronchus, duodenum, pancreas)
	Lymphoma
	Thymoma
	Bronchial carcinoid
CNS disorders	Meningitis
	Encephalitis
	Subarachnoid haemorrhage
	Guillain–Barré syndrome
	Acute intermittent porphyria
	Brain abscess
	Acute psychosis
	Tumours
Drugs	Nicotine
	Thiazides
	Chlorpropamide
	Carbamazepine
	Vincristine
	Cyclophosphamide
	Phenothiazines
	Tricyclic antidepressants
	Clofibrate
Endocrine	Hypothyroidism
	Glucocorticoid deficiency
Pulmonary	Pneumonia
	Tuberculosis

Thyroid disorders

The thyroid gland lies in front of the neck with its base usually at the level of the fourth or fifth tracheal ring. It consists of two lobes joined by a narrow isthmus and weighs 15–20 g. Remnants of thyroid tissue may be found along the course of the embryological descent of the gland. Lingual thyroid tissue may be seen as a swelling at the foramen caecum and may rarely represent the only functioning thyroid tissue. The main histological features of the gland are the rounded follicles containing colloid.

Thyroid hormones, thyroxine (T4) and triiodothyronine (T3), are stored within the colloid bound to a glycoprotein, thyroglobulin. The thyroid gland takes up iodide avidly which is then oxidized and bound covalently to tyrosine residues to form iodotyrosines, the precursors of the thyroid hormones. The thyroid peroxidase enzyme is important in these processes. Although T4 is the major hormone secreted by the gland, T3 is the more active hormone and is produced mainly by the extra thyroidal deiodination of T4. The conversion of T4 to T3 is inhibited in conditions such as starvation and systemic disease. Thyroid hormones are bound to the carrier protein thyroxin binding globulin in plasma and less than 1 per cent of the hormones are 'free'.

The receptors for thyroid hormone are located in cell nuclei and bind the hormones with high affinity. Over 90 per cent of receptor bound hormone is T3. Following receptor binding T3 induces the formation of messenger RNA coding for various proteins including the enzymes sodium/potassium ATPase, NADP-linked malate enzymes and α-glycerophosphate dehydrogenase enzyme, growth hormone and β-adrenergic receptors. There are also important direct effects on some membrane functions including calcium uptake, amino acid transport and cyclic AMP concentrations. Thyroid hormones are essential for normal growth and development having multiple effects on carbohydrate, protein and fat metabolism. Perhaps the best known action of the hormones is the stimulation of cellular oxygen consumption seen as an increase in basal metabolic rate.

Hormone production by the thyroid gland is controlled by the glycoprotein thyroid stimulating hormone (TSH) which is produced in the thyrotrophs of the anterior pituitary. TSH binds to specific receptors on thyroid cell membranes and stimulates thyroid hormone synthesis acting through the adenyl cyclase enzyme. Both the release and synthesis of TSH are inhibited directly by T4 and T3. TSH secretion is stimulated by the tripeptide thyrotrophin releasing hormone (TRH) which is formed in the hypothalamus.

Hyperthyroidism

Hyperthyroidism or thyrotoxicosis is the syndrome resulting from excess circulating levels of free thyroxine (T4) and/or triiodothyronine (T3). Grave's disease is the commonest cause of thyrotoxicosis. The thyroid gland is stimulated by a circulating IgG autoantibody (thyroid stimulating immunoglobulin) which binds to the TSH receptor on the thyroid cell with consequent prolonged production of thyroid hormone. In toxic multinodular goitre, hyperthyroidism results from multiple autonomous nodules with secondary suppression of extranodular tissue. A solitary hyperfunctioning thyroid nodule (toxic adenoma) may also lead to thyrotoxicosis. These three conditions account for approximately 90 per cent of cases. The remaining 10 per cent are caused by a number of unusual causes (Table 4.22).

Table 4.22   Causes of thyrotoxicosis

Graves' disease
Toxic multinodular goitre
Toxic adenoma
Viral thyroiditis (de Quervain's thyroiditis)
Iatrogenic – inappropriate replacement therapy
Factitious – self-administration
Drugs (amiodarone)
Tumours (TSH secreting pituitary adenoma;
    hydatidiform mole producing TSH)

Clinical features

The incidence of hyperthyroidism in most studies probably reflects that of Grave's disease, which is the predominant cause of hyperthyroidism. A careful study from the Mayo Clinic, has reported the annual incidence of Grave's disease to be 19.8/100 000 inhabitants. Among Swedish women aged 44–64 years, the annual incidence was noted to be 130/100 000 and the prevalence 2 per cent. In Britain, the annual incidence is 9/100 000 for men and 35/100 000 for women. Grave's disease

Table 4.23   Clinical features of hyperthyroidism

Weight loss
Increased appetite
Increased irritability
Fatigue
Excessive sweating
Heat intolerance
Palpitations (sinus tachycardia, atrial fibrillation)
Heart failure
Diarrhoea
Tremor
Proximal myopathy
Oligomenorrhoea/amenorrhoea
Infertility
Gynaecomastia
Pruritis
Palmar erythema
Goitre

is rare before the age of 20 but its incidence rises to reach a peak in the 4th decade and then remains at a plateau until the age of 70. The condition usually develops insidiously though there is great individual variation. Typical symptoms are listed in Table 4.23. It is important to remember that in the elderly atrial fibrillation and/or heart failure may be the sole manifestation of thyrotoxicosis.

A goitre is usually palpable but this is not invariable. In Grave's disease, this is typically diffuse and auscultation may reveal a bruit. Other features of Grave's disease include periorbital oedema, exophthalmos and ophthalmoplegia. The ophthalmopathy is present in 17–60 per cent of patients and is due to swelling of the retro-orbital muscles. It is probably due to an immune reaction: a circulating antibody which binds specifically to a retro-orbital antigen, has been described. This opthalmopathic immunoglobulin does not cross-react with other thyroid antibodies. Five to ten per cent of patients with dysthyroid eye disease remain euthyroid but TRH testing may reveal a suppressed TSH response. CT scanning of the orbits shows the thickened muscles typical of Grave's ophthalmopathy. Rare features of Grave's disease include pretibial myxoedema (found in 4 per cent of adults with thyrotoxicosis) which consists of asymptomatic thickened raised pink lesions on the feet and shins, and thyroid acropachy (frequency 1 per cent) with finger clubbing and new bone formation classically found on the ulnar side of the 5th metacarpal.

Investigations

The clinical diagnosis of thyrotoxicosis can usually be made with confidence, but must be confirmed with elevated serum levels of T4 and T3. Until recently, the total circulating hormone was measured and the decisive free hormone was calculated indirectly. However, methods for direct assay of the total and active, free hormone have now become widely available. Total serum T3 and T4 are now measured by radioimmunoassay with antibodies towards triiodothyronine and thyroxine respectively. Since total T3 and T4 values are influenced by the concentration of binding proteins, misleading results may be obtained when binding proteins are abnormal (e.g. high in pregnancy, contraceptive pill use, viral hepatitis, acute intermittent porphyria; low in general hypoproteinaemia, salicylate ingestion). In borderline cases, a flat TSH response to the injection of TRH is a useful confirmatory test as is the failure of T3 suppression of radio-iodine uptake. In some centres a new, very sensitive assay is available for TSH which renders the TRH test virtually redundant. Using this assay TSH will be undetectable in cases of thyrotoxicosis. Scanning with radio-iodine or technetium demonstrates the classical diffuse toxic goitre of Grave's disease. It is also useful in delineating toxic adenoma and toxic multinodular goitre. Sometimes in cases of thyrotoxicosis the T4 remains within the normal range and T3 concentrations are selectively raised. It is very important therefore to measure T3 as well as T4 if thyrotoxicosis is suspected.

Management

There are three main therapeutic options for the treatment of thyrotoxicosis, medical, surgical and radio-iodine therapy. Opinions differ as to the most appropriate form of treatment and it is best to consider each patient individually.

Medical management

Drug treatment may be used as the sole management for thyrotoxicosis or render the patient euthyroid prior to surgery. It is generally the preferred form of therapy in the young or adults not wishing to undergo surgery. Antithyroid drugs (carbimazole, propylthiouracil) act by blocking the synthesis of thyroid hormone. High doses are given (carbimazole 45 mg/day; prophylthiouracil 300 mg/day) until the patient is euthyroid (approx 4–8 weeks); thereafter a maintenance dose is used for up to 2 years. Adverse effects include skin rashes and arthralgia and, rarely, agranulocytosis.

β-blockers are a helpful adjunct to therapy in the early stages of treatment and block the β-adrenergic mediated actions of thyroid hormones, such as anxiety, tremor and palpitations. Propranolol has been the most popular agent used for this purpose. It decreases the peripheral conversion of thyroxine to triiodothyronine, but this effect is relatively trivial and of doubtful significance.

Surgery

Subtotal thyroidectomy is indicated in patients who cannot be controlled adequately (generally due to side-effects or non-compliance) by anti-thyroid drugs. In addition it is necessary in patients with large goitres causing pressure symptoms and the treatment of choice in cases of solitary toxic adenoma. Surgery is contraindicated in hyperthyroidism in the early stages of de Quervain's thyroiditis.

Preoperative preparation The patient should be rendered euthyroid prior to surgery to reduce the vasculartiy of the gland and to prevent thyrotoxic crisis. Antithyroid drugs are the mainstay of treatment. This normally, takes around 6 weeks and progress must be monitored with frequent serum T4 and T3 estimations. β-blocking drugs given in conjunction with carbimazole are of proven value in the immediate control of the severely thyrotoxic patient. Indeed some surgical units have advocated the use of propranolol alone in the preoperative period; in these case, however, it is essential that the drug is continued for 5 to 7 days postoperatively, as thyroid crisis is otherwise a risk.

Other essential investigations prior to surgery include indirect laryngoscopy to exclude a unilateral cord paralysis and estimation of serum calcium levels because of the unusual association with a parathyroid tumour (though thyrotoxicosis *per se* may be a cause of hypercalcaemia) and also to assist in the postoperative diagnosis of inadvertent parathyroid damage during surgery.

Postoperative care The recovery room staff must be alerted to any sign of laboured breathing, neck swelling, or excessive volume in the drainage bottle. Haemorrhage may result in laryngeal oedema and subsequent respiratory obstruction. It is wise therefore to prop the patient up as soon as possible after the operation to relieve venous congestion, and also to intubate the patient who develops inspiratory stridor.

In the event of parathyroid gland damage, symptoms of hypocalcaemia (i.e. parasthesiae and tetany) usually occur within 36 hours. This complication occurs in approximately 3–4 per cent of cases but is permanent only in about 1 per cent of cases. Adults requiring urgent treatment can be given 10–20 ml of 10 % calcium gluconate i.v. over 10 minutes. (In patients on digitalis, rapid i.v. administration of calcium may be hazardous). In a less urgent situation, i.v. calcium gluconate may be administered slowly i.v. over 4–8 hours to alleviate symptoms. Chronic treatment with calcium supplements may be necessary together with a vitamin D preparation (e.g. dihydrotachysterol calcitriol).

Thyrotoxic crisis

This extreme form of thyrotoxicosis with a high mortality is fortunately rare because hyperthyroidism is diagnosed earlier and treated effectively. However, continued awareness is necessary to avoid precipitatory factors such as infection, surgical injury and major stress in the untreated or partially treated thyrotoxic patient. The major clinical features include high fever, tachycardia, marked tremor, dehydration and cardiac failure.

Thyrotoxic crisis is an acute medical emergency requiring urgent diagnosis and treatment. Large doses of antithyroid drugs are required either orally or by nasogastric tube, e.g. propylthiomal 250 mg 6 hourly. Large doses of iodine are also given by mouth, e.g. potassium iodide 10 mg 4 hourly. β-blocking drugs are very useful given intravenously to control cardiac and neuromuscular manifestations, e.g. propanolol-2 mg 6 hourly. Other supportive measures include dexamethasone, parenteral fluids and treatment of associated hyperpyrexia.

Results of surgery Surgery for an autonomous toxic adenoma is straightforward and complications are rare but removal of a toxic multinodular goitre is associated with significant postoperative hypothyroidism. Partial thyroidectomy for Grave's disease has a 15–20 per cent incidence of thyroid insufficiency and a 5 per cent incidence of relapse.

Table 4.24 Causes of hypothyroidism

Primary hypothyroidism
 Hashimoto's (autoimmune) thyroiditis
 Destruction of thyroid tissue (surgery,
  radioiodine, external irradiation)
 Drugs (thionamide drugs, perchlorate, lithium
  iodine)
 Iodine deficiency
 Inborn errors of thyroid hormone synthesis
 Aplasia of thyroid tissue
Secondary hypothyroidism
 TRH deficiency
 TSH deficiency (panhypopituitarism, isolated)

Radio-iodine therapy

It is simple to administer and is generally reserved for those over the age of 45; it is particularly useful in patients over the age of 60 but is contraindicated in children and pregnancy. Relative contra-indications are large diffuse and large nodular goitres which require unusually high doses of radioactivity.

Potential risks of radioiodine therapy include a carcinogenic effect on the thyroid gland itself or the induction of leukaemia due to irradiation of the bone marrow. However several long-term studies have confirmed the long-term safety of radioactive iodine administration. The incidence of hypothyroidism is high after radioactive iodine treatment rising to almost 50 per cent after 15 years.

Hypothyroidism

Hypothyroidism is the clinical syndrome resulting from reduced secretion of T3 and T4 from the thyroid gland. The majority of cases are due to an autoimmune process and thyroid failure following radioiodine or surgical ablation, though the commonest cause world-wide is iodine deficiency (Table 4.24). Recent epidemiological studies have shown a high prevalence of hypothyroidism, with levels ranging between 0.5 and 3 per cent. Women predominate in all surveys by ratios, varying from 4:1 to 20:1. It usually presents between 40 and 50 years of age, though it may occur at any age. Secondary hypothyroidism which is much less common is caused by failure of TSH production resulting from disease of the pituitary or hypothalamus.

Autoimmune thyroiditis (Hashimoto's thyroiditis) which may or may not be associated with goitre is the commonest form of spontaneous hypothyroidism in the adult. The thyroid is infiltrated with lymphocytes and antibodies to thyroid tissue (thyroid microsomes and thyroglobulin) are found in over 80 per cent of patients. Patients with this disorder often give a family history; indeed euthyroid relatives have an increased incidence of serum antibodies to thyroid tissue.

Women are afflicted with autoimmune hypothyroidism at least five times as frequently as men.

In addition to the causes of hypothyroidism listed in Table 4.24 some causes of Grave's disease progress to hypothyroidism and de Quervain's thyroiditis (viral thyroiditis) occasionally causes hypothyroidism, but this is permanent only in rare cases.

Clinical features

Hypothyroidism affects most systems of the body. It has an insidious onset and is often diagnosed on routine testing. The clinical features listed in Table 4.25, are due both to slowing down of cellular metabolism and the infiltration of body tissues by mucopolysaccharides.

Investigations

Measurement of serum T4 has been the most convenient single test, but the diagnosis of primary hypothyroidism must be confirmed by the demonstration of a raised TSH. Recently supersensitive immunoradiometric assays for TSH have been developed which are capable of detecting TSH

Table 4.25   Clinical features of hypothyroidism

Goitre
Weight gain
Tiredness
Cold intolerance
Bradycardia
Cardiac failure, pericardial effusion
Hypercholesterolaemia
Carpal tunnel syndrome
Deafness
Hoarseness
Slow relaxing tendon reflexes
Anaemia
Dry flaky skin, coarse hair, alopecia
Carotenaemia
Infertility, menorrhagia
Constipation
Ascites
Hyperprolactinaemia

values down to 0.1 MU/litre. Low T4 values may be found in low-protein states, in patients with deficient thyroxine binding globulin (TBG), and altered TBG binding due to competition from drugs. They may also be low in the so-called 'sick euthyroid syndrome' in which a severe illness results in increased conversion of T4 to reverse T3. In these circumstances serum TSH is normal. Measurement of 'free' plasma hormone levels are becoming increasingly available which help in the assessment of patients with altered TBG levels.

Treatment

Hypothyroidism is treated with L-thyroxine in an initial dose of 50 μg daily, increasing 3 to 4 weekly to an average maximum dose of 150–200 μg or until the serum T4 and TSH are within the normal range. In the presence of coronary artery disease, or in the elderly, caution must be exercised starting with 25 μg or alternatively using triiodothyronine which has a shorter half-life. Thyroxine replacement therapy must be continued for life.

Myxoedema coma

Myxoedema coma constitutes a medical emergency and carries a very grave prognosis, particularly in elderly patients. Precipitating factors such as exposure to cold, intercurrent infections and treatment with phenothiazines or barbiturates must be avoided. Severe electrolyte and body fluid disturbances are always present, especially hyponatraemia and hypoglycaemia. Pleuropericardial effusions may be found and the tendon reflexes show extremely slow relaxation.

Primary myxoedema may be difficult to differentiate from secondary myxoedema (due to hypopituitarism) but the presence of thin atrophic skin, scanty pubic and axillary hair and atrophic testes point to pituitary disease. In a clinical context, differentiation is irrelevant to the emergency treatment. Management includes assisted respiration if necessary, and after blood has been drawn for the later estimation of glucose, electrolytes, cortisol and thyroid function corticosteroids and triiodothyronine (12.5 μg every 12 hours) are administered intravenously. Hypoglycaemia is corrected with 50 % dextrose, and hyponatraemia may be treated with hypertonic saline infusion or fluid restriction, depending on the state of hydration. Arterial hypotension requires therapy with slow i.v. infusions of plasma or plasma expanders; pressor amines should only be used with great caution. Drainage of pericardial or pleural effusions may be necessary.

Thyroid swellings

Thyroid swellings (goitres) are very common and may or may not be complicated by hypo- or hyperthyroidism. An enlarged thyroid is referred to as a simple goitre in the absence of inflammatory or neoplastic processes and with normal hormone levels. There are probably many causes of simple goitre perhaps with a common pathophysiology involving increased effective TSH activity resulting in hypertrophy, hyperplasia and increased vascularity of the gland. At a later stage the gland may become fibrotic and nodular – the multinodular goitre.

The major cause of thyroid swelling world-wide is dietary iodine deficiency leading to endemic goitre. These goitrous subjects are generally euthyroid but hypothyroidism does occur if the iodine deficiency is severe and is a particular problem in infants producing cretinism. Goitrogens may be present in the diet; an active substance has been isolated from cassava and in parts of Japan goitre is associated with a dietary excess of iodide from seaweed ingestion. This interferes with organification of iodide in the thyroid gland and impairs release of thyroid hormones.

Investigation of thyroid swelling

It is important to assess both the anatomy of the gland as well as thyroid hormone production (this has been described previously). X-ray of the thoracic inlet will demonstrate retrosternal extension and tracheal compression. Isotope scanning with iodine[131] or technetium[99] demonstrates the consistency of the gland in terms of the uptake of isotope. Thyroid malignancy has to be excluded if there is no uptake of isotope – 'cold nodule'.

Ultrasound examination of the thyroid will show whether the 'cold nodule' is solid or cystic. Percutaneous needle biopsy may be performed in doubtful cases, or cysts aspirated.

Thyroid malignancy

Malignant tumours arising from the thyroid gland are rare (1 per cent of cancer deaths) and secondary involvement of the gland by other carcinomas, particularly lung, breast and kidney is more

Table 4.26   Thyroid carcinoma

Type	Frequency (%)
Papillary	60
Follicular	25
Anaplastic	10
Medullary	5

common. Primary tumours are more common in women (3:1) and are of four types (Table 4.26). There is no evidence that pre-existing goitre predisposes to thyroid malignancy and in fact most tumours arise in otherwise normal glands. Follicular carcinoma is more common in iodine-deficient areas while papillary carcinoma is more common in areas of high iodine intake. Papillary carcinoma is occasionally familial and shows an increased incidence following external irradiation to the head and neck.

Medullary carcinoma of the thyroid arises from the parafollicular cells which are neural-crest in origin. Although very rare (5 per cent of thyroid carcinomas) it is of interest because of its production of calcitonin and other important biochemical mediators such as serotonin and prostaglandins. Approximately 15 per cent of medullary carcinomas are familial and are inherited as an autosomal dominant as part of multiple endocrine adenomatosis (Sipple's syndrome) type II. In this syndrome medullary carcinoma may be associated with phaeochromocytoma and parathyroid adenoma. A variant of the syndrome is also associated with cutaneous and mucosa neuromas on the face, lips and tongue. Other causes of thyroid nodules are shown in Table 4.27.

Table 4.27   Causes of solitary thyroid nodule

Cyst
Colloidal nodule
Degenerative changes
Thyroiditis
Lymphoma
Granuloma formation
Infection

Viral thyroiditis (de Quervain's thyroiditis)

The clinical features include a preceding systemic upset with fever, thyroid gland tenderness and often, a history of thyrotoxic symptoms. The ESR is elevated and thyroid function tests may reveal transient hyperthyroidism in the early stages. Radioactive iodine uptake studies show low iodine uptake in the early phase, but high uptake during recovery.

The natural history of viral thyroiditis is recovery over a few months. The transient hyperthyroidism settles and the use of anti-thyroid drugs is usually unnecessary. This is often followed by a short period of biochemical hypothyroidism with gradual return to normal hormone levels. Occasionally there is a persistent hypothyroidism. Treatment is symptomatic and aspirin is useful. Severe cases with continuing pain and fever respond to corticosteroids.

Parathyroid glands

In normal circumstances four parathyroid glands (approximately 5 mm diameter) are located on the posterior surface of the four poles of the thyroid gland. The upper pair of glands is derived embryologically from the 4th branchial pouch and the lower pair from the 3rd branchial pouch. The total weight of tissue is approximately 120 mg.

The parathyroid glands secrete a single chain polypeptide hormone (84 amino acids, MW = 9500) named parathyroid hormone which is produced by enzymatic cleavage of large precursor polypeptides. The amino terminal third of parathyroid hormone contains the active sequence and the 1–34 amino acid sequence possesses full biological activity.

The secretion of parathyroid hormone which is stimulated by a lowering of plasma ionized calcium concentrations and inhibited by a high ionized calcium has direct effects on calcium and phosphate transport in the kidney. Calcium absorption from the distal convoluted tubule is increased and the reabsorption of phosphate by the proximal renal tubule is inhibited.

The hormone action appears to be mediated via the adenylate cyclase system. Parathyroid hormone, through complex direct effects on bone (including the resorption of bone by osteoclasts, the formation of new osteoclasts, the stimulation of osteocytic osteolysis and the inhibition of collagen biosynthesis and osteoblast function) leads to mobilization of calcium from bone and the elevation of plasma calcium. In addition the absorption of calcium from the small intestine is increased through effects of parathyroid hormone on the hydroxylation in the kidney of 25-hydroxycholecalciferol to 1:25-dihydroxycholecalciferol, the physiological active vitamin D.

Hyperparathyroidism

Excessive secretion of parathyroid hormone may be primary due to a parathyroid adenoma, hyperplasia of the parathyroid glands or parathyroid carcinoma. Chronic renal failure, rickets or osteomalacia may result in secondary hyperparathyroidism and tertiary hyperparathyroidism is characterized by the development of parathyroid autonomy in the hypertrophied glands of secondary hyperparathyroidism.

Primary hyperparathyrodism is a relatively common condition (approximately 1:1000; males: females 1:3). It may result from solitary adenoma (80–90 per cent), primary hyperplasma of all parathyroid glands (10–15 per cent) or carcinoma (4 per cent). Parathyroid adenomas may be composed of chief cells, transitional forms between chief and oxyphil cells, and, rarely, solely of oxyphil cells. Adenomas vary from 500 mg to several grams in weight and may be multiple but these probably represent part of the spectrum of chief cell hyperplasia.

In hyperplasia all parthyroid glands are enlarged with the histological appearance of chief cell (or clear cell) hyperplasia. Parathyroid carcinoma is a rare cause of primary hyperparathyroidism. The lesion may be palpable with regional lymph node involvement and distant metastasis to lung or liver has been described. Adenomas or more frequently glandular hyperplasia may occur as part of multiple endocrine neoplasia (MEN). Hyperparathyroidism with adrenal, thyroid, pancreatic and pituitary adenomas comprises MEN I and with medullary carcinoma of the thyroid and phaeochromocytoma comprises MEN II.

The manifestations of primary hyperparathyroidism (Table 4.28) are largely due to hypercalcaemia. In a milder form however the patient may remain asymptomatic and the diagnosis is made on routine measurement of serum calcium. Rarely the patient may present with hypertension, peptic ulcer, pancreatitis or a mass in the neck. Renal stone disease is the presenting complaint in approximately 50 per cent of patients. Most stones are calcium oxalate, but calcium phosphate stones also occur.

Bone disease is a common feature in primary hyperparathyroidism. Bone pain, pathological fractures and localized bone swellings ('brown tumours') occur; this bony involvement is reflected biochemically by an elevated alkaline phosphatase. Non-specific arthralgias, usually in the hands may be reported in primary hyperparathyroidism, and gout and chondrocalcinosis occur

Table 4.28   Clinical features of primary hyperparathyroidism

Causative factor	Clinical feature
Due to hypercalcaemia	Anorexia
	Polyuria and polydipsia
	Constipation and abdominal pain
	Muscle weakness
	Mental changes
Due to resorption	Bone pain
	Bone deformity, pathological fractures
Due to hypercalciuria	Renal stones
	Nephrocalcinosis

Table 4.29   Causes of hypercalcaemia

Primary hyperparathyroidism	
Neoplasia	Osteolytic secondary carcinoma
	Multiple myeloma
	Humoral hypercalcaemia of malignancy
	Reticuloses involving bone
Medication	Milk-alkali syndrome
	Vitamin D overdosage
	Lithium
	Thiazide diuretics
Sarcoidosis	
Bone disease	Paget's disease during immobilization
Endocrinopathies	Thyrotoxicosis
	Adrenal insufficiency

in greater frequency than they do in the general population.

Diagnosis

The finding of an elevated serum calcium in the presence of hypophosphataemia suggests the diagnosis of primary hyperparathyroidism. (The blood sample should be taken without venous stasis with the patient fasting and at rest). The calcium level is corrected for the albumin concentration and nomograms are available for this. The urinary excretion of calcium is often but not always raised. Radioimmunoassay for PTH is available and this together with hydrocortisone suppression test enables accurate diagnosis in the majority of cases. Hydrocortisone (40 mg t.d.s. for 10 days) fails to lower plasma calcium in the majority of patients with primary hyperparathyroidism but usually does so in hypercalcaemia due to other causes. (Table 4.29).

The characteristic radiological changes are now seen in less than 10 per cent of patients with primary hyperparathyroidism because of earlier diagnosis. Renal calculi and nephrocalcinosis may be evident on abdominal radiographs but the commonest change is the subperiosteal resorption of bone best seen in the radial aspect of the middle phalanges of the hand. Chondrocalcinosis and loss of the lamina dura around the tooth sockets, subperiosteal erosions in the skull (the 'pepper-pot skull') and 'brown tumours' may also be detected radiologically.

The search for parathyroid tumour or hyperplasia may be difficult, particularly if previous neck surgery has been undertaken or if the tumour is ectopically sited. Preoperative localization may therefore be necessary. Methods available include ultrasound scanning, arteriography, selective venous sampling and radioisotope subtraction imaging. CT scanning has not proved very successful with small adenomas.

Surgery to remove abnormal parathyroid tissue represents the best therapeutic approach, and, in experienced hands, success rates approach 90 per cent. Elderly patients with minor symptoms are best treated conservatively with regular checks on serum calcium. There is no effective drug therapy.

Transient hypocalcaemia may occur 2–4 days after surgery. This is due to mild hypoparathyroidism and recovers as the remaining previously suppressed glands recover function. The patient may complain of digital and circumoral tingling, and Trousseau's and Chvostek's signs may be positive. Spontaneous tetany is uncommon but usually seen in patients with severe osteitis fibrosa cystica. Severe symptoms may require intravenous calcium in the acute situation. Persistent hypocalcaemia postoperatively is managed with vitamin D preparations such as dihydrotachysterol or lα-hydroxycholecalciferol ('one-alpha').

Treatment of severe acute hypercalcaemia

Occasionally hypercalcaemia may become severe leading to mental deterioration, severe weakness, coma and even death. The electrocardiogram may reveal a shortened QT interval. Aggressive intervention is required to allow stabilization of the clinical state pending the search for the cause of the hypercalcaemia and definitive treatment.

Patients with serum calcium concentrations in excess of 3 mmol/litre are commonly dehydrated; dehydration in turn lowers the glomerular filtration rate and reduces renal calcium excretion. Rehydration with intravenous physiological saline solution is an important first step in managing such patients. Loop diuretics such as frusemide increase urinary calcium excretion and, provided hydration is adequate, provides an effective short term therapy for hypercalcaemia of any aetiology but caution must be exercised in patients with cardiac or renal impairment. Thiazide diuretics should be avoided because these increase renal tubular absorption of calcium.

Additional agents used in the management of acute hypercalcaemia include those which reduce mobilization of calcium from bone by specifically inhibiting osteoclastic activity. Calcitonin (100–200 units subcutaneously or intravenously) is safe and has a rapid onset of action. The effects of calcitonin wear off after 48–72 hours, possibly due to down regulation of receptors, but may be prolonged by the simultaneous use of glucocorticoids. Glucocorticoids themselves are effective in less than 50 per cent of patients, but may be usefully employed (e.g. prednisolone 40–100 mg/day) in the hypercalcaemia of reticuloendothelial disorders and of sarcoidosis.

Diphosphonates such as etidronate are stable analogues of pyrophosphate. They probably act by a direct effect on osteoclastic resorption of bone and may be administered both orally and intravenously. The cytotoxic antibiotic mithramycin (0–25 µg/kg i.v.) is uniformly effective but its duration of action is unpredictable and its hepatic, renal and bone marrow toxicity preclude its routine use. Intravenous phosphate can be a very effective treatment for severe hypercalcaemia if other therapy is ineffective or contraindicated. However it should be reserved for dire emergenices only, as severe hypocalcaemia and ectopic calcification may result.

Secondary hyperparathyroidism

In chronic diseases associated with hypocalcaemia (e.g. malabsorption, chronic renal failure and vitamin D deficiency) the prolonged stimulus to PTH results in hyperplasia of all four parathyroid glands. Typical radiological features, including osteitis fibrosa cystica, are found, and are accompanied by a rise in the serum alkaline phosphatase. The condition can be prevented by the administration of vitamin D metabolites.

Tertiary hyperparathyroidism

This condition supervenes when the parathyroid glands become autonomous by the development of an adenoma after prolonged stimulus to PTH. Serum calcium is elevated and subtotal parathyroidectomy is required.

Hypoparathyroidism

Impaired parathyroid activity is rare but most commonly occurs after surgical damage during surgery for thyroid disease. Idiopathic hypoparathyroidism may occur as an isolated abnormality or may be associated wtih autoimmune diseases such as Addison's disease – these patients are usually short and suffer from cataracts, moniliasis, calcification of the basal ganglia and impaired dental and nail development.

Clinical features are those of hypocalcaemia, i.e. paraesthesiae, tetany, psychiatric disturbances and epileptic seizures. Trousseau's and Chvostek's signs may be positive. Serum calcium is low with a high phosphate and the alkaline phosphatase is normal.

Treatment is usually with vitamin D or its analogues (e.g. 'one-alpha', 1–2 mg/day or dihydrotachysterol 0.25–2.0 mg/day). Intravenous calcium may be needed in acute hypocalcaemic states.

Pseudohypoparathyroidism

Pseudohypoparathyroidism is a rare inherited disorder due to an insensitivity of the kidney, and sometimes bone, to the action of PTH; the defect lies at the PTH receptor level. In addition to the features of hypocalcaemia, patients with this condition have distinctive skeletal defects, particularly shortening of the 4th and 5th metacarpals and metatarsals.

Adrenal glands

The two adrenal glands (each approximately 5 g) lie retroperitoneally at the upper poles of the kidneys. Each gland is approximately 2.5 cm wide and 5 cm long and consists of medulla and cortex which have separate embryological origins. The adrenal cortex develops from mesoderm but the medulla arises from the neural crest tissue of the ectoderm.

The adrenal cortex

The cortex comprises approximately 90 per cent of the adrenal tissue. The principal steroid hormone products of the cortex are the mineralocorticoids (e.g. aldosterone) and the glucocorticoids (e.g. cortisol) but well over fifty different steroids are produced. The glucocorticoids are essential for many important metabolic effects including carbohydrate metabolism which gives them their name. Aldosterone is an important regulator of sodium, potassium and water balance. The adrenal cortex also produces sex hormones. Small amounts of oestrogen are produced in both sexes and in women the cortex is the site of androgen production but in men less than 10 per cent of androgen production takes place in the adrenal. Corticosteroids, androgens and oestrogens are produced in the zona fasiculata and reticularis whereas aldosterone is produced in the outermost zone, the zone glomerulosa.

The adrenal production of glucocorticoid hormones is stimulated by adrenocorticotrophic hormone (ACTH) from the anterior pituitary. This trophic hormone is itself regulated by corticotrophin-releasing factor (CRF) from the hypothalamus. Adrenal cortisol reduces ACTH production by feedback inhibition of the hypothalamus. Plasma cortisol is highest in the morning and falls during the day. This diurnal rhythm is disturbed by stressful stimuli such as surgery, trauma and other physical and psychological factors.

In contradistinction to the glucocorticoids, mineralocorticoid secretion is controlled principally through the renin/angiotensin system. Renin is secreted by the cells of the juxtaglomerular apparatus (located close to the afferent glomerular arteriole) in response to volume depletion, sodium depletion, cardiac failure and hypoalbuminaemia. Renin which has a molecular weight of 3500 acts as a proteolytic enzyme converting angiotensinogen to the decapeptide angiotensin I. This is in turn converted to the octapeptide angiotensin II by angiotensin converting enzyme in lung and blood. Angiotensin II stimulates aldosterone secretion from the zona glomerulosa and has a direct vasoconstrictor effect.

Adrenocortical disease: Cushing's syndrome

This syndrome which bears the name of the American neurosurgeon who first described pituitary-dependent or Cushing's disease has several causes. It is characterized by an inappropriate excess of glucocorticoid hormones which leads to characteristic physical and metabolic findings.

Clinical features

The main clinical features of Cushing's syndrome are shown in Table 4.30. Centripetal obesity is the classical but not invariable finding and often generalized obesity is present. The 'buffalo hump' and the 'moonface' result from alterations in the distribution of body fat, the mechanism of which is not fully understood. The muscle wasting and weakness is related to the promotion by cortisol of protein catabolism resulting in a negative nitrogen balance. The myopathy tends to be proximal in distribution. Osteoporosis and vertebral collapse may cause backpain and the effects of cortisol on collagen synthesis results in thinning of the skin, bruising and purple striae. Glucose intolerance is common secondary to the anti-insulin actions of cortisol. Hypernatraemia, hypokalaemia, hypertension and ankle swelling results from excess mineralocorticoid activity. In women with Cushing's syndrome, hirsuties, acne, greasy skin and menstrual irregularities result from excess adrenal androgen production. Severe virilization with cliteromegaly and temporal recession is suggestive of adrenal carcinoma. Psychiatric manifestations may affect as many as 70 per cent of patients. Depression is common but hypomania and frank psychosis are also seen. It can be seen that many of the symptoms and signs of Cushing's syndrome are non-specific although bruising,

Table 4.30   Clinical features of Cushing's syndrome

Centripetal obesity
Purple striae
Weakness, proximal myopathy
Bruising, thin skin
Hypertension
Osteoporosis
Moonface, facial plethora
Buffalo hump
Impaired glucose tolerance
Acne, hirsuties
Amenorrhoea, impotence
Infection
Psychiatric disturbances
Poor wound healing

nyopathy, hypertension and plethora appear to have the highest discriminatory value in diagnosis.

Causes of Cushing's syndrome

The assay of ACTH in cases has proved to be very helpful in the differential diagnosis of cases of Cushing's syndrome and the syndrome is best thought of as secondary ACTH-dependent causes or ACTH-independent causes.

ACTH-dependent Cushing's syndrome and pituitary-dependent (Cushing's disease) This is the commonest cause of spontaneous Cushing's syndrome accounting for approximately 70 per cent of affected adults. Women are more commonly affected than men and the peak incidence is in the 4th and 5th decade. Over production of ACTH results from an adenoma of the anterior pituitary gland. The majority of tumours are less than 10 mm in diameter and are generally located in the central core of the gland. In most cases of Cushing's disease, therefore, the pituitary fossa is not enlarged as seen on the lateral skull X-ray. Approximately 10 per cent of patients present with larger tumours and suprasellar extension.

The majority of ACTH-producing tumours are basophilic and unencapsulated but chromophobe adenomas may also occur. Immunostaining reveals positive reactions for ACTH. Some patients have diffuse hyperplasia of corticotroph cells without a discrete adenoma and occasional patients have been described with ectopic production of CRF.

Excess ACTH production leads to bilateral adrenal cortical hyperplasia and occasionally nodules develop – 'nodular hyperplasia'.

Ectopic ACTH syndrome Ectopic ACTH production accounts for approximately 10 per cent of cases of Cushing's syndrome. A wide variety of tumours, both benign and malignant, may produce ACTH including small cell carcinoma of the bronchus, bronchial adenomas, carcinoid tumours of the lung, gut, thymus, pancreas and liver, phaeochromocytomas and paragangliomas, ovarian tumours and medullary thyroid carcinoma.

Fully developed clinical characteristics of Cushing's syndrome are rare in patients with highly malignant tumours producing ACTH such as carcinoma of the lung as death ensues rapidly. However biochemical abnormalities are severe often with profound hypokalaemia. An important diagnostic problem is that the benign slowly growing tumours producing ectopic ACTH may mimic pituitary-dependent disease.

ACTH-independent Cushing's syndrome

Adrenal tumours Autonomous production of cortisol by a benign adenoma is responsible for approximately 10 per cent of cases of Cushing's syndrome. ACTH production is suppressed with consequent shrinkage of the contralateral adrenal gland. Malignant adrenal tumours are a common cause of Cushing's syndrome in children but only account for 10 per cent of cases overall. These tumours often secrete large amounts of androgens resulting in marked virilization in women.

Other causes of Cushing's syndrome

Iatrogenic Chronic administration of ACTH or glucocorticoids will produce Cushing's syndrome. The important point to remember is that if this medication is suddenly stopped acute hypo-adrenalism will occur. Occasionally sufficient glucocorticoid may be absorbed from topical steroid applications to suppress the pituitary adrenal axis.

Pseudo Cushing's syndrome Alcohol abuse may produce the clinical features of Cushing's syndrome. In addition there may be high basal levels of cortisol with loss of the normal diurnal rhythm and failure of suppression with dexamethasone. However these changes revert on abstention from alcohol.

Diagnosis and management

Biochemical tests The diagnosis and management of Cushing's syndrome involves demonstration of excessive glucocorticoid production and loss of the normal diurnal rhythm, determining the cause of the syndrome and localizing the pathological tissue (Table 4.31).

The most useful index of glucocorticoid overproduction is 24-hour urinary free cortisol but this should be measured on at least three occasions as cortisol secretion may be episodic. Normal values depend on whether the fluorometric assay or radioimmunoassay is used. Plasma cortisol measurements at 0900 hours and 2400 hours may demonstrate the loss of the normal diurnal circadian rhythm but factors such as depression or admission into hospital may result in elevated 2400-hour cortisol. It is important that the patient is not warned of the intention of performing the

Table 4.31 Diagnosing Cushing's syndrome

Test	Normal	Cushing's disease	Ectopic ACTH syndrome	Adrenal adenoma	Adrenal carcinoma
Plasma cortisol	Circadian rhythm	High, no rhythm	High, no rhythm	High, no rhythm	High, no rhythm
Plasma ACTH	Normal	High	Marked increase	Low	Low
Response to 8 mg dexamethasone	Suppression	Partial	Absent	Absent	Absent
Response to metyrapone	2–4 fold rise	Exaggerated	No fall	No fall	No fall
Response to CRF test	Present	Present	Absent	Absent	Absent

midnight test. Anomalous results may be obtained in patients taking phenytoin and in rare patients who fail to metabolize dexamethasone normally. Depression may be distinguished from Cushing's syndrome by measuring plasma cortisol response to insulin-induced hypoglycaemia (blood glucose less than 2.2 mmol/litre). In Cushing's syndrome but not in depression, there is failure of the cortisol to rise.

A further test indicating cortisol over-production is the low-dose dexamethasone suppression test where 0.5 mg dexamethasone is administered 6-hourly for 48 hours. In normal subjects, plasma cortisol should be suppressed to less than 170 mmol/litre (by fluorimetry) while patients with Cushing's syndrome show no suppression. One situation that may pose diagnostic problems is the so-called 'cyclical Cushing's syndrome' in which test results may at times be normal.

Once the diagnosis of Cushing's syndrome is confirmed the cause of the excessive corticosteriod production has to be found. This involves biochemical and radiological studies. Plasma ACTH levels are extremely high in the ectopic ACTH syndrome, high or in the normal range in Cushing's but suppressed in adrenal lesions.

In the high dose dexamethasome test plasma cortisol is measured before and after giving 2 mg of dexamethasone 6-hourly for 2 days. Urinary steroids may be suppressed by 50 per cent or more in some patients with pituitary-dependent Cushing's disease, but only rarely in other causes of Cushing's syndrome. The metyrapone test is useful in the differential diagnosis of Cushing's syndrome. The drug inhibits the 11 β-hydroxylase enzyme which catalyzes the final step in cortisol synthesis resulting in a rise in 11-deoxycortisol and other precursors. These can be measured as 17-oxygenic steroids in the urine before and after administering of 750 mg of metyrapone 4-hourly for 24 hours. In pituitary dependent disease there is an exaggerated rise in metabolites following metyrapone administration.

Recently CRF (a 41-amino acid peptide isolated from bovine hypothalami) has become available for diagnostic use. Blood samples for corticotrophin are collected before and after injecting CRF. A rise in plasma ACTH is seen in patients with Cushing's disease; patients with an adrenal adenoma or carcinoma are characterized by undetectable baseline corticotrophin levels unresponsive to CRF, whereas patients with ectopic ACTH secretion have raised basal corticotrophin levels also unresponsive to CRF. The diagnostic accuracy of the CRF test is comparable to that of the high dose dexamethasone test.

Imaging techniques Biochemical techniques to diagnose Cushing's syndrome are sometimes inconclusive and various radiological techniques are useful in localizing the cause. Plain chest X-ray may detect some pulmonary tumours and should be performed in every patient. Clinical findings may indicate the need for barium studies, bronchoscopy and biopsy in individual cases. Only a minority of cases have pituitary fossa abnormalities on plain skull X-ray or even tomography but the advent of CT scanners has enabled the identification of intrasellar pituitary microadenomas. Whole body CT scanning may be necessary to localize small ACTH-secreting tumours in the lungs, mediastinum, pancreas and elsewhere which are not visualized by routine radiology.

If primary adrenal disease is suspected, pyelography to detect renal displacement ultrasound and CT examination of the adrenal areas should be performed. The affected adrenal is enlarged and the contralateral adrenal is small. If indicated, adrenal arteriography or venography is used to further localize the lesion. At venography, adrenal vein sampling for cortisol confirms localization. Venous sampling from major systemic veins may also help to localize ectopic ACTH secretion. In addition sampling from the inferior petrosal vein for ACTH helps in the identification of pituitary disease in equivocal cases.

Treatment

There are three approaches to the management of Cushing's syndrome: surgery, radiotherapy and drug therapy. The choice of treatment depends on the cause.

Successful resection of an adrenal adenoma will result in complete cure. The operative mortality can be as high as 2–5 per cent, pulmonary embolism being a common cause of death. This mortality can largely be avoided by prior induction of normo-cortisolaemia and clinical remission with metyrapone. Preoperatively, pulmonary and cardiac function must be optimized and hypo-kalaemia, hypertension and diabetes mellitus corrected. Extreme care must be taken when moving the patient because of thin skin and osteo-porotic bones; venous access may be difficult and infection must be avoided at all costs. If malignancy is not suspected, several weeks therapy with the drug metyrapone will allow correction of many of the metabolic abnormalities.

Full glucocorticoid cover is required during surgery. A typical regimen would be to give 200 mg of hydrocortisone intramuscularly the day before the operation and again with the premedication.

Postoperatively, the patient should be nursed in a high dependency unit as assisted ventilation may be required. Electrolyte disorders and signs of hypocortisolism may occur and must be corrected. Intramuscular hydrocortisone 100 mg t.d.s. is given for three days, followed by oral corti-costeroid replacement for several months or even years. Often the contralateral adrenal fails to recover and life long replacement therapy is required. Treatment of adrenal carcinoma involves surgery and postoperative radiotherapy. In metastatic disease adrenolytic drugs may be helpful as discussed later.

Treatment of ectopic ACTH syndrome involves removal of the tumour source of ACTH if possible.

Metyrapone therapy may be beneficial to control symptoms. If no primary tumour can be found adrenalectomy causes excellent remission in some cases.

Microsurgical removal of a pituitary adenoma by the trans-sphenoidal route is now the treatment of choice. In experienced hands, the mortality and complication rates are very low and satisfactory remission is seen in about 85–95 per cent of patients. Larger tumours causing radiologically visible sellar enlargement are considered for more radical surgery. Transient diabetes insipidus is common in the early postoperative period and full endocrinological assessment is needed post-operatively to assess the need for hormone replacement therapy.

Radiotherapy to the pituitary by implantation of either by conventional techniques or radioactive Yttrium seeds is an alternative procedure for those with pituitary tumours. However response to radiotherapy is slow and may take up to several years for a full effect, so that metyrapone therapy is needed in the interim. Ultimately, however, approximately half the patients are cured, though some abnormalities of dynamic testing of pituitary-adrenal axis may persist.

Long term medical treatment of Cushing's syndrome requires close supervision by the endo-crinologist with frequent measurements of plasma cortisol. The following drugs are available.

Metyrapone, in an initial dose of 250 mg t.d.s. after meals inhibits the conversion of 11-deoxy-cortisol to cortisol. Control is usually reached within a few weeks on 2–4 g a day depending on the underlying lesion. It is most effective for the restoration of normocortisolaemia prior to adrena-lectomy, transphenoidal surgery or during investi-gation of suspected ectopic ACTH. Metyrapone is also suitable as emergency treatment in severely hypercortisolaemic patients with acute physical or psychiatric complications. Inoperable pituitary, adrenal or ectopic ACTH-producing tumours, or failure of surgery are also indications for the use of metyrapone. Side-effects include nausea, dizziness, rashes, hirsuties and acne. A dangerous fall in cortisol often occurs and this may be preven-ted by giving dexamethasone in a dose of 0.25 mg twice daily.

Aminoglutethimide inhibits the conversion of cholesterol to pregnenolone. Its side-effects are more troublesome, but may be used in combina-tion with metyrapone if adrenal blockade is un-satisfactory when used alone. Trilostane blocks the enzyme 3β-hydroxysteroid dehydrogenase required in the conversion of pregnenolone to progesterone. However it is probably not as effective as the first two drugs.

Nelson's syndrome In approximately one-third of patients who undergo bilateral adrenalectomy for Cushing's disease, the pituitary adenoma continues to grow resulting in rising levels of ACTH and 'Addisonian' pigmentation. This syndrome may be prevented by giving pituitary irradiation following adrenalectomy.

Primary hyperaldosteronism

Primary hyperaldosteronism was first described in 1955 by Conn and results from overproduction of the mineralocorticoid hormone, aldosterone, by the zona glomerulosa of the adrenal cortex. In approximately 60 per cent of cases there is a unilateral adrenal adenoma: other cases are due to bilaterial hyperplasia of the zona glomerulosa. The cause of the bilateral hyperplasia is as yet undetermined but is subject to intense research in an attempt to isolate a stimulating factor probably of pituitary origin.

Aldosterone acts on the distal renal tubules promoting sodium, chloride and water reabsorption and potassium and hydrogen ion secretion. Therefore in aldosterone excess there is an increase in total body sodium, hypokalaemia and alkalosis.

Clinical features

This condition should be considered in hypertensive patients especially when there is associated hypokalaemia. The incidence in unselected hypertensives is approximately 2 per cent. Symptoms will depend on the degree of hypokalaemia. If this is marked with associated alkalosis, symptoms of thirst, polyuria and paraesthesiae may be present. Flaccid paralysis due to severe hypokalaemia is very rare. Trousseau and Chvostek signs may be positive due to low ionized calcium levels secondary to the alkalosis. Despite the expanded extracellular fluid, oedema is rare: hypertension is seldom severe. It is not unusual for women presenting with primary hyperaldosteronism to give a history of hypertension in a previous pregnancy. An electrocardiogram may show left ventricular hypertrophy and the characteristc changes of hypokalaemia with T-wave flattening and U-waves.

Diagnosis and management

The demonstration of hypokalaemia is the first critical step in the diagnosis. Previous treatment with diuretics is the commonest cause of hypokalaemia in patients with hypertension and electrolyte status should be assessed prior to the use of these drugs. In patients already taking diuretics these drugs should be stopped for at least 3 weeks prior to workup. Sodium intake can markedly effect serum and urinary potassium levels and on a low sodium intake the potassium abnormalities may not be apparent. However in Europe the average sodium intake (110 mEq/day) is high enough for the potassium abnormalities to develop. The hypokalaemia is associated with an inappropriately high urinary potassium excretion (50 mEq/24 h). The diagnosis is confirmed by the presence of a high plasma aldosterone level with a suppressed plasma renin concentration.

Once the diagnosis of primary hyperaldosteronism has been made it is important to identify the cause, (adenoma or hyperplasia) as the management of these two conditions is different.

CT scanning of the adrenals is of only limited use as aldosterone producing adenomas are often less than 1 cm in diameter. Bilateral adrenal vein sampling for aldosterone can be helpful in localizing an adenoma as can iodocholesterol scanning. The most useful biochemical procedure for differentiating adenoma from hyperplasia depends on measuring aldosterone in response to changes in posture. In patients with an adenoma plasma aldosterone levels remain unchanged or fall when measured at 8 a.m. when the patient is recumbent and again at 11 a.m. with the patient standing. This is in contrast to normals and patients with bilateral hyperplasia where plasma aldosterone levels rise.

The treatment of choice for a patient with primary hyperaldosteronism due to an adrenal adenoma is surgery. The majority of these patients will become normotensive postsurgery. The potassium depletion seen in patients with an adenoma puts them at risk from anaesthesia but this can be overcome by pretreatment for 3–4 weeks with the specific aldosterone antagonist, spironolactone and a low sodium diet. Some physicians advocate potassium supplementation (4–6 g of potassium chloride) in the week prior to surgery. In the postoperative period the plasma potassium must be carefully monitored.

Patients with primary hyperaldosteronism due to bilateral hyperplasia of the zona glomerulosa are treated medically with spironolactone (300 mg/day). Important side-effects of this drug in men (up to 50 per cent) are decreased libido and tender enlargement of the breasts. Alternative drugs are triameterene and amiloride. Often other hypotensive agents are required to render the patient normotensive. Some success in the treatment of primary hyperaldosteronism has been reported with trilostane, a selective inhibitor of the enzyme 3-β-hydroxysteroid dehydrogenase/△⁵-3-oxosteroid isomerase. This agent reduces mineralocorticoid production.

Addison's disease

Addison's disease, or primary adrenocortical failure, results from destruction of the adrenal cortex by various pathological processes (Table 4.32).

Formerly, the principal cause of Addison's disease was tuberculosis but autoimmune adrenalitis is now responsible for more than 80 per cent of cases. This may be associated with other autoimmune conditions such as pernicious anaemia, Hashimoto's disease, diabetes mellitus, hypoparathyroidism and primary ovarian failure. Women are affected twice as often as men. There is lymphocytic infiltration of the adrenal cortex and circulating autoantibodies against adrenal cortex are detected in the majority of patients.

Table 4.32 Causes of adrenocortical failure

Primary adrenal disease		Secondary disease
Idiopathic/autoimmune	≈ 80 %	Pharmacological
Tuberculosis	≈ 20 %	use of
Other causes	≈ 1 %	corticosteroids
(metastasis, amyloid,		Pituitary disease
sarcoid, surgery, adrenal		Hypothalamic
haemorrhage,		disease
haemochromatosis, fungal		
infections, congenital		
enzyme deficiencies,		
irradiation)		

Clinical features

Addison's disease may present with the patient shocked and hyponatraemic (Addisonian crisis) or insidiously, depending on the severity of the glucocorticoid and mineralocorticoid deficiency.

Initial symptoms include lassitude and muscular weakness, anorexia, abdominal pain, nausea, vomiting and weight loss. Dizziness due to postural hypotension results from either aldosterone or cortisol deficiency. Lack of aldosterone results in impaired ability to conserve sodium and excrete potassium. This results in a decrease in extracellular fluid and plasma volume, weight loss, decrease in renal blood flow and uraemia. The reduced plasma volume leads to increased ADH secretion which causes water retention and low serum sodium. Potassium on the other hand is retained by the renal tubules resulting in elevated serum levels. Other biochemical features include occasional hypercalcaemia of unknown aetiology, hypoglycaemia and high blood urea.

The typical feature of Addison's disease which most often leads to diagnosis is pigmentation. Pigmentation is directly caused by the very high circulating level of ACTH. The whole body may become diffusely pigmented but pressure areas, recent scars, palmar creases and especially the nipples, buccal mucosa, scrotum and labia are preferentially affected. Less common features of Addison's include nocturia, impotence, amenorrhoea, depression and diarrhoea.

Investigations

The characteristic abnormalities include hyponatraemia, hyperkalaemia and an elevated blood urea (Table 4.33). Anaemia and a raised ESR may be present but are non-specific. Serum cortisol will be inappropriately low in severe cases. In less severe cases a morning cortisol may not be unequivocally low and confirmation of the diagnosis with a short Synacthen test is required (250 mg). Of the synthetic 1–24 N-terminal sequence of ACTH (tetracosactrin Synacthen) is injected intramuscularly between 0800 and 0900 hrs and the plasma cortisol response measured at 0, 30 and 60 minutes. Failure of the cortisol to rise (mean increment in normal subjects ≅ 600 nmol/litre) is consistent with a diagnosis of hypoadrenalism. ACTH levels will be high in primary adrenal

Table 4.33 Laboratory findings in Addison's disease

Normochromic normocytic anaemia
Relative lymphocytosis
Eosinophilia
ESR is often raised
Hyponatraemia
Hypochloraemia
Hyperkalaemia
Hypercalcaemia

failure but its measurement is not usually necessary as the diagnosis can be made on cortisol measurements which are much simpler. Additional investigations in the diagnosis of Addison's disease include abdominal X-ray which may reveal tuberculous calcified adrenals and chest X-ray which may show TB lesions or malignancy. Adrenocortical auto-antibodies may also be demonstrable.

Management

In severely ill patients fluid replacement is essential and this should be in the form of physiological saline, one litre given in the first hour and then 500 ml hourly for the next 3 hours. Several litres may be required in the first 24 hours. Hydrocortisone is given in a dose of 50–100 mg every 6 hours. At these doses, no mineralocorticoid is required because the intrinsic mineralocorticoid properties of hydrocortisone are sufficient. Oral hydrocortisone can usually be commenced after 24–36 hours and life-long therapy is required.

An attempt is made to mimic the normal daily cortisol rhythm by hydrocortisone, giving 20 mg in the morning (on rising) and 10 mg in the afternoon. More or less cortisol may be required in different patients. Mineralocorticoid replacement with aldosterone is impracticable because it is not absorbed and therefore fludrocortisone, in a dose of 0.05–0.2 mg daily is used. The dose may be adjusted by measuring plasma renin which should be suppressed into the normal range. All patients should carry a steroid card and should be advised to double their dose and seek immediate medical advice during intercurrent illness.

Surgery, pregnancy and Addison's disease

Minor surgery must be covered with 100 mg of hydrocortisone sodium succinate intramuscularly 6-hourly starting with the premedication. This should be continued for 24 hours or until the normal oral replacement dose can be restarted. During major surgery the same regime is recommended except parenteral hydrocortisone should be continued for at least 72 hours post-operatively. If oral medication is delayed because of unforeseen complications, 50 mg of i.m. hydrocortisone should be administered 8-hourly.

During pregnancy, the dose of oral hydrocortisone need not be adjusted unless there is an intercurrent illness, but in labour parenteral hydrocortisone must be given as for major surgery.

The adrenal medulla

The cells of the adrenal medulla which act as sympathetic post-ganglionic neurones without axons, receive their preganglionic nerve supply (cholinergic) via the greater splanchnic nerve from the sympathetic chain. The adrenal medulla unlike other sympathetic tissue contains the enzyme phenylethanolamine N-methyl transferase and so is

Table 4.34 Major alpha and beta adrenergic receptors and their response to stimulation in various tissues

Cardiovascular
  Heart
    beta ↑ heart rate
        ↑ atrial and ventricular contractility and conduction velocity
        ↑ A-V node conduction velocity
  Arterioles
    skin   alpha ↑ constriction
    skeletal muscle alpha ↑ constriction;
                  beta ↑ dilatation
    abdominal viscera alpha ↑ constriction;
                  beta ↑ dilatation
  Veins
    alpha ↑ constriction
Pulmonary
  Bronchial musculature beta ↑ dilatation
Genitourinary
  Urinary bladder alpha ↑ trigone and sphincter contraction
                beta ↑ detrusor relaxation
  Male sex organs alpha ↑ ejaculation
Gastrointestinal
  Stomach and intestine
    alpha ↑ sphincter contraction
    beta ↓ motility
Exocrine pancreas
  alpha ↓ secretion
Skin
  sweating
    alpha ↑
Salivary glands
  alpha ↑ potassium and water secretion
  beta ↑ amylase secretion
Eye
  alpha ↑ contraction of radial muscle of iris
Metabolic
  Fat
    beta ↑ lipolysis
  Liver
    beta ↑ glycogenolysis and gluconeogenesis
  Skeletal muscle
    beta ↑ glycolysis
    beta ↓ proteolysis

able to synthesize adrenaline. Adrenaline is a hormone in the traditional sense whereas noradrenaline and dopamine are primarily neurotransmitters which may have hormonal functions in certain situations.

Noradrenaline and adrenaline are secreted by the adrenal medulla in response to various stimuli such as emotional stress, fear, hypoglycaemia, exercise and trauma. Their actions are mediated through α, β and dopaminergic receptors (Table 4.34). The principal source of plasma noradrenaline is the sympathetic nerve endings whereas most of the noradrenaline is from the adrenal.

The enzyme catechol-o-methyl transferase which is found principally in the liver and kidney is responsible for the breakdown of catecholamines to normetadrenaline and metadrenaline. These substances are further catabolized to vanillyl mandelic acid by monoamine oxidase.

If both adrenal glands are removed the rest of the sympathetic nervous system appears to compensate for lack of the adrenal medulla and replacement therapy is only required for the adrenocortical hormones. However hyperfunction of the adrenal medulla, although very rare, gives rise to a very interesting and taxing clinical condition known as phaeochromocytoma.

Phaeochromocytoma

The term phaeochromocytoma is derived from the histological characteristics of this rare tumour of chromaffin tissue leading to a dusky colour on staining with chromium salts (Greek i-phaios = dusky; 'chroma' = colour). The majority of these tumours are adrenal in origin (90 per cent) though they may occur anywhere in the sympathetic chain. Ten per cent are histologically malignant. The true incidence is unknown but large autopsy studies and screening studies within hypertensive populations estimate an incidence of between 0.1 and 0.3 per cent. It generally occurs in adults aged 25–55 and has an equal sex distribution.

Clinical features

The clinical manifestations of a phaeochromocytoma are the result of excessive catecholamine secretion from the tumour (Table 4.35). These will vary somewhat depending on whether adrenaline (α and β receptor stimulation) or noradrenaline (predominantly α activity) is predominant. Extra-adrenal tumours secrete noradrenaline only.

Table 4.35 Clinical features of phaeochromocytoma

Palpitations
Hypertension
Angina
Anxiety, sweating
Headaches
Facial pallor
Flushing
Fever
Nausea/vomiting
Glycosuria

The main clinical presentation is hypertension, more often sustained than paroxysmal, but with superimposed hypertensive crises. Sweating is a common symptom and may be continuous or episodic and associated with profound flushing or blanching. Weight loss, tremulousness and tachycardia are also the direct result of increased production of catecholamines. Catecholamines may produce myocarditis and myocardial necrosis in patients with phaeochromocytoma and in severe cases the presenting symptoms may not be hypertension but congestive heart failure. Owing to their small size these tumours do not present with an obvious mass and therefore diagnosis may be difficult unless there is a high index of suspicion.

Neurofibromatosis (Von Recklinghausen's disease) occurs in 5 per cent of patients with phaeochromocytoma. Patients with the Von Hippel–Lindau syndrome (cerebello-retinal haemangioblastomatosis) also have a high incidence of phaeochromocytoma, as do patients with Sturge–Weber disease, hereditary cerebellar ataxia and tuberous sclerosis.

Sipple's syndrome consists of medullary carcinoma of the thyroid and adrenal phaeochromocytoma. These patients also have an increased incidence of hyperparathyroidism; the thyroid tumour which arises from the 'C' cells synthesizes calcitonin but may also produce prostaglandins, serotonin and ACTH. Sipple's syndrome is one of the multiple endocrine neoplasia syndromes (MEN) and has been classified as MEN Type II.

Diagnosis

A firm diagnosis of phaeochromocytoma depends on the demonstration of overproduction of catecholamines. 24-hour urine specimens are collected for assays of adrenaline and noradrenaline or one of their metabolites: normetadrenaline, metadrenaline and vanillylmandelic acid (VMA). The excretory products of various drugs and foods may affect urinary assays and therefore should be withdrawn before urine specimens are collected. These include methyldopa, phenothiazines, MAOI's, coffee, vanilla, chocolate, tea, bananas, citrus fruits and various vegetables. In patients with paroxysmal hypersecretion of catechols, diagnosis may be difficult and thus repeat testing is required, particularly immediately after symptomatic attacks. Concentrations of catecholamines in plasma can now be accurately ascertained and are very useful in diagnosis.

After definitive diagnosis of phaeochromocytoma is made, the ratio of noradrenaline to adrenaline in the urine may aid in localizing the tumour. The N-methylating enzyme for the conversion of noradrenaline to adrenaline is located in the adrenal medulla and the Organ of Zuckerkandl and therefore, if adrenaline constitutes more than 20 per cent of the total urinary catecholamines, the tumour is almost invariably located within either of these two organs. If noradrenaline alone is increased the tumour may be found within the adrenal gland, possibly in intra-abdominal sites or occasionally outside the abdomen.

Provocative tests for the diagnosis of phaeochromocytoma have largely been discarded but the pentolinium suppression test has improved the accuracy of diagnosis. This ganglion-blocking drug will inhibit catecholamine release from the adrenal medulla while having no effect on the autonomous secretion by phaeochromocytoma which lacks a pre-ganglionic nerve supply. In the test, plasma adrenaline and noradrenaline levels are measured before and 10 minutes after 2.5 mg pentolinium intravenously. Levels are suppressed in patients without a phaeothcomocytoma, but there is no suppression in patients with a tumour.

When the diagnosis is established, localization of the growth is essential prior to surgery. Many techniques are available but their use varies from centre to centre depending on availability. Ultrasound, plain abdominal X-ray, computerized tomography, selective venous sampling and arteriography have all been used, but the latter two require preparation as for surgery. The most significant contribution has been the development of a specific radionuclide (^{131}I-metaiodo-benzylguanidine, MIBG) for isotopic imaging of the tumours.

Treatment

Phaeochromocytoma should be surgically excised wherever possible. It must be emphasized that, as with invasive localization procedures, surgical exploration might stimulate a phaeochromocytoma to release potentially fatal amounts of catecholamines, and thus careful preoperative management is essential.

Preoperative management

It is customary to initiate blockade with a noncompetitive alpha adrenergic blocker such as phenoxybenzamine in a dose of 10 mg t.d.s. before surgery. This dose is increased gradually until postural hypotension is noted. The contracted plasma volume is thus allowed to respond, and any anaemia corrected with whole blood transfusions. Unopposed β-adrenergic effects, more likely if the tumour is a predominantly adrenaline-secreting one, are controlled with a β-blocking drug such as propranolol. By restoring normal blood pressure, euglycaemia and reducing ventricular extrasystoles, alpha and β-blockade have reduced operative mortality from approximately 20 per cent to 2 per cent.

During surgery

Surgery for phaeochromocytoma constitutes a very critical period and a team of experienced anaesthetists is essential. Intense preoperative monitoring with arterial and central venous pressure lines is essential because major disturbances in blood pressure may occur despite preoperative blockade. Episodes of hypertension may occur during intubation, induction of anaesthesia, peritoneal incision and manipulation of the tumour. Such episodes can be readily managed by injections of 1–5 mg of phentolamine. Hypertensive crises are best managed with sodium nitroprusside which exerts its short-lived arterial and venous dilatation independently of α and β-adrenergic receptors. The early postoperative period may be complicated by hypotension and hypoglycaemia. Removal of the tumour is usually straightforward though the possibility of malignant spread must not be forgotten. Malignant tumours are removed if possible. If resection is incomplete then radiotherapy is given. Hypertension can be controlled with the combined α and β blocking drug labetalol. The malignant phaeochromocytomas are often very slowly growing.

Carcinoid syndrome

The clinical carcinoid syndrome occurs in about 5% of patients with carcinoid tumours and is more likely to occur with tumours arising from the ileum. For tumours arising from the gut it appears that the presence of hepatic secondaries is a necessary pre-requisite for the clinical carcinoid syndrome. This is likely to be due to the fact that the secondary tumour secrets active substances into the peripheral circulation. Carcinoid syndrome has also been described in rare extra-gut tumours, e.g. bronchus and ovary in the absence of metastases in the liver.

The appendix is the most common site for carcinoid tumours, the jejunum and rectum being the other important sites. There appears to be a strong correlation between the size of the primary tumour and the metastasis; tumours less than one centimeter rarely metastasize whereas those tumours which are above two centimeters in dia-meter are almost certainly metastatic, usually involving the regional lymph nodes and the liver.

The clinical carcinoid syndrome is due to the secretion of vasoactive and other substances from the tumour. Serotonin, 5-hydroxytryptophan, bradykinin, prostaglandins and histamine are the commonest secretory products. Symptoms include diarrhoea and abdominal cramps, broncho-constriction, right sided valvular heart disease but the commonest symptom to occur is the typical episodic cutaneous flushing. The flush usually affects the upper trunk, face and neck and may last up to ten minutes. This is generally spontaneous but triggering factors include emotion, intake of food, alcohol and mechanical stimulation of the tumour such as liver palpation. Cardiac lesions, in particular tricuspid regurgitation, occurs in about a third of patients although pulmonary stenosis is not uncommon. The involvement of the heart is due to the presence of the carcinoid plaque which consists of smooth muscle cells, reticulum fibres and mucopolysaccharides. The aetiology of this lesion is unknown. Bronchoconstriction occurs in about a fifth of patients. An important practical point is not to use sympathomimetic amines for treatment as these agents can lead to increased release of chemical mediators from the tumour.

A useful diagnostic measure is by urine analysis for 5-hydroxyindole acetic acid (5HIAA, normal 2–9 mg/24 hours) which is the major excretory end-product of the tryptophan/serotonin pathway. Imaging techniques also help to confirm the diagnosis.

Many pharmacological agents such as anti-serotonin drugs, aprotinin, steroids, adrenergic blockers, antihistamines have been advocated without success prior to operation. Surgical removal of the tumour may be hazardous because of profound hypotension secondary to the stress response releasing chemical mediators by the tumour. Hepatic artery occlusion has been used in some patients. Chemotherapy with agents such as 5 fluorouracil and adriamycin has been singularly disappointing. For long term therapy perhaps the somatostatin analogues currently on trial may prove more successful.

Further reading

Besser, G.M. and Cudworth, A.G. (Eds). (1987). *Clinical Endocrinology – An Illustrated Text.* Chapman and Hall, London.

Ellenberg, M. and Rifkin, H. (Eds). (1983). *Diabetes Mellitus – Theory and Practice.* Third Edition. Medical Examination Publishing, New York.

Felig, P., Baxter, J.D., Broadus, A.E. and Frohman, L.A. (Eds). (1981). *Endocrinology and Metabolism.* McGraw-Hill, New York.

Keen, H. and Jarrett, J. (Eds). (1982). *Complications of Diabetes.* Second Edition. Edward Arnold, London.

Marble, A., Krall, L.P., Bradley, R.F., Christheb, A.R. and Soeldner, J.S. (Eds). (1985). *Joslin's Diabetes Mellitus.* Twelfth Edition. Lea and Febiger, Philadelphia.

Taylor, K.G. (Ed). (1987). *Diabetes and the Heart.* Castle House Publications, Tunbridge Wells.

Wilson, J.D. and Foster, D.W. (Eds). (1985). *William Textbook of Endocrinology.* Seventh Edition. W.B. Saunders, Philadelphia.

5
Neurology

Peter Bradbury

Introduction

Medical students and qualified practitioners are often intimidated by neurology and the 'neurological patient'. Whilst the complexities of function and integration of any system with an estimated 10–50 billion operational sub-units (neurones) may well defy comprehension, in clinical practice careful history taking and methodical, rather than exhaustive, techniques of examination will usually allow the examiner to localize the neurological lesion(s) and reach a sensible differential diagnosis. The clinical observations and deductive reasoning of the great neurologists (Charcot, Friedreich, Jackson and others) have to a large extent stood the test of time; however, the advent of the newer technologies of neuroradiology, magnetic resonance imaging, neurophysiology and neuropharmacology have greatly increased our understanding of the nervous system, both in sickness and health. Furthermore, these techniques have greatly facilitated the ease of diagnosis of many neurological conditions, and have allowed a steady decrease in the morbidity associated with previous invasive techniques of investigation.

As with other branches of medicine, the effective diagnosis and management of the neurological case depends to a great extent on the doctor's ability to communicate with and elicit information from the patient. All too often a misunderstood question or imprecise instruction will lead to errors in the interpretation of a subtle history or sign and in turn lead to inappropriate management.

History taking and examination

A complete account of the complexities of neurological examination is beyond the scope of this chapter. However, the taking of a careful history, both from the patient, family and any suitable witnesses may well indicate a specific diagnosis in the neurological patient.

This chapter attempts to indicate some of the potential pit-falls in assessing the neurological patient.

History taking

In neurology perhaps more than any other speciality, the subtleties and nuances of the patient's history are likely to help in differentiating between common presenting features or symptoms (for example funny turns or headaches). Great care must be taken to avoid the confusion that may arise from the patient's use of common terms or expressions such as 'numbness' (the term numbness may be used to describe anaesthesia, dysaesthesia, paraesthesia or even pure motor weakness). In assessing the history, account must be taken of the patient's cultural, educational and occupational background. Many seemingly more sophisticated patients may offer half rationalized symptoms, or use inappropriate jargon in describing their problems.

Socio-economic factors may not only be relevant in making a diagnosis, but may be of profound importance once that diagnosis is reached – for example, the diagnosis of epilepsy may have completely different implications for the livelihood of a bus driver as compared to that of a home-based freelance graphic designer. Furthermore, whilst many patients may have no recall for major or minor fits, others, aware of the medico-legal implications of the diagnosis, may alter their accounts or even lie when giving their history. In such situations a witness account may be invaluable.

When considering the history offered by the patient, the interviewer must remember that the patient may be confabulating. Whilst obvious nonsensical confabulation may rapidly alert the examiner, when offered by a charming socially articulate dement, the history may seem eminently, if transiently, plausible.

Patients may be reluctant to declare certain symptoms for fear of seeming stupid or, at worst, mad. The highly variable presenting symptomatology associated with temporal lobe epilepsy may dissuade the patient from portraying his symptoms to the doctor e.g. attacks of irrational fear or the hearing of disembodied voices.

Even with the most assiduous care in history taking, the causal sequence of events associated with a symptom or attack may remain unclear – for example a vasovagal attack may lead to a secondary hypoxaemic fit, or an epileptic attack may be preceded by palpitations or epigastic discomfort.

Neurological examination

No attempt will be made here to detail the intricacies of a complete neurological examination. The reader is directed to the excellent accounts in Brain (1978) and Patten (1977). However, certain common pit-falls can be avoided with a little effort:

- The neurological examination begins as the patient walks into the consulting room, or as the doctor approaches the bedside. The loss of arm swing on one side, the scuffing of one shoe front or the food-stained city suit, may all provide valuable clues as to the underlying disorders (hemi-Parkinsonism, spastic hemiparesis and dementia respectively). Conversely apparently obvious signs may be misleading (for example in polyglots, cerebral insults of various kinds may cause the patient to return to their first language. The author has diagnosed severe expressive dysphasias in patients speaking perfect Polish and Welsh!). Furthermore, whilst some changes in higher intellectual function and motor performance may be clear and sustained, others may be transient, forgotten by the patient or potentially misleading (for example postictal confusional states or Todd's pareses).
- A full assessment of higher intellectual function is impossible in the clinic or at the bedside. Whilst some impression of intellect and learning will be gained from the history, bedside tests of cognitive function may be misleading, as for example in the case of a demented chartered accountant who remained able to perform 'serial 7's' rapidly, even in the presence of severe Alzheimer's disease.
- The neurological examination must be interpreted in the light of the findings on general examination, be it in the stroke patient with previous rheumatic heart disease, or in the severely cachetic individual presenting with glove and stocking sensory loss suggestive of a non-metastatic peripheral neuropathy.
- In the neurological examination it is possible to obtain some objective assessment of the motor system and reflexes. However, sensory testing may be extremely difficult to interpret as the examiner is largely dependent upon the subjective reporting of the patient. It is important that patients understand the nature of any stimulus that is to be applied, and, that not only are they expected to report if they feel the stimulus, but also whether they perceive the stimulus as being of a similar nature at all sites. However, a brisk routine sensory examination including assessment of fine touch, pain, vibration, joint position and temperature senses may localize a neurological lesion. Remember that *subjective* sensory changes may well be significant, (for example pin prick sensation may be detected on both sides of the body, but associated with dysaesthesiae on the affected side).

Diseases of the nervous system

Epilepsy

Many patients present to the neurological clinic complaining of 'funny turns' or episodes of loss of consciousness. In either case it is important, wherever possible, to obtain a witness account of the attacks. In many cases the primary problem is the differentiation between epilepsy and syncope. In some cases the diagnosis may be straight-forward, for example when the patient falls to the ground without warning and proceeds to a tonic/clonic grand mal seizure with tongue biting and incontinence. However, fainting with a full bladder may lead to incontinence. Syncopal attacks are often preceded by feelings of weakness, dizziness, nausea and sweating. The patient usually sinks to the ground and seldom injures himself. He may be observed to be pale, and his pulse to be of small volume or impalpable.

The concept of the epilepsies as recurrent disorders resulting from abnormal neuronal discharges within the central nervous system was proposed by J Hughlings Jackson over 100 years ago. However, it should always be remembered that epilepsy is in itself a symptom and not a disease, and that it may reflect congenital or acquired neuronal dysfunction, or may be secondary to systemic metabolic disorders or other structural brain disease.

The incidence of epilepsy shows two peaks, firstly in childhood and secondly after the age of 40. The average annual incidence rate for seizures starting over the age of 20 is approximately 15–18/100 000 population. However, between the ages of 60–75 years this rises to 40–80/100 000 population. A prevalence rate of 3.3/1000 of the total population has been determined in England. The incidence of idiopathic grand mal epilepsy decreases with age in contrast to the rise in secondary attacks in the elderly. (There is five times the expected incidence of epileptic seizures [2.7 per cent of the population] in near relatives of patients suffering from epilepsy).

The electrophysiological stability of neurones is dependant upon the physical and chemical structure of their cell membranes.

An epileptic fit results from the abnormal paroxysmal discharge of cerebral neurones. The nature of the attack resulting from such a discharge depends upon its site and any spread to surrounding brain. The commonest form of fit is the partial seizure. This may be

- simple – without the impairment of consciousness, (including Jacksonian, temporal lobe and psychomotor attacks);
- complex—with impairment of consciousness, or;
- may become secondarily generalized.

Generalized seizures may be grand mal convulsions, absences (petit mal in children), myoclonic episodes, or tonic and akinetic attacks. Secondary epilepsy, whether due to metabolic disturbance or structural brain disease may show a picture of focal or generalized attacks or a mixture of both. A list of metabolic disorders associated with epilepsy is shown in Table 5.1.

Almost any structural abnormality in the brain may act as an epileptogenic focus. Truly inherited

Table 5.1   Metabolic disorders associated with epilepsy

Hyper- and hypoglycaemia
Hypocalcaemia
Hypomagnesaemia
Uraemia

forms of epilepsy are extremely rare, however an increased incidence amongst first degree relatives is recognized. In the new born, cerebral birth injury and developmental abnormalities of the brain are the most common associations wtih the onset of epilepsy. In later life cerebral tumours (both primary and secondary), cerebrovascular disease and the degenerative disorders are increasingly common causes of epilepsy. At any age, intracranial infection, cerebrovascular accident or head trauma may be followed by the onset of epilepsy. Similarly seizures at any age may be associated with the use of drugs, both therapeutic and illicit (Table 5.2).

Table 5.2   Drugs associated with epileptic fits

Alcohol
Anticonvulsants
Antidepressants
Amphetamines
Barbiturates

It may be that, when the patient is first seen, the diagnosis of epilepsy is apparent from the description of the attack. However, the differential diagnosis of 'funny turns' is wide (Table 5.3), and in a significant proportion of cases it remains impossible to confirm a diagnosis of suspected epilepsy either clinically or after investigation.

Table 5.3   Differential diagnosis of funny turns

Fits (major and minor)
Syncope
Cardiac arrythmias (tachy and bradycardias)
Metabolic disorders (e.g. hypoglycaemia)
Panic attacks
Drop attacks in the elderly
TIAs

Investigation of epilepsy

Causes of secondary epilepsy are numerous, and initial assessment of the patient should include full blood count, ESR, biochemical screening (including liver function tests and calcium studies) and syphilis serology. A chest X-ray should be performed to exclude infective or neoplastic lesions, particularly in the elderly. Routine 12-lead electrocardiography and 24-hour ECG ambulatory monitoring may be helpful in the detection of syncopal atacks secondary to cardiac lesions and arrhythmias.

An EEG may be useful in demonstrating paroxysmal activity or other changes suggestive of underlying epilepsy: however, it should be borne in mind that up to 40 per cent of interictal EEGs in patients with undoubted epilepsy show no epileptic activity. Twenty-four hour EEG monitoring may provide useful further evidence for or against the diagnosis of epilepsy, as may the technique of telemetry in which a video recording of the patient is made over a set period whilst his EEG is simultaneously recorded, allowing the potential correlation of clinical events with changes in the EEG. Photic stimulation, sleep recording, sleep deprivation and short acting barbiturate (e.g. methohexitone) administration may be employed to enhance the detection of epileptic abnormalities on EEG study.

CT scanning may reveal structural abnormalities such as tumours, infarcts, abscesses or degenerative changes. The detection of such lesions is higher in those patients with focal EEG abnormalities; however, only a small percentage of such lesions will be either potentially treatable by surgery or will result in alteration in the management of the patient's epilepsy.

Treatment of epilepsy

In considering the treatment of epilepsy the first decision to take is as to whether the patient's seizures are of a severity and frequency to require any active intervention. It would seem reasonable to treat children, as there is now evidence that seizures in childhood may predispose individuals to epilepsy in later life. However, only a small proportion of children suffering from febrile convulsions continue to have fits in later life. Having decided to treat a patient, it should be remembered that polypharmacy only rarely has any advantage over monotherapy. The drugs of choice in the management of both major and partial seizures are phenytoin (100–600 mg *nocte*) and carbamazepine (100 mg bd–600 mg t.d.s.). Whilst phenobarbitone and mysoline are highly

effective anticonvulsants, both tend to be associated with sedation, and may cause behavioural problems in both young and old. Sodium valproate would seem to be effective in major epilepsy, but less so for minor attacks (dosage 600 mg–2.5 g daily in divided doses). (However, in petit mal sodium valproate is the drug of choice, although ethosuximide remains an effective alternative).

At the start of treatment it should be explained to the patient that it may not prove possible to abolish the fits completely, only to decrease the frequency of attacks. Routine monitoring of drug levels is not appropriate; however when control of attacks worsens the estimation of serum anticonvulsant levels may firstly, allow the detection of toxicity (which may be associated with an increase in frequency of seizures), secondly, indicate poor compliance, and thirdly, give an indication as to any possible change in drug therapy. It should be remembered that there are many interactions between anticonvulsants and other drugs. It is particularly important to advise young women on the contraceptive pill that they should be on 'high' rather than 'low dose' preparations. Some phenytoin treated patients may become intolerant of alcohol. Conversely, chronic alcohol ingestion may lead to a reduction in serum phenytoin level. Many patients find that they are more likely to have a fit the morning after a night of high alcohol ingestion.

Female patients of child-bearing age must be warned that there is a slight increase in the incidence of minor congenital abnormalities in patients on anticonvulsant drug therapy. Whenever possible, patients are withdrawn from their anticonvulsant therapy during pregnancy; however, often both patient and baby may be more at risk from frequent seizures than from the minor teratogenic risks of continued anticonvulsant therapy. Carbamazepine may be the safest anticonvulsant to use in pregnancy.

Phenytoin has other unsatisfactory side-effects in some patients. Acne and hirsutism are a particular problem in women, whilst gingival hyperplasia may be a source of embarrassment to both sexes. In cases where phenytoin seems to provide satisfactory control, rather than change drugs, it is often advisable to refer the patient to their dental surgeon for treatment of their gum hypertrophy. Long-term administration of phenytoin may be associated with some coarsening of facial features.

Idiosyncratic reactions occur to all anti-convulsant drugs, varying in severity from mild skin rashes to severe liver dysfunction. All anti-convulsants may induce a degree of sedation. Phenytoin toxicity usually presents with a picture of cerebellar ataxia, dysarthria and nystagmus, but these features may be seen with poisoning from other anticonvulsants.

Status epilepticus

Somewhat surprisingly, patients with the various forms of epilepsy rarely injure themselves severely. Status epilepticus, however, is a life-threatening condition. 'Status' must be differentiated from 'serial' epilepsy. Patients are often referred to hospital having had numerous attacks in the course of a few hours, but having regained consciousness between the attacks – this constitutes serial epilepsy. In status epilepticus, the patient may have numerous attacks, or be in a continuous seizure without regaining consciousness. An EEG will show continual epileptic activity. On admission to hospital in status epilepticus, it may be worth a trial of 10 mg diazepam given intravenously. Facilities for cardiopulmonary resuscitation must be available if this approach is tried. It is usually not worth repeating the dose if the first bolus is unsuccessful in controlling the attacks, further injections tending only to cause respiratory depression without improvement in the epilepsy. Status may be brought under control by the use of infusions of chlormethiazole (0.7 g/hour i.v. not more than 50 mg/minute i.v. with ECG control) or phenytoin. Whilst unpleasant to use, paraldehyde may be highly effective in gaining control of the seizures. In severe cases, the patient may need to be paralysed and ventilated during administration of thiopentone and a muscle relaxant. Status epilepticus remains a potentially lethal condition.

The aim of any anti-epileptic treatment regime must be the control of seizures in the absence of systemic or neurological toxicity. For several decades there has been controversy as to whether drug resistant complex partial seizures might be affected by cortectomy or lobectomy. Clearly any proposed neurosurgical procedures should only be carried out without undue risk to life and without producing serious neurological deficits. The criteria for selection for neurosurgical treatment of epilepsy are not clearly defined at present, but it would seem most appropriate in those patients with a clear temporal lobe focus associated with mesial temporal sclerosis.

Socio-economic complications of epilepsy

Whilst in many cases it is possible to get complete or at least satisfactory control of seizures, the diagnosis of epilepsy may have profound implications for the patient with regard to his family and his livelihood. Any patient who is diagnosed as suffering from epilepsy must be instructed by his doctor that he is not eligible to drive for the time being and that he must inform the Driving Vehicle Licensing Centre (DVLC) of this as soon as possible. The British regulations at present state that the patient must be fit-free for a period of 2 years, or only have had nocturnal seizures for a period of 3 years before the DVLC may consider whether they can drive again. No patient can hold a heavy good vehicle (HGV) or public service vehicle (PSV) licence after a fit of any kind above the age of 50 years.

Whilst patients with epilepsy should be encouraged to lead as normal a life as possible, a fair measure of common sense must be applied about the potential risks of indulging in dangerous sports such as rock climbing or parachute jumping, and workers may be in particular danger if they use heavy equipment or cutting gear. Female patients of child bearing age should be advised that the taking of anticonvulsant drugs decreases the effectiveness of the contraceptive pill (due to hepatic enzyme induction) and that they should not be on low-dose preparations.

Headache

Headache is one of the commonest presenting symptoms in neurology. Whilst in the majority of cases a careful history and examination will reveal the nature of the headache, in many cases further investigation, particularly plain radiology and/or CT scanning are required in order to reassure both patient and physician. It should not be forgotten that headache may be symptomatic not only of intracranial disease, but also of disorders of the neck, sinuses, teeth, eyes and psyche. Of particular importance are those pains secondary to diseases of the eye and optic nerve. In the older age group ocular pain may be associated with glaucoma, and patients in whom this is suspected should be referred to the ophthalmologists as a matter of urgency. Similarly, in patients of 50 years or more the diagnosis of giant cell arteritis should not be forgotten as, although it is readily excluded by the finding of a normal ESR and if undetected patients may experience the sudden, onset of uniocular or binocular blindness, stroke or myocardial infarction.

Tension headache

Nuchal, frontal, temporal or occipital muscle contraction probably represents the commonest cause of headache. Typically patients describe a constant band-like ache or tight cap over the skull. The pain may be made worse by emotional stress or strain. It is often worse in the evening, but does not usually prevent sleep. Examination reveals no abnormality, although there may be some tenderness over the scalp and neck.

The management of tension headaches is frequently difficult and leads to much patient dissatisfaction. Often the triggers to these headaches are sources of stress in the patient's life which they are unable or unwilling to alter. Many will find temporary relief in analgesics such as aspirin or paracetamol. In those cases where a clear depressive component is identifiable, specific antidepressant therapy may be useful. In some individuals relaxation therapy classes, acupuncture or yoga may be appropriate.

Migraine

Migraine may be defined as recurrent attacks of headache, commonly unilateral in onset, usually associated with anorexia and sometimes with nausea and vomiting. Some may be preceded or associated with visual, sensory, motor or emotional disturbance. There is often a positive family history.

Migraine may begin at any time of life, but its onset is less common after middle-age. It has been suggested that up to 19 per cent of men and 29 per cent of women will experience migrainous headaches at some time: however the epidemiology is difficult to interpret in view of the wide range of definitions offered for migraine.

The aetiology of migraine is unknown, but the alternative description, vascular headache, would seem wholly appropriate. The aura experienced by some patients is due to focal cerebral ischaemia associated with intracranial vasoconstriction. The development of the headache would seem to be related to extracerebral vasodilatation. In many patients there are clearly identifiable trigger factors (Table 5.4).

Table 5.4 Common trigger factors in migraine

Stress
Relaxation after stress
Head injury
Menstrual cycle
Food (cheese, oranges, chocolate, wine, etc)
Menopause

Classical migraine

In classical migraine the development of lateralized headache is preceded by an aura which may be visual, taking the form of positive scintillations or fortification spectra, or negative scotomata or field defects. Some patients may experience paraethesiae and numbness in the limbs or face prior to the onset of headache. The visual aura usually lasts between 15 and 45 minutes, and is usually followed by the development of a unilateral headache. Whilst patients may describe their headache as typically occurring on either the right or the left side of the head, should a patient report that he or she *never* experiences pain on the other side, then they should be investigated further. The development of the headache is often associated with nausea, vomiting, photophobia and facial pallor. The duration of attacks may vary considerably, but patients often report a duration of up to a week.

Management

Many patients find that the routine use of analgesics is of no benefit at all once the headache is established. Wherever possible they should avoid identifiable trigger factors. Patients often report that their headache is relieved if they manage to sleep for a period of time. In severe attacks, it may be possible to provide relief with a cocktail of drugs such as codeine phosphate, diazepam and an antiemetic. In patients troubled by frequent and severe attacks, ergotamine may be extremely useful, particularly if used during the aura. Ergotamine may be administered by inhaler, injection or suppository. Patients should be advised that they should not use total doses greater than 12 mg per week in view of the risk of limb gangrene. Ergotamine preparations are not appropriate in patients with hemisensory or hemiplegic symptoms before or during their attacks.

Prophylaxis

The prophylaxis of migraine often requires changes in the patient's life-style, particularly either with regard to their diet or work and home stress. However, many people cannot alter their life pattern, and patients with severe and frequent attacks of migraine may demand further help. The most commonly used prophylactic drugs are propranolol, pizotifen and clonidine. In very severe cases methysergide may be used for periods of up to 3 months. Longer periods of treatment with methysergide may result in the development of retro-peritoneal fibrosis.

Common migraine

Although classical migraine constitutes the most recognisable form of vascular headache, the majority of patients suffer from common migraine. Typically in these attacks, the headache is not preceded by an aura and is not usually localized. There is often associated nausea and vomiting.

Rarer forms of vascular headache

Hemiplegic migraine Hemiplegic migraine is characterized by the development of hemisensory, or, less often, hemiplegic weakness at the onset or during the headache. Such patients need further investigation including a CT scan. Hemiplegic migraine is usually worthy of prophylactic treatment, as whilst the hemisensory or hemiplegic picture usually resolves after the headache, on occasion, permanent deficits result (which on CT scanning have been shown to be due to cerebral infarction).

Basilar migraine In basilar migraine patients may suddenly lose consciousness without epileptic features. They may also complain of inco-ordination, bilateral sensory disturbances, dizziness and double vision.

Migraine equivalents Migrainous aura may occur without the subsequent development of headache or vomiting – these are termed migraine equivalents.

Migrainous neuralgia Migrainous neuralgia or cluster headache is a particular distressing form of pain, which shows a male/female ratio of approximately 6:1. Typically the patient develops a severe pain around one eye, which may radiate to the forehead, cheek and temple. It may occur at a similar time of day or night for several weeks. Associated with the headache, there may be conjunctival injection, nasal stuffiness, lacrimation, facial flushing, partial ptosis and miosis. Attacks may be provoked by the ingestion of alcohol. This particularly distressing form of vascular headache warrants active treatment, as the recurrent episodes of pain may lead to suicide. Standard anti-migrainous preparations such as propranolol and methysergide may be useful in preventing clusters ocurring. However, resistant cases may require treatment with corticosteroids or lithium carbonate.

Trigeminal neuralgia

Trigeminal neuralgia usually presents over the age of 50, in females more than males. The typical pain is lancinating in nature, and may occur in any or all divisions of the trigeminal nerve on one side. Common triggers reported by patients include wind on the face, talking, smiling, laughing, chewing, washing, brushing teeth, shaving and most commonly, touching trigger points in the distribution of the pain.

Examination is usually normal, although specific trigger points may be discovered in the course of the examination.

Posterior fossa lesions and multiple sclerosis may cause trigeminal neuralgia, but in the majority of cases no cause is found. Recently it has been suggested that many idiopathic cases may be secondary to irritation of the trigeminal nerve near the pons by tortuous branches of the superior cerebellar artery.

The treatment of choice in trigeminal neuralgia is carbamazepine (initally 100 mg b.d.) which may be steadily increased until symptoms are controlled or side-effects develop (up to 1.8 g daily). Alternative but usually less effective treatments are phenytoin, clonazepam and baclofen. Surgery or injection of the nerve may be necessary in intractable cases.

Post-herpetic neuralgia

The trigeminal nerve is a common site for shingle infections due to herpes zoster, and such attacks are often followed by prolonged and agonising post herpetic neuralgia. Although many cases do slowly improve with time, many patients become desperate for pain relief. As routine analgesics are usually ineffectual in this condition, it is often useful to attempt treatment with antidepressants (e.g. amitriptyline 50 mg nocte increasing as required). Neurosurgical intervention may be helpful.

Atypical facial pain

Atypical facial pain has often been a 'dustbin' diagnosis for patients in whom careful examination and investigation have failed to identify a cause for chronic facial pain. Often these patients have been seen in numerous surgeries and clinics without gaining relief from their symptoms. The patients are often depressed, and their pain frequently labelled as psychogenic; however, it is interesting to note how frequently there is a history of dental manipulation prior to the onset of the original pain. Patients often obtain a measure of relief from anti-depressant therapy.

Glossopharyngeal neuralgia

Glossopharyngeal neuralgia shares many characteristics with trigeminal neuralgia, but is considerably rarer. The pain is usually triggered by swallowing or coughing, and often responds to carbamazepine.

Headache due to cranial infection or inflammation

Giant cell arteritis

Giant cell arteritis should be excluded in all patients presenting with headaches over the age of 50. Patients often complain of severe generalized pain, but may also describe specific scalp tenderness and pain in the jaw on chewing (jaw claudication). In some unfortunate patients, the first indication of this condition may be the sudden onset of unilateral or bilateral blindness. There may be a history suggestive of polymyalgia rheumatica.

The condition can be rapidly excluded or suggested by the estimation of the ESR. Temporal artery biopsy may reveal typical changes of giant cell arteritis: however, the institution of corticosteroid therapy should not be deferred pending biopsy as the patient could be rendered blind at any time if untreated. Temporal artery biopsies often show no specific abnormalities as there are frequently 'skip' lesions along the lengths of the arteries.

Treatment with high dose corticosteroid should be started immediately the diagnosis is suspected. Patients often describe a diagnostically significant relief of pain within hours of the institution of steroid therapy.

Intracranial infection

Features of meningeal irritation, whether secondary to the chemical meningitis following a subarachnoid haemorrhage or due to bacterial or viral meningitis are similar, i.e., neck stiffness and photophobia. It is now desirable to perform a CT scan of the head prior to lumbar puncture wherever this will not significantly delay the further management of the patient. Should the patient describe focal symptoms or demonstrate focal neurological signs on examination, then a CT scan is mandatory to exclude space occupying lesions and raised intracranial pressure prior to lumbar puncture. Patients continue to die as a result of inappropriate lumbar punctures being performed in the presence of raised intracranial pressure.

Post lumbar puncture headache

This low pressure headache may follow lumbar puncture. It is treated by bedrest, simple analgesics (especially codeine phosphate) and time. This complication would seem less likely to occur if a small gauge needle is used for lumbar puncture.

Raised intracranial pressure

Headache, papilloedema and vomiting are classic features of raised intracranial pressure: however, the relative severity of these varies greatly. Many patients presenting with headache fear the presence of a brain tumour and may in consequence develop further muscle tension headache or migraine. In raised intracranial pressure, the headache is often present on waking, may be worse on lying down and may be intensified by exertion or straining. None of these features, however, are exclusive to raised intracranial pressure. The presence of cranial nerve signs, especially third and sixth nerve palsies may be useful indications of intracranial masses, but may be 'false localizing signs'.

Multiple sclerosis

Multiple sclerosis is the commonest potentially disabling disease of young adults in the United

Kingdom. It demonstrates a peak age of onset of around 30 years, cases under the age of 10 being rare, and the incidence declining after the age of 45. Multiple sclerosis (MS) affects women compared to men in a ratio of 3:2. It is a disease of temperate climates, the prevalence being low in the tropics. In the United Kingdom, the prevalence ranges between 50–80/100 000 in England, climbing to 300/100 000 in the Shetlands and Orkneys.

The characteristic lesion in multiple sclerosis is destruction of myelin in the CNS leaving axons intact. The most characteristically affected sites are the periventricular structures, optic nerves, brainstem and cervical spinal cord. In a typical case, the lesions are disseminated both in the central nervous system and in time.

Clinical features

In the majority of patients, the onset is at one site, the most typical presentations being:

- optic neuritis
- lower limb weakness
- sensory disturbance affecting the trunk and limbs and
- brainstem symptoms including ataxia and diplopia.

Many patients present with a history of visual disturbance in one eye, which may vary between slight blurring to no perception of light. On examination there may be a marked reduction in visual acuity associated with a central scotoma. Fundoscopy may appear normal, or there may be swelling of the disc or optic atrophy.

Typically vision begins to improve within a few days to a few weeks. It is impossible to predict the level of recovery in any particular attack, although usually patients will comment that their vision has returned to normal.

Spinal cord lesions

Plaques of demyelination in the spinal cord may result in upper motor neurone lesions affecting the limbs and/or alteration in sensation (which may be dissociated) in the limbs or trunk. In cervical cord lesions patients may describe a feeling 'like an electric shock' passing down the back and into the limbs on flexing the neck. Lhermitte's sign however, is not pathognomonic of MS, but may occur in association with other abnormalities of the cervical cord.

Brainstem lesions

The involvement of the brainstem may result in diplopia, ataxia, sensory disturbance over the face and tongue, and dysarthria. Patients may present with a picture of trigeminal neuralgia.

Natural history

In approximately two-thirds of patients with MS the disease will take a relapsing/remitting form, whilst in the remaining third it is progressive without remission. Although it can be stated that there is a mean relapse rate of approximately one attack every 2 years, the disease behaves in a highly individual way in different patients, and clusters of attacks may be followed by long periods in remission. However, in general terms the younger the onset and the more frequent the attacks, the greater the likelihood of significant residual neurological deficit. Some patients with the relapsing/remitting form of MS may later develop the chronic progressive form. After 10–15 years, many patients will show a spastic paraplegia of variable severity associated with some disturbance of micturition. Impotence in men is common and may be the presenting symptom of MS. There may be dysarthria, ataxia and nystagmus. Optic atrophy may be seen on fundoscopy as evidence of previous clinical or sub-clinical retrobulbar neuritis.

In many earlier texts euphoria was described as the characteristic mental change seen in patients with MS. In fact, many patients with MS are clearly depressed. A picture of euphoria is only usually seen in those patients who have become demented and have lost insight into their condition.

Severely disabled patients may die of hypostatic pneumonia or urinary tract infections. Rarely, plagues may effect the vital centres in the brainstem leading to respiratory failure.

Whilst the severe cases of MS are conspicuous both to the general public and doctors, many mildly affected patients do not present at the surgery or clinic. In view of this fact, the epidemiology of multiple sclerosis is sometimes difficult to interpret. Most neurological clinics will have on their lists patients with undoubted multiple sclerosis who, after 20 years or more, show little or nothing in the way of residual disability. At the time of initial diagnosis, there would seem to be no specific indicators as to the prognosis of the disease in any indiviual patient.

Investigation

There is no specific diagnostic test for multiple sclerosis. In recent years the development of visually evoked, brainstem and somatosensory evoked potentials has allowed the diagnosis of often unsuspected demyelinated lesions in optic nerves, brainstem and spinal cord. In those patients, particularly middle-aged and older, who present with a picture of a spinal cord lesion, a myelogram is often the only way to exclude a compressive lesion. Examination of the spinal fluid may show an increase in total protein, an increase in the IgG as a proportion of the total CSF protein, and/or an increase in lymphocytes up to 50 × 10⁶/litre. Electrophoresis of the CSF may reveal oligoclonal bands in more than 95 per cent of patients. CT scanning may reveal intracranial lesions, which when first seen may be indistinguishable from secondary deposits. The most typical CT change is of low attenuation at the tips of the lateral ventricles. The advent of magnetic resonance scanning has allowed the detection of clinically silent plaques in patients, in whom the diagnosis is unclear.

Whilst the cause of MS remains unclear, it would seem that the incidence is increased in patients with certain HLA types (particularly DRW2 in the UK).

Differential diagnosis

Whilst multiple sclerosis is clearly the commonest cause of multiple neurological lesions in young adults, other rarer causes should be considered including: neurosarcoid, neurosyphilis, Behçet's disease, SLE, polyarthritis nodosa, multiple emboli and multiple secondaries.

Treatment

There is no specific treatment for MS.

Steroid therapy

Steroid therapy either as prednisolone, dexamethasone or ACTH may shorten the duration of an acute relapse: however, the use of steroids does not effect the degree of recovery or the extent of any residual disability.

Immunosuppression

Several authorities have claimed that the use of immunosuppresant drugs confers some protection from relapse in MS and may also slow down the rate of deterioration in those patients with the chronic progressive form of the disease. Cyclophosphamide and azathioprine have been used, both requiring frequent checks of the full blood count and liver function tests.

Diet

Whilst numerous diets have been proposed in the management of MS, there is no evidence from controlled trials to indicate that any one diet gives particular advantage.

Hyperbaric oxygen

Unfortunately the recent enthusiasm for hyperbaric oxygen treatment has proved unjustified, and controlled trials have shown no benefit to patients.

Anaesthesia

There is no evidence that anaesthesia or surgery precipitates relapses of MS.

Pregnancy

There would seem to be a slightly increased risk of relapse in the puerperium.

Brain tumours

The incidence of brain tumours in the United Kingdom is approximately 5 per 100 000 population per year. In children, 70 per cent of intracranial neoplasms occur below the tentorium cerebellae, but in adults most arise above the tentorium. Primary intracranial tumours are found in approximately 1 per cent of post mortems. A break down of the most commonly occurring intracranial tumours is shown in Table 5.5.

Table 5.5 Common brain tumors

Gliomas	47 %
Meningiomas	19 %
Pituitary	10 %
Schwannomas	9 %
Congenital	5 %
Vascular	5 %
Metastatic	5 + %

Presentation

Brain tumours may present:

- with an increase in intracranial pressure
- as a result of focal neurological deficit or
- with generalized, focal or partial epilepsy.

Slow growing tumours such as meningiomas may grow to a considerable size before producing any symptoms at all.

Gliomas

Gliomas constitute the commonest type of intracranial tumour, their behaviour depending upon their degree of histological differentiation (grade I indicating highly differentiated tumours and grade IV highly malignant tumours consisting of poorly differentiated cells). The apendymomas and medulloblastomas found in children usually in the posterior fossa, are both highly malignant, the former metastasizing throughout the ventricular system and the latter spreading both within and without the central nervous system.

Meningiomas

Intracranial meningiomas are commonly situated along the major dural venous sinuses but may also arise from the falx and tentorium. The peak incidence is between 40 and 50 years of age. Although usually histologically benign, they are often large at the time of presentation, and there is a significant morbidity associated with their removal.

Pituitary tumours

Most pituitary tumours are histologically benign. Patients may present with symptoms and signs resulting from reduced pituitary hormone secretion (decreased libido, amenorrhoea, weight gain, intolerance of cold, reduction in body hair) or with symptoms secondary to enlargement of the tumour within and outside the pituitary fossa (headache, bitemporal hemianopias). Patients may also present with symptoms secondary to increased hormone secretion from the pituitary (amenorrhoea and galactorrhoea in prolactin secreting tumours, and gigantism and acromegaly in growth hormone secreting tumours).

Management

Well differentiated gliomas and some meningiomas may require intervention beyond symptomatic treatment of resulting epilepsy. Some authorities have recommended radical surgery in combination with chemo- and radiotherapy in the management of gliomas, but there is little evidence that this approach significantly enhances or prolongs life. Although usually histologically benign, the resection of large meningiomas is often complicated by the development of serious neurological deficits thought to be due to infarction. Transcranial or trans-sphenoidal surgical approaches are employed for the removal of pituitary tumours. Whilst bromocriptine may be highly effective in the management of prolactin secreting adenomas, large or rapidly increasing visual field defects are an indication for surgery.

Movement disorders

Parkinson's disease

James Parkinson's essay on the shaking palsy was first published in 1817. Advanced cases of this slowly progressive degenerative disease of the basal ganglia are characterized by resting tremor, bradykinesia, paucity of voluntary movement and rigidity. Over the age of 65 the disease would seem to affect approximately 1 per cent of the population. (Above the age of 85 the figure rises to 2.6 per cent of the population). Men are more commonly affected than women in a ratio of 3:2. The aetiology of the condition remains unknown, but there would seem to be no clear genetic inheritance. In recent years viral and auto-toxic agents have been proposed as significant factors in the development of the disease, but in contrast to the clear viral aetiology of postencephalitic Parkinsonism in the 1920s, the cause of idiopathic Parkinson's disease remains unclear. The condition would seem to be less frequent amongst tobacco smokers.

On neuropathological examination the most striking changes seen in this condition are loss of the pigmented neurones in the substantia nigra, and the presence of eosinophilic inclusion bodies (Lewy bodies) and neuro fibrillary tangles. Whilst neuropharmacological studies, and more recently the use of Positron Emission Tomography (PET) scanning have clearly demonstrated a significant decrease in dopamine within the cells of the basal ganglia, levels of noradrenaline, 5-hydroxy-tryptamine, and gamma-aminobutyric acid are also altered. The significance of these changes is poorly understood at present.

Clinical features

In its early stages, Parkinson's disease may be extremely difficult to diagnose. Patients may offer vague symptoms, such as fatigue, or depression which may be misleading. The most characteristic onset is with a unilateral resting tremor.

The full blown clinical picture of Parkinson's disease usually offers no problems in diagnosis. The typical resting tremor may not only affect the hands and upper limbs, but also the legs, jaw and tongue. In addition to the lead-pipe rigidity found when examining the limbs, there may also be cog-wheeling rigidity, most often present at the wrists. Although tremor may be the most apparent and often the most distressing feature of the condition leading to considerable embarrassment for the patient, the most disabling features are the difficulty in initiating movement (bradykinesia) and rigidity. In addition to the classic diagnostic triad of tremor, rigidity and bradykinesia, other common features are a flexed posture, impassive parkinsonian facies, seborrhoaeic skin and a rapid and short paced (festinant) gait. There may be a positive glabella tap on examination. Although the disease tends to be slowly progressive, patients may describe marked diurnal variations in their performance at presentation.

The differential diagnosis of idiopathic Parkinson's disease is shown in Table 5.6. Of particular relevance are the postencephalitic and drug-induced parkinsonian syndromes. Atheromatous disease does not, itself, cause parkinsonism, but multiple lacunar infarcts may produce a picture of 'pseudo-parkinsonism'.

Table 5.6 Differential diagnosis of Parkinson's disease

Idiopathic Parkinsonism
Drug induced Parkinsonism
Pseudo-Parkinsonism (multi-infarct)
Cerebral tumour (especially frontal)
Neurosyphilis
Postencephalitic Parkinsonism
Carbon monoxide poisoning
Manganese poisoning

Treatment

The average time from diagnosis to death is 9 years, most patients dying of pneumonia. Modern drug therapy has improved the outlook in this disease, the treatment of choice being levodopa combined with a peripheral dopa-decarboxylase inhibitor (carbidopa or benserazide). In the early days of levodopa therapy, treatment was initiated early and at a high dose. However, the ideal time to start treatment remains unclear, as, with prolonged therapy all patients seem to run into side-effects.

The role of anticholinergic drugs would now seem to be limited. Benzhexol is the most effective of these drugs, and is perhaps best used to treat young patients with a unilateral tremor. Amantadine would seem to give little benefit. If Parkinson's disease coexists with depression, then it is reasonable to try amitriptyline or nomifensine.

Levodopa is usually given in submaximal doses. Side-effects such as nausea, vomiting, hallucinations, confusion and postural hypotension may occur with small doses. It is best to start with a small dose (50 mg t.d.s.), which may subsequently be increased until benefit is obtained, or until side-effects restrict further increases in dosage. From the outset of treatment, patients on higher doses may develop peak-dose dyskinesias, which can be improved by reduction in total dose or giving small doses more frequently. Unfortunately increasing experience of long-term therapy with levodopa preparations has indicated that many patients will eventually run into drug related side-effects. With advancing disease, the duration of benefit from each individual dose is likely to decrease. However, the patient may become increasingly troubled by end-dose dyskinesias, dystonic spasms and, less frequently, the on/off effect (an effect where patients swing rapidly and unpredictably between parkinsonian and dyskinetic states with little or no useful time between). With increasing doses of levodopa preparations patients frequently develop visual hallucinations which, in conjunction with the picture of dementia sometimes appearing in association with Parkinson's disease, can cause a particular problem of management.

The dopamine receptor agonist, bromocriptine has similar effects to treatment with levodopa. Occasionally, partial substitution of bromocriptine (15–75 mg/day) may smooth out wild swings between the parkinsonian and dyskinetic states.

Selegiline hydrochloride is a selective type β-monoamine-oxidase inhibitor, whose action potentiates the effects of levodopa and may improve end dose deterioration (initially 5 mg daily).

Whilst the vogue for sterotactic surgery in which lesions were placed in the ventro-lateral thalamic nucleus in order to relieve severe tremor has now passed, there has been further interest in such procedures recently in patients with severe refractory unilateral tremor.

Death is usually from pneumonia secondary to reduced respiratory function.

Other movement disorders

Drug induced movement disorders

Table 5.7 illustrates some of the common movement disorders induced by drugs. Several forms of involuntary movement may coexist in the same patient (athetosis, chorea, akathisia, hemiballismus). When considering any patient presenting with a parkinsonian syndrome, it is essential to take a history of previous drug use. The major tranquillizers, in particular the phenothiazines, may all produce a picture indistinguishable from ididopathic Parkinsonism. The prolonged use of phenothiazines and butyrophenones may result in the development of tardive dyskinesias, in which withdrawal of the appropriate drug may actually precipitate or worsen symptoms. The picture of akathisia, in which the patient is beset by uncontrollable motor restlessness resulting in constant movement, may be associated with use of these drugs. Many drugs may induce acute dystonic reactions (phenothiazines, metoclopramide) consisting of trismus, blepharospasm, torticollis and oculogyric crises. Patients presenting with trismus may be diagnosed as suffering from tetanus: however, the taking of a careful drug history and treatment with diazepam

Table 5.7   Drug-induced movement disorders

Phenothiazines
Butyrophenones
Reserpine
Tetrabenazine
Contraceptive pill
Amphetamines
Phenytoin
Alcohol

or anticholinergic drugs will rapidly reverse the dystonic reaction.

Essential tremor

In certain families a fine or coarse tremor, found with hands outstretched and on active movement, demonstrates an autosomal dominant pattern of inheritance. Whilst often only an embarrassment to the patient, the more severe forms may lead to problems in motor activity. Such tremor may be helped by propranolol, primidone or ethyl alcohol.

Sydenham's chorea

This form of chorea occurs commonly in association with rheumatic fever. Although spontaneous recovery is the rule, recurrences can occur.

Chorea gravidarum

Choreiform movements may develop during pregnancy and may be of sufficient severity to warrant abortion. A similar picture may be seen in patients taking the contraceptive pill.

Huntington's chorea

Huntington's chorea is characterized by progressive dementia and chorea. The development of the chorea may precede that of the dementia and vice versa. The condition demonstrates an autosomal dominant inheritance with a mean age of onset of 45 years. There is no known cure for this condition, but affected families may require genetic counselling.

Idiopathic torsion dystonia

This condition commonly occurs in childhood or adolescence often resulting in extreme torsion deformity of the spine and limbs. The treatment of choice is high dose benzhexol. In some cases of late onset, dystonia is restricted to one body segment.

Spasmodic torticollis

In this condition the head turns involuntarily to one side. Whilst initially intermittent, the spasm may become continual, resulting in hypertrophy of the contracted muscles.

Writer's cramp

Writer's cramp has often been regarded as a neurotically based disorder. It is now recognized that writer's cramp may now be the earliest sign of other movement disorders such as Parkinson's disease.

Kernicterus

Children who have had neonatal jaundice may subsequently develop athetoid posturing of the limbs between the ages of 5 and 15. This disorder may be prevented by exchange transfusion in rhesus-negative babies and by *in utero* immunization techniques.

Wilson's disease

In Wilson's disease abnormal copper metabolism results in the metal being deposited in the basal ganglia and liver. The clinical picture is of a range of involuntary movements in association with a Kayser–Fleischer ring at the edge of the limbus of the cornea. The patient may show stigmata of liver disease. The serum copper and caeruloplasmin are decreased. The disease is treatable with penicillamine.

Postencephalitic Parkinsonism

This diagnosis should only be made where there is a clear history of encephalitis before the development of an extra-pyramidal syndrome. Postencephalitic parkinsonism often shows the additional features of oculogyric crises, seborrhoea, sialorrhoea and behavioural disturbance.

Ballism

Vascular lesions of the subthalamic nucleus are the commonest cause of usually unilateral violent involuntary flinging movements of the arm and leg. The long-term prognosis is often good, but early symptomatic relief may be obtained by treatment with tetrabenazine.

Head injury

Approximately 100 000 patients are admitted to general hospitals in the United Kingdom per annum with head injuries. Of the estimated 15 000 or so who leave hospital with significant brain damage, half will be disabled to the extent of never being able to work again. In addition to the clear personal tragedy of these serious head injuries, much distress and morbidity is associated with many of the lesser head injuries with their medico-legal and socio-economic considerations. Road traffic accidents are responsible for more than half of the head injuries leading to death, with significant numbers resulting from accidents at work, sporting injuries and assaults. It is important to note that 50 per cent of patients presenting to hospital with head injuries are below the age of 20 years.

The significance of head injury

Whilst the severity of a head injury may be apparent on a patient's arrival in hospital, the complications of seemingly trivial head injury may be life-threatening and all patients require careful observation with regard to the often rapid and calamitous deterioration that may be associated with complications such as extra-dural haemorrhage. It is a disturbing fact that one-third of patients dying in hospital of their head injuries have, in fact, been lucid for a period following their injury. In many of these patients an intracerebral or extradural haematoma is found at post-mortem. Others die from raised intracranial pressure associated with contusion of the brain or infection secondary to penetrating injury.

Many patients dying after head injury do so as a result of hypoxic brain damage. On arrival in the Accident Department, initial efforts must be directed at resuscitating patients with evidence of cardiovascular or respiratory insufficiency. Hypoxic problems may arise from hypotension, blood loss, loss of central respiratory drive or chest injury resulting in poor respiratory effort.

Whilst head injuries associated with unconsciousness, no matter how brief, are more likely to be associated with structural brain injury resulting in short and long-term problems, it is clear that head injuries without loss of consciousness can be associated with brain damage. Should the patient regain consciousness, a useful guide to the severity of the head injury is the duration of retrograde and posttraumatic amnesia. Penetrating head injuries may result in focal signs such as limb paresis or a focal seizure rather than loss of consciousness.

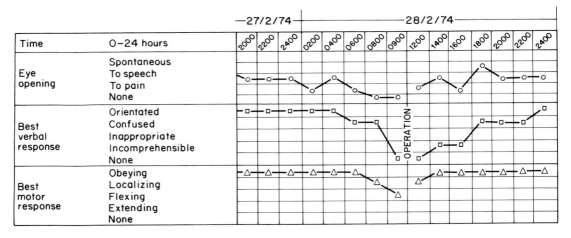

Fig 5.1 Glasgow Coma scale – Parameters assessed and grading of response. (a) Eye opening (b) Verbal response (c) Motor response.

Initial management

In many cases, confusion or coma limits the available information about the nature of the original injury and details of the duration of unconsciousness and any associated features such as fits. Whilst many patients show evidence of ingestion of alcohol or other intoxicating drugs, confusion or coma may be secondary to head injury. Scalp laceration may indicate an underlying depressed skull fracture, or may be associated with significant blood loss. It should not be forgotten that head injury may be secondary to other intracerebral insults such as seizures, strokes or primary intracranial haemorrhages.

In assessing patients' initial conscious level and subsequent progress the Glasgow coma scale has proved consistently useful (Teasdale and Jennett, 1974). The Glasgow coma scale takes account of a patient's response to standard set of specific stimuli (Fig. 5.1), thereby allowing a reproducible assessment of conscious level, and the monitoring of subsequent change. The initial total score has been found to have prognostic importance. While monitoring the patient's condition, particularly the level of consciousness, care must be taken not to administer drugs which will result in sedation, cardiac or respiratory depression, or which disturb pupillary reactions.

After initial resuscitation and full examination the patient may be investigated further. Skull fractures may be apparent in cases with scalp lacerations, exposed skull or when CSF rhinorrhoea or otorrhoea is detected. Similarly, a peri-orbital haematoma without evidence of trauma in that area usually indicates a skull fracture in the anterior fossa, and post auricular bruising may indicate a petrous fracture.

Plain skull X-ray may demonstrate a fracture with its implications for possible subsequent intracranial infection, evidence of intracranial air is rarely seen. Any skull fracture should alert medical staff to the possibility of intracranial haematoma and possible infection.

The widespread use of CT scanning has clearly shown that significant haematomas may be found in patients without signs of raised intracranial pressure, or haematoma. It is essential that patients with serious head injuries should be referred early for CT scanning and neurosurgical advice. Further deterioration in comatose patients may be less readily detected than that in conscious patients in whom confusion may increase, or who may complain of specific motor and sensory symptoms.

Further management

CT scanning may demonstrate the presence of intracerebral haemorrhage. Small intracerebral and subdural haemorrhages may be managed conservatively although larger collections may require neurosurgical evacuation. The finding of an extradural haematoma necessitates urgent neurosurgical intervention. The management of patients in whom no clear haemorrhage is demonstrated, but in whom local or generalized cerebral contusion is found, is largely conservative.

Several series have now shown that steroid therapy, the use of hyperosmolar solutions and surgical decompression have little to offer, in comparison with a high standard of general medical care. The primary purpose of treatment must be to prevent secondary damage from hypoxia, be it due to respiratory or cardiovascular causes. In those patients managed conservatively, neurosurgical intervention may be precipitated by evidence of increasing intracranial pressure, particularly signs suggestive of lateral brain shift associated with tentorial herniation (coning) and midbrain distortion. It is essential that such changes are detected early, as by the time the patient shows extensor spasms and pupillary dilatation, the outlook is grim, no matter what intervention is undertaken. These observations apply particularly to the rapid deterioration that may be associated with an extradural haematoma. Even in the best hands the surgical mortality for an extradural haematoma is up to 20 per cent.

Chronic subdural haematoma

Chronic subdural haematoma may be particularly difficult to diagnose, due in part to the fact that many patients cannot remember any head injury. Patients may present with headache and/or changes in higher intellectual function which sometimes run a fluctuating course. Similarly, the patient may experience variable drowsiness. The presence of focal signs or symptoms, such as hemiparesis or dysphasia should alert the examiner to the possibility of a chronic subdural haematoma. Whilst CT scanning will often reveal the lesion, the inexperienced should beware the bilateral isodense sub-dural haematomas which may be difficult to visualize on the scan.

Long-term complications of head injury

The most feared complication of serious head injury is that which sometimes results from assiduous general medical care, i.e. a chronic vegetative state. However, for the majority of patients a clear degree of recovery may occur although this may take many months or years.

Whilst many of the physical problems resulting from head injury may be readily identified and managed (motor weakness, ataxia etc) it is often the mental symptoms that are most distressing both to patients and relatives alike. Changes in personality, memory and cognitive function may be particularly disabling. Patients often exhibit emotional and personality problems which make them unsuitable for management in general rehabilitation units. Whilst many patients may be left with permanent problems of personality and higher intellectual function, it should be stressed to both patients and relatives that it is possible for improvement to take place over a long period of time. Expectations for rapid recovery are often unrealistic, particularly amongst relatives and employers.

Of particular importance is the so-called 'post-traumatic syndrome'. Whilst the clinical picture may vary from patient to patient, the symptoms of irritability, impaired concentration, poor memory and depression are remarkably constant. These problems may be associated with more specific physical symptoms, such as headache and dizziness. In general the milder the initial head injury, the better the prognosis for recovery long-term, although many patients continue to be troubled by such symptoms long-term. Many patients affected by the post-traumatic syndrome become increasingly depressed as a result of their slow progress and the reaction of family, friends and employers to the apparent slowness of their recovery. Malingerers do present from time to time in the clinic in an attempt to obtain damages in medico-legal proceedings.

Post-traumatic epilepsy

Approximately 5 per cent of patients presenting with head injuries have a seizure in the first week. Such fits are associated with an increased likelihood of epilepsy in later life. So-called late epilepsy (after the first week) occurs in approximately 5 per cent of patients admitted to hospital. In 50 per cent the epilepsy will develop within one year of the injury. Epilepsy is more likely to develop in patients sustaining depressed fractures and intracranial haematomas.

Mortality

Many deaths attributable to head injury occur before the patient is admitted to hospital. For patients in prolonged coma (greater than 6 hours) mortality is about 50 per cent, the death rate increasing above 60 years of age.

Dementia

Approximately 10 per cent of the population over 65 years of age show features suggestive of dementia characterized by a decline in intellect, behaviour and personality. All forms of dementia have profound implications both with regard to the patient and family, and it is important to differentiate between true dementia and pseudo-dementia, as found for example in association with depression. Furthermore, whilst most patients with dementia are found to suffer from Alzheimer's disease it is important to exclude treatable causes (Table 5.8). It is reasonable to make the distinction between presenile (less than 60 years of age) and senile dementia (greater than 60 years of age). However, whilst there are differences in the typical aetiologies of dementia in the two groups, treatable dementias do occur in the elderly and Alzheimer's disease may occur in the young.

Table 5.8   Potentially treatable causes of dementia

Sub-dural haematoma
Neurosyphillis
Vitamin B_{12} deficiency
Pellegra
Thiamine deficiency
Drug intoxication – alcohol, barbiturates, solvents, amphetamines
Hypothyroidism
Hypopituitarism
Hypercalcaemia
Cushing's disease
Communicating hydrocephalus
Multi-infarct dementia
Depression

Spinal cord disease

The spinal cord extends from the base of the skull to the first or second lumbar vertebrae. In making any assessment of apparent disease of the spinal cord, it is useful to remember the classical differentiations between congenital and acquired lesions, and intrinsic or extrinsic lesions of the cord.

Congenital spinal cord lesions

Congenital bony abnormalities at the base of the skull or the spine may result in compression of the

spinal cord. The clinical picture at presentation will depend both upon the level of the lesion and the severity of compression. Patients of all ages presenting with symptoms in the legs and disorders of bladder control should be examined with particular regard to possible spina bifida (dimpling of the skin or hair tufts over the spine). Congenital tethering of the cauda equina may not present until puberty. Tubular cavitation of the spinal cord (syringomyelia) may be congenital or acquired. Extradural or intradural arachnoid cysts may cause spinal cord compression.

Spino-cerebellar degenerations

Friedreich's ataxia

Patients with Friedreich's ataxia usually present in their teens with a variable picture of ataxia, cardiac problems and diabetes mellitus. On examination they may show cerebellar ataxia, peripheral sensory loss, nystagmus, optic atrophy, loss of reflexes with extensor plantars, and kyphoscoliosis.

Familial spastic paraplegia (FSP)

FSP causes paraparesis without sensory or sphincter disturbances, often in association with pes cavus.

Cord compression

Cord compression may result from the congenital lesions previously described or may result from other acquired compressive lesions. The characteristic clinical presentation, is of spastic weakness below the level of the lesion associated with sensory loss with an identifiable sensory level on examination, loss of normal bladder control and impotence. Any patient presenting with bladder symptoms should be treated as a medical emergency as loss of bladder control secondary to cord compression is unlikely to improve if the cord is not decompressed within 24 hours of the onset of retention.

The commonest cause of spinal cord compression is cervical spondylosis in which osteophyte formation in combination with bony sclerosis and disc prolapse can result not only in compression of the spinal cord and myelopathy, but also radiculopathy, most typically at levels C5/6 and C6/7. Spondylitic myelopathy tends to occur in the older age groups, but may occur in earlier life, particularly in patients who have sustained previous neck injuries.

Particular problems may arise around the atlanto-axial joint. Patients with developmental anomalies at this level or with rheumatoid arthritis are prone to potentially lethal subluxation of the atlanto-axial joint. These patients may present with a tetraplegia of acute or subacute onset. They require emergency fixation of the atlanto-axial joint. In recent years the transoral approach for removal of pannus from the joint in rheumatoid arthritic patients has proved successful.

Acute herniation of an intervertebral disc in the neck or dorsal region is often secondary to trauma.

Whilst mild symptoms from cervical spondylosis may require no invasive investigation, patients with clear evidence of cord compression (particularly bladder disturbance) should be investigated further with regard to possible neurosurgical intervention. Myelography has been the traditional method for demonstrating spinal cord compression, but CT scanning and magnetic resonance imaging have proved useful in detecting both extrinsic and intrinsic spinal cord lesions.

Vertebral collapse

Vertebral collapse may occur in association with generalized osteoporosis, but possible infective or malignant causes must be remembered. Often these patients present with a history of pain in the back localized to the level of the lesion. Vertebral collapse may be demonstrable on plain spinal X-rays before proceeding to myelography. Remember that even in patients with diffuse secondary spread of carcinoma, it is worth considering laminectomy if symptoms of spinal cord compression develop as, no matter how limited their life expectancy, they are better able to cope if continent and ambulant. If such a diagnosis is suspected these patients should be referred as a matter of urgency to a neurosurgical unit.

Epidural lesions

Epidural haematomas resulting from trauma or an overdose of anticoagulants may result in the rapid onset of cord compression. Similarly, epidural abscesses may be the cause of acute or subacute cord compression. If demonstrated by myelography, these lesions require urgent surgical evacuation as there is a high morbidity. Epidural lesions may result from epidural anaesthetic techniques.

Neurofibromatosis

Neurofibromas most characteristically occur at the foramen magnum and in the upper dorsal spine. Whilst many in the dorsal region may result lin radiculopathy, there may be associated cord compression. Such patients may demonstrate other features of Von Recklinghausen's disease (subcutaneous neurofibromas, cafe au lait patches, axillary pigmentation).

Meningiomas

Meningiomas may cause cord compression at the foramen magnum or in the mid-dorsal region. The CSF protein levels are often raised both with neurofibromatosis and meningiomas.

Intrinsic lesions

Perhaps the commonest intrinsic lesion of the spinal cord in the United Kingdom is the demyelinating plaque: however, as with extrinsic lesions affecting the cord, patients presenting with a typical picture of spastic weakness below the level of the cord lesion in association with sensory loss may require urgent investigation. In contrast to extrinsic lesions of the spinal cord, detection of a dissociated sensory loss of examination is highly suggestive of an intrinsic cord lesion (for example as in syringo-myelia with loss of pain and temperature sensation, and preserved fine touch, vibration and joint position sense). Lesions affecting half the spinal cord may result in the Brown–Séquard syndrome with an ipsilateral spastic paraparesis and loss of position sense, and contralateral loss of pain and temperature sense below the lesion. At or just below the lesion on the same side there may be lower motor neurone signs and a band of spinothalamic loss.

Vascular disease of the spinal cord

A water shed area exists in the upper thoracic region (about T4) between the supply from the anterior spinal artery and the upward flow in the great spinal artery of Adamkiewicz. There are two posterior spinal arteries. Whilst occlusion of one posterior spinal artery rarely results in persistent sensory loss, occlusion of the anterior spinal artery may cause infarction of the anterior horn cells, the corticospinal tracts and, to a lesser extent, the spinothalamic tracts.

The main predisposing factors for a spinal cord infarction are those of atheromatous disease elsewhere. The auto-immune arteritides may also result in spinal cord infarction. Hypotension for any reason is a potential source of cord ischaemia, and the author has encountered three cases in whom infarction in the anterior spinal artery territory had occurred in associated with hypotension at the time of anaesthetic induction.

Arteriovenous malformations

These lesions are characteristically situated in the thoracolumbar cord and may present either due to their mass effect or with spinal subarachnoid haemorrhage, causing back pain, radicular pain, spinal cord signs, and meningism.

Bleeding into the substance of the cord (haematomyelia) may result from AV malformations, clotting disorders or trauma.

Inflammatory disorders

Multiple sclerosis

Multiple sclerosis is a common cause of spinal cord lesions. A previous history of other CNS lesions, disseminated in space and time (for example optic neuritis or brainstem signs), will help clarify the diagnosis.

Transverse myelitis

Transverse myelitis tends to occur in young people. It may be seen as part of the background picture of multiple sclerosis, but may occur as a separate entity. Possible aetiologies for transverse myelitis are auto-immune disease, viral infection, post vaccination, embolism and trauma. Typically the patients develop a flaccid weakness with loss of bladder and bowel control. It is usually impossible to exclude compression of the cord clinically, and such patients should undergo myelography. The CSF may show an increased white count and protein level.

In transverse myelitis, corticosteroids are the treatment of choice. Occasionally the disease progresses to necrosis and cavitation of the cord.

Intrinsic tumours

The clinical picture of any intrinsic spinal cord tumour may mimic syringomyelia and previously,

cord lesions such as ependyomas and gliomas were often difficult to differentiate from syringomyelia even at myelography. The advent of CT scanning and magnetic resonance imaging has helped in the diagnosis of such intrinsic lesions.

Surgery to intrinsic tumours of the spinal cord is usually not indicated, but it may be that laminectomy may slow the progression of neurological symptoms and signs.

The surgical treatment of syringomyelia is contentious. Some authorities maintain that the insertion of a shunt into the syrinx may help prevent progression of the disease. When syringomyelia is present with the Arnold–Chiari malformation, decompression of the foramen magnum may be indicated.

Other spinal cord disease

Motor neurone disease

Motor neurone disease is characterized by progressive deneration of both upper and lower motor neurones. Patients present with three classical syndromes:

- Wasting in the upper limbs associated with spasticity in the lower limbs (amyotrophic lateral sclerosis).
- Progressive muscular atrophy.
- Bulbar palsy.

The aetiology of motor neurone disease is unknown. Most patients present over the age of 60 and the mean survival is 3–4 years.

The diagnosis may be apparent when the patient first presents, especially if there is a mixed picture of upper and lower motor neurone signs in the absence of any sensory disturbance. However, in view of the poor prognosis associated with the diagnosis of motor neurone disease, most neurologists investigate patients fully to exclude alternative diagnoses. Cervical spondylosis may present with a predominantly motor picture, often with mixed upper and lower motor neurone signs, however the finding of sensory abnormalities is against the diagnosis of motor neurone disease.

Although the diagnosis of motor neurone disease may be painfully apparent in the outpatient clinic, it may be appropriate to admit patients to hospital to perform a myelogram to exclude a high cervical lesion. CSF examination is necessary to exclude the diagnosis of neurosyphilis. Neurophysiological investigation, particularly surface EMG, may uncover widespread fasciculation.

The prognosis varies considerably. Patients often finally succumb to pneumonia secondary to their bulbar problems. Patients with a predominant picture of progressive muscular atrophy or amyotrophic lateral sclerosis may deteriorate slowly and, with the use of suitable aids at home, may live for many years.

Vitamin B₁₂ deficiency

Vitamin B_{12} deficiency may result in peripheral neuropathy, spinal cord disease, optic atrophy or dementia. Subacute combined degeneration of the posterior and lateral columns of the spinal cord is typified by Rombergism, loss of position sense, spasticity and extensor plantar responses. It is important that this diagnosis is made early, as replacement therapy with hydroxocobalamin may not result in complete recovery.

Spino-cerebellar degenerations

The most recognizable clinical picture is of Friedreich's ataxia, characterized by ataxia, nystagmus, kyphoscoliosis, areflexia with extensor plantars, diabetes mellitus and cardiomyopathy. Patients often die suddenly as a result of their cardiomyopathy.

Familial spastic paraplegia is usually easy to differentiate clinically from Friedreich's ataxia, as it presents with a picture of spastic paraparesis often in association with pes cavus. There is often a clear family history. Familial spastic paraplegia must be differentiated from multiple sclerosis, cervical spondylosis and other cord diseases.

Peripheral nerve lesions

It must be remembered that the spinal roots constitute part of the peripheral nervous system. Whilst many lesions of peripheral nerve are easily recognizable (sciatica or carpal tunnel syndrome), others may be insidious in their onset.

Intervertebral disc lesions

The commonest cause of time lost from work in the UK is backache. Lumbar disc prolapse may be associated with backache and symptoms of root compression (sciatica). Patients may complain of sensory disturbance in the distribution of the affected nerve root. On examination there may be weakness and wasting in the distribution of the nerve root in association with loss of the appropriate tendon reflexes.

Cervical and dorsal disc prolapse

Prolapse of cervical and dorsal discs is usually associated with pain which may be of acute onset. In the young, symptoms are often triggered by trauma. In older patients cervical disc prolapse may be associated with the chronic degenerative changes of cervical spondylosis.

Lumbosacral disc prolapse

The most frequent presentation of lumbosacral disc prolapse is with backache and pain radiating down the leg.

Central disc prolapse in the lumbosacral region may result in the acute disturbance of sphincter control. Patients who present in such a manner require urgent investigation, with a view to surgical decompression of the cauda equina.

Plain X-rays may show degenerative changes in the spine in addition to narrowing of the disc spaces and slippage of adjoining vertebrae.

Management

Many patients with acute intervertebral disc lesions can be managed conservatively, either by wearing a cervical collar or by a period of enforced bedrest. Whilst manipulation of the spine may produce symptomatic relief, it is contraindicated in the presence of neurological signs.

In the presence of bladder disturbance or clear neurological signs, myelography is indicated. This should only be performed in units with ready access to neurosurgical facilities. CT scanning or magnetic resonance imaging may be useful in detecting intervertebral disc lesions.

Surgery for cervical lesions is usually indicated in the presence of myelopathy or if there is clear evidence of root entrapment. In Cloward's procedure, the prolapsed disc is removed through an anterior or antero-lateral approach. A decompressive laminectomy may be appropriate in the presence of multiple cervical lesions.

Decompressive laminectomy of the lumbar lesions is indicated if the pain does not respond to conservative management or in the presence of clearly demonstrable signs of root compression (including bladder disturbance).

Epidural injections of lignocaine may give pain

relief and extradural injections of a corticosteroid may be helpful.

Chemonucleolysis with the proteolytic enzyme chymopapan has proved less effective than at first thought.

Other spinal root lesions

Malignancy

Spinal roots may be compressed by primary and secondary tumours. Benign lesions are rare, but careful examination may reveal features suggestive of neurofibromatosis.

Infective lesions

Spinal root lesions may occur due to compression from extradural collections of pus or as a result of secondary vertebral collapse (for example Pott's disease).

Plexus lesions

Asymptomatic cervical ribs may be found on many plain X-ray films of the cervical spine. Elongated cervical ribs may result in vascular or neurological symptoms in the upper limbs. Patients may complain of pain in the arm, wasting of small hand muscles or progressive sensory loss.

Investigation of cervical rib is extremely difficult, but nerve conduction studies may be useful. Intractible pain resulting from the presence of cervical ribs may lead to the patient undergoing surgery. In many cases a fibrous band is found at the tip of the cervical rib and adherent to the nerves.

Lumbar sacral plexus lesions

Whilst pain in the back radiating down the leg is usually secondary to prolapsed intervertebral disc, retro or intraperitoneal masses, (both neoplastic and infective) may result in pressure upon the lumbar sacral plexus. The diagnosis is often difficult to make clinically, but the advent of CT scanning and ultrasound of the abdomen has aided detection of such lesions.

Classical peripheral nerve lesions

A detailed knowledge of the motor and sensory distribution of all peripheral nerves is unnecessary, and it is interesting to note the number of neurologists who carry the HMSO *Guide to Peripheral*

Nerve Injuries in their cases. Certain classical syndromes are common, however, and should be readily diagnosed.

Carpal tunnel syndrome

Typically patients present with pain and paraesthesiae in the arm and hand particularly at night. The patients may report sensory sparing of the ring and little finger. Symptoms may be aggravated by using the hand, but most typically awaken the patients from sleep.

Examination may reveal sensory loss in a median distribution over the palmar surface of the hand, sparing the little finger and frequently the ulnar border of the ring finger. There may be weakness and wasting of abductor pollicis brevis.

Nerve conduction studies are useful in making the diagnosis. The carpal tunnel syndrome may be associated with rapid weight gain, pregnancy, the contraceptive pill, working with vibrating equipment and myxoedema.

Ulnar nerve lesions

The ulnar nerve is most characteristically damaged at the elbow, and is particularly common in patients with arthritic or post-traumatic bony changes at the joint, or in patients who tend to rest their elbows on desks or tables for long periods of time. Patients usually describe pain and paraesthesiae in the forearm and hand. On examination, sensory loss affecting the ulnar half of the ring finger and the little finger may be found in addition to wasting of the small muscles of the hand with the exception of abductor pollicis brevis. The ulnar nerve may suffer compression injury at operation, especially at the elbow. The diagnosis may be confirmed by nerve conduction studies.

The nerve may be surgically decompressed or transposed at the elbow.

Radial palsy

The classic, 'Saturday night' palsy occurs when patients fall asleep with their arm hanging over the sides of chairs. The radial nerve is compressed as it winds down the shaft of the humerus, resulting in paralysis of the muscles distal to the triceps, and a dropped wrist. There may be a small area of sensory disturbance at the base of the thumb.

Many radial nerve palsies improve spontaneously, although in severe lesions recovery may take place over many months or even years.

Lateral popliteal nerve palsy

This nerve is usually damaged as it winds around the neck of the fibula. Patients present with foot drop and sensory loss over the outer border of the foot. This nerve palsy is common after orthopaedic or gynaecological surgery.

It is sometimes difficult to distinguish between a lateral popliteal nerve lesion and an L5 root lesion. Nerve conduction studies may help in the differential diagnosis.

Recovery is usually spontaneous, but occasionally surgical decompression is required.

Meralgia paraesthetica

The lateral cutaneous nerve of the thigh may be compressed as it passes under the inguinal ligament, particularly in patients who have rapidly gained weight (as in pregnancy). The characteristic symptoms of burning pain over the anterolateral thigh may respond to weight reduction, although on occasion decompression of the nerve in the groin may be required.

Herpes zoster

Shingles is characterized by the development of the painful vescicular rash in the sensory distribution of peripheral nerves (including the trigeminal nerve with potential ocular involvement). Involvement of motor neurones may also occur, resulting in paralysis. On recovery, patients may be left with permanent sensory disturbance in the distribution of the rash, and post herpetic neuralgia is a particularly distressing problem in the elderly.

It has been shown that local application of the antiviral agent idoxuridine at the onset of the rash or oral administration of acyclovir may decrease the incidence of post herpetic neuralgia. In severe post herpetic neuralgia unresponsive to analgesics, neurosurgical intervention may be attempted.

Neuralgic amyotrophy

This condition is characterized by the acute onset of severe pain in a limb or limbs. Characteristically the arms are affected. As the pain settles, the limb may become wasted and weak. There is no specific treatment, but recovery may be prolonged and on occasion incomplete.

Diabetic amyotrophy

In diabetic amyotrophy the patients may develop severe pain in the thighs, followed by marked wasting and weakness. This complication usually occurs in poorly controlled diabetics. There is often a good recovery following improved control of blood glucose levels. (*See* section on diabetes.)

The Guillain-Barré syndrome

The Guillain-Barré syndrome is characterized by the development of a polyneuropathy following a flu-like illness. Motor symptoms are usually more striking than sensory disturbance. Many patients initially complain of paraesthesiae in the extremities. Whilst in some patients sensory and motor disturbance is mild, in others there may be a relentless progression to total paralysis with respiratory failure and bulbar weakness. Such patients usually require tracheostomy and ventilation. The most useful bedside test to detect potential respiratory failure is the forced vital capacity as patients may maintain their blood gases until there is rapid deterioration into respiratory failure.

There are no specific diagnostic tests, although CSF examination usually shows an increased protein, without cellular response. Nerve conduction studies may show evidence of peripheral neuropathy.

There is no specific treatment for this condition. Steroid therapy is contraindicated, and may in fact prolong recovery time. Management should be supportive with particular attention to respiratory function, nutrition and passive physiotherapy. Approximately 5 per cent of patients are left with some neurological disability longterm.

Other peripheral neuropathies

Perhaps the commonest peripheral neuropathy is that associated wtih diabetes mellitus. Characteristically patients are affected by numbness in the hands and feet, often associated with unpleasant burning dysaesthesiae. Similar uncomfortable sensations may be experienced by heavy drinkers. In all cases of peripheral neuropathy Vitamin B_{12} levels should be checked.

Porphyria may result in an asymmetrical polyneuropathy. Patients may give a history of abdominal pain and mental disturbance suggestive of acute porphyric attacks.

Carcinoma may be associated with a non-metastatic peripheral neuropathy and causes of peripheral neuropathy may include heavy metals, solvent abuse and exposure to certain insecticides.

Bell's palsy

Bell's palsy is an idiopathic acute lower motor neurone facial palsy of unknown aetiology. Typically the onset of a lower motor neurone picture of facial weakness is preceded by post-auricular pain. In association with the facial weakness there may be ipsilateral loss of sense of taste, hyperacusis and excessive lacrimation of the eye on the affected side.

There is no specific diagnostic test for Bell's palsy: however, alternative causes of acute facial palsy should be excluded, such as otitis media, shingles, sarcoidosis and multiple sclerosis.

Management is essentially conservative. Failure of eye closure may result in corneal damage and if the eye becomes red or uncomfortable, tarsorrhaphy may be indicated. The use of steroids is contentious, but it may be that there is some place for them if used within a few days of onset of the facial weakness.

Many patients find the acute onset of facial weakness extremely alarming. It is possible to reassure them that in 80 per cent or more cases a full spontaneous recovery occurs.

Mononeuritis multiplex

Many patients present with the picture of disease of several individual nerve trunks (mononeuritis). Table 5.9 shows a list of potential causes. Although diabetes mellitus is probably the commonest cause of peripheral nerve lesions in the UK, leprosy is a frequent cause in other countries.

Table 5.9   Causes of mononeuritis multiplex

Diabetes
Polyarteritis nodosa
SLE
Rheumatoid arthritis
Wegener's granulomatosis
Leprosy
Sarcoid
Malignant infiltration
Non-metastatic syndromes
Amyloid
Post-vaccination

Genetically determined neuropathies

The commonest inherited disorder of peripheral nerve is Charcot–Marie–Tooth disease. Typically, patients develop distal wasting associated with pes cavus between the ages of 10 and 30 years. Two common forms of Charcot–Marie–Tooth disease are recognized:

- The hypertrophic type (hereditary motor and sensory neuropathy type I), in which peripheral nerve demyelination occurs.
- The neuronal type (hereditary motor and sensory neuropathy type II) in which axonal degeneration occurs.

Nerve biopsy

In many chronic polyneuropathies of unknown aetiology, diagnostic information may be obtained by biopsy of the sural or radial nerves.

Diseases of muscle

In recent years our understanding of neuro-muscular disease has been greatly aided by development of sophisticated biochemical and histochemical techniques.

In patients presenting with muscle disease, it is vital to obtain a clear family history. The patient should also be asked about any episodic weakness of the muscles and associated pain and discomfort.

Inherited diseases of muscle

Duchenne's muscular dystrophy

Duchenne's muscular dystrophy shows a sex-linked recessive pattern of inheritance and is almost exclusively limited to males. Affected boys demonstrate delayed motor development and by the age of 4 to 6 years show a symmetrical, proximal myopathy of the upper and lower limb girdles with hypertrophy of the muscles of the calf. There follows a relentless progression of the muscle disease. There is an associated cardiomyopathy. The patients usually die in cardiorespiratory failure or of pneumonia between 18 and 22 years.

Investigation, typically shows a raised CPK level in the early stages, which tends to revert to normal as the muscle wasting progresses. EMG study may reveal a myopathic pattern. Muscle biopsy may reveal progressive replacement of muscle tissue by fibrosis and fatty change. There is no specific treatment, but the patients and parents may be helped by the numerous aids for daily living now available to the disabled.

Becker muscular dystrophy

Becker muscular dystrophy show the similar clinical and pathological features of Duchenne muscular dystrophy, but follows a benign course.

Spinal muscular atrophy

Werdnig–Hoffman disease In this condition babies show profound hypotonia, weakness and respiratory embarrassment. Examination may reveal total areflexia and fasciculation of tongue. There is no cure and the patients usually die in the first year of life.

Kugelberg–Welander disease This condition shows an autosomal recessive pattern of inheritance with a marked variation in clinical severity. Muscular atrophy occurs secondary to anterior horn cell death. The patients usually succumb between the ages of 20 and 30 years due to respiratory failure.

Myotonic dystrophy

This extraordinary condition is inherited in an autosomal dominant pattern. Most patients present in adult life with distal weakness and wasting in the upper or lower limbs. On examination the clinical features consist of impassive facies, frontal balding, ptosis, atrophy of the temporalis, masseter and sternomastoid muscles, and myotonia. Patients may have a severe dysarthria. The deep tendon reflexes are usually absent.

The EMG may show a myopathic picture with characteristic myotonic discharges.

The condition may progress slowly. Evidence of cardiomyopathy is usually present, particularly intracardiac conduction abnormalities. Patients may die suddenly in a Stokes–Adams attack.

Vital capacity and maximum expiratory pressure are often impaired and patients tolerate general anaesthesia poorly and may develop hypersomnia.

Death is usually from respiratory infection or cardiac failure or arrhythmias.

Myotonia congenita

Myotonia congenita is usually present from birth. It frequently occurs as an autosomal dominantly inherited condition and presents with generalized myotonia which is made worse by rest or cold. The myotonia may be relieved by exercise. Diffuse muscle hypertrophy may be found.

Inflammatory myopathies

Auto-immune myopathies

Polymyositis/dermatomyositis (PM/DM) The aetiology of PM/DM is unknown. Patients usually present with slowly progressive weakness in a limb girdle distribution, accompanied by muscle pain and cramps. In patients with dermatomyositis there may be a heliotrope rash around the eyes and over the extensor surfaces of the hands. Examination of the limb muscles may reveal tenderness.

The serum creatinine kinase is usually moderately elevated, and muscle biopsy may reveal necrotic changes, with or without inflammatory infiltrates.

Steroid therapy with or without associated immuno-suppression is the treatment of choice.

Polymyalgia rheumatica Polymyalgia rheumatica usually presents with muscle pain and tenderness in patients over the age of 55. The symptoms may be associated with low grade fever and general malaise. There may be associated symptoms suggestive of giant cell arteritis. The condition responds to steroid therapy.

Infective myopathies

Viral myositis is usually a benign self-limiting illness in children, characterized by transient pain and weakness in the calf muscles.

Myositis secondary to coxsackie infection (Bornholm's disease) may cause severe muscle pain, and variable degrees of weakness. The associated viral cardiomyopathy may be lethal. There is no specific treatment.

Metabolic myopathies

Present day histochemical and biochemical techniques have allowed the classification of many inherited muscle diseases, secondary to identifiable biochemical defects.

• **Glycogen storage disorders** In these inherited disorders, one or more of the enzymes involved in the synthesis or breakdown of glycogen is deficient. Muscle biopsy and histochemical staining may allow specific differentiation between the glycogen storage diseases.

• **Lipid disorders** The oxidation of fatty acids is a major source of energy for skeletal muscle. Two disorders of lipid metabolism have been identified: carnitine palmityl transferase deficiency and carnitine deficiency.

- **Mitochondrial myopathies**   This group of rare muscle diseases is characterized by abnormalities of mitochondrial structure and function, the myopathy often being associated with disorders of other systems.

- **Periodic paralyses**   These rare disorders show a dominant pattern of inheritance. Patients complain of episodes of flaccid weakness which may last for hours to days. Respiratory muscles are usually spared, except in severe attacks. The attacks may be precipitated by cold. Two forms are recognized; the hyperkalaemic and hypokalaemic forms. In hypokalaemic periodic paralysis attacks may be triggered by excessive carbohydrate ingestion.

- **Malignant hyperpyrexia**   The tendency to malignant hyperpyrexia is inherited as an autosomal dominant character. Affected individuals may show a clear myopathy or merely a raised serum creatinine kinase. Attacks may be triggered by exposure to inhaled anaesthetic agents, particularly halothane, and are characterized by unstable blood pressure, metabolic acidosis, rapid respiration, ventricular arrhythmias and skin cyanosis. Fever is a relatively late feature, sometimes rising to 46° C. Treatment consists of rapid cooling, correction of acidosis and administration of intravenous dantrolene to decrease muscle rigidity. Recovery depends on early recognition of the condition with prompt treatment, otherwise patients may die from renal failure.

Toxic myopathies

Steroid myopathies

Both chronic steroid administration and Cushing's syndrome may be accompanied by wasting and weakness in proximal muscles. Patients usually recover on withdrawal of steroid therapy or treatment of the underlying endocrine abnormality.

Thyroid myopathy

The commonest picture of myopathy associated with thyroid disease is that of chronic proximal weakness in association with hypothyroidism. Myxoedema may also be associated with pain, cramps and stiffness in the muscles and occasionally with associated weakness.

Toxic myopathies

Painful proximal myopathies may result from administration of certain drugs (for example, vincristine, lithium carbonate, salbutamol, propranolol and cimetidine).

Chronic alcoholic myopathy

Drinking bouts may be followed by the onset of generalized muscle weakness and pain. There may be associated cardiomyopathy. If alcohol is withdrawn, recovery usually follows.

Myasthenic syndrome (Eaton–Lambert syndrome)

The myasthenic syndrome is usually associated with bronchial carcinoma, being characterized by muscle fatiguability resulting from impaired released of acetylcholine from the presynaptic nerve terminal. It is now believed to have an auto-immune aetiology. The myasthenic syndrome may also follow the administration of D-penicillamine or aminoglycosides.

Myasthenia gravis

Myasthenia gravis is an acquired auto-immune disorder characterized by fatiguability and weakness of skeletal muscle. Patients may present between childhood and old age. The condition is associated with the production of acetylcholine receptor antibodies, which bind to the postsynaptic membrane of the neuromuscular junction.

The clinical presentation may be with generalized weakness or highly specific weakness (for example localized to one extra-ocular muscle). Whilst many patients give a history suggestive of fatiguability of skeletal muscle, others may report a non-specific weakness. In approximately two-thirds of cases, the ocular muscles are the first to be involved, resulting in diplopia or ptosis. Other patients may present with distal or proximal limb weakness. Of particular importance with regard to life expectancy is the development of bulbar and respiratory muscular weakness, (the former may lead to difficulty in speech, chewing and swallowing and the latter to shortness of breath and respiratory failure).

Anti-acetylcholine receptor antibodies may be

detected in the majority of patients with generalized myasthenia, and in most with disease confined to the ocular muscles. Anti-striated muscle antibodies are found in 90 per cent of patients with associated thymomas and 30 per cent of other myasthenic patients. The edrophonium chloride (Tensilon) test has previously been used to demonstrate reversibility of fatiguable weakness in affected patients.

In this test an initial intravenous test dose of 1 mg of edrophonium chloride is followed by the injection of a further 5–8 mg. The result is deemed positive if an improvement in muscle weakness, be it ocular, limb or respiratory is noted within 1 minute. The response does not last longer than five minutes (often to the distress of the patient!). It should be emphasized that the Tensilon test should only be performed where facilities for cardio-pulmonary resuscitation are immediately available. EMG study may reveal characteristic changes. Chest X-ray and CT scanning of the chest may reveal abnormalities of the thymus gland. Myasthenia gravis is associated with benign thymic hyperplasia and benign/malignant thymomas).

The management of patients with myasthenia gravis will depend in part upon the severity and distribution of the affected muscles. In many cases with ocular problems, moderate doses of anti-cholinesterases (neostigmine or physostigmine) may be sufficient to control the symptoms. In patients with severe weakness, prednisolone treatment may be affective, although some patients will become weaker before improving. In patients who require long-term steroid therapy, immuno-suppression may be introduced as a steroid sparing manoeuvre. In patients with demonstrable thymic lesions, thymectomy may be followed by an improvement in myasthenic symptoms. However, in patients with thymomas, surgery may be followed by a temporary deterioration in muscle power, sometimes leading to hypoventilation. *Remember* that both under and over-treatment with anti-cholinesterase drugs may result in weakness, although over-dosage is often accompanied by abdominal pain and diarrhoea.

Plasma exchange seems to have a role in the management of acute relapses of myasthenia gravis.

Myasthenia gravis may show spontaneous relapses and remissions. Any complaint of increasing weakness or malaise from a myasthenic patient should be treated seriously. It is not

Table 5.10   Drugs likely to increase weakness in Myasthenia gravis

Streptomycin
Gentamicin
Kanamycin
Neomycin
Polymyxin
Curare
Quinine
Quinidine
Procainamide

uncommon for respiratory function to deteriorate extremely rapidly. Whilst it is often possible to monitor and predict such deterioration by the frequent measurement of forced vital capacity, occasionally acute upper airways obstruction due to bulbar problems may result in sudden respiratory arrest.

Certain drugs should be avoided in patients with myasthenia gravis as they are likely to increase weakness (Table 5.10).

Neonatal myasthenia

Neonatal myasthenia is seen in approximately one in seven of children born to myasthenic mothers. Those who survive recover within 1 week to 3 months of birth.

Infections of the nervous system

Rapid and accurate diagnosis of infections of the nervous system is vital in order to prevent death or significant morbidity.

Bacterial meningitis

The three main causative organisms of bacterial meningitis in the UK are *Haemophilus influenzae* (commonest under age 4), *Neisseria meningitidis* (commonest between 4 and 45 years) and the *pneumococcus* (commonest over the age of 45). It must, however, be borne in mind that in the neonatal period, and in immunocompromized patients the range of potential causitive organisms is wide. In any patient presenting with meningism, a careful past medical history must be taken, including details of illness amongst family or friends, and recent travel abroad.

Patients with bacterial meningitis typically

present with a history of 'flu-like' symptoms associated with headache, photophobia, neck stiffness and various degrees of drowsiness: however, meningitis may present with coma or stroke-like events, particularly in older patients infected with the pneumococcus. In some patients with meningococcal infections the clinical picture at presentation may be of the purpuric rash and circulatory shock associated with the Waterhouse–Friedreichsen syndrome.

Investigation

Whilst there may be clear indications as to any possible organism causing meningitis (for example, previous middle ear infections in children with *Haemophilus influenzae* infections) initial investigation will only allow limited information about the cause of a particular patient's illness. On admission the patient should be carefully examined with regard to any potential source of infection (skin, ears, throat, chest etc). It is important to try and culture possible organisms, and therefore blood cultures, throat swabs and urine should be sent for microbiological examination before antibiotic treatment is commenced (however this should not delay the initiation of an effective antibiotic regime). A full blood count may reveal evidence of systemic infection and chest X-ray may show a pulmonary source of infection.

The most useful information with regard to potential treatment may be obtained from CSF examination. Wherever possible it is important to obtain a CT scan of the head before performing lumbar puncture on patients with suspected meningitis. This is particularly so in any patient with focal neurological signs suggestive of a possible cerebral abscess. Neurological examination may, in fact, fail to reveal evidence of raised intracranial pressure due to cerebral abscesse(s) (for example there may be no papilloedema). If the CT scan shows a normal ventricular system and no obvious abscess it is safe to proceed to lumbar puncture. The CSF obtained may be turbid on visual inspection, suggesting purulent meningitis: however, more specific information will be obtained on biochemical and microbiological examination. Whilst the classic alterations in CSF may be useful in differentiating between bacterial and viral meningitides (high protein and neutrophil count in the former, and raised protein with high lymphocyte count in the latter), these patterns may

be misleading. Of particular importance in this respect is the CSF in tuberculous meningitis, which may show no cellular response, or high lymphocyte and/or high neutrophil counts. The CSF picture may also be altered by previous antibiotic treatment, often leading to a predominantly lymphocytic response. It is vital that the blood sugar should be estimated at the time of estimation of the CSF sugar, in order to determine whether there is a significant difference between these values suggestive of bacterial meningitis. Routine staining of the CSF may allow the microbiologist to immediately identify the causitive organism, but the laboratory should be warned in advance if unusual organisms such as fungi or yeasts are suspected causes, or if there is a history of neoplastic disease or immunosuppression.

Treatment

Opinions vary as to the ideal treatment of an undiagnosed meningitis. The author prefers a regime of benzylpenicillin 2 mega units i.v. every 2 hours and chloramphenicol 1 g i.v. 6-hourly as initial treatment. The role of intrathecal therapy is not clear. Corticosteroids are contraindicated in bacterial meningitis unless there is evidence of developing circulatory collapse or cerebral oedema.

Meningitis is a notifiable disease, and patient contacts should be assessed as soon as possible with regard to appropriate prophylactic antibiotic therapy.

Viral meningitis

Viral meningitis requires no specific treatment, although patients may be quite unwell in the acute phase. Certain forms of viral meningitis, particularly mumps, are often associated with a prolonged postviral syndrome.

Tuberculous meningitis

Tuberculous meningitis has a high mortality and morbidity rate, due in part to delayed diagnosis in many cases. The classical picture is of a subacute meningitis, but the CSF findings may be initially misleading. It must be stressed that in view of the potential high mortality, early treatment with standard regimes such as streptomycin, isoniazid and PAS may be life saving, and can be easily altered if microbiological cultures reveal an alternative organism. Some authors have proposed initial therapy with five antibiotics. (Rifampicin and ethambutol may be substituted for drugs in the standard regime). It must be stressed that patients' colour vision should be carefully checked and monitored if treated with ethambutol.

Some patients with tuberculous infections of the CNS present with symptoms secondary to intracranial tuberculous granulomas, (i.e. symptoms suggestive of space occupying lesions).

Other forms of meningitis

Generalized systemic disease may predispose patients to unusual forms of meningitis (diabetes, neoplasia, immunosuppression and AIDS).

Cryptococcal meningitis tends to occur in debilitated immunosuppressed patients. It presents with a picture of meningoencephalitis. The organism may be readily identified in the CSF in some cases by staining with Indian ink. Amphotericin-B may provide effective treatment, particularly if started early.

Viral encephalitis

The viral encephalitides vary in severity between mild and lethal. An encephalitis may follow systemic viral infections such as measles, mumps or chicken pox, but perhaps the most feared infection is that with herpes simplex. Patients often present with a picture of meningism associated with disturbance of level of consciousness, and sometimes features suggesting temporal lobe disturbance. Patients with herpes simplex encephalitis may have raised intracranial pressure, and a CT scan is mandatory before considering CSF examination. Although, previously associated with severe disability and death, the prognosis in herpes simplex encephalitis has been markedly improved by the use of acyclovir.

Brain abscess

As previously indicated, lumbar puncture should not be performed in patients in whom a brain abscess is suspected. Affected patients typically present with fever and progressive neurological deficits. Such patients must have a CT scan performed, and if necessary be referred to a neurosurgical unit for further management. Treatment involves surgical aspiration or resection and antibiotic therapy, (usually including metronidazole to combat anaerobic organisms). Chloramphenicol

is particularly useful in view of its excellent penetration of the blood/brain barrier.

Subacute sclerosing panencephalitis

This rare condition affecting children is characterized by deterioration of behaviour and intellectual performance, ultimately leading to a decorticate state associated with myoclonus prior to death. The cause is the measles virus.

Progressive multifocal leucoencephalopathy

The JC polyoma virus causes multiple demyelinating lesions in the brain. Most patients die within a year. The condition is associated wtih immunosuppression, either due to intercurrent neoplastic disease or drug therapy.

Creuzfeld–Jakob disease

In Creuzfeld–Jakob disease, patients show a mixed picture of progressive dementia, akinetic rigidity and myoclonus. There is no known treatment.

Neurosyphilis

If untreated approximately 10 per cent of infected patients develop tertiary neurosyphilis.

Three main forms are seen:

- *Meningovascular syphilis* – characterized by stroke, cranial nerve palsies, deafness and optic nerve swelling.
- *General paralysis of the insane* – with dementia, headaches, behavioural change, psychoses, fits and motor weakness.
- *Tabes dorsalis* characterized by lightning pains, sensory disturbance (postural loss), loss of bladder control, visual failure.

Patients may show evidence of more than one form of disease. Argyll Robertson pupils may be found in any patient with neurosyphilis.

In active neurosyphilis positive VDRL, TPHA and FTA-ABS will be found in blood and CSF. In treated cases the blood TPHA and FTA-ABS tests may be negative.

Although the neurological lesions in neurosyphilis may be relentlessly progressive, it is still appropriate to give patients antibiotic treatment (for example Procaine penicillin 600 000 units daily for 3 weeks with initial steroid cover against Herxheimer reactions).

Poliomyelitis

The polio virus causes disease of the anterior horn cells of the spinal cord and the motor nuclei of the brainstem. Exposure to the virus may lead to immunity without illness or neurological complications. In other patients, however, a flu-like illness is associated with the clinical picture of a mild meningoencephalitis. This may be followed by pain in the back and limbs and may be associated with muscle tenderness. Some cases progress to the paralytic phase, characterized by pain in the limbs and muscles in association with weakness and fasciculation. In severe cases, the paralysis may be wide-spread affecting the neck, trunk and all four limbs. Involvement of the respiratory and bulbar musculature may threaten life. Fortunately only a proportion of affected muscles remain permanently paralysed. CSF examination may show a picture of a mild meningitis with between 50 and 250 white blood cells per mm^3, usually a mixture of neutrophils and lymphocytes. Later in the illness the CSF is characterized by a lymphocytosis.

Patients with a respiratory paralysis may need respiratory support for weeks and occasionally indefinitely.

Tetanus

Tetanus results from the effects on the nervous system of the exotoxin produced by the anerobic bacillus *Clostridium tetani*. This organism is widely distributed in soil and as a result even trivial injuries may result in the organism entering the body. Whilst many patients may specifically describe an injury over the week or so prior to the illness, in many patients the injury may be so trivial as not to have been noticed. A prodromal phase of restlessness and flu-like symptoms may be followed by a clinical picture characterized by trismus, muscle rigidity and later paroxsymal exacerbations of rigidity associated with severe cramp-like pain. Spasm of the larynx and respiratory muscles may occur leading to dyspnoea and/or respiratory arrest. The paroxysms may be elicited by external stimuli. Death occurs from asphyxia, exhaustion or associated autonomic disturbances.

On presentation if the diagnosis of tetanus is suspected certain pit-falls may be readily avoided. Firstly, a history of previous drug taking should be elicited from the patient as dystonic reactions may mimic tetanus (e.g. after metoclopramide).

Secondly, if possible remove the patient's dentures prior to the development of severe trismus as oral manipulation at a later stage may trigger life-threatening spasms.

Initial management consists of wound débridement, and administration of tetanus antitoxin. Increasing numbers of physicians now doubt whether administration of antitoxin has any specific value, its only possible role being the neutralization of circulating toxin. Moderate degrees of muscle spasm may be treated with the administration of diazepam. Should the rigidity become severe or the patient develop severe spasms, then the patient should be paralysed and ventilated. Autonomic storms consisting of hyper- or hypotension and tachy- or bradycardias should be managed as appropriate. The nutrition and food balance of the patient must be watched carefully. Patients often become rapidly dehydrated due to massive insensible fluid loss associated with autonomic disturbance. The patient may be weened from the muscle relaxant as the spasms decrease.

On full recovery the patient must be formally inoculated against tetanus as the disease itself does not confer the same degree of immunity as immunization.

Cerebrovascular disease

An estimated 30 000 people die each year in England and Wales of stroke. Between 10 to 30 per cent of stroke patients give a previous history of transient cerebral ischaemic attacks (TIAs). Life expectancy is reduced after both stroke and TIA, the usual cause of death being myocardial infarction.

The epidemiology of stroke has been confused in the past, not least by the difficulty in differentiating between intracerebral haemorrhage and infarction. At the present time it would seem that approximately 80 per cent of strokes are caused by infarction, 10 per cent by primary intracerebral haemorrhage and 10 per cent by subarachnoid haemorrhage. The advent of CT scanning has shown that in some patients diagnosed clinically to have had a TIA (their neurological deficit improving within 24 hours) their CT scan shows an abnormality suggestive of permanent cerebral damage.

The incidence of stroke is greatly increased after a first TIA (15 per cent in the first year), but even after one year the incidence is approximately 5 per ent per year (i.e. 5 times the incidence in the normal population). There is no difference between the sexes in the incidence of cerebral infarction, but males are more likely to suffer subsequent myocardial infarction.

Risk factors

The most important risk factor for stroke is hypertension. However, diabetes mellitus, peripheral vascular disease and heart disease of any kind are also identifiable risks. Less clear associations have been reported for cigarette smoking, blood lipid disorders and the oral contraceptive.

Pathogenesis

Whilst considerable attention in recent years has been focused on the role of platelet embolism as the cause of stroke and TIA, it must not be forgotten that cerebral ischaemia may result from other mechanisms. The potential sources of embolism from the heart are listed in Table 5.11. Arteritides other than atherosclerosis may also be sources of embolism.

'Haemodynamic crisis' seems to be a potent cause of transient cerebral ischaemia, particularly in the vertebrobasilar rather than the carotid circulation. The commonest clinical presentation of focal cerebral ischaemia with a haemodynamic cause is the aura or hemisensory disturbance

Table 5.11   Cardiac sources of embolism

Paradoxical embolism
Left atrium
  thrombus
  myxoma
Mitral valve
  rheumatic change
  infective endocarditis
  annulus calcification
  mitral valve prolapse
  prosthetic valves
Left ventricle
  mural thrombus
  cardiomyopathy
  sino-atrial disease
Aortic valve
  rheumatic change
  infective endocarditis
  aortic sclerosis
  prosthetic valves
  syphilis

Table 5.12   Causes of 'Haemodynamic crisis'

Hypotension
  drug induced
  haemorrhage
  arrhythmias
  postural
Steals-subclavian
  carotid A-V fistulae
Migraine

experienced by some patients with migraine. A list of potential haemodynamic causes of focal cerebral ischaemia are shown in Table 5.12.

Differential diagnosis

Whilst the clinical picture of stroke may be all too apparent at presentation, the features of TIAs may be extremely subtle, (for example consisting of only minimal disturbances of sensation or function in the limbs, or transient disturbances of higher intellectual function).

Visual disturbance may occur as a result of vascular lesions in both carotid and vertebrobasilar territories, its nature being of particular diagnostic significance. In the anterior circulation, retinal artery occlusion or embolism results in transient or permanent uniocular visual loss. In vertebrobasilar events, there is usually a binocular and often congruent homonymous visual field disturbance. The differential diagnosis for the aetiology of stroke and TIA is given in Table 5.13. There may be more than one pathogenic factor operating in any given patient.

Table 5.13   Differential diagnosis for stroke and TIA

Migraine
Epilepsy
Raised intracranial pressure
Tumour
Haematomas
Polycythaemic
Hyperviscosity syndromes
Sickle cell disease
Anaemia
Hypoglycaemia
Hypotension
Hypertension
Multiple sclerosis
Hysteria

Of particular importance are those patients with raised intracranial pressure who present with transient neurological disturbances. These patients may complain of obscuration of vision impossible to differentiate from embolic amaurosis fugax or vertebrobasilar TIAs: however failure to reach the true diagnosis may result in irreversible blindness. These patients should have a CT scan as a matter of urgency.

Investigation

Any patient presenting with a history of TIA should be investigated further in view of the implications for possible stroke. A scheme for investigation is given in Table 5.14.

Table 5.14   Investigation of TIA or stroke

FBC
ESR
Urea and electrolytes
Blood sugar
WR
ECG
Chest X-ray
CT scan
Ultrasound of heart and carotids
Angiography
Optional
Cervical spine
Blood cultures
Autoimmune screen
Lipids
Protein electrophoresis
EEG
Temporal artery biopsy
Cardiac catheterization

In the older age group giant cell arteritis may be associated with cerebrovascular events. Whilst patients often present having suffered a stroke or gone blind, any elderly patient presenting with headache associated with scalp tenderness, musculoskeletal aching and/or malaise, should have an urgent ESR performed to exclude this diagnosis.

The role of invasive investigation such as carotid arteriography is under review at present. Unfortunately it is not clear which, if any, patients with a demonstrable carotid stenosis should be considered for vascular surgery. It may be that the increasing use of non-invasive techniques such as Duplex scanning will allow clearer evaluation of such patients and their suitability for surgery.

Treatment

There is no specific treatment for stroke. Rarely in the presence of a large intracerebral clot, neuro-surgical evacuation is indicated.

It would seem that it is reasonable at present to treat patients with TIAs with soluble aspirin. However, TIA is a 'lumping' diagnosis and mechanisms other than platelet embolism may be the cause of the patient's symptoms.

Anticoagulation is not usually indicated in the management of stroke. In addition to the risks of inducing bleeding into infarcted brain tissue, there is evidence that patients are at significant risk of primary intracerebral bleeding in the long term.

If clear risk factors are identified, then these may be treated. Hypertension may be cautiously brought under control, but it must be remembered that over-zealous lowering of the blood pressure may, in fact, compromise the cerebral circulation. Patients should be encouraged not to smoke and, if appropriate, be taken off the contraceptive pill. Polycythaemic patients may require regular venesection.

Subarachnoid haemorrhage

Patients may present with a clinical picture of stroke with meningism as a result of bleeding from cerebral aneurysms, arteriovenous malformations or ruptured arteriosclerotic vessels.

The development of aneurysms may be associated with hypertension and diffuse vascular disease. The majority are located on the Circle of Willis and its major branch points. Micro-aneurysms are often situated on deep perforating vessels, particularly in hypertensive patients. Mycotic aneurysms are rarely seen, but are often associated with evidence of systemic infection.

Presentation

The clinical picture will vary according to the extent and location of the bleeding. Typically the patient will experience the sudden onset of symptoms sometimes associated with loss of consciousness. In many patients death is immediate. In those who rapidly recover consciousness or do not pass out the cardinal symptom is of severe headache, often associated with nausea, vomiting, photophobia and neck stiffness. If the haemorrhage is due to rupture of an aneurysm. In addition to the neurological picture secondary to intracerebral damage, here may be associated cranial nerve signs resulting from the mass effect of the original unruptured aneurysm.

Management

Patients suspected as having had a subarachnoid haemorrhage should be admitted to hospital for further investigation.

It is advisable to obtain a CT scan on admission. This will allow possible visualisation of any aneurysm, large haemorrhagic collection and features of raised intracranial pressure.

If not contra-indicated by the CT scan findings, it is important to confirm the diagnosis by examination of the CSF which is characteristically uniformly blood stained fluid and/or xanthochromic.

In patients under the age of 50 further angiographic investigation is advisable. Formal angiography in the early stages may be associated with the risk of cerebral artery spasm, and result in deterioration of the patient's condition. The timing of angiographic study varies from neurosurgical unit to unit, some performing angiography within hours of admission, and others several days later.

Surgical treatment

Whilst many patients may survive a first bleed from an aneurysm, they remain at risk of further catastrophic bleeding, particularly over the 2 weeks following the first bleed. Where aneurysms are accessible to neurosurgical approach, the treatment of choice is to place a clip over the neck of the aneurysm. Infraclinoid aneurysms may be treated by carotid ligation.

Conservative management

In patients in whom no obvious source of bleeding is identified, or those in whom surgically untreatable arteriovenous malformation are demonstrated, the risk of recurrent haemorrhage may be reduced by a period of a minimum of 4 weeks' bedrest. Many patients with arteriovenous malformations do not present with subarachnoid haemorrhage, but may complain of epilepsy or headache. There may be an intracranial bruit heard over the skull, or in Sturge–Weber disease a port wine stain in the trigeminal territory overlying an arteriovenous abnormality on the brain surface.

Surgical removal of AV malformations is often

contra-indicated, as there is a significant morbidity.

Coma

No matter what the cause of coma, an immediate cardiorespiratory assessment is mandatory and resuscitation should begin immediately if appropriate. Thereafter, the cause of coma will require investigation. The more important causes of coma are listed in Table 5.15. Whilst useful information can be rapidly gained from general examination, certain treatable causes of coma are sometimes overlooked, often resulting in significant morbidity and mortality. (For example, losing consciousness due to hypoglycaemia a brittle diabetic may fall striking his head). The blood sugar of all patients presenting in coma should be checked within minutes of arrival, in order to exclude the possibility of hypoglycaemia which, if untreated, may rapidly lead to significant brain damage. Similarly, bacterial meningitis may present with a classical picture of meningism, but can also present with seizures or stroke-like events (particularly pneumococcal meningitis).

In the present author's opinion, urgent CT scanning is justifiable in almost all cases presenting in coma. For most CNS causes and the majority of

Table 5.15   Common causes of coma

Systemic causes	Central nervous system causes
Drugs	Intracranial infections
therapeutic	bacterial, viral, fungal
of abuse	Meningitis, encephalitis,
electrolyte disturbance	brain abscess
Metabolic	Epilepsy and postictal
encephalopathies	states
hypoglycaemia,	Head injury
diabetic ketoacidosis,	cerebral contusion
hepatic failure, renal	Extradural or subdural
failure, myoedema,	haematomas
Addison's disease.	Stroke
Shock	subarachnoid
septic	haemorrhage
haemorrhagic	ischaemic infarction
	primary intracerebral
	haemorrhage
	Tumours
	Postanoxic
	encephalopathy

systemic causes of coma, rapid intervention may prevent significant brain damage or death. However, it should be remembered that in some situations investigation itself can be potentially hazardous. Any patient presenting with focal neurological features, or symptoms suggestive of raised intracranial pressure should not undergo lumbar puncture (even in the presence of neck stiffness). It is often difficult to differentiate clinically between primary meningitis or meningo-encephalitis and the decreased conscious level and neck stiffness associated with cerebral masses and early coning. Should a CT scan fail to demonstrate any evidence of cerebral abscess or raised intracranial pressure due to any other cause, then lumbar puncture may be attempted in safety.

Infections

If an infective cause of coma is suspected, an attempt should be made to ascertain any factors which might predispose the patient to the rarer causes of meningoencephalitis (immuno-suppression, intravenous drug abuse, possible HTV infection, foreign travel, previous ENT problems, head injury).

Whilst *Haemophilus influenzae*, meningococcus and pneumococcus remain the commonest causes of bacterial meningitis, possible tuberculous meningitis should never be forgotten. This often presents insidiously and may be associated with isolated cranial nerve palsies rather than presenting with a picture of florid meningism. An early chest X-ray may suggest the diagnosis in 80 per cent or more of patients. The differential white blood cell count can give valuable information as to the possible nature of CNS infections. Similarly throat swaps, blood, urine and faeces culture may be useful in determining the aetiology of CNS infections.

Encephalitis tends to produce greater alteration in conscious level than meningitis. The management of herpes simplex encephalitis, previously a devasting illness with high mortality and frequent severe neurological consequences, had been radically improved by the use of the anti-herpetic agent acyclovir. However, treatment is often begun on the basis of the clinical picture possibly supported by the findings on CT scan (oedema in the temporal lobes) or on EEG (characteristic high voltage complexes). The common causes of viral encephalitis are given in Table 5.16.

Table 5.16 Common causes of viral encephalitis

Herpes simplex
Herpes zoster
Coxsackie
Poliomyelitis
Echo
Mumps
Rabies
Measles
Rubella
Varicella
Vaccina
Influenza

Epilepsy and postictal states

Fits of all kinds, particularly grand mal seizures, may result in significant periods of altered consciousness. Whilst focal weakness on recovery may be attributable to postictal paralysis (Todd's paralysis) failure to recover quickly after an apparent seizure is an indication for an urgent CT scan. Patients with epilepsy often sustain significant head injuries during their attacks and other potentially lethal causes of coma must be excluded and rapidly and effectively treated (for example extradural and subdural haemorrhages or meningitis).

Drugs

Wherever possible, a drug history should be obtained from a relative or friend. The patient should be carefully examined for evidence of drug abuse and the patient's effects rapidly checked for evidence of long-term drug therapy (insulin, steroid) or drug abuse.

Other systemic causes

A wide biochemical screen should be performed on patients on admission with particular regard to potential hepatic or renal failure.

Postanoxic encephalopathy

It may be apparent from the history available that the patient has sustained a cardiopulmonary arrest. Circumstantial evidence as to the cause may be rapidly found on examination or investigation (e.g. ECG changes suggestive of myocardial infarction) but other possible causes of cardiorespiratory failure should not be forgotten.

Table 5.17   Investigation schedule for patients in coma

Blood	Radiology	Other investigations
Sugar	Chest X-ray	Urine analysis
Full blood count	CT Scan	EEG
and		Blood, urine
differential		and gastic
white count		aspirate for
Electrolytes		toxicology
Calcium studies		screen
Liver		
function		
tests		
Thyroid		
function		
tests		
Blood cultures		
Blood gases		

An investigation regime for patients in coma is given in Table 5.17.

Brain death

Assessment of recovery from coma

Certain features have been identified as of prognostic significance with regard to potential recovery from coma. Absence of pupillary light and corneal reflexes six hours after the onset of coma due to cardiopulmonary arrest is generally incompatible with survival. Deep and prolonged coma carries a universal poor prognosis whatever the cause. Whether coma is due to head injury or not, absent pupillary light, corneal, caloric or oculocephalic reflexes in the first 24 hours result in a one in 20 chance of recovery. The outlook is worse when coma is due to a structural cerebral lesion rather than ischaemia or metabolic disturbance.

Diagnosis

The current approach to diagnosing brain death is based upon the work of Plumb (1972) whose recommendations formed the basis of the assessment regime suggested by the Conference of the Medical Royal Colleges and Faculties of the U.K. (Lancet 1981).

The factors proposed were:

- The nature and duration of coma:
  1. the cause being structural or clearly anoxic;
  2. the possibility of drugs or hypothermia contributing to the picture being excluded;
  3. absent brain function being present for at least 12 hours under observation.
- Absent cerebral cortical function:
  1. behavioural or reflex responses above the foramen magnum must be absent when painful stimuli are applied anywhere on the body;
  2. the EEG should be isoelectric for 60 minutes at an amplitude of 50 microvolts per cm.
- Brainstem function must be absent:
  1. the pupils must be fixed in the absence of peripheral burden of injury;
  2. the oculo-vestibular response must be absent;
  3. no evidence of motor activity in the cranial nerves;
  4. no spontaneous respiration;
  5. intact circulation;
  6. spinal reflex responses may be retained.

The British Criteria recommend that the clinical tests should be carried out independently by two doctors, both achieving consistent results. In Britain the EEG is not regarded as essential. Other investigations may be arranged as appropriate (cerebro-angiography, CT scanning, evoked potentials and cerebral blood flood measurements).

The British Criteria would seem to be reliable as in one series not one of 1003 survivors of severe head injury would have been suspected of being brain dead.

Porphyria

The porphyrias are characterized by disordered metabolism of porphyrins and porphyrin precursors. They may be divided in the three varities of hepatic porphyria; acute intermittent porphyria and coproporphyria. The first two forms are inherited as autosomal dominant traits. In acute intermittent porphyria, acute attacks are often precipitated by drugs, particularly barbiturates. Light sensitivity does not occur. In hepatic porphyria attacks are always precipitated by drugs and are often fatal. Light sensitivity is found in many individuals, particularly males. Coproporphyria is less common. In acute attacks neurological dysfunction may be precipitated by the administration of barbiturates. Other precipitants would seem to be chlordiazepoxide, chloroquine, phenytoin, phenylbutazone, tolbutamide and others.

The pathological changes found in the nervous system are characterized by demyelination in the peripheral nerves and changes in the anterior horn cells. The mental disturbances observed in acute attacks seem to be of metabolic origin and no pathological appearances have been found in brain. The neuropathy seen is primarily axonal but there is often secondary demyelination.

Early symptoms of nervous involvement include restlessness, emotional instability and mood disorder sometimes associated with a confusional state. Fits may occur. In severe cases patients may present in coma or status epilepticus.

Systemic symptoms may precede the attacks particularly abdominal pain, nausea and vomiting. There may be associated hypertension and impairment of renal function. In hepatic porphyria skin may show erosions or bullous eruptions and brown pigmentation and hirsutism are often seen.

In an attack the urine contains large amounts of delta-amino-laevulinic acid and porphyrobilinogen. The urine is not invariably abnormal in colour although the patient may have noticed a darkening. The typical port wine colour occurs on standing.

Sufferers should be advised to avoid the drugs known to precipitate attacks. Treatment is primarily symptomatic. Bulbar and respiratory problems may require supportive management in an acute episode.

Chronic pain

Chronic pain syndromes may result from damage to the sensory system at any point between the pain endings and the thalamus. Chronic pain may result from a variety of pathological processes in different sites (for example diabetes mellitus affecting peripheral nerves, cerebrovascular disease resulting in thalamic strokes). Management of chronic pain syndromes is often poorly executed. Simple analgesics on a regular basis may be quite sufficient to alleviate if not to eliminate pain. However, in many such syndromes routine analgesics are ineffectual. The use of antidepressants (for example amitriptyline 75 mg nocte) may modify the nature of the pain experienced and make it more bearable. Counter stimulation techniques such as transcutaneous nerve stimulation and the use of Pifco vibrators may give benefit. Similarly, the use of hot water bottles and ice packs may provide relief. Whilst most effective in paroxysmal pin (for example trigeminal neuralgia) patients sometimes benefit from the use of anticonvulsants such as tegretol and phenytoin. In severe pain neurosurgical intervention may offer some relief (for example section or injection of the trigeminal nerve or its ganglion, or tractotomy for postherpetic pain). Doctors are often resistant to the long-term administration of opiates, but this should be considered in any case with pain.

Intrathecal or extradural opiates may be administered via implanted reservoirs, either by intermittent injection or by syringe pump.

Further reading

Bannister, R. (1978). *Brain's Clinical Neurology*. Fifth Edition. Oxford University Press, Oxford.

The Lancet. (1981). Braindeath, *Lancet* **i**, 363.

Patten, J. (1977). Neurological Differential Diagnosis. Harold Starke, London.

Plum, F. (1972). *Organic Disturbances of Conciousness in Scientific Foundations of Neurology*. Heinemann, London.

Teasdale, G.B. and Jennet, B. (1974). Assessment of coma and impaired consciousness. *Lancet* **ii**, 81–3.

6

Acid–Base Balance

Bryan Walton

Introduction

An understanding of acid–base physiology and ready interpretation of the results of blood gas analysis are fundamental requirements for safe anaesthetic practice. A practical approach to acid–base balance will therefore be presented – based on the various diagrammatic representations in common use – and the implications of acid–base abnormalities in anaesthesia will be discussed.

Fundamentals

Acids and bases

An acid is a substance which ionizes (dissociates) in solution to raise the concentration of protons (hydrogen ions, H^+). *Strong* acids (e.g. HCl, H_2SO_4) dissociate almost completely, with equilibrium shifted far to the right, whereas with *weak* acids (e.g. H_2CO_3), the shift is less pronounced. Conversely, a base is a proton acceptor.

- $$Acid \rightleftharpoons H^+ + Base$$

Acidity

The acidity of a solution is an expression of the hydrogen ion concentration $[H^+]$. In order to encompass the very wide variations in $[H^+]$ found in body fluids and in chemistry generally, the pH scale was introduced; pH is merely a convenient mathematical manipulation of otherwise unwieldy numbers, and is defined in the following expression.

- $$pH = -\log_{10}[H^+], \text{ or } \frac{1}{\log[H^+]}$$

Table 6.1 Relationship between $[H^+]$ and pH

$[H^+]$ (nmol/litre)	pH	Example
10^8	1	Gastric acid
100	7	Pure water
80	7.1	
40	7.4	Arterial blood
20	7.7	
10	8	Pancreatic juice

The characterization of pH 7 as 'neutral' relates to the H^+ concentration in pure water (10^{-7} mol/litre, or 100 nmol/litre)*, and the reciprocal element of the pH manipulation means that the addition of H^+ will lower the pH. Table 6.1 gives some relevant examples of typical $[H^+]$ and pH values and also demonstrates that, in this conversion from a linear $[H^+]$ to logarithmic (pH) scale, doubling or halving $[H^+]$ results in an *approximate* change of 0.3 pH units.

Purists distinguish between hydrogen ion *concentration* ($[H^+]$, or number of hydrogen ions present) and hydrogen ion *activity* ((H^+), or apparent concentration). $[H^+]$ and (H^+) are related by an activity coefficient which only *approximates* to unity at biological concentrations, but, although pH measurement techniques estimate (H^+) rather than $[H^+]$, in practical, clinical terms such differentiation is irrelevant.

Buffers

A buffer tends to resist a change in the acidity of the environment. Thus, in response to 'insult' with acid or base, the resulting change in pH will be less in the presence of a buffer than in its absence. The

*pH 7.35 = 45 nmol
pH 7.40 = 40 nmol
pH 7.46 = 35 nmol

Table 6.2   Buffers (total about 1000 mmol)

Intracellular fluid (70 %)	Extracellular fluid (30 %)
Proteins Phosphate	(Plasma) proteins Haemoglobin Phosphate Bicarbonate

main buffers are listed in Table 6.2. For the purposes of this practical discussion, bicarbonate may be considered exclusively extracellular.

A buffer, which is a mixture of a weak acid and its conjugate (strong) base, is at its most efficient when present half in its acid and half in its basic forms. The pK of a buffer is the pH at which this balance exists. Thus, the closer the pK of a buffer is to its operating pH, the more efficient it is. For example, proteins (quantitatively most important) have an average pK of 7.0. They are therefore considered more efficient intracellular buffers (where the pH is 7.0) than in the extracellular fluid (ECF – pH 7.4). Haemoglobin (Hb) has a pK of 7.4 and, in addition to operating at its optimal pH, has variable buffering capability related to the capacity of imidazole groups to accept more or less H^+, depending on whether the haemoglobin is reduced or oxygenated. Thus, as Hb is reduced during its passage through the tissues, it becomes a more avid acceptor of H^+ (generated by metabolic activity in those tissues).

The bicarbonate buffer system – the constituents of which are related by the Henderson–Hasselbalch equation:

$$\bullet \; pH = pK + \log \frac{[HCO_3^-]}{H_2CO_3} \; \text{or} \; \log \frac{Base}{Acid}$$

would appear to be a rather ineffective buffer, as the ratio $\dfrac{Base}{Acid}$ is 20:1, log 20 is 1.3 and:

$$\bullet \qquad pH(7.4) = pK(6.1) + \log \frac{20}{1} \; (1.3)$$

In other words, the pK of the bicarbonate buffer system (6.1) is some way from its operating pH. However, this system is considered to be the most important for several reasons. Firstly, it is the system which "connects" the two pairs of acid excreting organs, the lungs and kidneys, and,

indeed, the respiratory and metabolic aspects o[f] acid–base homeostasis (see below). Secondly concentrations of various components can b[e] altered physiologically; and, finally, the system lends itself to clinical measurement and therefor[e] forms the basis for diagnosis and treatment.

$$\bullet \quad \underset{\substack{CO_2 \\ \text{Respiratory} \\ \text{acid}}}{\underbrace{\text{Lungs}}} + H_2O \rightleftharpoons H_2CO_3 \rightleftharpoons \underset{\substack{H^+ \\ \text{Non-respiratory} \\ \text{(or metabolic)} \\ \text{acid}}}{\underbrace{\text{Kidneys}}} + HCO_3^-$$

Normal acid–base homeostasis

Under normal circumstances, the alkaline ECF i[s] being constantly bombarded with acid products o[f] cellular carbohydrate and fat metabolism: som[e] 15 000 + mmol/day excreted as CO_2 by the lungs[.] In addition, normal intake provides about 7[0] mmol/day and protein catabolism results in [a] similar quantity of so-called 'fixed' acid[s] (phosphoric and sulphuric) which are normall[y] excreted by the kidneys. Clearly, in any give[n] period, the overall production (+ intake) of aci[d] must be balanced by the combined excretor[y] efforts of the lungs and kidneys. The buffe[r] systems absorb minor variations in acid load an[d] keep the pH of the ECF within normal limit[s] (7.36–7.44).

The vast majority of hydrogen ions generated i[n] the renal tubular cells (under the influence o[f] carbonic anhydrase) pass into the proximal tubul[e] and combine with filtered bicarbonate ions. Th[e] resultant carbon dioxide diffuses back into the cell[s] and, by this mechanism, base is conserved. Som[e] hydrogen ions are excreted into the urine i[n] combination both with mono-hydrogen phosphat[e] and ammonia:

$$\bullet \; HPO_4^{--} + H^+ \rightleftharpoons H_2PO_4^-$$
$$\bullet \; NH_3 + H^+ \rightleftharpoons NH_4^+$$

By these mechanisms, some 75 mmol/day o[f] hydrogen ions are excreted by the kidneys – [a] figure which can increase to about 750 mmol/da[y] in the face of severe acidosis. It is interesting t[o] contrast the maximum figure excretable by th[e] kidneys under extreme 'duress' with the 15 000 [+] mmol/day excreted as CO_2 by the lungs, even [at] rest.

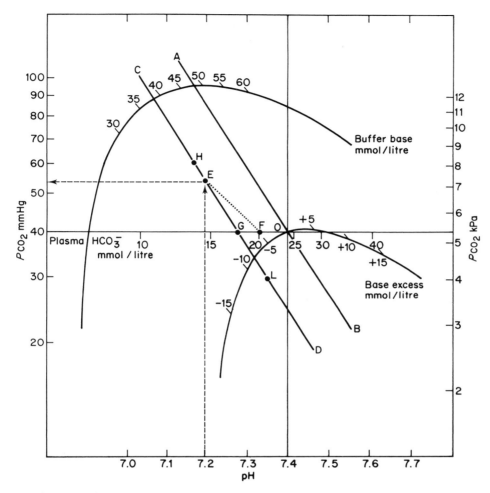

Fig 6.1 Interpolation method, using pH electrode and equilibration tonometry. **Line AB**: Normal *in vitro* buffer line for fully oxygenated blood, passing through buffer base scale at 48 mmol/litre, plasma bicarbonate scale at 24.5 mmol/litre and base excess scale at zero (i.e. normal metabolic status). **Line CD**: *In vitro* buffer line for a blood sample, drawn after equilibration of fully oxygenated sample with known high and low P_{CO_2} gas mixtures. **Points H and L**: Plots of pH values of blood sample after equilibration. **Point E**: Plot of actual pH of blood sample (without equilibration, pH 7.19) on buffer line. P_{CO_2} can be read from ordinate (53 mmHg, 7.1 kPa). Buffer line passes through *buffer base* and *base excess* scales at 39 mmol/litre and −8 mmol/litre respectively. **Point G**: Point of intersection of buffer line with plasma HCO_3^- scale (18 mmol/litre) is, by definition, *standard* bicarbonate (i.e. bicarbonate concentration *if* P_{CO_2} were normal (40 mmHg, 5.3 kPa). **Point F**: *Actual* bicarbonate can be determined by drawing a line at slope of −45° from point E to intersect plasma HCO_3^- scale (20 mmol/litre). Note that *actual* bicarbonate is greater than *standard* bicarbonate, as the actual value reflects extra bicarbonate resulting from buffering of the raised P_{CO_2} (*see* text). In this example (point E), both a respiratory acidosis (P_{CO_2} 53 mmHg, 7.1 kPa) and a metabolic acidosis (*standard* bicarbonate 18 mmol/litre, base excess −8 mmol/litre) are present.

Assessment of acid–base status

Early assessment of the P_{CO_2} of a blood sample involved the use of a pH electrode to measure the effect on the pH of a blood sample of equilibration with two gas mixtures with known high and low P_{CO_2} values. The resultant pH values were entered on a pH/log P_{CO_2} diagram (Siggaard–Andersen & Engel, 1960; Astrop et al., 1960) and an in vitro

CO_2 titration line was plotted (line CD, Fig. 6.1). By interpolation of the pH of the unequilibrated blood sample on to the line (point E, Fig. 6.1), the P_{CO_2} could be read from the ordinate.

The in vitro buffering capacity of a blood sample is dependent on the Hb concentration. Equilibration of normal blood samples with varied Hb concentrations with known P_{CO_2} gas mixtures produces a 'family' of in vitro buffer lines, as shown in Fig. 6.2. The point of intersection of the buffer lines for the normal blood samples (point 0 Fig. 6.2) at pH 7.4, P_{CO_2} 40 mm Hg and norma

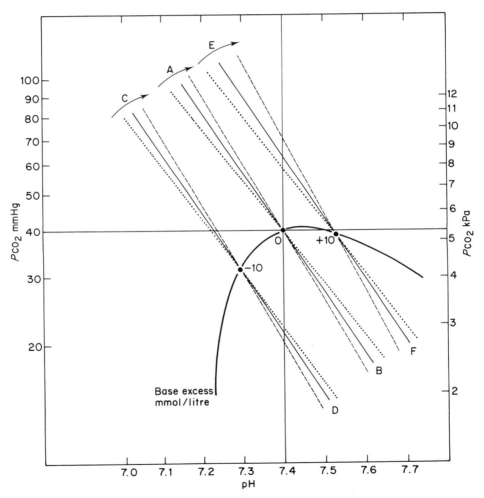

Fig 6.2 Construction of base excess scale. **Line AB**: In vitro buffer lines for fully oxygenated normal bloo with differing Hb concentrations. **Lines CD, EF**: Families of buffer lines for fully oxygenated blood sample with differing haemoglobin concentrations to which 10 mmol/litre acid (CD) or base (EF) had been added.

Arrows indicate, within each family, better buffering of P_{CO_2} changes (i.e. steeper slope and therefore les pH change) as Hb increases. Points of intersection of each family form basis of Hb independent base exces scale.

metabolic (non-respiratory) status represents the base excess zero position, which is irrespective of Hb concentration. If known amounts of base or acid are added to blood samples with varied Hb concentrations, and the *in vitro* buffer lines are plotted as before, sets of buffer lines result, with the points of intersection of each 'family' representing the induced metabolic status of the blood samples (points + 10, − 10, Fig. 6.2), in each case irrespective of the Hb concentration (Astrup *et al.*, 1960; Siggaard–Andersen, 1963). By this means a 'base excess' curve was plotted on the pH/log PCO_2 diagram. Within each 'family', the slopes of the buffer lines increase with increasing Hb concentration. Thus, changes in PCO_2 produce less marked changes in pH, or, in other words, the buffering capacity of blood improves. As the base excess points were constructed by adding known quantities of acid or base to normal blood samples, the term 'base excess' could be defined at that stage as the amount of acid or base needed (per litre of *blood*) to return the pH to 7.4 if the PCO_2 were normal. This term thus became an assessment of the metabolic status of the blood.

Using the pH/log PCO_2 diagram, construction of the *in vitro* buffer line for a blood sample (line CD, Fig. 6.1) allows the metabolic status of the sample to be read at the point the line crosses the base excess curve. In addition, the Siggaard–Andersen curve nomogram (Siggaard–Andersen 1960; 1962; 1963) includes both bicarbonate and buffer base scales. The plasma bicarbonate scale, entered along the normal PCO_2 (40 mmHg, 5.3 kPa) isobar was derived from consideration of the Henderson–Hasselbalch equation. The point at which the *in vitro* buffer line crosses the bicarbonate scale represents the '*standard* bicarbonate' – another expression of the metabolic status of the blood sample which will be discussed more fully later. Clearly, the *actual* bicarbonate concentration of a blood sample reflects not only the metabolic status, but also changes imposed by the bicarbonate buffer system attempting to resist alterations in PCO_2. The distinction between standard and actual bicarbonate will be made clear later with consideration of Figures 6.7 and 6.8. The *actual* bicarbonate of the sample can be derived by the construction of a line with a slope of − 45° from the pH point of the sample on its *in vitro* buffer line (point E, Fig. 6.1) to cross the bicarbonate scale at point F (Fig. 6.1). The slope of this line is derived by further rearrangement of the Henderson–Hasselbalch equation and is fully discussed elsewhere (Siggaard–Andersen, 1971).

The *in vitro* buffer line of the sample could also be extended upwards to cross a scale indicating total buffer base. This somewhat outmoded concept was intended to indicate the total concentration of all buffers in the blood sample (Hb, HCO_3^-, phosphate and plasma proteins – normal 48–50 mmol/litre). This value is no longer usually considered and is included only for historical interest. In recognition of the fact that haemoglobin becomes more alkaline as it is reduced, minor corrections could be applied to the position of the *in vitro* buffer line for samples with significantly reduced haemoglobin oxygen saturation.

The above discussion relates to the *in vitro* buffering capacity of blood samples. However, blood is a better buffer *in vitro* than *in vivo*. *In vivo* blood is 'operating' in direct inter-relationship with the interstitial fluid with which it comprises the ECF. Interstitial fluid (about twice the blood volume) is devoid of haemoglobin, so the *in vivo* buffering capacity of blood is said to approximate to blood *in vitro* with a haemoglobin concentration of 5 g %. If, in animals or man, PCO_2 levels are altered, the resultant pH changes do not correlate with those seen *in vitro*. The slope of the *in vivo* buffer line drawn as a result of such experiments approximates to an *in vitro* buffer line adjusted to a haemoglobin of 5 g % (line AB, Fig. 6.3). If, in animals, metabolic acidosis or alkalosis is induced by the administration of acid or base, the pH changes then induced by alterations in PCO_2 produce a 'family' of *in vivo* buffer lines – each with a constant base deficit or excess (lines P, Q, R and S, Fig. 6.3). Note that all these *in vivo* buffer lines have somewhat 'flatter' slopes than line AB in Fig. 6.1 – reflecting *less* effective buffering *in vivo*.

In practical terms, *in vivo* considerations are of greater value, and, therefore the original Siggaard–Andersen nomogram was modified with, as shown in Fig. 6.3, almost parallel *in vivo* (constant base excess) buffer lines drawn and a new base excess scale (Siggaard–Andersen, 1971). The base excess is now redefined per litre of ECF (*see* p. 198) – in practice a more relevant concept than consideration of blood alone.

The process of blood sample analysis has been simplified by the introduction of the PCO_2 electrode, enabling both the pH and the PCO_2 of a blood sample to be readily determined. The results can then be plotted on, for example, the Siggaard–Andersen acid–base chart (ref. 5, from which Fig. 6.3 is derived). Using the plotted results (point E, Fig. 6.3), an *in vivo* buffer line (roughly

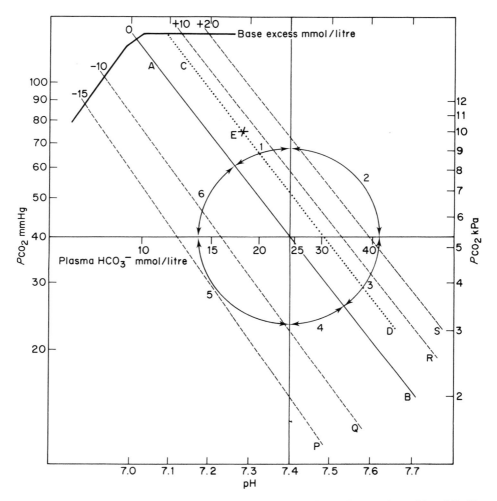

Fig 6.3 Modified PCO_2/pH diagram, showing plot of measured pH and PCO_2 values. **Line AB**: Normal *in vivo* buffer line for fully oxygenated blood. Slope is less steep than normal *in vitro* buffer line in Fig. 6.1 and in fact, approximates to an *in vitro* buffer line for blood with a haemoglobin concentration of 5 g % (*see* text). This line intersects base excess scale (mmol/litre ECF) at zero and plasma HCO_3^- scale at 24.5 mmol/litre. As this latter scale is drawn along the normal PCO_2 isobar, the value is, by definition, *standard* bicarbonate. **Lines P, Q, R, S**: Selection of *in vivo* buffer lines, each with a constant base excess (i.e. constant metabolic (non-respiratory) acid-base status). **Point E**: Plot of results of measurement of pH (7.27) and PCO_2 (75 mmHg, 10 kPa) of patient blood sample. **Line CD**: *In vivo* buffer line for patient blood sample drawn through point E and parallel to the nearest constant base excess line (R). Line intersects base excess scale at +7 mmol/litre ECF and plasma HCO_3^- scale at 31 mmol/litre (by definition, *standard* bicarbonate).

Position of point E allows deductions to be made regarding acid-base status, given that: (a) pH 7.4 line separates acidosis (to the left) from alkalosis (to the right); (b) normal PCO_2 isobar separates respiratory acidosis (above) from respiratory alkalosis (below); (c) line AB (normal *in vivo* buffer line, base excess zero) separates metabolic acidosis (below and to the left) from metabolic alkalosis (above and to the right). Six areas can be identified with, in some cases, conclusions drawn regarding the primary abnormality – assuming that the patient is untreated (*see* text): **Area 1**: respiratory acidosis, metabolic alkalosis (pH acidotic, therefore respiratory acidosis primary). **Area 2**: respiratory acidosis, metabolic alkalosis (pH alkalotic, therefore metabolic alkalosis primary). **Area 3**: respiratory and metabolic alkaloses. **Area 4**: respiratory alkalosis, metabolic acidosis (pH alkalotic, therefore alkalosis primary). **Area 5**: respiratory alkalosis, metabolic acidosis (pH acidotic therefore acidosis primary). **Area 6**: respiratory and metabolic acidoses.

Point E falls into area 1 (primary respiratory acidosis, compensating metabolic alkalosis).

parallel to the nearest constant base excess line) can be drawn (line CD, Fig. 6.3), with the base excess and '*standard bicarbonate*' being read at the points where the buffer line crosses the respective scales.

In Fig. 6.3, the pH 7.4 line, the normal P_{CO_2} (40 mmHg, 5.3 kPa) isobar and the normal *in vivo* buffer line (line AB – base excess zero) can be seen to divide the log P_{CO_2}/pH chart into six areas (*see* legend, Fig. 6.3). The position of the P_{CO_2}/pH plot can indicate the acid-base status. Thus, point E (pH 7.27, P_{CO_2} 75 mmHg, 10 kPa) lies above the normal P_{CO_2} isobar (i.e. respiratory acidosis) and above and to the right of the zero base excess buffer line (i.e. metabolic alkalosis). The position of point E in relation to the pH 7.4 line will indicate (in the *untreated* patient) the likely *primary* problem, as the pH is always abnormal in the direction of the primary problem (*see* p. 198).

Understanding acid–base problems

All acid–base abnormalities, however complex, can be reduced to analysis of one or more of four fundamental disorders, each implying an 'insult' too great for the buffers to 'contain'. These disorders can easily be defined with reference to the bicarbonate buffer system:

- $CO_2 + H_2O \leftrightarrows H_2CO_3 \leftrightarrows H^+ + HCO_3^-$

The pair of dynamic equilibria interlink the two 'compartments' of acid–base physiology, with respiratory acid (CO_2) on the left and metabolic acid (H^+) on the right. Primary *respiratory* problems (acidosis or alkalosis) *directly* raise or lower the P_{CO_2} (with, as the above equation shifts to the right or left, a *secondary* change in $[H^+]$). On the other hand, primary *metabolic* disorders *directly* affect components at the right hand end of the above equation.

The terms acidaemia and alkalaemia refer *specifically* to the pH of the blood, and are not necessarily interchangeable with the terms acidosis and alkalosis. For example, in an acute primary metabolic *acidosis*, by definition the pH of the blood will fall below 7.36 (the lower limit of normal) and the patient will also have (again by definition) an *acidaemia*. Subsequently, as longer term compensating mechanisms (in this case a compensating respiratory alkalosis ($P_{CO_2}\downarrow$) return the pH towards normal, the *acidaemia* will be (by definition) abolished, although the patient

obviously still has a chronic (well compensated) metabolic *acidosis*.

The term 'compensation' can, in some ways, be used to describe two distinct processes. Firstly, it can be applied to the (for all practical purposes) immediate attempts by buffers to minimize primary alterations in various components. For example, in the equation above, the bicarbonate buffer system will respond to an initial acute rise in arterial P_{CO_2} (primary respiratory acidosis) by *immediately* converting some of the extra CO_2, via H_2CO_3, to H^+ and HCO_3^-. This shift from left to right, by raising the level of HCO_3^-, will partially compensate for the initial rise in P_{CO_2} – in so far as the pH will not deviate as much as it otherwise would have done. Secondly, as the patient comes to terms with a chronic problem, the longer term 'compensation' resulting from, in this example, retention of HCO_3^- and excretion of H^+ by the kidneys, will slowly return the pH towards the normal range. These two 'compensations' will be diagrammatically illustrated later.

To appreciate the simplicity of the practical interpretation of acid–base abnormalities, it may be helpful to return to the Henderson–Hasselbalch equation relating the various components of the bicarbonate buffer system:

- $$pH = pK + \log \frac{[HCO_3^+]}{[H_2CO_3]}$$

As the equilibrium $CO_2 + H_2O \leftrightarrows H_2CO_3$ is *very* far to the left, $(CO_2:H_2CO_3 \approx 1000:1)$, we can rewrite the above as follows:

- $$pH = pK + \log \frac{[HCO_3^-]}{\alpha \, pCO_2}$$

where α is the solubility coefficient of CO_2 in plasma (0.03 mmol/litre/mmHg, or 0.23 mmol/litre/kPa) and, when the arterial P_{CO_2} is normal, 1.2 mmol of CO_2 is carried per litre of plasma. By removal of various constants, one can reduce this equation to:

- $$pH \propto \frac{[HCO_3^-]}{PCO_2}$$

The pH is proportional to the ratio of $[HCO_3^-]/P_{CO_2}$, and the two constituents of this ratio are all one needs to study in patients with acid–base abnormalities. With this approach, each of the four fundamental problems of acid–base

Table 6.3 Alterations in PCO_2 and $[HCO_3^-]$ in acid–base disorders

	Acute		Chronic (compensated)	
	PCO_2	$[HCO_3^-]$	PCO_2	$[HCO_3^-]$
Respiratory acidosis	1 ↑↑	↑	2 ↑↑	↑↑
Respiratory alkalosis	3 ↓↓	↓	4 ↓↓	↓↓
Metabolic acidosis	5 ∼→	↓↓	6 ↓↓	↓↓
Metabolic alkalosis	7 ∼→	↑↑	8 ↑↑	↑↑

Key

Arrows refer to direction and relative magnitude of changes in acute and chronic disorders listed.

Numbers refer to arrows diagrammatically representing the changes in Figs. 6.4, 6.5 and 6.6.

balance can be viewed *primarily* as an upward or downward movement of either $[HCO_3^-]$ or PCO_2. Clearly, *respiratory* acidosis and alkalosis will result from, respectively, PCO_2 rising or falling. By exclusion (and, of course, because HCO_3^- is at the metabolic end of the bicarbonate buffer system), metabolic acidosis and alkalosis will result in movement of $[HCO_3^-]$ downwards or upwards respectively.

Furthermore, if the pH depends on a ratio ($[HCO_3^-]/PCO_2$) and the primary problem involves, say, a rise in the numerator ($[HCO_3^-]$), then, if the ratio is to return towards normal, the compensating mechanism *must* involve a rise in the denominator (PCO_2). In other words, if the constituents of the ratio move at all, they always move in the same direction (Table 6.3).

Diagrammatic representation of acid–base disorders

The four fundamental disorders – respiratory acidosis and alkalosis, metabolic acidosis and alkalosis – can be represented satisfactorily in several ways. Some texts favour the pH/P_{CO} diagram of Sigaard–Andersen, others the pH/HCO_3^- diagram of Davenport or the PCO_2/HCO_3^- diagram of Campbell. Any of these diagrams can be used as a basis for discussion, and for completeness this review includes all

three approaches (Figs. 6.4, 6.5 and 6.6). It could be argued that, as pH and PCO_2 are actually measured, the diagram with those variables as ordinate and abscissa·is the most logical. Alternatively, if pH $\propto \dfrac{[HCO_3^-]}{PCO_2}$, it also seem logical to refer to a diagram with those axes. The present author has found the Campbell diagram (*see* Fig. 6.6) most easily understood.

Each of the four acid–base disorders can be somewhat artifically divided into acute and chronic phases. This separation of the acute rapid deviation of pH from normal, from the longer term compensatory attempt by the untreated patient to return the pH to within the normal range, does not, of course, imply that, for example, acute bronchitis suddenly becomes chronic. In fact, the acute changes are gradually modified by the longer-term compensating mechanisms. Nonetheless, the separation does allow illustration of several fundamental concepts.

The legends relating to Figs. 6.4, 6.5 and 6.6 describe the changes represented in the diagrams, but several points may be worth stressing.

Acute changes in PCO_2 seen in primary respiratory acidosis and alkalosis are resisted by the bicarbonate buffer system with resultant changes in $[HCO_3^-]$. These changes are in *actual* $[HCO_3^-]$, rather than *standard* $[HCO_3^-]$ (which, by definition, eliminates the effect of buffering changes in PCO_2). Note that, as a result of this movement of the bicarbonate buffer system (equation p. 193) from left to right in acute respiratory acidosis (arrow 1, Fig. 6.6) or right to left (acute respiratory alkalosis – arrow 3, Fig. 6.6), the pH remains closer to the normal range than would otherwise have been the case (for example, as in arrow C, Fig. 6.7).

Similarly, one would have expected acute changes in $[HCO_3^-]$ to be accompanied by short-term alterations in PCO_2. For example, in acute metabolic acidosis (arrow 5), a rise in $[H^+]$ should be resisted by a shift of the bicarbonate buffer system from right to left (equation p. 193). The expected corollary of a rise in PCO_2 is, in practice, resisted by the respiratory centre responding to the rise in CSF PCO_2 (and therefore the fall in CSF pH) by increasing ventilation, even in the short term. ECF and CSF PCO_2 levels change together, whereas the 'blood-brain-barrier' ensures that changes in ECF $[HCO_3^-]$ are *not* immediately associated with similar changes on the other side of the barrier – in the CSF.

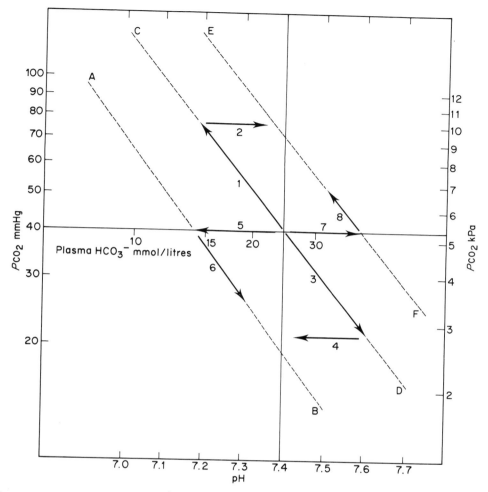

Fig 6.4   Representation of acute and chronic acid–base disorders on the P_{CO_2}/pH diagram. **Lines AB, CD, EF:** *In vivo* buffer lines of constant base deficit, base normal (zero) and base excess respectively. **Arrow 1:** Acute respiratory acidosis. P_{CO_2} rises and pH falls. Patient initially moves up *in vivo* buffer line (constant base excess zero), implying that, in the acute phase, metabolic status is unchanged. **Arrow 2:** Chronic respiratory acidosis. Compensating mechanism for established respiratory acidosis is a metabolic alkalosis. Thus renal compensation returns pH towards normal and base excess rises. **Arrow 3:** Acute respiratory alkalosis, with movement down normal *in vivo* buffer line (base excess stays zero). **Arrow 4:** Chronic respiratory alkalosis, with compensating metabolic acidosis reducing base excess (or more correctly, inducing a base deficit) to return pH towards normal. **Arrow 5:** Acute metabolic acidosis. Plasma bicarbonate, by definition *standard* bicarbonate (as P_{CO_2} remains normal) falls. P_{CO_2} remains normal, as tendency for P_{CO_2} to alter as bicarbonate buffer system attempts to limit pH change is resisted by the respiratory centre (*see* text). **Arrow 6:** Chronic metabolic acidosis, with compensating respiratory alkalosis and patient moving down line AB (constant base deficit *in vivo* buffer line) towards normal pH. **Arrow 7:** Acute metabolic alkalosis, with plasma *standard* bicarbonate rising and P_{CO_2} remaining constant (for reasons stated above). **Arrow 8:** Chronic metabolic alkalosis, with compensating respiratory acidosis. As P_{CO_2} rises, patient moves up constant +ve base excess *in vivo* buffer line, returning pH towards normal.

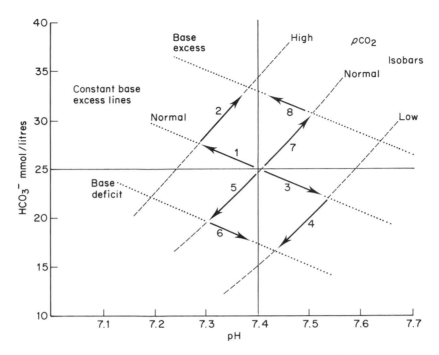

Fig 6.5   Representation of acute and chronic acid–base disorders on the pH/HCO$_3^-$ diagram. **Arrow 1**: Acute respiratory acidosis. Patient moves up normal constant base excess line towards high PCO$_2$ isobar. Metabolic status unchanged. **Arrow 2**: Chronic respiratory acidosis. pH returns towards normal as *compensating metabolic alkalosis* moves patient along high PCO$_2$ isobar towards a + ve base excess line. **Arrow 3**: Acute respiratory alkalosis. Patient moves down normal constant base excess line towards low PCO$_2$ isobar. Metabolic status unchanged. **Arrow 4**: Chronic respiratory alkalosis. *Compensating metabolic acidosis* moves patient down constant low PCO$_2$ isobar towards base deficit (− ve base excess) line (due to renal excretion of HCO$_3^-$) and normal pH. **Arrow 5**: Acute metabolic acidosis. Patient moves down constant normal PCO$_2$ isobar to new base deficit (− ve base excess) buffer line. PCO$_2$ initially kept constant by respiratory centre. **Arrow 6**: Chronic metabolic acidosis. *Compensating respiratory alkalosis*, with hyperventilation shifting patient down constant base deficit line towards normal pH. **Arrow 7**: Acute metabolic alkalosis. pH rises as patient moves along constant normal PCO$_2$ isobar towards new + ve base excess buffer line. PCO$_2$ kept normal initially by respiratory centre. **Arrow 8**: Chronic metabolic alkalosis. *Compensating respiratory acidosis*. Hypoventilating patient moves up new + ve base excess buffer line towards high PCO$_2$ isobar and normal pH.

If pH is proportional to the ratio of [HCO$_3^-$]/PCO$_2$, then if, for example, the primary abnormality is a rise in PCO$_2$, the compensating mechanism *must* be a rise in [HCO$_3^-$]. Thus, in Table 6.3, movements of PCO$_2$ and [HCO$_3^-$] are always in the same direction, in an attempt to keep the ratio (and therefore the pH) as close to normal as possible.

In the untreated patient, compensating mechanisms (arrows 2, 4, 6 and 8 in Figs. 6.4, 6.5 and 6.6) whilst frequently returning the pH to within the normal range, never quite return it to 7.4, let alone overcompensate. In other words, arrows 2, 4, 6 and 8 never cross the pH 7.4 line. This

means that, in the *untreated* patient, the pH always remains deviated in the direction of the primary problem.

Interpretation of blood-gas results

Although assessment of acid–base status must depend, in the final analysis, on clinical judgement, interpretation of the results of blood-gas analysis should be among the fundamental skills of the anaesthetist – both in the operating theatre and intensive therapy unit. Measured pH and PCO$_2$ values can, of course, be plotted on any of the

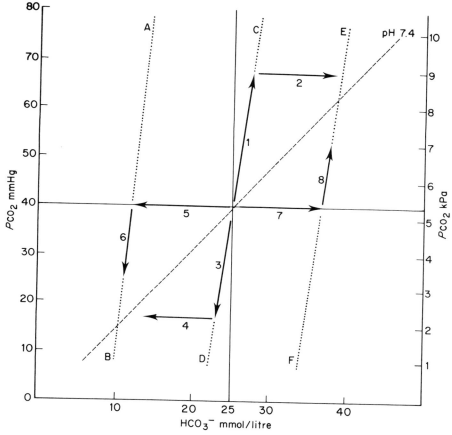

Fig 6.6 Representation of acute and chronic acid–base disorders on the P_{CO_2}/HCO_3^- diagram. **Lines AB, CD, EF:** Low (deficit), normal, and high (excess) constant base excess buffer lines. **Arrow 1:** Acute respiratory acidosis. As P_{CO_2} rises, *actual* bicarbonate rises (abcissa is *actual* bicarbonate), reflecting movement of bicarbonate buffer system from left to right (*see* text). However, patient moves up constant normal base excess line, implying that, initially, metabolic status is unchanged. **Arrow 2:** Chronic respiratory acidosis. *Compensating* metabolic alkalosis. [HCO_3^-] rises further, as renal compensating mechanisms return pH towards normal. **Arrow 3:** Acute respiratory alkalosis. Hyperventilation reduces P_{CO_2} and patient moves down constant normal base excess line. Actual bicarbonate falls reflecting movement of bicarbonate buffer system from right to left. Metabolic status is unchanged. **Arrow 4:** Chronic respiratory alkalosis. *Compensating* metabolic acidosis. Renal mechanisms excrete HCO_3^- and patient moves towards normal pH and lower (base deficit) constant base excess line. **Arrow 5:** Acute metabolic acidosis. [HCO_3^-] falls as patient moves towards new low (base deficit) base excess line. P_{CO_2} is initially kept approximately constant by respiratory centre (resisting changes imposed by bicarbonate buffer system). **Arrow 6:** Chronic metabolic acidosis. Hyperventilation lower P_{CO_2} (*compensating* respiratory alkalosis) and patient moves down low (base deficit) constant base excess line towards normal pH. **Arrow 7:** Acute metabolic alkalosis. [HCO_3^-] rises, with P_{CO_2} remaining constant (for reasons stated above). pH rises and patient moves towards new high base excess buffer line. **Arrow 8:** Chronic metabolic alkalosis. Hypoventilation raises P_{CO_2} and moves patient up new constant high base excess buffer line towards normal pH. (Reproduced by kind permission of Blackwell Scientific Publications. Taken from *Clinical Physiology*, 4 E, by Campbell, EJM).

acid–base diagrams discussed earlier (Figs. 6.3, 6.4, 6.5 and 6.6), and conclusions drawn from the sector into which the plot falls (*see* legend, Fig. 6.3). Indeed, commercially available acid–base charts facilitate interpretation further by designating areas into which with, say, 95 per cent confidence, plots from patients with various abnormalities can be expected to fall. However, appreciation of the essentials of acid–base physiology and the development of the various approaches to analysis should allow ready interpretation of results of blood-gas analysis produced by automated analysers without the need for 'artificial aids'.

In general, interpretation is quite simple, with analysers measuring pH and PCO_2 and deriving a variety of values aimed at diagnosis and treatment. Various machines deliver results in differing formats, and relevant definitions may bear repetition here.

- **pH** Normal range 7.36–7.44 (equivalent to 44–36 nmol/litre H$^+$). The pH of the sample (temperature corrected if appropriate). In the *untreated* patient, the pH is always deflected in the direction of the primary problem (reflecting the 'rule' that a patient never quite fully compensates for a primary acid–base problem, let alone overcompensates). Thus, if, as in most patients, there are two 'opposing' acid–base abnormalities, say respiratory acidosis and metabolic alkalosis, the pH will indicate which of the two abnormalities is primary (and which, by exclusion, is compensating).
- **PCO_2** Normal range 35–45 mmHg (4.5 –6 kPa). Again, temperature corrected if appropriate, the PCO_2 indicates the respiratory component of acid base status. By definition, values above and below the normal range imply respiratory acidosis and alkalosis respectively.
- **HCO_3^-** *Actual* bicarbonate concentration, normal range 22–26 mmol/litre. This figure reflects both the metabolic status *and* effects of buffering of abnormal PCO_2 levels, and is of little value in practical interpretation.
- **TCO_2** Total CO_2, normal approximately 26.2 mmol/litre. This is a somewhat outmoded assessment of total CO_2 carriage, both as bicarbonate and in solution in the plasma. It is merely the sum of the bicarbonate concentration (say 25 mmol/litre and α PCO_2 where α is the solubility coefficient for CO_2 (0.03 mmol/litre/mmHg, 0.23 mmol/litre/kPa).
- **BE** Base excess, normal 0 ± 2 mmol/litre

defined as the number of mmol of HCO_3^- which must be added to (or theoretically removed from) each litre of ECF to return the ECF pH to 7.4 – if the PCO_2 were normal. As this derived value is standardized to normal respiratory function, it both identifies the metabolic status of the patient and provides a basis for treatment – *if* the metabolic aspect of the condition requires treatment. Originally defined 'per litre of blood' but now more pragmatically applied 'per litre of ECF' (throughout which bicarbonate is distributed), some analyses differentiate between these two concepts by delivering BE and SBE ('standard' BE) figures respectively. In practice this is irrelevant and 'base excess' should remain defined per litre of ECF and discussed as such. By definition, a negative base excess (or, perhaps, more properly a base deficit) implies a metabolic acidosis, and a positive value a metabolic alkalosis. Whether or not the base excess figure is seen as a basis for treatment depends, of course, on whether the metabolic abnormality is the primary problem or the compensating mechanism. In the *untreated* patient, reference to the pH will identify the direction of primary change (*see* above).

- **SBC** Standard bicarbonate, normal 22–26 mmol/litre. Defined as the ECF bicarbonate concentration the patient *would* have *if* the PCO_2 were normal, the SBC is a further (some say superfluous) index of metabolic status. By definition, values below and above the normal range indicate respectively metabolic acidosis or alkalosis. Diagrammatic representations of the differentiation between standard and actual bicarbonate are shown in Figs. 6.7 and 6.8.
- **PO_2 and O_2 saturation** Arterial PO_2 (normal $\approx$ 100 mmHg, 13 kPa breathing air, and decreasing with age) and percentage saturation of haemoglobin with oxygen will, with knowledge of the inspired oxygen concentration (F_IO_2) provide evidence of respiratory status.

Temperature correction for blood-gas analysis

All blood-gas analyses are carried out at 37° C, but pH, PCO_2 and PO_2 are all temperature dependent (Burnett and Nooman, 1974). Therefore, temperature corrections should be applied to the

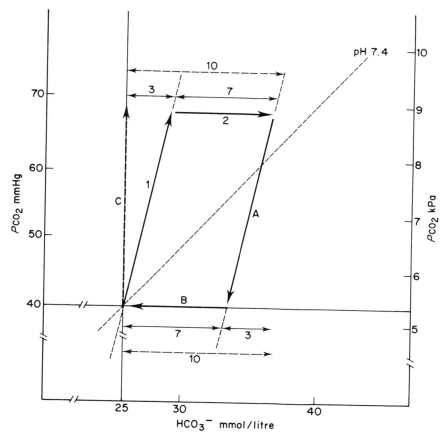

Fig 6.7 Representation of standard and actual bicarbonate levels on the PCO_2/HCO_3^- diagram. Arrows 1 and 2 represent acute and chronic respiratory acidosis as in Fig. 6.6. **Arrow 1**: As PCO_2 rises, *actual* bicarbonate rises from 25 to 28 mmol/litre, shown as an initial rise of 3 mmol/litre. Note that, by this means, pH is kept closer to 7.4 than would have been the case without the rise in bicarbonate for buffering reasons (arrow C). **Arrow 2**: Compensating metabolic alkalosis raises *actual* bicarbonate by a further 7 mmol/litre to 35 mmol/litre. Total rise in [HCO_3^-] is 10 mmol/litre, of which 3 mmol/litre represents the result of buffering the rising PCO_2 by the bicarbonate buffer system and 7 mmol/litre results from renal metabolic compensation.

As *standard* bicarbonate (SBC) is *defined* as the bicarbonate concentration the patient would have if the PCO_2 were normal, this expression eliminates effects of bicarbonate buffering of abnormal PCO_2 levels. Therefore, at the end of arrow 2, while the *actual* bicarbonate is 35 mmol/litre, the *standard* bicarbonate is 3 mmol/litre less (i.e. 32 mmol/litre).

This may be further clarified by following the changes imposed on a patient with established chronic respiratory acidosis by mechanical ventilation (IPPV) down to a normal PCO_2. **Arrow A**: The patient is moved *across* the pH 7.4 line, down a constant high base excess buffer line, and thus loses the 3 mmol/litre bicarbonate related solely to buffering the high PCO_2. Arrow A meets the normal PCO_2 isobar at a bicarbonate level of 32 mmol/litre (which, by definition, is *standard* bicarbonate). Note that, as the respiratory acidosis has now been mechanically corrected, the patient is left with a compensating metabolic alkalosis without the initial respiratory acidosis for which it was compensating! Over several hours, the now superfluous metabolic alkalosis is abolished by the kidneys, and the patient moves along arrow B towards pH 7.4.

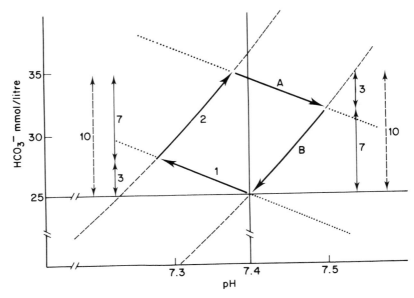

Fig 6.8 Representation of standard and actual bicarbonate levels on the pH/HCO$_3^-$ diagram. **Arrows 1 and 2** represent acute and chronic respiratory acidosis as in Fig. 6.5, and are explained in the legend for Fig. 6.7.

Arrow A describes the patient with established chronic respiratory acidosis mechanically ventilated down to a normal PCO$_2$ and moving down a high constant base excess buffer line to the normal PCO$_2$ isobar (*see* Fig 6.5). Note that, as the PCO$_2$ is returned to normal, the actual bicarbonate falls from 35 to 32 mmol/litre and the value 32 mmol/litre is, by definition, the *standard* bicarbonate.

Arrow B represents the patient, mechanically ventilated to a normal PCO$_2$, excreting the now superfluous excess HCO$_3^-$ and passing down the normal PCO$_2$ isobar towards pH 7.4.

results if the patient is not normothermic. The pH of whole blood changes by approximately 0.015 units per degree Celsius, rising as temperature falls. The solubility coefficient (α) of any gas rises as temperature falls (i.e. the gases become more soluble) and for any given content of gas, the pressure falls. The simple relationship of α to temperature is complicated by, for example, the equilibrium of CO$_2$ with H$_2$CO$_3$, or the equilibrium between oxyhaemoglobin and dissolved oxygen. Some approximate correction factors for relevant patient temperatures are given in Table 6.4,

although a slide rule has been devised to facilitate correction (Severinghaus, 1966) and modern blood-gas analysers can be programmed to produce corrected data.

The implications of acid–base abnormalities

Respiratory abnormalities

Acidosis

The commonest causes in this country are acute and chronic bronchitis. A rise in PCO$_2$ is associated with increased levels of circulating catecholamines. The circulation is 'hyperdynamic', with increased myocardial contractility, rate and output, and dilatation of peripheral vessels. The tendency for catecholamine-related peripheral constriction is countered by the direct vasodilating action of carbon dioxide. Carbon dioxide is a potent vasodilator, and hypercarbia is associated with a

Table 6.4 Correction factors for pH, PCO$_2$ and PO$_2$

Temp. °C	pH	PCO$_2$ (% correction)	PO$_2$ (% correction)
40	− 0.04	+ 12	+ 19
37	−	−	−
35	+ 0.03	− 8	− 13
32	+ 0.07	− 19	− 30
30	+ 0.10	− 26	− 39
26	− 0.16	− 37	− 54

rise in cerebral perfusion and intracranial pressure – to be avoided at all costs in patients with even a suspicion of intracranial problems. There is a tendency towards increased surgical bleeding, even seen in routine anaesthetic practice as the P_{CO_2} is allowed to rise towards normal (either by reducing IPPV or even administering a low concentration of carbon dioxide) to encourage the return of spontaneous respiration as muscle relaxants are reversed.

As a result of direct effects on the myocardium, dysrhythmias are common, with a tendency towards atrio-ventricular block, brachycardia and ventricular ectopics (often dangerously multi-focal). This tendency is exacerbated by hypoxia or the presence of anaesthetic agents such as halo-thane and cyclopropane (said to 'sensitize' the myocardium to circulating catecholamines). It appears that both enflurane and, especially, isoflu-rane have much less dysrhythmogenic potential under these circumstances.

An increase in P_{CO_2} initially stimulates respiration (both centrally as a result of a fall in CSF pH and peripherally via chemoreceptors in the aortic and carotid bodies), but this is followed by CNS depression, with confusion, eventual unconscious-ness and further hypoventilation.

Even under well-managed anaesthesia, the spontaneously breathing patient tends to become hypercarbic. Alterations in ventilation/perfusion relationships under anaesthesia may impede gaseous exchange and all anaesthetic/sedative drugs tend to depress respiration further. This tendency will be exacerbated by the use of inappropriate anaesthetic circuitry or inadequate fresh gas flows – allowing unacceptable degrees of rebreathing and carbon dioxide accumulation.

Alkalosis

The commonest causes are hysteria and iatrogenic (IPPV in anaesthesia). A fall in P_{CO_2} is associated with increased cerebral vascular resistance and a reduction in blood flow. Cardiac output falls and peripheral vasoconstriction may produce periphe-ral cyanosis.

Without routine on-line end-tidal or arterial P_{CO_2} monitoring, in patients for whom muscle relaxation is necessary, there is a sensible tendency for anaesthetists to hyperventilate moderately – using alveolar minute volumes somewhat greater than those generally accepted as 'adequate'. The

resulting tendency towards vasoconstriction is usually of little consequence (except, perhaps, in patients with barely adequate cerebral perfusion at best). Indeed, modern 'hypotensive' anaesthesia can often achieve a satisfactory surgical field, without the necessity for potentially dangerously low pressures, by moderate hyperventilation and resultant reductions in P_{CO_2}, cardiac output and blood flow at the surgical site.

Metabolic (non-respiratory) disorders

Acidosis

There is general cardiovascular depression, with decreased myocardial contratility and cardiac output. Increased sympathetic tone is associated with intense peripheral vasoconstriction and reduction in hepatic and renal blood flow. Pulmonary vascular resistance may rise. Dysrhyth-mias are common, often exacerbated by too rapid correction of the acidosis and the associated hyper-kalaemia. Hyperkalaemia reflects a shift of K^+ from the ICF (as H^+ moves in the opposite direction). Close monitoring is essential.

Initially of course, a metabolic acidosis will stimulate respiration, as the patient attempts to compensate with a respiratory alkalosis. Even-tually, however, a continuing severe metabolic acidosis will centrally depress respiration and reverse the trend.

Essentially, metabolic acidosis can be catego-rized with regard to whether or not the aetiology involves the generation of acids, such as ketoacids in diabetes or lactic acid in lactic acidosis. Such acids can be detected by consideration of the 'anion gap'. The normal anion gap:

- $([Na^+] + [K^+]) - ([Cl^-] + [HCO_3^-])$

is < 15 mmol/litre and reflects the presence of phosphate, sulphate, proteins and other anions which are not usually measured.

Lactic acidosis (levels > 5 mmol/litre) has been classified into Type A (related to inadequate peripheral tissue perfusion (shock) and anaerobic metabolism) and Type B (without clinically obvious inadequate perfusion but related to, for example, hepatic insufficiency, diabetes, phen-formin, methanol or ethylene glycol intoxication). Type B lactic acidosis would be associated with an increased anion gap. However, in most patients with Type B lactic acidosis, the picture is likely to be complicated by a degree of circulatory insufficiency and thus a contribution by Type A. Conversely, in patients with severe shock, inadequate hepatic blood flow may cause lactate production by the liver (rather than, physiologically, lactate uptake and metabolism).

The treatment of metabolic acidosis with, perhaps, multiple aetiologies, will partly be directed at improvement of peripheral tissue perfusion by the administration of fluids (when appropriate), vasodilators and inotropes, with, at the same time, the administration of appropriate amounts of sodium bicarbonate. In general, an acidotic myocardium responds poorly to inotrope infusions, so at least partial correction of the acidosis is usually advisable. The negative base excess (or base deficit) figure is used as a rough guide to the amount of bicarbonate needed. A result of, say, -10 suggests that 10 mmol bicarbonate are required *per litre of ECF* to return the pH to normal. ECF volume is commonly taken as some 25 per cent of body weight (i.e. 60 per cent of bodyweight is water, of which 35 per cent is ICF and 25 per cent ECF). Thus, a man weighing 80 kg with a base excess of -10 requires approximately 200 mmol of bicarbonate. The usual concentration of bicarbonate used is 8.4 per cent (which contains 1 mmol HCO_3^-/ml), but several practical points are worth remembering. As 8.4 % $NaHCO_3$ is grossly hypertonic (osmolality 2000 mosm/kg), very alkaline and therefore very irritant to small veins, let alone extra-vascular tissues, it should always be administered via large antecubital or, even better, central veins. If such veins are inaccessible, 1.4 % $NaHCO_3$ (one sixth molar) is available, but, of course, large volumes are required. The base excess figure is only an approximate guide to base requirements at the time of sampling. If, as bicarbonate is being administered, steps are being taken to improve oxygenation and peripheral tissue perfusion, rather less than the calculated amount may be necessary. In these circumstances, it may be thought advisable to administer, say, half the apparent requirement over 30 minutes and then reassess the acid–base status. Over-correction, by shifting the haemoglobin-oxygen dissociation curve unnecessarily far to the left, reduces oxygen delivery to the tissues. The very rapid administration of bicarbonate is inadvisable except in emergency circumstances for two reasons. Firstly, carbon dioxide will be generated by the bicarbonate buffer system shifting further to the left – and more ventilation will be necessary. The extra carbon dioxide may diffuse into cells (much faster than bicarbonate can do) and exacerbate intracellular acidosis. Secondly, the rapid correction of an acidosis (with its usual corollary, hyperkalaemia) may, by rapidly reducing potassium levels, encourage dysrhythmias.

It should be noted that bicarbonate is not usually advocated in the treatment of diabetic ketoacidosis (unless the pH is low enough to embarrass myocardial function) because such treatment would involve the administration of a grossly hypertonic fluid to an already hyperosmolar patient, and also because such patients usually respond to the administration of saline and insulin and correct the acidosis themselves.

Furthermore, as implied above, correction of the acidosis with bicarbonate may well adversely affect tissue oxygenation – at least in the short term. Tissue oxygenation in acidosis reflects a balance between two opposing forces. Firstly, the acidosis shifts the haemoglobin-oxygen (HbO_2) dissociation curve to the right. This Bohr effect raises the P_{50} of Hb (i.e. the PO_2 at which Hb is 50 per cent saturated with O_2) or, in other words, decreases the saturation of Hb with O_2 at any given PO_2 and thus increases oxygen availability to the tissues. On the other hand, the reduction in 2,3-diphosphoglycerate (2,3-DPG) seen in acidosis, by shifting the HbO_2 dissociation curve to the left (back towards normal), tends to reverse these changes. The beneficial results of the Bohr effect are, to some extent, nullified by the reduction in 2,3-DPG.

Following rapid correction of the acidosis with bicarbonate, as regeneration of 2,3-DPG takes at least several hours, the shift of the HbO_2 dissociation to the left results in a period of reduced tissue oxygenation – the clinical significance of which is uncertain.

Alkalosis

The common causes are persistent vomiting (e.g. in pyloric stenosis), self-administration of alkali by patients with peptic ulcer (the milk–alkali syndrome) and iatrogenic (overadministration of bicarbonate when treating metabolic acidosis). Potassium depletion (perhaps diuretic-induced) is also associated wtih a metabolic alkalosis, as the kidney excretes H^+ while retaining K^+. This is an example of so-called paradoxical aciduria, with inappropriately *acid* urine in the face of a metabolic *alkalosis*. It is rarely necessary to treat metabolic alkalosis directly (by the intravenous infusion of NH_4Cl or even HCl) as it is usually more appropriate to treat the cause – for example, the correction of potassium depletion.

Iatrogenic metabolic alkalosis is, in some respects, invited by the availability of 8.4 % sodium bicarbonate in 200 ml containers. In emergency circumstances, it is all too easy to administer 200 mmol of bicarbonate as a routine. It seems that, if the circulation is *quickly* restored following cardiac arrest, such treatment is unnecessary. In any event, as a simple rule, it seems that 100 mmol will suffice in an adult in emergency circumstances until the acid–base status can be assessed.

Anaesthesia for patients with metabolic acidosis

Patients with severe metabolic acidosis must be approached with great care. Not only is there compromise and instability of the cardiovascular system when they present for operation, but their response to ostensibly 'normal' doses of commonly used agents may be disastrous. Monitoring of electrocardiogram and arterial pressure is mandatory. Clearly, if time allows, assessment and treatment of the acidosis and hyperkalaemia, and at least partial correction of contributory factors such as hypovolaemia, inadequate peripheral tissue perfusion and hypotension is advisable. In addition, the importance of careful monitoring (of blood gases, potassium and blood sugar levels, and urine output) and reliable venous access (including, if possible, a central venous cannula) cannot be over-emphasized. Acidosis is associated with insulin resistance and blood sugar may be difficult to control.

Changes in pH may affect the ionization and availability of drugs. For example, in the acidotic patient, thiopentone is less protein-bound, more 'available' and thus more potent than usual.

The diffusion of a drug across cell membranes and its renal excretion depend on the degree of ionization – which in turn is a function of the dissociation constant (pKa) of the drug in relation to the ambient pH. If the pKa of the drug is the same as the pH, the ionized and unionized forms of the drug are present in equal proportions.* In

general, cell membranes are permeable only to a drug in its unionized (lipid soluble) form. A fall in pH will decrease ionization of acidic drugs and increase ionization of basic drugs, with weakly ionizing drugs being most affected by alterations in pH. Weak acids such as thiopentone will become less ionized as the ECF pH falls, more lipid soluble and perhaps more effective.

Urinary excretion of weak electrolytes may be profoundly affected by alterations in urinary pH. Thus alkalinization of the urine may increase the excretion of weak acids such as aspirin and phenobarbitone. Once such drugs have diffused across tubular cells in their unionized form, they ionize in the relatively alkaline environment within the lumen, become non-diffusible and are excreted. This forms the basis of forced alkaline diuresis in the treatment of overdosage.

Poor hepatic and renal blood flow may hinder metabolism and excretion of drugs. As non-depolarizing muscle relaxants may last longer and reversal may be difficult, smaller doses are wise, at least initially. Perhaps atracurium, which degrades spontaneously at body temperature, may be useful in these patients. The dose of *any* drug, be it induction agent, sedative or analgesic, must be reduced to minimize unnecessary additional myocardial depression and, as in all 'difficult' anaesthetic circumstances, drugs such as induction agents should be *slowly* 'titrated' against patient response. It is clearly more important to choose the anaesthetist than the anaesthetic drugs themselves! All current inhalational agents depress myocardial function to some degree and, perhaps, should be avoided. Halothane sensitizes the myocardium to circulating catecholamines, and therefore enflurane and isoflurane are probably less dysrhythmogenic in acidotic patients. Isoflurane seems less depressant to the myocardium than either halothane or enflurane but has been reported to cause 'steal phenomenon' from the damaged myocardial. Intermittent positive pressure ventilation may severely exacerbate hypotension in the hypovolaemic patient by decreasing venous return – further underlining the importance of preanaesthetic rehydration. A ventilatory pattern which minimizes the rise in mean intrathoracic pressure (and therefore the decrease in venous return) is advisable i.e. infrequent large tidal volumes with a short inspiratory phase.

Appropriate resuscitation drugs should be readily available to allow urgent treatment of dysrhythmias and hypotension. Infused inotropes in general seem less effective in the presence of

---

*pKa of thiopentone = 7.6
 pKa of lignocaine = 7.9
 pKa of tubocurarine = 14

acidosis, and it is said that dopamine is more readily converted to nor-adrenaline and is more likely to constrict perpherally – even at low doses. None the less, a low dose infusion of dopamine (≈ 3 μg/kg/min) throughout the perioperative period may encourage renal blood flow and urine output.

Careful monitoring of all the parameters mentioned must, of course, be extended well into the postoperative period.

References and further reading

Diagrammatic representations of acid–base changes

Log PCO_2 / pH diagrams (on which Figs. 6.1, 6.2, 6.3 and 6.4 are based)

Astrup, P., Jorgensen, K., Siggaard-Andersen, O. and Engel, K. (1960). The acid-base metabolism. A new approach. Lancet, **1**, 1035.

Siggaard-Andersen, O. (1962). The pH, log PCO_2 blood acid–base nomogram revised. *Scandinavian Journal of Clinical and Laboratory Investigation* **14**, 598–604.

Siggaard-Andersen, O. (1963). The acid–base status of the blood. *Scandinavian Journal of Clinical and Laboratory Investigation* **15**, Suppl. 70.

Siggaard-Andersen, O. (1971). An acid–base chart for arterial blood with normal and pathophysiological reference areas. *Scandinavian Journal of Clinical and Laboratory Investigation* **27**, 239–45. (The Siggaard-Andersen Curve Nomogram and Acid–Base Chart have been distributed under copyright (1959, 1962, 1967, 1970, 1974) by Radiometer A/S, Copenhagen, Denmark).

Siggaard-Andersen, O. and Engel, K. (1960). A new acid–base nomogram. *Scandinavian Journal of Clinical and Laboratory Investigation* **12**, 177–86.

Blood–gas alignment nomogram

Siggaard-Andersen, O. (1963). Blood acid–base alignment nomogram. *Scandinavian Journal of Clinical and Laboratory Investigation* **15**, 211–17. (The Siggaard-Andersen Alignment Nomogram has been distributed under copyright (1962, 1967) by Radiometer A/S, Copenhagen, Denmark).

pH / HCO_3^- diagram (on which Figs. 6.5, and 6.8 are based)

Davenport, H.W. (1974). *The ABC of acid–base chemistry*. Sixth edition (revised). University of Chicago Pres, Chicago.

pCO_2/HCO_3^- diagram (on which Figs. 6.6 and 6.7 are based)

Campbell, E.J.M. (1974). *Hydrogen Ion (Acid–Base) Regulation in Clinical Physiology*. Fourth Edition, pp. 232–58. Blackwell Scientific Publications, London.

Review of correction factors for blood gases
(on which Table 6.4 is based)

Burnett, R.W. and Noonan, D.C. (1974). Calculations and correction factors used in determination of blood pH and blood gases. *Clinical Chemistry* **20**, (12), 1499–1506.

Blood-gas and temperature correction slide rule

Severinghaus, J.W. (1966). Blood-gas calculator. *Journal of Applied Physiology* **21** (3), 1108–16.

7
Nephrology

Gwyn Williams

Measurement of renal function

There are many tests designed to measure the various functions of the kidneys, some of them complex and invasive. In this section only those performed in general medical and surgical wards are considered.

Tests of renal function are designed to answer the following questions:

- Is glomerular filtration rate normal?
- Is the filtrate itself correctly formed within the glomeruli?
- Is the filtrate handled correctly by the tubules?

The various tests will be described in ascending order of complexity or invasiveness.

Urinalysis by dipstick testing and microscopy

The detector square on Labstix contains methyl red, bromthymol blue and buffering salts. These dissolve when dipped into urine and stabilize the pH of the paper at a level which keeps the colour of the indicators a pale yellow-green. Protein in the urine lowers the pH at which these indicators change colour, so the detector becomes increasingly green in proportion to the protein concentration. Albustix contains bromphenol blue and works similarly. False positives occur in very alkaline urine, as in urinary infection. Labstix is most sensitive to albumin, i.e. the main constituent of most pathological proteinurias, but it is not sensitive to some other proteins, especially Bence–Jones protein.

If proteinuria is detected it should be investigated further as described on p. 220. The dextrose detector on Labstix uses glucose oxidase so it is specific to dextrose. Glycosuria is found in

hyperglycaemia, but also in some patients with heavy proteinuria due to functional changes in the proximal tubular cells, in tubular disorders, and as an isolated congenital abnormality. Labstix detects free haemoglobin or myoglobin in urine. Haematuria is usually accompanied by lysis of red cells and therefore commonly produces a positive chemical reaction for haemoglobin. However a positive chemical test should always be confirmed by urinary microscopy.

Microscopy

This is a very powerful tool for investigating renal disease, but is too often neglected. The following abnormalities may be readily seen after only moderate experience:

- Heavy contamination with bacteria, indicating urinary tract infection.
- Leucocytes are easily recognized by their granular cytoplasm and lobed nuclei. Mononuclear cells are rarely seen. Leucocytes appear in the urine in large numbers during acute renal failure, in toxic nephropathies and in the first 24–48 hours after consumption of aspirin and other analgesics. Heavy pyuria, causing cloudy urine, is found almost exclusively in acute urinary infection. Less impressive leucocyturia is found in analgesic nephropathy, renal stones and chronic pyelonephritis with uninfected urine. Leucocyturia is common in several forms of glomerulonephritis.
- Red Cells. Red cell morphology depends on the origin of the cells. Red cells from the glomeruli are irregular in size and shape whilst red cells from the renal pelvis, ureter or bladder are of uniform shape apart from a few red cell ghosts.
  It has been found that the number of red cells in the urine rises after exercise.
- Casts. Casts are protein precipitate formed

within tubules, i.e. they are a 'cast' of a part of the urinary system. They have a variety of appearances depending upon their other constituents.

Hyaline casts are close to the refractive index of urine and are best observed in low illumination or under phase contrast. They consist of Tamm–Horsfall mucoprotein. A small number are excreted by normal individuals. Numerous hyaline casts are seen after very strenuous exercise, during febrile illnesses and after the administration of loop diuretics. They are found in most forms of chronic renal disease, usually with the other types described below and persist for years in the urine of patients with essential hypertension.

Densely granular casts are always pathological and are found in all forms of glomerulonephritis, in diabetic nephropathy and in amyloid. They accompany the accelerated phase of essential hypertension but disappear with effective treatment. The granules contain various proteins which have leaked through the glomerulus.

Cellular casts are hyaline or granular casts with tubular epithelial cells on their surface. Those with few cells are common in many forms of renal disease. Casts covered with many tubular cells are characteristic of acute tubular necrosis and rapidly progressive and acute types of glomerulonephritis.

Red cell casts are extremely important, as they are pathognomonic of glomerular bleeding. Numerous red cell casts are seen in acute nephritis and in rapidly progressive nephritis. Scantier red cell casts are found in the more active forms of other proliferative glomerulonephritides. They are virtually never seen without haematuria.

White cell casts are very uncommon. They are seen in acute pyelonephritis.

- Crystals. Cystine crystals are found in the urine of homozygous cystinurics. Oxalate crystals in fresh specimens indicate liability to oxalate stone formation, particularly if found in aggregates. Sulphonamide and other crystals are now rarely seen.

Measurement of plasma urea and creatinine concentrations

Urea clearance is about 35 per cent of glomerular filtration rate (GFR) at maximum urinary concentration and rises to about 70 per cent of GFR with a water diuresis over 2 ml/minute. If fluid intake and urea production are constant, plasma urea rises and falls with GFR. It is still used as an indicator of GFR, but has several disadvantages. Urea production varies with protein intake and with net catabolism of body protein, so the plasma urea rises disproportionately for a given GFR if the patient has a high protein intake or is catabolizing protein due to surgery, trauma, infection or treatment with corticosteroids or tetracyclines. Urea clearance falls, out of proportion to GFR, during sodium depletion producing a high plasma urea in relation to plasma creatinine. Conversely plasma urea is disproportionately lower for GFR during the anabolism of pregnancy and in hepatic disease.

Creatinine is a superior guide to GFR. Its production rate is almost independent of diet, although a heavy meal of cooked red meat can raise the plasma creatinine. Production rate depends on muscle mass, so is lower in women then men, falls with age and varies appropriately between individuals of the same age and sex. The normal range is large but a rising or falling plasma creatinine usually reflects a rising of falling GFR. Serial measurement of plasma creatinine is the most convenient means of following the progress of chronic renal disease. The rise in plasma creatinine with falling GFR is hyperbolic. Considerable renal function is lost in the early stage of the disease for a slight rise in plasma creatinine, whereas a rapid rise occurs during the later stages of the disease. This problem can be partly overcome by plotting the reciprocal of plasma creatinine against time. The fall in the reciprocal of plasma creatinine parallels the decline in GFR.

Because of the wide normal range plasma creatinine is less satisfactory in confirming normal renal function – hence the need for accurate measurements of GFR.

Creatinine clearance

When carefully performed creatinine clearance correlates closely with inulin clearance except in the few circumstances where creatinine secretion is important e.g. late renal failure and following renal transplantation. However it has several errors and a low reproducibility. The commonest source of error is loss of part of the urine collection. Some authors state that creatinine clearance should be measured only if calculation of GFR from serum creatinine is likely to be erroneous (wasting, obesity, pregnancy, oedema) and if other methods described below are inapplicable (oedema, pregnancy) or inconvenient. It is performed on 24-hour urine collections, and a single blood sample. Inulin clearance, the standard method of measuring GFR in research, is inapplicable as it requires bladder catheterization. Several radio-active markers behave more or less like inulin i.e. they are filtered at the glomerulus but not secreted or reabsorbed by the tubule. Chromium-51-labelled EDTA is the most popular. It is usually employed as a single dose technique. After intra-venous injection, the concentration of the tracer in blood, measured in serial venous samples or by external counting over the heart, falls rapidly as it is distributed through extracellular fluid, then drops exponentially at a rate which depends on GFR. The test is accurate to about 5–8 per cent.

Tubular function

The simplest test of concentrating ability is to check the osmolality of all urine samples for 24 hours. Water deprivation tests are uncomfortable and have been largely abandoned. If no spontaneous urine sample reaches an osmolality of 800 mosmol/litre, desmospressin is administered intra-muscularly, after an overnight fast. Osmolality is measured on all urine passed over the next 9 hours or until a sufficiently concentrated sample is obtained earlier. An osmolality of 800 mosmol/kg is normal but most healthy young adults can achieve 900 mosmol/kg whilst many elderly healthy subjects cannot improve on 700 mosmol/kg.

Urinary acidification

For the diagnosis of classical distal renal tubular acidosis the short test of Wrong and Davies is employed. If there is a significant acidosis, shown by an abnormally low plasma bicarbonate, and urine pH is above 5.5, there is no need to proceed further i.e. urinary acidification is inadequate. If plasma bicarbonate is normal, ammonium chloride 100 mg/kg body weight is given. A urinary pH of 5.3 or less should be detected on at least one sample during the following 8 hours.

Measurement of renal function by imaging techniques

The IVU gives a rough guide to the relative contribution of each of two kidneys to the total GFR; it is not very accurate because it depends upon the observer's visual assessment of radio-graphic density. Much more accurate is the assessment of relative function by injection of radionuclide and subsequent counting of the renal images, e.g. by using radioactive technetium-labelled diethylene triamine penta acetic acid (DPTA). Scanning the kidneys with labelled DTPA also gives information on the arterial perfusion of the kidneys, therefore being useful in detecting renal artery stenosis and rejection in the transplanted kidney.

Changes in renal function with age and pregnancy

Age The infant kidney is immature, not reaching the maximum powers of concentration until approximately one year of age. From the age of thirty years, a steady and almost linear decline in GFR begins, so that at age 70 years the mean and range of GFR for males is 80, 60–120 ml/min, and for females 90, 65–120 ml/min. It is important to realize that this fall in GFR does not mean a rise in plasma creatinine – this remains constant owing to the diminution in muscle mass with age. The ability to concentrate and acidify the urine also reduces from the age of thirty onwards.

Pregnancy GFR and renal plasma flow both increase by approximately 50 per cent during the first and second trimesters of pregnancy, and fall during the last month. Despite the rise in GFR, salt and water retention occurs, with eventual retention *in toto* of approximately 900 mol of sodium causing the well known physiological hyper-volaemia of pregnancy.

Acute renal failure

Acute renal failure is a serious condition which, despite the fact that dialysis can substitute for the kidneys' failure to function, still carries a mortality rate of 50 per cent.

Acute renal failure (ARF) may be defined as a sudden fall in glomerular filtration rate (GFR) sufficient to cause uraemia. It may occur when previous renal function was completely normal, or may be a presentation of chronic renal failure when the patient suffers an illness which precipitates acute renal failure but which would have been innocuous in a person with normal renal function.

There are several terms used in the condition of acute renal failure which merit explanation.

Oliguria   This is the urine volume below which, with maximal urine concentration, the body fails to excrete metabolic products. This volume is 400 ml/day for a body weight of 70 kg.

Anuria   Anuria is the complete absence of urine.

Prerenal uraemia (reversible renal hypoperfusion): hypovolaemia and/or a low cardiac output lead to renal vasoconstriction. This is a physiological response of previously normal kidneys causing a reduced volume of concentrated urine with a low sodium and a high urea concentration. In its earlier stages the oliguria is reversible if the renal hypoperfusion is corrected.

Acute tubular necrosis (vasomotor nephropathy) is a sequel of renal hypoperfusion or of nephrotoxic drugs or chemicals, and leads to renal failure. The urine is isotonic or hypotonic with a high urinary sodium and a low urinary urea concentration. Oliguria is usual though some patients with acute tubular necrosis continue to pass large volumes of urine. This non-oliguric form of acute tubular necrosis is more common following burns, aminoglycoside administration and prolonged methoxyflurane anaesthesia. It must be emphasized that absence of oliguria does not exclude acute renal failure.

Causes

The causes of acute renal failure (ARF) may be divided into prerenal, renal and post-renal factors. This classification although frowned on by some, is extremely useful for diagnosis and management. The causes of ARF are extensive; Table 7.1 outlines some of them. More than one cause may operate and it is important not to cease seeking for causes when the first is found e.g. a patient with acute obstruction may have hypovolaemia due to vomiting due to uraemia and septicaemia arising from an obstructed urinary tract – the primary cause of acute renal failure.

Effects

The early effects of acute renal failure are simple and lethal.

- *Hyperkalaemia* results from failure of urinary excretion of potassium, and is exacerbated in hypercatabolic states e.g. trauma and sepsis.

Table 7.1   Main causes of acute renal failure

• *Prerenal*	
Extracellular volume loss	Gastrointestinal
	Urinary
	Burns
Intravascular volume loss	Sepsis
	Haemorrhage
	Hypoalbuminaemia
Decreased cardiac output	Heart failure
	Cardiac tamponade
Other causes of decreased glomerular filtration rate	Hypercalcaemia
	Hepatorenal syndrome
• *Renal*	
Nephrotoxic agents	Antibiotics
	Analgesics
	Contrast media
	Heavy metals
	Solvents
Glomerulonephritis	
Acute interstitial nephritis	Antibiotics
	Analgesics
	Leptospirosis
	Viral infections
Vasculitis/polyarteritis	Myeloma
Intratubular obstruction	Urate
Coagulopathies	Haemolytic uraemic syndrome
	Thrombotic thrombocytopenic purpura
	Postpartum renal failure
• *Postrenal*	
Renal tract obstruction	Stones
	Tumour (prostatic or pelvic)
	Periureteric fibrosis
	Bladder dysfunction
Major vessel occlusion	Renal artery thrombosis
	Renal vein thrombosis

- *Acidaemia* similarly results from failure of obligate urinary excretion of H^+ ions and is also **heightened** in trauma and sepsis.
- *Fluid overload* leading to pulmonary oedema results from failure to adjust the fluid intake to oliguria, and unfortunately is a frequent iatrogenic insult.

Presentation

Table 7.1 shows that acute renal failure can come in many guises, and the salient presenting features may be those of the underlying primary condition, overshadowing the features of renal failure, e.g. multiple trauma, or systemic lupus erythematosus.

Whatever the cause of acute renal failure, the patient may present with symptoms arising directly from the deficient kidney function:

- Oliguria, which may be noted by the patient himself or by alert nursing or housestaff.
- The symptoms of uraemia.
- Dyspnoea due to fluid overload.

Other presenting features may briefly be considered according to the type of acute renal failure.

Prerenal uraemia   The setting in which prerenal uraemia occurs, e.g. oliguria in a patient following surgery, burns, haemorrhage, provides clues to its cause. The signs of hypovolaemia include: postural hypotension, low internal jugular venous pressure, and cool extremities. These signs are confirmed by measuring the central venous pressure (CVP). A weight chart is usually a more accurate measurement of fluid balance than many fluid charts. In cardiac failure the signs of peripheral hypoperfusion occur with raised atrial pressures.

Acute tubular necrosis   Persistence of renal hypoperfusion leads to acute tubular necrosis. Several factors predispose to acute tubular necrosis such as complicated surgery, nephrotoxic drugs and septicaemia. A careful history of drug intake and of occupational exposure to chemicals should be taken. Muscle damage secondary to trauma, severe exercise, heat stroke, viral infections and alcohol may lead to rhabdomyolysis and acute tubular necrosis.

Glomerulonephritis   Haematuria or a history of pre-existing oedema or of a nephrotic syndrome suggests the possibility of a glomerulonephritis. A vasculitic rash or arthralgia indicates that the renal failure may be due to a systemic disorder such as systemic lupus erythematosus or polyarteritis and haemoptysis is suggestive of Goodpasture's syndrome.

Acute interstitial nephritis   A fever and a rash in a patient who has taken drugs such as antibiotics, diuretics, or NSAIDs raises the possibility of an allergic interstitial nephritis.

Postrenal uraemia   Anuria or alternating periods of oliguria and polyuria suggest an obstructive uropathy. A poor urinary stream suggests bladder neck obstruction from prostatic disease in elderly men, or posterior urethral valve obstruction in young boys. Anorexia and weight loss and, in women, vaginal bleeding may suggest pelvic malignancy with ureteric obstruction. All patients with ARF should have a rectal or pelvic examination. A distended bladder is easily missed in the obese patient and bladder catheterization should be considered.

Ureteric colic raises the possibility of obstruction by calculi or papillae; these must be bilateral or occur in a solitary kidney to cause renal failure. Obstruction from uric acid crystallization in the renal tubules occurs in patients with a leukaemia or lymphoma, usually following cytotoxic therapy.

Acute-on-chronic renal failure   Acute deterioration of pre-existing chronic renal failure is common and this is often due to dehydration or infection. Many patients are previously asymptomatic.

Diagnosis

There are two stages in the diagnosis of acute renal failure – first, establishing that acute renal failure is present, as opposed to oliguria due to prerenal uraemia, and second, defining the cause of the acute renal failure.

Diagnosing acute renal failure

Biochemistry   In oliguria due to renal hypoperfusion, the urine: plasma ratios of urea and osmolarity are raised and urine sodium is low, while in acute tubular necrosis the reverse is true. A considerable degree of overlap is seen with these measurements. An important practical point is that treatment with diuretics invalidates urine sodium measurements and radiographic contrast media interfere with the accuracy of urinary osmolarity.

Diagnosing the cause of acute renal failure

The precipitating cause of the acute renal failure can be obvious e.g. in a patient with postoperative sepsis, or obscure. Some form of visualization of the renal tract is essential to exclude obstruction when the diagnosis is uncertain, and should be performed even when the diagnosis seems clear to exclude underlying chronic disease. Ultrasound examination is now widely available and in practised hands gives reliable information on the number of kidneys present, their size, the presence of obstruction, whether stones or prostatic hypertrophy are present. In the absence of ultrasound facilities an intravenous urogram should be performed, using a high dose injection. The demonstration of a nephrogram 5–10 minutes after injection of the contrast medium shows whether the renal vasculature is intact and demonstrates the size of the kidneys. An early nephrogram which persists for hours or days suggests acute tubular necrosis. Bilateral small kidneys are indicative of chronic renal failure. With good tomography the pelvicalyceal system and ureters can be seen thus defining whether obstruction is present or not.

Urine microscopy proteinuria and haematuria with typical glomerular red cells – greater than 1×10^9/litre (1000/mm^3) – and red cell casts indicate glomerulonephritis. Eosinophiliuria may be seen in drug-induced interstitial nephritis.

Bacteriology Infections, especially when accompanied by septicaemia, are an important cause of acute renal failure. Aerobic and anaerobic cultures of blood, urine and sputum should be performed routinely.

Haematology Anaemia develops rapidly in acute renal failure and this is more marked in patients with massive intravascular haemolysis or with disseminated intravascular coagulation (DIC). A reticulocytosis and diminished haptoglobins are seen in both conditions and in DIC there is thrombocytopenia, raised fibrinogen degradation products and a blood film showing fragmented red cells.

Other investigations Many other tests may be suggested by the clinical picture, e.g. serum creatine kinase for rhabdomyolysis, serum and urine protein electrophoresis for myeloma, and anti DNA antibodies for SLE. Renal perfusion may be examined by radionuclide techniques or by arteriography. Renal arteriography or venography are needed to diagnose renal artery occlusion or renal vein thrombosis. In polyarteritis, aneurysms may be seen on the renal vessels though it is more usual to diagnose this condition by biopsy.

Renal biopsies are necessary in patients who present with unexplained acute renal failure or in whom there is clinical evidence of a glomerulonephritis or of a drug-induced interstitial nephritis. The prognosis of rapidly progressive or crescentic nephritis can be improved by treatment making it of the utmost importance that renal biopsy is performed as early as possible so that there is no delay in making the diagnosis.

Management

After the history is taken and clinical examination performed, the urine, if available, should be examined microscopically. If urine microscopy suggests a glomerulonephritis a renal biopsy should be carried out without delay. Blood and urine are sent for culture and for urgent measurements of urea, creatinine, sodium and osmolarity. A bladder catheter is passed and a CVP line inserted. A chest radiograph and intravenous urogram or ultrasound, if available, are performed. Within a few hours the initial biochemical and radiological results should be available; these and the clinical assessment will indicate the need for acute dialysis. The two major indications for urgent dialysis are hyperkalaemia and pulmonary oedema. By this stage a reasonable assessment of the cause of the renal failure should have been established, and plans for further investigations and management made.

Prerenal failure Hypovolaemia is corrected with the fluid that has been lost (i.e. saline, plasma or blood). The adequacy of the volume replacement is monitored by the usual clinical signs and by CVP measurements, and its success by an increase in urine volume. The treatment of renal hypoperfusion from myocardial failure varies with the haemodynamic status of the patient. Management of these patients is made easier with left atrial pressure measurements, either direct (e.g. after cardiac surgery) or with a wedged pulmonary artery catheter. Injudicious fluid administration in a patient with renal failure leads to pulmonary oedema, which can be relieved only by dialysis.

Diuretics are widely used in patients with renal hypoperfusion though the evidence that they can prevent the development of acute tubular necrosis is inconclusive. Hypovolaemia must be corrected before diuretics are given. If frusemide is given the dose should not exceed 4 mg/minute for an adult weighing 70 kg for a larger dose can cause deafness. Mannitol, 10–20 g i.v., has also been used; higher doses may increase extracellular fluid osmolarity and volume and thus precipitate pulmonary oedema. Occasionally a gratifying diuresis is produced, in which case the urine volume and composition must be carefully monitored and replaced by the appropriate fluid.

Dopamine   At low rates of infusion (1–5 ug/kg/minute) dopamine is a renal vasodilator and has been reported to reverse oliguria in patients with renal hypoperfusion.

Obstructive uropathy   Relief of the obstruction may simply require bladder catheterization. Often, however, cystoscopy and retrograde or antegrade ureteropyelography are necessary to define the site of obstruction. Patients who are ill or hyperkalaemic may need dialysis prior to these procedures. In such patients percutaneous nephrostomy allows drainage of the kidneys and enables a definitive surgical procedure to be deferred until renal function improves.

Established acute renal failure

The principles underlying the treatment of established renal failure are the same regardless of its cause. However, several causes of ARF (e.g. SLE and crescentic glomerulonephritis) may need treatment with steroids, immunosuppressive drugs and plasma exchange.

Infections   Infections are an important cause of ARF and a major cause of death in patients with ARF. If septicaemia is suspected treatment with antibiotics must be started 'blindly' (i.e. before results of bacteriological studies are available).

Drugs   Many drugs normally excreted by the kidneys accumulate in patients with renal failure, often with toxic effects although haemodialysis and peritoneal dialysis affect the clearance of drugs to a variable extent. Before prescribing any drug for a patient with ARF, the clinician must know its precise pharmacokinetics. It is a sound principle to avoid unfamiliar drugs unless the dosage and side-effects are checked.

Fluid and electrolyte balance   The amount and type of fluid given to a patient with ARF is based on regular clinical assessment of the state of hydration and on accurate measurements of weight and fluid intake and output. In general, fluids are restricted to about 500 ml plus measured or estimated losses (in urine, gastrointestinal and third space fluid). Dietary sodium and potassium intake are restricted to less than 60 mmol/day.

Hyperkalaemia   The serum potassium can rise very rapidly, especially in patients who are hypercatabolic. Hyperkalaemia is usually asymptomatic, but leads to electrocardiographic abnormalities culminating in cardiac arrest. The serum potassium must, therefore, be measured at least daily in patients who are hyperkalaemic. In patients with a potassium level less than 6 mmol/litre cation exchange resins may be used to increase the faecal excretion of potassium. A calcium based resin (30g b.d. orally or as an enema) is preferred to the sodium based resin, as, with the latter, sodium overload may occur. Potassium levels of greater than 6 mmol/litre are an absolute indication for dialysis and all other measures must be regarded as temporary.

Acidaemia   In itself acidaemia is rarely a problem though it worsens hyperkalaemia. The treatment must be dialysis and not hypertonic sodium bicarbonate which may lead to pulmonary oedema in the oliguric patient.

Nutrition   There is little value in restricting dietary protein in patients with AFR. Such a restriction leads to a negative nitrogen balance particularly in hypercatabolic patients, and to malnutrition which, by depressing the immune response, worsens sepsis. We now attempt to give a diet containing at least 1 g/kg protein and 14 400 kJ/day (3000 cal/day). The nausea and poor appetite of renal failure often makes this impossible. In these patients enteral or parenteral feeding is essential. A major problem of both types of feeding is the large amount of fluid that is required; in oliguric patients either daily dialysis or ultrafiltration will be necessary.

Dialysis   The indications for dialysis are as much clinical as biochemical. Most nephrologists would start dialysis when the blood urea reaches 30 mmol/litre (180 mg/100 ml) or if there is hyperkalaemia or pulmonary oedema. It seems sensible to dialyse patients early and frequently and, if possible, before they become ill from uraemia, though the value of this in reducing the mortality from ARF remains to be established. Peritoneal dialysis may be used for patients with milder degrees of renal failure, but haemodialysis is required for hypercatabolic patients. Efficient ultrafiltration of water and small molocular weight components from plasma is now possible and this had made fluid management in ARF much easier.

This process, also known as haemofiltration, can be performed continuously, as an alternative to intermittent dialysis.

Gastrointestinal bleeding Because of the high incidence of gastrointestinal bleeding in ARF many units now give patients antacids or H_2 antagonists (e.g. cimetidine) prophylactically. Magnesium-containing antacids must be avoided as they can lead to hypermagnesaemia.

Diuretic phase of acute tubular necrosis This occurs after a variable period of oliguria averaging 11 days. At this stage, urine volume increases to several litres daily and urine excretion of sodium and potassium rises. Losses may be sufficiently high to require frequent estimations and appropriate replacement of fluid, sodium and potassium.

Prognosis

The prognosis is largely dependent on the cause of renal failure. Patients with ARF from obstetric causes have the lowest mortality (10–20 per cent) while postoperative and posttraumatic ARF still carries a mortality of 40–70 per cent. In most series older patients fare worse than younger patients. Sepsis remains the single most important cause of death in patients with ARF, other causes being gastrointestinal haemorrhage, respiratory failure and myocardial failure.

In patients who survive, recovery of renal function is good with about 80 per cent of the expected glomerular filtration rate being attained by 6 months.

Chronic renal failure (CRF)

Definition CRF is a permanent impairment of glomerular filtration due to loss of nephrons; uraemia or a raised plasma creatinine does not suffice as a definition. Uraemia is used as a synonym for the later stage of CRF during which plasma urea and creatinine concentrations rise.

Epidemiology The incidence of CRF rises with age, particularly over the age of 60 years, and an annual incidence of 150 cases per million up to the age of 70 years has been suggested. For various reasons not all these patients can be treated for end stage renal failure (ESRF); a conservative estimate of the incidence of patients requiring treatment of ESRF is 50/million/annum.

Aetiology Most conditions described in this section can cause CRF; the major diagnostic groups in patients requiring dialysis and transplantation are glomerulonephritis (30 per cent), chronic infections and reflux, hypertension and cystic disease.

Pathophysiology As GFR falls, urea and creatinine plasma concentrations eventually rise. These alone have very little or no toxicity; it is other molecules, still mainly unidentified, which are toxic in renal failure. The gradual loss of nephrons leads to an inability to concentrate urine due to the increased solute load in the remaining nephrons. Consequently urine osmolality becomes constant at about 300 mosmol.

In the later stages of CRF, sodium retention occurs after the maximum filtration fraction of sodium is reached. In some diseases, before this stage is reached, there may be excessive sodium loss in the urine due to involvement of the medulla and tubules. As disease progresses there is eventual failure to excrete potassium, hydrogen, phosphate and urate, loss of the kidney's endocrine functions, the most important of which are the production of erythropoietin and the hydroxylation of vitamin D.

Effects and complications The metabolic abnormalities induced by CRF are complex and not fully understood. From a clinical point of view the effects and complications of CRF are closely intertwined, and may be conveniently considered as abnormalities arising from the disordered physiology, the diminished endocrine function, and the effects of the uraemic/toxic state on various organs in the body.

Disordered physiology The failure of urinary concentration produces the characteristic polyuria and thirst of CRF, with the added inability to compensate for states of salt and water loss, e.g. vomiting. Sodium retention leads to peripheral and pulmonary fluid retention and systemic hypertension. Acidaemia may be asymptomatic at first, but eventually causes the effects of metabolic acidosis. Hyperkalaemia can cause cardiac arrhythmias and uric acid retention can cause gout. Phosphate retention plays an integral part in the development of renal osteodystrophy (*see* below).

Diminished endocrine function   The lack of functional erythropoietin is a major cause of the chronic anaemia so typical of CRF. Hypereninaemia occurs in a proportion of patients and contributes to hypertension.

The failure by the kidneys to effect hydroxylation of vitamin D from the 25–OH form to the 1–25 OH form coupled with phosphate retention is the basis of the renal osteodystrophy occurring in CRF. This disorder is not completely understood, but is essentially due to hyperparathyroidism, induced by hypocalcaemia due to phosphate retention. This results in bone resorption, inadequate provision of vitamin D and osteomalacia. In time the excess parathyroid function may increase and become autonomous, causing hypercalcaemia and metastatic calcification.

Effects of uraemia on organs and tissues   Apart from the understandable effects described above, uraemia causes malfunction in many organs and tissues presumably by the action of the retained toxic metabolites. The majority of these effects do not begin to become apparent until quite late in the course of CRF i.e. when the GFR is 10 ml/min or less.

Nervous system   Lethargy, diminished powers of concentration and mental effort, clumsiness, fits and coma are well recognized. A change of mood consisting of depression and irritability is not uncommon. In the peripheral nervous system peripheral neuropathy and tremor occur; EMG will demonstrate conduction abnormalities in most patients even though there are no symptoms or signs of disease.

Gastrointestinal tract   Anorexia, nausea and vomiting are universal symptoms of CRF. There is also an increased incidence of peptic ulceration, related to raised gastrin levels and an increased bleeding tendency. Uraemic colitis is very rare.

Blood and bone marrow   In addition to erythropoietin deficiency a normocytic normochromic anaemia is produced by a general depression of bone marrow function, and decreased red cell survival. There is an increased bleeding tendency due in part to platelet dysfunction; this is partly correctable by dDAVP, which releases Factor VIII from vascular endothelium.

Skin   The anaemia plus retained urochomes gives the skin its characteristic colour. Itching is a distressing problem which is largely but not completely explained by phosphate retention. The much quoted uraemic frost is extremely rare.

Endocrine   Disturbance of hypothalamic – pituitary – gonadotrophic function results in loss of libido, impotence in the male, and infertility in both sexes. An abnormal glucose tolerance test can be found due to insulin resistance.

Lipids   Hypertriglyceridaemia, hypercholesterolaemia and increased LDL but reduced HDL are characteristic of uraemia, and may be related to the increased incidence of atheromatous disease in patients with CRF.

In addition to the above well-defined effects, two very common generalized disturbances occur; malaise and, in children, failure to thrive. The latter, coupled with bone disease, contributes to the stunted growth of children with CRF.

Presenting features of CRF   CRF can present in many different ways, and, in practice, patients with CRF may present to many different medical or surgical specialities under many different guises, e.g. anaemia resistant to iron therapy, carcinoma of the stomach, and even, in children and adolescents, behavioural disturbances. Briefly, from a practical point of view, the presentations of CRF can be grouped as follows.

- *Asymptomatic.* Patients may be found at routine medical examination to have proteinuria, haematuria or hypertension.
- *Typical symptoms of CRF.* Many patients do not present until late CRF, when they develop fatigue, anorexia, weight loss, nausea and vomiting and, frequently, itching and fluid retention.
- *Other effects and complications of CRF.* These arise from the many effects of diminished kidney function and uraemia, described above, and may occur in many different combinations.
- *Acute renal failure.* As CRF is so often aymptomatic, the first sign of renal disease may be acute renal failure superimposed upon the chronic damage, the latter only being revealed when investigations are performed. A relatively slight insult may precipitate the acute renal failure, e.g. a chest infection, or an episode of diarrhoea and vomiting.

- *Features of the underlying disease.* The primary cause of the renal failure may declare itself and investigations show permanent renal damage, e.g. a patient may present with pain and haematuria due to stones, or with a nephrotic syndrome due to nephritis.

Diagnosis   The diagnosis of CRF is relatively easy to make. Plasma biochemistry, or a measurement of GFR if the plasma creatinine or urea are not yet significantly elevated, will define the functional impairment. Imaging techniques i.e. intravenous urography, ultrasound or radionuclide scanning will reveal whether there are any gross structural changes e.g. obstruction, bilateral shrunken kidneys, polycystic disease. If the kidneys appear grossly normal and if analysis or microscopy of the urine suggests glomerular disease, renal biopsy is indicated.

The underlying cause of CRF must be sought as it may require treatment in its own right, to prevent progression if possible of renal disease, and, if transplantation is to be contemplated in the future, it is important to be aware of the possibility of recurrent disease in the graft.

Management of chronic renal failure

The management of chronic renal failure takes place in two stages; conservative management during the period of stable or declining impaired function, followed by end-stage renal failure, when dialysis or transplantation become necessary for survival.

Conservative management   This has two aims – preventing decline in renal function, and preventing complications.

Preventing decline   Manoeuvres for preventing decline in renal function consist of treating reversible factors which if left untreated would accelerate decline, and using less well-proven treatments aimed at reducing the work performed by the surviving nephrons.

Reversible factors

Hypertension

Even if not a primary factor causing renal failure, hypertension develops in nearly all patients as a complication of renal disease. Therefore blood pressure must be regularly measured in patients with chronic renal failure. Treatment relies on the drugs used for essential hypertension, as follows.

Diuretics – loop diuretics may be used. As there is a dose-response relationship with GFR, the dose of frusemide can be increased to 250–500 mg/day, but at lower values of GFR diuretics become ineffectual.

β-blockers and vasodilators – in most cases, hypertension can be controlled using conventional therapy, such as β-blockers (e.g. propranolol) and vasodilators (e.g. prazosin or hydralazine) administered in increasing doses as necessary. Atenolol should be avoided when the GFR falls below 15 ml/min as it is renally excreted and therefore accummulates.

Calcium antagonists– nifedipine has proved to be relatively free of side effects in chronic renal failure.

ACE inhibitors – captopril and enalapril have proved to be useful, but caution in their use is necessary as they can cause deterioration in renal function if renal artery stenosis is present.

Electrolyte and fluid depletion   Gross dehydration is easily detectable, but negative salt and water balance may develop slowly, especially in patients with analgesic nephropathy, chronic pyelonephritis, polycystic disease or when there has been inappropriate diuretic use or dietary salt restriction. The only signs of dehydration may be postural hypotension and a low jugular venous pressure associated with a rise in blood urea.

Obstruction   Obstruction resulting in functional deterioration usually occurs due to papillary necrosis in analgesic nephropathy, renal calculi, and prostatic hypertrophy.

Infections   Urinary tract infections should always be excluded and, if present, treated vigorously but with the dangers of nephrotoxic drugs always borne in mind. Infections elsewhere, e.g. chest, can also cause a reversible change in renal function.

Drugs   Inappropriately used nephrotoxic drugs are a depressingly common factor diminishing GFR in patients with already impaired renal function.

Exacerbation of primary cause of renal failure This usually refers to an inflammatory cause such as nephritis due to systemic lupus or polyarteritis.

Other factors

Attempts to slow the rate of deterioration of GFR by dietary means have recently been the subject of much interest and some controversy.

Protein restriction Varying degrees of protein restriction have been used in the treatment of chronic renal failure for many years. In the 1960s, very low protein diets of 20 g/kg or less (the Giovannet diet) were commonly used. Although these diets caused an improvement in uraemic symptoms, there was no convincing evidence of better survival and many patients became severely malnourished.

More recently there has been a renewed interest in low protein diets as a means of reducing the decline in renal function. An increase in protein intake increases renal blood flow and GFR both in experimental animals and man and causes glomerular hyperfiltration and hypertension. Conversely, a reduction in protein intake reverses these changes and results in prolonged survival and a reduction in proteinuria and glomerulosclerosis in animals. Retrospective studies of protein restriction in man have shown a reduction in the rate of decline in renal function. However, the use of protein restriction is controversial and a number of controlled trials are being undertaken to establish the role of this approach.

A typical low protein diet provides a daily intake of 40 g of protein (0.6 g/kg), which will not lead to a negative nitrogen balance. The stage of renal failure at which protein restriction should be introduced has yet be established. Low protein diets are usually commenced when the serum creatinine is 400–500 μmol/litre. The protein must be of high biological value and the total caloric intake must exceed 1800 kcals/day, using carbohydrate supplements if necessary. Care must be taken when giving these diets to children in order to ensure maximal growth velocity – supplementation is often essential.

Phosphate Experimental data suggest that a reduction in dietary phosphate intake is associated with less rapid decline in renal function and prolonged survival. However, satisfactory phosphate restriction is difficult to achieve in man as it also causes decreased calcium intake, which can accelerate the development of renal osteodystrophy. Excessive use of aluminium-containing oral phosphate binders (aluminium hydroxide) should be avoided as increases in serum aluminium cause neurological and skeletal problems in later life (e.g. dialysis dementia and osteodystrophy in patients on regular haemodialysis).

By contrast, some centres use no dietary restrictions other than phosphate binders and sodium and potassium restriction. Their approach is that when mild mild uraemic symptoms appear or when creatinine clearance is less than 15 ml/minute, definitive treatment for end-stage renal failure should commence.

Preventing complications

Hypertension The ubiquity of hypertension and its treatment in chronic renal failure have been referred to above.

Renal osteodystrophy Normalization of serum phosphate should be attempted by dietary restriction and use of aluminium hydroxide in gel, tablet or capsule form. Alternatively, calcium carbonate may be used, with the advantage of increasing calcium intake and also correcting acidaemia. Magnesium hydroxide should be avoided as it is a less efficient phosphate binder and can cause hypermagnesaemia. The serum calcium should be maintained in the normal range by synthetic vitamin D analogues, such as 1-hydroxy-cholecalciferol, 0.25 μg/day, or the vitamin D metabolite, 1,25-dihydroxy-cholecalciferol, 1–2 mg/day. Frequent estimation of the serum calcium is required for early detection of hypercalcaemia, which would further decrease renal function and cause pruritus and vomiting.

Acidaemia Most patients will tolerate mild acidaemia, but when the plasma bicarbonate falls to 15 mmol/litre or less, careful correction with sodium bicarbonate, 600–1200 mg b.d. or t.d.s., is indicated. The increased sodium load may, however, worsen oedema and reduce blood pressure control.

Pruritus Pruritus is a common symptom of chronic renal failure. It is distressing, and difficult to treat. Some patients will excoriate the skin so that bleeding and secondary infections result. Correction of serum calcium and phosphate levels may improve matters, as will some antipruritic agents (e.g. chlorpheniramine maleate, hydroxyzine hydrochloride).

Peripheral neuropathy   If peripheral neuropathy has developed before the patient's GFR falls below 25 ml/minute, other factors, such as drugs (e.g. nitrofurantoin) or alcohol, may be responsible. If uraemia is the cause, dialysis should produce an improvement.

Anaemia   Blood transfusion has been the only effective method of reversing the anaemia of chronic renal failure, with the disadvantage of its short-lived effect, and its possibility of sensitizing prospective recipients of a transplanted kidney. The recent production of erythropoetin by DNA technology has revolutionized this aspect of these patients' care.

Management of end-stage renal failure (ESRF)

End-stage or terminal renal failure is that point when the patient will die without treatment by dialysis or transplantation. Following presentation, this point may be reached very rapidly, or gradually over a period of several years.

The choices of treatment are haemodialysis, either in the home or in a dialysis unit, chronic ambulatory peritoneal dialysis (CAPD) or transplantation. During the course of treatment a patient may move from one form of treatment to another, as circumstances dictate. A brief description of each form of treatment follows, concluding with comments on the various strategies employed in their use.

Dialysis   The principle of dialysis is simple, being the transfer of solute from high concentration to low concentration across a semi-permeable membrane without free mixing of fluid. In haemodialysis, the blood, in an extra-corporeal circulation, is exposed to dialysis fluid separated by an artificial semi-permeable membrane. In peritoneal dialysis, the peritoneum, a naturally occuring semi-permeable membrane, separates the blood from dialysis fluid in the peritoneal cavity.

Modern haemodialysis equipment consists of a machine that generates dialysis fluids from a concentrate, has blood and anticoagulant pumps, safety checks and alarms. Artificial kidneys are now very small and disposable, and contain the equivalent of approximately 1 m² of semi-permeable membrane in the form of hollow fibres or layered plates.

Successful haemodialysis requires removal of blood at 200 ml/minute. The favoured form of access is the arteriovenous fistula, created in the forearm by joining a major artery and vein. Arteriovenous shunts, which consist of permanent cannulae in an artery and vein are less commonly used for long-term dialysis because of the problems of infection and vascular stenosis. In patients with diseased blood vessels various forms of prosthetic grafts or access catheters can be used.

Most patients require 12–15 hours of haemodialysis each week in two or three sessions. Treatment schedules can be organized for individual patients according to body size, type of access to the circulation, residual renal function, compliance with dietary and fluid restrictions, and the patient's employment.

Home-based haemodialysis   Patients can be trained to perform haemodialysis themselves with the help of a relative or helper. It is chosen mainly for patients for whom early transplantation is not planned. The advantage of home dialysis is the independence from hospital gained by the patient and the reliability of the technique. There are disadvantages, such as the cost of home conversion to provide suitable facilities, and the inefficient use of the dialysis equipment because it is dedicated to one user. In addition, the stresses placed on the patient and family can be considerable.

Dietary restrictions are necessary for most patients. The diet should consist of high quality protein, 0.8 g/kg body weight, with a restriction in potassium intake to 60 mmol/day. Sodium and fluid restriction vary according to urine output (not all patients on dialysis are anuric).

Complications of haemodialysis

Salt and water   Excess fluid and salt intake will cause weight gain, oedema, hypertension and pulmonary oedema. The need to remove excess fluid may lead to unpleasant side-effects, such as cramp and hypotension.

Hypotension and cramp   Some patients suffer severe cramps and hypotension during haemodialysis sessions. These may be corrected by:

increasing the sodium concentration in the dialysis fluid; dialysing with a bicarbonate buffer instead of acetate; or removing solutes and fluids separately by haemodialysis without fluid removal, followed by ultrafiltration without dialysis to remove fluid.

Hypertension The blood pressure in dialysis patients is largely salt and water dependent, and dialysis will usually allow hypotensive drugs to be reduced or stopped. Some patients may have renin-angiotensin driven hypertension and require drug treatment. Rarely patients may have severe hyper-reninaemia and extreme thirst, and hypotension following fluid removal may occur. In these patients and others in whom control of blood pressure is difficult, bilateral nephrectomy may be necessary, but with the availability of modern anti-hypertensive drugs this procedure is now rarely performed.

Anaemia invariably occurs and its severity is influenced by the nature of the renal disease. Patients with cystic renal disease have a higher haemoglobin level than those with chronic paren-chymal disease and those that have undergone bilateral nephrectomy. Most haemodialysis patients are not iron deficient; serum ferritin levels will indicate the need for iron supplements. Measures to correct anaemia have been disappointing. Some patients may respond to androgenic steroids, but virilization in the female and drug-induced cholestatic jaundice make this form of treatment unattractive. Regular blood transfusions may be required, as there is a beneficial immunological effect of transfusion on transplantation: dialysis units more readily transfuse patients with symptomatic anaemia. Over transfusion can cause haemosiderosis.

Renal osteodystrophy This problem continues in patients on dialysis, its treatment being as described above.

Hyperlipidaemia Type II hyperlipidaemia with elevated triglyceride and very low density lipo-protein occurs in maintenance dialysis patients. As there is a cardiovascular morbidity and mortality in long-term dialysis and transplant patients, more active steps to correct hyperlipidaemia would be appropriate but are seldom used.

Aluminium toxicity Together with other trace metals, aluminium is retained in renal failure, and serum and tissue concentrations can reach toxic levels by using dialysate made from water rich in aluminium and by the use of aluminium containing phosphate binders. Aluminium toxicity causes a fracturing osteodystrophy and a potentially fatal encephalopathy. The treatment of water supplies by reverse osmosis will reduce the aluminium level in the dialysate, and aluminium can be removed by infusions of desferrioxamine.

Acquired cystic renal disease Long-term dialysis patients develop cystic degeneration of the kidney whatever the original renal disease. These may cause haematuria and develop into benign or malignant renal tumours.

Socio-psychological problems The development of renal failure and its long-term treatment may cause considerable social and psychological stress in the patient and relatives. An increased suicide rate has been reported in dialysis patients.

Continuous ambulatory peritoneal dialysis

After insertion of the permanent dialysis catheter, patients can be trained within 7–10 days to conduct their daily exchanges of dialysis fluid by themselves. The fact that this form of dialysis is speedily learnt, conducted at home and without complicated equipment, is beneficial both to the patient and family and to the dialysis centre, which avoids expensive machinery and home adaptations.

The number of daily exchanges of dialysis fluids required is three or four, with the longest dwell time being 8–10 hours overnight.

Contraindications

- Intraperitoneal adhesions from previous surgery or infection may have reduced the surface area available for dialysis, or prevent drainage.
- Hernias may be exacerbated by, or develop during, CAPD and can be associated with fluid extravasation. They should be surgically corrected before CAPD is begun.
- Bowel pathology (e.g. inflammatory bowel disease, diverticulitis) may cause an increased transmural spread of pathogenic bowel organisms. Some centres therefore exclude patients with diverticulosis.
- Visual handicap was initially thought to be a contraindication, but many centres now successfully train blind patients.

- Arthritic diseases that reduce manual dexterity may be a relative contraindication, but modern mechanical aids to CAPD have mostly solved this problem.
- Comprehension and compliance are essential to the success of CAPD. Some patients are unable or unwilling to perform the comparatively simple aseptic bag exchanges.

Complications

- Peritonitis – bacteria can enter the peritoneal cavity via the lumen of the catheter, along the catheter track, via the bloodstream or across the intestinal wall. The commonest organisms are *E. coli*, *Enterobacter* spp., *Klebsiella* spp., and *Staphylococci*.
Peritonitis presents as a cloudy dialysis effluent with or without abdominal pain and fever. A neutrophil leucocyte count of 10×10^9/litre within the fluid confirms the diagnosis. Treatment is with antibiotics according to bacteriological sensitivities. Severe cases, may require hospital admission and parenteral antibiotic treatment. Fungal peritonitis is an uncommon but serious complication, and altogether intra-peritoneal and systemic antifungal therapy may be effective, removal of the dialysis catheter is often necessary.
- Infections of the exit site and catheter track – these infections can be difficult to eradicate with antibiotics and can cause peritonitis. Removal of the catheter may be necessary.
- Sclerosing peritonitis – a progressive sclerosing fibrosis of the peritoneum, resulting in bowel obstruction and a high mortality, is a rare complication.
- Loss of ultrafiltration – damage to the peritoneum due to infection or toxins (e.g. plasticizers or other ingredients within the dialysis fluid), can lead to the rapid absorption of glucose from the dialysis fluid and loss of the osmotic gradient required for ultrafiltration. Ultrafiltration can also be lost as a result of adhesions limiting the available surface area.
- Catheter displacement and obstruction – migration of the catheter out of the pelvis can lead to poor drainage. The omentum may occlude the catheter tip causing blockage or one-way dialysis flow. The catheter may therefore need repositioning or replacement.

Renal Transplantation

Renal transplantation remains the treatment of choice as it allows the patient to resume a normal life-style, without restrictions in diet and fluid intake. All patients should be assessed for suitability for transplantation; two types of renal transplantations are available.

Living donor transplantation   First degree blood relatives (i.e. siblings, children or parents) are suitable, providing the donor is ABO compatible and has at least a one haplotype antigen match with the recipient. Donor nephrectomy has no long-term detrimental effect on renal function, though there is some evidence of an increased incidence of mild hypertension.

Cadaveric transplantation

Most patients achieve transplantation from cadaveric donors.

Patient Selection

Age limits for transplant recipients are constantly revised and with the increasing success of transplant programmes, both younger patients (under the age of 5 years) and older patients (over the age of 65 years) are being transplanted successfully. Some patients will refuse transplantation and others are unsuitable for medical reasons, such as:

- age
- associated conditions that might deteriorate with immunosuppression (e.g. bronchiectasis or marked cardiovascular disease)
- the presence of high titres of cytotoxic antibodies to transplant antigens.

Management of transplanted patient

The graft functions immediately following operation in most patients, but, especially in the cadaveric group, delayed function occurs due to tubular necrosis. During this period dialysis will be necessary. Graft function is assessed by measurement of urine output, plasma urea and creatinine concentration, and, particularly in the graft with acute tubular necrosis, by radionuclide scanning techniques, which provide measurements of renal perfusion and excretion. Successful immunosuppression is the key to transplantation, success meaning graft survival without inducing complications which are lethal or causing a high morbidity. At present the main means of immunosuppression are:

- prednisolone, which reduces the numbers of circulating T and B cells and is anti-inflammatory;
- azathioprine, which inhibits the primary antibody response, cyclosporine A, which prevents activation of T helper cells, antilymphocyte sera, which may be polyclonal or monoclonal, and which eradicate subpopulations of lymphocytes.

These drugs are used in various combinations for maintenance immunosuppression and for treatment of rejection episodes; each renal unit by a process of trial and error creates its own regime and there is no agreed 'best treatment'. Cyclosporine A appears to have produced an improvement in graft survival.

Complications of transplantation

Surgical Haemorrhage, ureteric obstruction, leakage of urine from the vesicoureteric junction, renal artery stenosis and the collection of lymph (lymphocoele) may occur. Impaired venous drainage or frank thrombosis may occur on the operated side.

Immunosuppressive The regime of immunosuppression puts the patient at risk of infection. The infections may be commonly occurring ones such as wound infections, urinary tract and chest infections with common organisms, or they may be rarer disorders due to infections with opportunistic organisms such as fungi, pneumocystis, cytomegalovirus. Post-transplant infections are the commonest cause of death in the early stages of transplantation, but the incidence has fallen in recent years due to better management of the infections and the use of lower doses of steroids. In the long term there is an increased risk of malignancy, comprising the common cancers and lymphomas.

Drug complications other than immunosuppression Prednisolone can cause all its well-known side effects, but prominent in transplant clinics are glucose intolerance, cataracts, and vascular necrosis of bone. Azathioprine's commonest complication is bone marrow suppression, but hepatotoxicity occurs rarely. Cyclosporine A is nephrotoxic, and this effect has caused much difficulty because of the need to differentiate it from rejection. The most satisfactory way of doing this is by renal biopsy, although whether abnormalities

are completely specific for cyclosporine A occur is not clear; the main use of renal biopsy in this context is excluding rejection. Other effects of cyclosporine A are hypertrichosis, gingival hyperplasia, and tremor. All these complications of cyclosporine A are dose dependent.

Rejection Rejection is the commonest cause of graft loss, and is most frequent during the first 2–3 months post transplant. It is usually manifest by a rising plasma creatinine or urea and hence the need for close supervision of patients during this period. More aggressive rejections cause oliguria, fluid retention, fever, malaise and pain and tenderness in the graft; rarely it may rupture. The diagnosis may be made clinically, but in the majority of episodes, i.e. clinically silent ones, when other causes of graft dysfunction have been excluded such as obstruction then a biopsy in indicated, as discussed above.

Rejections which lead to loss of a graft have the unfortunate effect in some instances of producing long-lasting antibodies which can make subsequent transplantation difficult or impossible.

Other complications Hypertension is common in transplanted patients, due to a number of causes such as steroids, rejection, and the primary renal disease. Gastrointestinal bleeding was a serious complication but is now much less common owing to lower doses of steroids and prophylactic use of H_2 antagonists.

Strategies for treating ESRF

Haemodialysis, CAPD and transplantation are not to be seen as rigid choices; during their management individual patients may move from one to the other depending upon the facilities available, the preference of the patient, as well as medical considerations. Space does not allow a full discussion of the approaches to selecting modes of treatment, but a few general statements outline the main principles involved.

The ideal treatment is transplantation because of the cure of uraemia, and the return to a normal lifestyle. Unfortunately there are not enough donor kidneys to satisfy the needs. Priority is therefore given to children, adolescents, and young adults, and particularly among the latter women who wish to bear children. The main use of CAPD is as a holding measure for these patients while they await transplantation. In addition it is used for treating the elderly, for whom it is much easier to learn and less disruptive than home haemodialysis. The latter is a very safe and reliable form of treatment, and, if a transplant is not a very likely event within the practice of the treating unit, is the method of choice. Hospital based haemodialysis is the least used form of treatment in the UK because it is in short supply; it is reserved for patients who cannot, for medical or social reasons, undergo any other form of treatment.

The outcome of treatment for ESRF

ESRF is a fatal condition. Survival rates for haemodialysis and transplantation are remarkably similar, and depend upon the age of the patient, being higher in younger age groups.

Proteinuria and the nephrotic syndrome

The presence of protein in the urine can range from very small but detectable quantities, which are normal, to larger amounts, which in themselves are not harmful but indicate disease, and gross amounts which lead to hypoproteinaemia and the nephrotic syndrome. As routine urine testing is part of a general medical examination chance findings of proteinuria are common. Proteinuria does not always indicate serious underlying renal disease and therefore it is important to decide whether patients have, or will develop, serious renal disease.

A positive test needs confirmation and should be repeated several times; transient positive tests are rarely important. Although much has been made of orthostatic proteinuria, it does not discriminate between benign or pathological proteinuria. Once proteinuria has been confirmed a 24 hour urine collection is necessary for quantitation. Normal protein excretion is 100 mg/m^2 body surface/24 hours; more than 200 mg/day is abnormal. Protein excretion of more than 2 g/day signifies glomerular disease.

Mechanisms Proteinuria is a result of either glomerular or tubular disorders.

Glomerular proteinuria results from increased permeability of the glomerulus. The urine may contain mostly albumin, when proteinuria is selec-

tive, or it may contain larger molecules as well, i.e non-selective. Glomerular proteinuria results from increase in pore size and loss of negative charge on the glomerular basement membrane – the normal negative charge repels most protein molecules which are themselves negatively charged.

Tubular proteinuria occurs when there is tubular damage or interstitial inflammation. Urine electrophoresis distinguishes glomerular from tubular proteinuria as proteins of tubular origin are predominantly alpha and beta globulins of low molecular weight.

Other causes of proteinuria include the following: overflow proteinuria which occurs when the plasma contains large amounts of protein that pass through the glomerular filter and saturate the reabsorptive capacity of the tubules, e.g. light chains in multiple myeloma; failure of normal tubular reabsorption of protein; loss of protein from the epithelium of the urinary tract below the glomeruli and tubules; drainage of lymph into the urinary tract.

Investigation of asymptomatic proteinuria

Persistent proteinuria requires quantitation and assessment of renal function with measurement of GFR. If these are normal no further investigations are required. If either or both are abnormal, then renal disease is present and must be diagnosed. A detailed history should be taken paying special attention to the family history (e.g. nephritis, polycystic disease, diabetes), and noting any features that might indicate systemic disease. Physical examination must include measurement of blood pressure, assessment of hearing, and fundoscopy.

The most helpful test is microscopic examination of the urinary sediment from fresh urine. Red cells in the absence of infection indicate glomerular disease and red cell casts are diagnostic of glomerulonephritis. An abnormal urinary sediment indicates that serious underlying renal disease is associated with the proteinuria. A renal biopsy is indicated in patients who have proteinuria with hypertension or impaired GFR, proteinuria greater than 1 g/24 hours, or when systemic disease is suspected.

Prognosis In significant proteinuria the prognosis depends upon the underlying disease. Long-term follow up of individuals with insignificant proteinuria shows no increased morbidity or mortality.

Nephrotic syndrome

The nephrotic syndrome is characterized by hypoalbuminaemia and oedema due to protein loss. Urinary protein loss usually exceeds 3 g/day before hypoalbuminaemia develops and salt retention sufficient to produce oedema is unusual unless plasma albumin falls below 30 g/litre. In patients with the nephrotic syndrome proteinuria often exceeds 10 g/day and plasma albumin may fall as low as 12 g/day. It is erroneous to define nephrotic syndrome on a level of proteinuria; such a level may easily be exceeded in young patients without oedema, whereas elderly patients may become nephrotic at a protein excretion below the usual figure.

Epidemiology

In the UK, the annual incidence of idiopathic nephrotic syndrome decreases from about 30/million in children under 5 years to 6–8/million in adults. Minimal change nephropathy accounts for 90 per cent of cases less than 5-years-old, but is less common in adults (20–25 per cent of cases, 2–3/million annually). All other causes are more common in adults than children.

In tropical countries, infections e.g. malaria, are much more common as causes of glomerular lesions so influencing the incidence and histopathology of the nephrotic syndrome.

Pathophysiology

In the normal glomerulus capillary blood is separated from the glomerular filtrate by several structures:

- The capillary endothelium which contains fenestrae, approximately 100 nm wide.
- The glomerular basement membrane (GBM), a continuous membrane made of collagen and glycoproteins. The glycoproteins are anionic and the surface of the basement membrane is therefore negatively charged.
- Lastly the epithelium, the cells of which extend processes (podocytes) over the glomerulus. Each podocyte extends small secondary processes from its lateral margins which interdigitate closely with those of an adjacent podocyte. The intervening spaces or pores are 10 nm wide.

Histologically, the glomerular wall forms a series of barriers to the passage of molecules. Experiments confirm that neutral molecules such as dextrans pass freely into the glomerular filtrate if less than 2.0 nm in radius but are excluded if greater than 4.5 nm. Between these sizes, the clearance of neutral dextrans depends on radius. In the case of charged molecules, anions are less well cleared than neutral molecules of similar size, while cations have enhanced movement through the GBM. The mechanism of the increase in glomerular permeability is multifactorial. Changes in the negative charge on the GBM, circulating or locally generated products which increase GBM permeability and/or damage to podocyte architecture are involved.

It is possible to determine the relative permeability of the damaged glomerular filter for different proteins by comparing their glomerular clearances. Compared to albumin, the clearance of other proteins bears a log-linear relation to molecular dimension. The steeper the slope of the line the more easy it is to determine glomerular protein selectivity by comparing the clearance of two proteins of different size, e.g. transferrin (molecular weight 38 000) and IgG, (molecular weight 150 000). The clearance (C) of the smaller protein is always greater and is used as the denominator. If the ratio C_{IgG}/C_{TF} is 0.1, proteinuria is termed 'highly selective'; if the ratio is 0.3, it is 'poorly selective'. In minimal change nephropathy (MCN), especially in children, highly selective proteinuria is the rule and this investigation can be used to predict the diagnosis of a steroid – responsive nephrotic syndrome.

Biochemical compensation for heavy proteinuria

Albumin comprises 90 per cent of daily protein excretion in glomerular disease. Up to 25 g/day may be lost, which is 15 per cent of the total plasma content. Since albumin maintains the plasma component of extracellular fluid, plasma volume would contract rapidly unless compensatory changes occurred. The mechanisms by which the plasma albumin pool is increased at the expense of the extravascular albumin store and by which hepatic protein synthesis is increased, are poorly understood. The liver normally has enough reserve capacity for protein synthesis to replace urinary protein loss of less than 3 g/day in a person on a normal diet. When protein loss exceeds 10 g/day it becomes increasingly difficult to compensate fully, even though hepatic protein synthesis increases at the expense of other tissues. The compensatory mechanism has priority over the utilization of amino acids for other body proteins which can become depleted.

If there is underlying liver disease, the capacity to increase protein synthesis is impaired, and even small daily protein losses produce hypoalbuminaemia.

Effects of protein loss

When compensation is inadequate, plasma albumin concentration falls. The accompanying hypovolaemia may cause prerenal uraemia or even acute oliguric renal failure.

The contraction in plasma volume which stimulates salt and water retention is due to the diminished plasma albumin pool. The retained salt and water passes into the extravascular space, there being no oncotic force to keep it in the circulation. Reduction in plasma volume promotes renal salt and water conservation. Renin levels are raised and aldosterone levels are high, but these are not the most potent factors in salt retention – large doses of the aldosterone antagonist, spironolactone do not produce natriuresis. Probably the most important factor is passive sodium resorption along the active chloride gradient produced in the loop of Henle. Diuretics, such as frusemide or ethacrynic acid acting on the loop of Henle are effective in inducing a natriuresis in the nephrotic syndrome. The mechanisms by which hypovolaemia stimulates chloride (and hence sodium) resorption at this site are not known.

Hyperlipoproteinaemia

Cholesterol is carried in plasma as a constituent of the lipoproteins, particularly the high and low density fractions (HDL, LDL). HDL are lost through the damaged glomerular filter, but LDL are not. The hypercholesterolaemia of nephrotic syndrome indicates that there is hyperlipoproteinaemia; LDL levels, in particular, are raised but all fractions except HDL are affected. The primary stimulus appears to be proteinuria, for hyperlipoproteinaemia occurs even if the plasma albumin level is normal. If proteinuria remits, the lipid pattern returns to normal. Hyperlipidaemia may contribute to an increased incidence of ischaemic heart disease in young patients with the nephrotic syndrome though there is no firm epidemiological evidence. Hyperfibrinogenaemia accompanies proteinuria contributing to the raised ESR seen in patients with the nephrotic syndrome. The raised

levels of these hepatic proteins, too large to escape the damaged glomerular filter reflect a rise in the rate of protein synthesis associated with the requirement for increased albumin production.

Renal tubular abnormalities

Very heavy proteinuria is accompanied by glycosuria, general aminoaciduria and phosphaturia. Hypocalciuria can occur in the nephrotic syndrome even when the GFR is normal but the reason is not known.

Causes   There are many causes; the main ones are shown in Table 7.2. The commonest in the UK are the primary forms of glomerulonephritis, diabetes mellitus, amyloidosis and drug reactions.

Table 7.2   Common causes of nephrotic syndrome

Primary forms of glomerulonephritis

Systemic diseases
Diabetes mellitus
Amyloidosis
Systemic lupus erythematosus
Henoch–Schonlein purpura
Cryoglobulinaemia
Polyarteritis

Infections
Malaria
Schistosomiasis
Hepatitis B
Streptococcal and staphylococcal infections
Syphilis

Drugs
Gold
Penicillamine
'Street' heroin
Anti-epileptics (e.g tridione)
Phenindione

Tumours
Carcinoma
Sarcoma
Leukaemia and lymphoma

Familial disorders
Fabry's disease
Congenital nephrotic syndrome

Miscellaneous conditions
Renal vein thrombosis
Allergic reaction to insect bites, pollen and vaccines

Presenting features The classical features are dependent oedema, and swelling of hands and, face in more severe cases. Patients frequently state that they have noted frothiness of the urine. Patients may also present with a complication of the nephrotic syndrome, or symptoms and signs of an underlying cause.

Complications

Thrombosis Hypercoagulability occurs for a number of reasons such as loss of antithrombin III in urine, and elevated plasma levels of factor VIII and fibrinogen. Haemoconcentration and immobility also contribute. Veins and arteries may thrombose, but there is a particular propensity for the renal veins to do so; pulmonary embolism is an obvious complication.

Infections Nephrotic patients are particularly susceptible to infections; the reasons are not entirely clear but may be in part due to IgG loss in the urine. Any infection may occur, but in children there is a particular tendency to pneumococcal infection, especially peritonitis.

Hypovolaemia and acute renal failure The hypovolaemia of nephrotic syndrome may lead to prerenal uraemia and eventual tubular necrosis.

Treatment Treatment of the nephrotic syndrome has two aims: removal, if possible, of the underlying cause, and measures designed to lessen the nephrotic state. Only the latter will be discussed here. The obvious problem to be overcome is the retention of salt and water, and diuretics are effective in most patients. Frusemide is most often used, and large doses up to 500 mg b.d. may be required. Amiloride or spironolactone are useful adjuncts. In grossly nephrotic patients intravenous plasma or albumin with concomitant intravenous frusemide can be employed. The mainstay of diuretic treatment can be supplemented by restriction of salt intake to 40–60 mmol/day, but this is not always necessary. The traditional high protein diet is usually prescribed, but there is no evidence that it is of benefit on top of a diet adequate in amino acids. In immobile patients prophylactic anticoagulattion is worthwhile.

A danger of the diuretic treatment which must be guarded against is the too rapid removal of salt and water which can precipitate circulatory collapse, renal failure, and even death.

Glomerulonephritis

Glomerulonephritis is a prime cause of morbidity and death from kidney disease and causes one-third of cases with end-stage renal failure. Many types of nephritis reflect immunological disturbances and more precise definition of these has contributed to our general understanding of immune-mediated disease.

Classification

The systems of classification are somewhat confusing as there is considerable overlap leading to lack of precision. The aetiology of nephritis is usually unknown; not enough is known about pathogenetic mechanisms for these to be used for classification. Morphological classification is limited because the glomerulus responds to injury in only a few ways. Nonetheless, the common use of percutaneous renal biopsy has led to a pragmatic histological classification. This approach has been useful and is in common usage as a working clinico-pathogical framework for clinical practice and research, despite its imperfections e.g. focal proliferative nephritis may be the first manifestation of anti GBM disease, SLE, or infective endocarditis.

Clinical syndromes

Glomerular disease may produce the following:

- *The nephritic syndrome* – reduction of glomerular filtration, retention of salt and water, expansion of the intravascular volume and hypertension. In severe cases acute renal failure occurs.
- *Haematuria* – macroscopic haematuria occurs in acute poststreptococcal nephritis and rapidly progressive glomerulonephritis. Recurrent macroscopic haematuria is a symptom of idiopathic focal nephritis and membranoproliferative glomerulonephritis. Microscopic haematuria is common in all glomerular disease.
- *Proteinuria* – this ranges from slight, when it is asymptomatic, to heavy, when it causes the nephrotic syndrome.
- *Loin pain* – this is usually only a feature of acute disease such as acute nephritis.
- *Chronic renal failure.*

Immunopathogenetic mechanisms in glomerulonephritis

The commonest mechanism is the glomerular deposition of antigen–antibody complexes i.e. immune complex disease which is recognized by deposits containing immunoglobulins and complement in the glomerular capillary walls. In some patients, circulating antigen–antibody complexes have been identified. However, only in a minority of diseases in man has the responsible antigen been

Table 7.3 Infectious organisms associated with human nephritis

Bacteria
Streptococcus (Group A haemolytic and viridans)
Staphylocuccus aureus and *Staph. albus*
Diplococcus pneumoniae
Meningococcus
Salmonella typhi
Klebsiella pneumoniae
Mycobacterium tuberculosis
Mycobacterium leprae
Treponema pallidum
Brucella spp.
Yersinia enterocolitica
Leptospira

Viruses
Hepatitis B
Epstein–Barr
Oncornavirus
Mumps
Measles
Rubella
Cytomegalovirus
Coxsackie
Variola
Varicella
Vaccinia
Guillain–Barré agent

Rickettsiaceae
Coxiella burnetti

Mycoplasma
Mycoplasma pneumoniae

Fungi
Candida albicans

Parasites
Plasmodium malariae and *P. falciparum*
Schistosoma mansonii and *S. haematobium*
Toxoplasma
Filaria spp.

Table 7.4 Drugs causing glomerulonephritis

Ampicillin
Methicillin
Rifampicin
Sulphonamides
Sodium diatrizoate
Gold
Penicillamine
Mefenamic acid
Probenecid
Phenindione
Doxorubicin
Potassium perchlorate
Tolbutamide
Troxidone

identified in the kidney or in circulating complexes. The largest group of antigens identified is found among infectious organisms, and examples are shown in Table 7.3. Other antigens have also been indirectly implicated e.g. drugs (Table 7.4), tumours, and a number of endogenous antigens e.g. the nuclear antigens of systemic lupus erythematosus, thyroglobulin in nephritis associated with Hashimoto's disease, and immunoglobulin itself in the mixed cryoglobulineamia. The second mechanism of injury is glomerular fixation of antibody against the GBM. This appears as smooth linear deposition of antibody in a continuous distribution along the glomerular basement. Finally, the occurrence of monocytes in the glomeruli, interstitium, and crescents of nephritic kidneys has been interpreted as evidence that cell-mediated immunity is contributing to tissue damage.

Glomerulonephritis is conventionally regarded as 'primary', in which the kidney alone is affected, or as "secondary" in which it is involved as part of a systemic disease. As this convention closely relates to clinical practice, it will be followed here. Space allows only brief descriptions of the clinical syndromes and their management.

Primary glomerulonephritis

Anti GBM nephritis

Anti GBM nephritis accounts for about 2–3 per cent of cases of nephritis. Most patients develop a severe nephritis rapidly progressive in type, and many patients have accompanying intraalveolar haemorrhage (Goodpasture's syndrome) due to fixation of antibodies on the alveolar basement membranes. Respiratory infection and sometimes exposure to hydrocarbons have been described as antecedent events. The diagnosis is made by demonstrating circulating anti GBM antibody or by the typical linear deposition of antibody on the GBM. Treatment with steroids, immunosuppressive drugs and plasma exchange is effective at removing the antibody and can diminish the renal and pulmonary damage. This approach to treatment has improved the prognosis, so that death is now uncommon. Whether renal function is regained depends on the degree of renal disease before treatment is begun.

Membranous nephropathy This is a disease mainly affecting adults, and it usually presents with proteinuria which may be severe enough to cause a nephrotic syndrome. Histologically the GBM is thickened and contains deposits of immunoglobulin and complement, due to immune complex deposition. In approximately one-third of patients the disease remits spontaneously, in one-third proteinuria continues, and in one-third there is a slow progression into chronic renal failure.

Because of the relatively high spontaneous remission rate assessment of treatment is difficult. A beneficial effect of course of steroids with immunosuppressive drugs has been reported, but awaits further evaluation.

Mesangiocapillary glomerulonephritis (MCGN; also known as membranoproliferative glomerulonephritis)

There are two types of this disorder, differentiated according to the histological characteristics of the glomerular deposits – subendothelial (Type I) and dense deposit disease (Type II). MCGN is a disease of teenagers and young adults and recent reports suggest that its incidence has fallen over the last 10–15 years. Its aetiology is unknown. Patients present with proteinuria, haematuria, nephrotic syndrome and occasionally with acute or chronic renal failure. There is a rare association of Type II with partial lipodystrophy. Histologically there is proliferation of the mesangial cells of the glomeruli with deposits of immunoglobulin and complement in the subendothelial position in Type I and of electron dense material between the layers of the GBM in Type II. A strikingly low serum concentration of complement (C3) is found in a large

number of patients. In approximately half, progression to end-stage renal failure occurs. There is no effective treatment.

IgA disease (Berger's disease)

This common form of nephritis gets its name from the deposition of IgA in the mesangium of the glomeruli which also exhibit focal proliferation. The main group affected are children and young adults who present with macroscopic haematuria, often preceded by upper respiratory tract infections. Other patients often present with hypertension with or without renal impairment. An association with alcoholic liver disease has been noted. Up to 10 per cent of patients eventually develop renal failure.

Acute glomerulonephritis

There are two basic types of acute glomerular inflammation:

Acute exudative proliferative nephritis

This is best exemplified by acute post streptococcal nephritis, but it can follow other recognized infections e.g. pneumococcal, meningococcal, but may occur without recognized antecedents.

The post streptococcal form has become uncommon in Northern Europe and Northern America but is still common in Third World countries where standards of health, general hygiene and housing are much less satisfactory. The typical clinical picture is the acute nephritic syndrome (see above) following pharyngitis or skin infection. Histologically there is proliferation of glomerular cells with infiltration of polymorphonuclear leukocytes, with deposition of immunoglobulins and complement in the subepithelial position. The disease is thought to arise as a result of immune complex formation due to antigen from the infecting organisms.

The prognosis is good, most patients recovering completely, although a minority may develop chronic renal disease later. Treatment is aimed at eliminating infections, correction of fluid and electrolyte imbalance, and dialysis if required for acute renal failure. Small amounts of proteinuria and haematuria may continue for months or years following the illness without ill effects.

Rapidly progressive or crescentic glomerulonephritis

This is so called because there is formation within the glomeruli of 'crescents' – a proliferation of cells in the capsular space around the glomerulus which surround it like a cap, and when cut in histological section give the appearance of a crescent. Clinically patients develop oliguric renal failure over days or weeks; loin pain, macroscopic haematuria and occasionally a nephrotic syndrome may occur. Although it can be an idiopathic disorder, this form of nephritis is often associated with systemic diseases (see below).

The prognosis for renal function is poor, many patients developing end-stage renal failure. Treatment with steroids, immunosuppressive drugs, with or without plasma exchange, anticoagulants and antiplatelet agents is employed, and undoubtedly remarkable improvements can occur, but these have to be seen against reported spontaneous improvements.

Minimal change nephropathy (MCN)

This glomerular disease is characterized by:

- no abnormality being detected on light microscopy – hence its name. Therefore, strictly speaking it is not a 'nephritis', and;
- the frequent loss of proteinuria on treatment with steroids – an enigmatic response in view of the complete lack of inflammation. It causes a nephrotic syndrome and occurs mainly in children, in whom it accounts for 90 per cent of cases of the nephrotic syndrome. It causes 10 per cent of cases in adults.

The pathogenesis is unknown, but there is circumstantial evidence which suggests that the lesion is caused by a product secreted by lymphocytes remote from the kidneys.

The proteinuria remits on treatment with steroids, but relapse is common, requiring further intermittent courses of steroids, continuous steroids, or an eight week course of cyclophosphamide. The eventual prognosis is good – chronic renal failure does not occur.

Focal glomerular sclerosis (FGS)

This type of nephritis causes proteinuria, frequently severe enough to produce the nephrotic syndrome. All age groups are affected, and a high proportion – up to 50 per cent – develop end-stage renal failure. Histology reveals a focal (affecting only a part) sclerosing lesion affecting some glomeruli. As not all the glomeruli may be affected it is possible to make a mistaken diagnosis of minimal change nephropathy. This is further compounded by the remission of proteinuria, albeit in only a small proportion of cases, by steroids and/or cyclophosphamide.

Recurrence of nephritis in transplanted kidneys

Anti GBM antibody nephritis, mesangiocapillary glomerulonephritis Type II (dense deposit disease), focal glomerulosclerosis, and mesangial IgA nephritis are the types of nephritis most likely to recur in grafted kidneys. Recurrence is less common in patients with mesangiocapillary glomerulonephritis Type I (subendothelial deposits) and membranous nephropathy. The risk of recurrence, which in most cases does not usually lead to rapid destruction of the graft, does not contraindicate transplantation, as graft survival in patients with nephritis as their original disease is not less when compared to other groups. However, in the case of anti GBM disease a transplant should be delayed until anti GBM antibody is absent from the circulation. The histological changes of membranous nephropathy have been found in transplanted kidneys in patients whose original disease was not this condition, and not nephritis of any kind. This new development of nephritis may be due to immune complex disease brought about by antibody formation against transplant antigens.

Interstitial nephritis

In contrast to glomerulonephritis, the pathological changes affect the interstitium and consist of an infiltration with lymphocytes. Interstitial nephritis is most commonly seen as a reaction to drugs, those most commonly involved being diuretics, antibiotics, and NSAID's; it may also occur as an accompaniment to glomerulonephritis (except minimal change nephropathy). Patients present with acute or chronic renal failure, with proteinuria and microscopic haematuria. Treatment consists of withdrawing culpable drugs, and using steroids to reduce the inflammation. Recovery is usual, although a minority of patients suffer permanent renal damage.

Renal involvement in systemic disease

A diseased kidney may be the only presenting feature of a systemic disease (e.g. nephritis in systemic lupus erythematosus). Investigation and management of other systems will be necessary accompaniments to management of the renal disease.

Systemic lupus erythematosus

Systemic lupus erythematosus (SLE) affects women more than men, and the black rather more than the white population. At presentation, 40 per cent of patients have clinical evidence of renal disease, but this figure becomes 100 per cent if all patients with SLE have a renal biopsy at presentation i.e. there are immunohistological abnormalities in patients without clinical evidence of disease.

Clinical features The renal disease may be the sole presenting feature of SLE (5 per cent of patients) or may be accompanied by any of the other features of the disease, arthritis and skin disease being the most common. Renal involvement can present in any of the ways in which kidney disease presents – asymptomatic proteinuria and/or haematuria, macroscopic haematuria, the nephrotic syndrome, rapidly progressive glomerulonephritis; varying degrees of renal failure may accompany each of these.

Pathology and pathogenesis The histological appearances range over the whole pattern of kidney disease; there is no diagnostic histological appearance for SLE. During the course of illness, the histological abnormalities may change from one type to another.

Although SLE has come to be regarded as a prototype of immune complex disease in man, the stimulus for the formation of antibodies to auto-antigens, particularly nuclear antigens is unknown. Factors associated with SLE are abnormal T and B cell function and experimentally, amelioration of the disease with androgens but a worsening with oestrogens. This effect of oestrogens is presumably related to the increased incidence of SLE in women during reproductive years. SLE is associated with complement deficiency, but how the latter predisposes to SLE is not known. Certain drugs e.g. hydralazine, procainamide and anti-convulsants (see p. 247) are associated with SLE which is usually reversible when the drug is stopped. Hydralazine has been most studied; the complication tends to occur in slow acetylators, with a female preponderance of 4:1, and in subjects with a tissue type of HLA-DR4.

Diagnosis The crucial diagnostic feature of SLE is a raised anti-DNA antibody titre. Rare exceptions occur when the anti-DNA titre is normal in the presence of a positive anti-nuclear factor test. Clinical pointers to the diagnosis of SLE are symptoms and signs in more than one system, a positive anti-nuclear factor test, and the presence in the renal biopsy of many immune reactants – e.g., IgG, IgM, IgA and complement (*Clq*, and C4 and C3).

Management and prognosis The treatment of SLE nephritis is not straightforward, and causes much controversy. The problem is worsened by the chronic and flucuating course of the disease, and the lack of controlled therapeutic trials, but guidelines can be offered. Severe acute renal disease is treated with high doses of steroids and either azathioprine or cyclophosphamide. Plasma exchange has been used in this group, but there is no evidence of its advantage. Less severe disease may require steroids if proteinuria is heavy or if extrarenal disease warrants it; immunosuppressive drugs are usually not used in this group. The patients with quiescent disease present a very difficult problem as it is not known whether treatment with steroids and/or immunosuppressive drugs influences the long-term outcome.

Although SLE remains a serious condition, its prognosis has improved, presumably due to the use of drugs and to the better management of infections.

Mixed connective tissue disease

Mixed connective tissue disease is a rare disorder with features of SLE, polymositis and systemic sclerosis. Patients may have asymptomatic proteinuria, the nephrotic syndrome and renal failure.

Polyarteritis

Polyarteritis is uncommon but life-threatening; its swift recognition is of great importance as treatment is effective. It occurs mainly in the elderly and is more common in men.

Clinical features

The onset of polyarteritis is accompanied by malaise, fever, sweating, myalgia, arthralgia and weight loss. These features can be acute, and often lead to a diagnosis of influenza and treatment with antibiotics. The nephritis usually presents silently, or with acute renal failure. Other systems involved are a vasculitic rash of the skin, the nervous system, with mononeuritis multiplex or strokes, the gut, with ischaemia and infarction, the liver, with hepatic failure; hypertension may be severe.

Pathology and pathogenesis   Inflammation of the arterial wall and surrounding tissue are characteristic. As these changes are usually patchy, normal vessels occur in biopsy tissue and therefore do not exclude the diagnosis. Polyarteritis resembles experimental serum sickness and there is some evidence that circulating immune complexes are pathogenic. Recently an antibody to cytoplasmic proteins in neutrophils has been found in patients' sera. Its pathogenicity has not yet been determined. Polyarteritis has been associated with hepatitis B antigenaemia and with various antibiotics, though the association with antibiotics is probably spurious as they are often prescribed for the prodromal symptoms.

The following types of polyarteritis are recognized:

- *Polyarteritis nodosa*, in which the medium sized vessels are affected. This often leads to gross infarction of tissues or organs.
- *Microscopic polyarteritis*, in which the vessels involved are much smaller and which is accompanied by a crescentic glomerulonephritis with ischaemic changes in the glomeruli.
- The Churg–Strauss type, in which renal involvement is rare and which is characterized by asthma and eosinophilia.

Diagnosis   Although precise diagnosis rests on histological evidence of arteritis this may prove impossible for the reason given above. The diagnosis may justifiably be made on clinical grounds alone, particularly in view of the need to institute speedy treatment.

Management and prognosis: although there are no controlled trials, early treatment with high-dose steroids for example, methylprednisolone, Ig i.v., daily for 3 days, and either cyclophosphamide or azathioprine is widely considered capable of halting and, in some patients, reversing the disease. For conserving renal function it is vital that treatment begins as soon as possible as recovery rarely occurs once oliguria has progressed to anuria. Plasma exchange, anticoagulants and drugs modifying platelet function are used, but there is no clear evidence to support their use. Once the acute illness has been treated, maintenance treatment with steroids and immunosuppression is usually required. The survival rate of treated patients is now 80 per cent at 5 years.

Wegener's granulomatosis

Wegener's granulomatosis is very similar to microscopic polyarteritis. Its distinguishing features are the granulomatous lesions in the airways and lungs, and the clinical features of epistaxis or haemoptysis. Intrapulmonary haemorrhage is a particularly serious event. Cyclophosphamide, with steroids, appears to be a particularly effective treatment.

Henoch–Schönlein purpura

Henoch–Schönlein purpura is a non-thrombocytopenic purpura and occurs mainly in children, being rare in adults.

Clinical features   The purpura usually affects the extremities and buttocks. Painful and swollen joints, gastrointestinal bleeding and haematuria are common. Sometimes acute renal failure is the main presenting feature. An infection or exposure to drugs antedates the illness. Attacks may be continuous or recurrent.

Pathology and pathogenesis   A variety of histological appearances are seen in the kidney. A hallmark of Henoch–Schönlein purpura is the deposition of IgA in the mesangial areas of the glomeruli. IgA is also found in the skin of affected and unaffected sites. The cause is unknown; no particular organism or drugs are associaed with this condition.

The diagnosis of Henoch–Schönlein purpura is easily made on clinical grounds.

Management and prognosis   No particular treatment has been shown to be effective; in patients with crescentic nephritis and acute renal failure rapid institution of high-dose steroids, azathioprine or cyclophosphamide, and plasma exchange have been effective in some cases.

Systemic sclerosis

The middle aged are affected by systemic sclerosis but it is an uncommon condition. Women are 3–4 times more commonly affected than men.

Clinical features Patients mainly present with involvement of the skin, gastrointestinal tract, lungs and heart. The kidneys become involved later with proteinuria, renal failure and hypertension. The hypertension is often very severe, and may be of the accelerated type.

Pathology and pathogenesis There is gross thickening of the arterial walls with narrowing or occlusion of the lumen. The glomeruli may be infarcted. The aetiology is unknown.

Diagnosis is usually easy with the typical involvement of several organs, and is confirmed histologically.

Management This relies on control of hypertension; steroids and immunosuppressive drugs are ineffective. The prognosis is poor. Plasma exchange has been used with some benefit in a small number of patients, but no controlled observations of this treatment have been made. Recently captopril has been reported in some patients to improve renal function, presumably by altering intrarenal haemodynamics.

Rheumatoid arthritis

Rheumatoid arthritis *per se* is rarely complicated by nephritis. Much commoner are membranous nephropathy, due to penicillamine or gold, and secondary amyloid.

Sjogren's syndrome Sjogren's syndrome may be accompanied by renal tubular acidosis, interstitial nephritis and, less commonly, glomerulonephritis.

Amyloidosis

The kidney is affected by both primary and secondary amyloid.

Clinical features Patients usually present with proteinuria, which in one-third causes a nephrotic syndrome. Uraemia at presentation occurs in a minority of patients. Hypertension is not common. In primary amyloid there is also involvement of other organs (e.g. heart, gastrointestinal tract and liver). In secondary amyloid there is evidence of the underlying disease – chronic infection (e.g. bronchiectasis or tuberculosis), neoplasia (e.g. myelomatosis) and features of the hereditary/familial forms (e.g. familial Mediterranean fever).

Pathology and pathogenesis Diagnosis is easy when renal disease involves other organs and the history suggests secondary amyloid.

Histology provides confirmation, but in a small number of patients, particularly those with primary amyloid, histology may be the only means of making the diagnosis. Tissue from the rectum, gum, or involved skin often contains amyloid, allowing a presumptive diagnosis without renal biopsy. Absence of amyloid in these extrarenal sites does not exclude renal involvement.

Management and prognosis Secondary amyloid can improve with treatment of the underlying cause, but otherwise treatment seems ineffectual. The exception is the use of colchicine in the treatment of familial Mediterranean fever. The prognosis of renal amyloid is that of the involvement of other organs and the underlying cause; dialysis and transplantation are effective.

Myeloma

Occasionally renal failure, which may be acute, or proteinuria, which may lead to the nephrotic syndrome, are the sole presenting features of myeloma. Usually however the patient also has typical features of myeloma i.e. bone pain, malaise, anaemia. Renal damage can arise from toxicity of light chains to tubular cells, obstruction due to intratubular precipitation of proteins, hypercalcaemia, the development of amyloid and hyperuricaemia due to therapy. The diagnosis is made by demonstrating the typical biochemical and bone marrow abnormalities of myeloma. Histology of the kidney shows a variety of appearances, the main diagnostic feature being the typical myeloma casts in the tubules, which are homogenous and eosinophilic.

The treatment is that of myeloma. If end-stage renal failure supervenes, dialysis and transplantation are appropriate, the prognosis being that of the myeloma itself.

Waldenstrom's macroglobulinaemia

In Waldenstrom's macroglobulinaemia the kidneys are affected by occlusion of glomerular capillaries by the IgM produced in this disease. Proteinuria and renal failure follow.

Mixed essential cryoglobulinaemia

Mixed essential cryoglobulinaemia is a disease of the middle-aged or elderly, rare in Northern Europe, but more commonly found in Mediterranean countries. Circulating cryoglobulins, usually consisting of a monoclonal IgM as antigen with IgG antibody, cause vascular disease which presents as purpura, especially on the legs, and Raynaud's phenomenon arthralgia, hepatosplenomegaly and nephritis. Histology of the kidney shows a proliferative nephritis and on electron microscopy there is a characteristic crystalline appearance. No treatment has been found to be effective, though plasma exchange has been reported to be beneficial.

Neoplasia

Carcinoma

There is an association between membranous nephropathy and carcinoma. The malignancies found are the common ones i.e. bronchus, pancreas, stomach, colon, uterus and ovary. The renal disease itself is indistinguishable from the idiopathic form. There is suggestive, but inconclusive, evidence that complexes of tumour antigen and antibody cause the nephritis.

Lymphoma

Minimal change nephropathy occurs with lymphomas. The nature of the association is not clear, but is of much interest as lymphocyte function is abnormal in both conditions when they occur separately. Treatment of the underlying neoplasia alone can cause remission of the proteinuria, indicating its causal role. The renal disease may recur, should the malignancy reappear.

Infections

Because infectious organisms are omnipresent and immunogenic it is not surprising that they should be implicated as causes of immune complex nephritis. The best known example is poststreptococcal nephritis, but there are many other organisms which cause nephritis (see Table 7.1). In most the renal lesion is glomerular, but in some an interstitial nephritis is the major lesion. Some of these conditions are now discussed in more detail.

Subacute bacterial endocarditis

The commonest finding in subacute bacterial endocarditis is asymptomatic proteinuria and haematuria; renal failure occurs in a minority of patients. A focal proliferative lesion is most often found, but a diffuse proliferative crescentic nephritis may occur. Immunoglobulins and complement are found in the glomeruli, and hypocomplementaemia is common. The nephritis is not confined to any particular organism causing the endocarditis. Improving the nephritis depends upon eradicating the endocarditis by antibiotics, or surgery, or both.

Shunt nephritis

In this case infection occurs on the shunt used for draining hydrocephalus. The pathogenesis is similar to that of nephritis complicating endocarditis (i.e. chronic infection producing a persistent antigenaemia with consequent immune complex formation). The organism is often *Staphylococcus albus*, and the histological appearance that of subendothelial mesangiocapillary glomerulonephritis. The renal manifestations range from haematuria and proteinuria to nephrotic syndrome and renal failure. Systemic symptoms and signs of infection and emboli may occur. As in endocarditis, removal of the infection is potentially curative of the nephritis.

Malarial nephropathy

There is an association between nephrotic syndrome and *Plasmodium malariae* infection as shown by epidemiological studies and by the demonstration of *P. malaria* antigen in glomeruli of affected kidneys. However, cure of malariae is not necessarily followed by an improvement in the nephropathy, the implication being that complexes containing malarial antigen are not causing the nephritis, or that the latter is due to some other mechanism.

Haemolytic uraemic syndromes

A number of syndromes are characterized by acute intravascular haemolysis and acute renal failure:

the haemolytic uraemic syndrome of childhood, a similar disorder occurring in adults, haemolytic uraemic syndrome in the puerperium, thrombotic thrombocytopenic purpura – Moschowitz's syndrome.

Clinical features These mainly are an acute haemolytic anaemia, bleeding due to thrombocytopenia and acute renal failure. In children there is often a preceding infection of the gastrointestinal or respiratory tract. In adults the only recognizable antecedent factors are parturition and oestrogens (usually the contraceptive pill). Other systems may be involved, especially the brain: indeed involvement of the brain is a central feature of Moschowitz's syndrome. Hypertension, which may be severe, often develops.

Pathology and pathogenesis Fibrin-like material occludes the arterioles which have fibrinoid necrosis in their walls. The glomeruli have ischaemic changes. The aetiology remains unknown, but the sequence is thought to be endothelial damage, coagulation with consumption of platelets and clotting factors, and haemolysis due to mechanical damage to red cells by the abnormal vessel wall and fibrin strands. This damage causes the fragmented and distorted erythrocytes characteristic of this condition, and has given rise to the term microangiopathic haemolytic anaemia. It has been suggested that in some patients there is a deficiency of plasma factor(s) necessary for the production of prostacyclin which prevents platelet aggregation.

Diagnosis The combination of microangiopathic haemolytic anaemia, thrombocytopenia, bleeding and renal failure, with or without the involvement of other organs, is unmistakable. Renal biopsy is not usually feasible because of the thrombocytopenia and indeed is not strictly necessary.

Management and prognosis There is a spontaneous remission rate, particularly in children which makes assessment of therapy difficult. However, other patients rapidly develop terminal renal failure, emphasizing the need for effective treatment. There is no convincing evidence that steroids, immunosuppressive drugs, and anticoagulants are useful. There have been reports that plasma infusion or plasma exchange produce improvement, presumably by correcting a deficiency of plasma factor(s). However, not all cases respond to this treatment.

Diabetes mellitus

Renal failure is an extremely important consequence of diabetes. Nephropathy develops within 20 years of diagnosis in 35–50 per cent of juvenile and maturity-onset insulin-dependent diabetics. Diabetes accounts for an increasing proportion of treated patients with end-stage renal disease.

Clinical features Patients develop proteinuria, nephrotic syndrome, and renal failure. Hypertension may not develop until a later stage. Almost all patients who develop diabetic nephropathy have diabetic retinopathy as well.

Pathology and pathogenesis Thickening of the basement membranes of the glomeruli, tubules and Bowman's capsule is the earliest change. The glomerular mesangium undergoes sclerosis which may be diffuse or nodular – the Kimmelstiel-Wilson lesion. Hyaline changes occur in the arterioles. The cause of the lesions is unknown. In experimental diabetes mellitus the nephropathy is reversible by transplantation of a diabetic kidney into a non-diabetic animal, i.e. the renal lesions are directly due to the diabetes. The crucial question is, therefore, the role of correctable factors such as defective insulin secretion, impaired insulin utilization and hyperglycaemia. New methods of insulin administration, such as continuous subcutaneous infusion by pump, have achieved better control of diabetes and it is clearly important to determine if this reduces the degree or frequency of diabetic nephropathy.

Diagnosis Proteinuria and renal failure in a diabetic of many years' standing who has retinopathy is virtually diagnostic. However, other forms of glomerular disease can occur in diabetes, and this may influence the need for a renal biopsy to confirm the diagnosis.

Management and prognosis Treatment in the early stages is that of the nephrotic syndrome and hypertension. Control of the high blood pressure is vital as hypertension has a markedly deleterious effect on diabetic vascular disease. Sudden deterioration in renal function suggests obstruction due to papillary necrosis. The treatment of end-stage renal failure in diabetics is now being practised more widely; until some years ago the results of chronic haemodialysis and transplantation were so poor that many renal units would not accept these patients. Although outcome has improved, the prognosis of treatment for end-stage renal failure in diabetics is still worse than for non-diabetics. Chronic ambulatory peritoneal dialysis has been very predictable especially as administration of insulin via the dialysis fluid has given good control of blood glucose levels.

Hyperuricaemic nephropathy

In patients with hyperuricaemia and/or hyperuricosuria, the renal consequences are gouty (chronic hyperuricaemic) nephropathy, acute hyperuricaemic nephropathy, and nephrolithiasis.

Gouty (chronic hyperuricaemic) nephropathy

Renal disease is the most common and most serious extra-articular complication of gout with reduced renal function in about 50 per cent of patients.

Clinical features Proteinuria occurs early but it is slight and occasionally absent. Pyuria and haematuria are uncommon unless kidney stones and infection are present. Loss of urine concentrating ability is the earliest functional disturbance, followed by slowly progressive renal insufficiency. Gouty nephropathy without a history of arthritis is unusual.

Pathology In gouty nephropathy the specific lesion is deposition of sodium urate crystals in the medullary interstitium, the pyramids and the papillae (i.e. in areas of highest concentration of sodium urate). Crystals are seldom seen in the renal cortex. Chronic interstitial nephritis, is commonly seen. Whether this results from chronic hyperuricaemia or from commonly associated conditions such as hypertension, diabetes, stone disease and ageing is still unclear.

Management Allopurinol, which reduces the formation of uric acid, can stop renal deterioration. There is little evidence to suggest that asymptomatic hyperuricaemia alone is associated with an increased incidence of kidney disease.

Acute hyperuricaemic nephropathy

Acute hyperuricaemic nephropathy is seen mainly in patients with lympho- and myeloproliferative disorders in whom hyperuricaemia and hyperuricosuria result from overproduction of uric acid due to increased cell turnover. This usually occurs after antimitotic treatment has begun. Uric acid crystals precipitate in the tubules and collecting ducts of the kidneys causing obstruction and acute renal failure.

Acute oliguria, often leading to anuria, with a rapidly rising serum creatinine level is the commonest form of presentation. Once renal failure has occurred, treatment should be directed at increasing the urine volume and the solubility of uric acid by raising the urine pH above 7 with sodium bicarbonate or a carbonic anhydrase inhibitor, and decreasing uric acid formation with allopurinol. It may be prevented by administering allupurinol for several days before chemotheraphy is given for the primary disease.

Urinary tract infection

Many terms, most of them applied to clinical subgroups under the general term 'urinary tract infection' are in use and require definition.

- Urinary tract infection is the presence of micro-organisms in the urinary tract.
- Bacteriuria is the presence of bacteria in the bladder urine.
- Asymptomatic or covert bacteriuria is significant bacteriuria detected in healthy individuals with no symptoms of infection. Cystitis consists of frequency, dysuria and sometimes haematuria.
- Urethral syndrome is frequency and dysuria in the absence of bacteriuria.
- Acute pyelonephritis is bacterial infection of the pelvis and parenchyma of the kidney.
- Chronic pyelonephritis is chronic interstitial inflammation due to longstanding or recurrent bacterial infection.

General comments

Urinary tract infection is common, accounting for a considerable degree of morbidity and absenteeism. The wide choice of effective antibiotics now available allows a reasonable chance of reducing morbidity and, in those patients with serious structural defects or infective damage to the urinary tract, diminishes or even halts progressive renal damage caused by the infection itself.

The diagnosis of urinary infection is critically dependent on specimen collection. Urine must be taken to the laboratory at once or refrigerated, to prevent multiplication of organisms.

Urine for microscopy and culture is obtained in most patients as a mid-stream urine. Alternative techniques are suprapubic aspiration, or, as a last resort, urethral catheterization. If infection is proven, then predisposing causes which can be treated must be excluded.

Aetiology and pathogenesis

Several factors predispose to the development of urinary tract infection.

- Anatomical structure of the female lower urinary tract. The shortness of the female urethra and its greater proximity to the perianal area and therefore to faecal flora allow easier colonization.
- Persistence of organisms in the urinary tract is due to the following:
  Renal – scars, papillary necrosis, stones.
  Ureter – vesicoureteral reflux, physiological dilation of pregnancy, duplex formation.
  Bladder – catheter, prolapse, neurogenic bladder, diverticulum, stones, tumour.
  Urethra – prostatomegaly and prostatitis, stricture, phimosis.
- Features of the bacteria themselves, such as resistance to phagocytes, production of mucinase, and adherence to mucosal surfaces.
- Organisms may be introduced by sexual intercourse, instrumentation (e.g. catheterization), enterovesical fistulae.

Clinical syndromes of infection

Asymptomatic bacteriuria

By definition this occurs without symptoms, and in practice is found in screening of healthy populations and of pregnant women. Women with normal urinary tracts have not shown progression to renal failure. However, some urea-splitting organisms (e.g. *Staphylococcus albus* and *Proteus* spp) may be associated with stone formation with all their associated complications. In non-pregnant women, no treatment is required; because pregnant women with asymptomatic bacteriuria have an increased incidence of pyelonephritis, they should receive appropriate antibiotics.

Non-specific urethritis

In the male this is a venereal disease, and is thought to be caused by *Chlamydia* and *Mycoplasmae*, occasionally *Trichomonas*. The symptoms are penile discharge and dysuria. This condition must be distinguished from gonococcal infection, and is treated by erythromycin or tetracycline.

In the female, non-specific urethritis is also known as bacterial cystitis, the urethral syndrome, or the frequency and dysuria syndrome. Sexual intercourse may precipitate the symptoms, which are dysuria, frequency and urgency. Urine cultures are repeatedly negative. Infection of the vagina or cervix should be excluded.

Cystitis

Although it is also known as bacterial cystitis to differentiate it from 'abacterial cystitis', other agents e.g. drugs, chemicals and X-rays may cause a similar disorder. It is characterized by frequency, dysuria, malodorous urine and often haematuria. The urine is purulent and, when bacteria are causative, cultures are positive for *E. coli* in the majority of patients.

In adult women, the urinary tract is nearly always normal, but in children associated abnormalities are frequently found; the prognosis will differ accordingly. Treatment of acute attacks is with appropriate antibiotics; trimethoprim, co-trimoxazole or ampicillin can be given pending the result of urine culture. If infections are frequent, due either to relapse or to reinfection, long-term treatment may be needed as proplylactic therapy, e.g. trimethoprim 100 mg nightly.

Acute pyelonephritis

The bacterial invasion of the kidney may be asymptomatic, but the typical symptoms are the combination of loin pain and fever; the urine may be foul smelling and macroscopic haematuria can occur, but these two symptoms are usually absent. Acute pyelonephritis can be a serious illness, producing septicaemia and shock, and occasionally, when bilateral or affecting the only functioning kidney, acute renal failure may occur.

The diagnosis is not difficult especially when accompanied by the physical sign of loin tenderness. The treatment consists of appropriate antibiotics, which may need intravenous administration in the severely ill patient. As the result of urine or blood cultures will not be known until

24–48 hours after the samples are taken, the initial period of antibiotic treatment is guesswork. Amoxycillin, ampicillin, or trimethoprim are reasonable first choices during this waiting period. When the acute infection has settled, the urinary tract must be investigated to exclude lesions predisposing to infection. If infections are recurrent, then prophylactic treatment, as above, is necessary.

Chronic pylonephritis

This disorder, defined above, accounts for 15–20 per cent of patients who develop end-stage renal failure. The majority of patients are thought to have developed chronic pylonephritis as a result of vesico-ureteric reflux during childhood; in others obstruction and/or stones are causative factors. Patients may present with hypertension, recurrent infection, or symptoms of chronic renal failure. Usually patients with chronic or end-stage renal failure present with a previously asymptomatic course. Although renal damage may have begun in childhood, the diagnosis rests upon the demonstration of scarred kidneys, which may be significantly and unequally reduced in size.

Treatment will obviously depend upon the stage at which the patient presents, and whether there are underlying correctable lesions in the urinary tracts. Without doubt the most important aspect of treatment, numerically speaking, is the prevention of infection and damage in children with vesico-ureteric reflux.

A number of other conditions require description under the general term of urinary tract infection.

Tuberculosis

This is much less common now in the more advanced countries of the world. The infection usually begins in the kidney, by haematogenous spread, and thereafter spreads to the ureter, bladder, and in men to the seminal vesicles, epididymes, and vasa deferentia. The most serious effect is formation of ureteric structures which cause obstruction and renal failure.

Patients do not present usually with systemic symptoms but with symptoms localized to the urinary tract such as dysuria, frequency, haematuria, renal colic and loin pain. The diagnosis is made by culture of mycobacterium tuberculosis from the urine. Treatment is with chemotherapy employing a mixture of drugs to prevent emergence of resistance. When the sensitivity of the organism is known, two appropriate drugs are continued for at least 1 year. Urological measures may be necessary to relieve obstruction; some centres recommend the use of corticosteroids to prevent cicatrization.

Prostatitis

Prostatic infection is a common cause of recurrent urinary tract infection. The symptoms are pain in the prostatic/perineal area, and dysuria. It can be diagnosed by the so-called 'three specimen test'. In sequence, a 'first 10 ml' specimen, which is an MSU, a prostatic secretion specimen after prostatic massage and a further 'first 10 ml' specimen are collected. The organism will be present in low numbers in the first specimen but in higher numbers in either the prostatic secretion or the 10 ml passed following massage. Treatment is straightforward for the acute stage, but treatment of chronic prostatitis is difficult, because antibacterial agents penetrate the non-inflamed prostate poorly. Three month courses of cotrimoxazole, trimethoprim, tetracycline or erythromycin can be effective since these drugs tend to penetrate satisfactorily.

Renal papillary necrosis

This may result from severe infection of the urinary tract as well as from diabetes mellitus and analgesic nephropathy.

Reflux nephropathy

Vesico-ureteric reflux (VUR) is caused by an incompetent vesico-ureteric junction. The condition is usually congenital but is also caused by trauma, mainly surgical, or inflammatory changes and scarring around the ureteric orifice. VUR may be classified in various ways – a classification using radiological findings is as follows

- *Grade 1*: incomplete filling of the urinary tract not reaching the kidney, with a normal ureteric oricie.
- *Grade 2*: complete filling of the urinary tract with little or no dilation of calyces.
- *Grade 3*: complete filling of the urinary tract with dilation of calyces.

Approximately 25 per cent of patients – adults and children – with urinary tract infection have scarred kidneys, and these in turn are related to the presence of VUR which is present in 35 per cent of infected children. This association probably arises because VUR allows organisms to ascend to the kidney and creates residual urine and so encourages bacterial multiplication. VUR may also produce mechanical kidney damage as a result of the back pressure of the column of urine. Although it is not known exactly how VUR causes kidney damage, tubular or calyceal rupture is probably necessary. The escape of Tamm-Horsfall protein from the ascending limb of the loop of Henle into the renal interstitium may also cause an inflammatory response which leads to interstitial damage.

Scarring due to VUR occurs very early in life, before the age of 4–5 years; if the kidneys are normal at this age they are very likely to remain so, whereas if they are already scarred, further scarring is likely. Both renal failure and hypertension may follow as a consequence of the scarring.

Management   In children with urinary tract infection (UTI) in whom the intravenous urogram is normal there is no indication for a micturating cystogram. All that is needed is simply prevention and/or treatment of symptomatic infection. When the intravenous urogram (IVU) in a child with urinary tract infection shows kidney scars a micturating cystogram should be performed. If VUR is found, the child may develop progressive kidney damage. Long-term treatment with a low dose of a suitable antibiotic is indicated, until the kidney growth can be improved and further scarring can be prevented. It is important to use long-term treatment as the reinfections which may follow short courses of treatment are particularly harmful. Surgical correction of VUR after the age of 4 years old is seldom indicated. In all patients blood pressure should be checked regularly, particularly in women when oral contraceptives are started or pregnancy occurs.

Renal Calculi

Epidemiology

Renal calculi are common but their incidence varies considerably between and within populations. Ureteric calculi are more likely to present during the summer. Calculi are most common between the ages of 30 and 60 years; the male to female ratio is 3:1.

Types of stones

There are four main types of kidney stones.

- Calcium oxalate stones account for approximately 80–85 per cent of all renal stones. They may be present in a pure form or as a mixture with calcium phosphate (usually hydroxyapatite).
- Triple phosphate stones, comprising 10 per cent or less of the total, are composed of a mixture of magnesium ammonium phosphate (struvite) and calcium phosphate.
- Uric acid stones comprise 5–10 per cent of all renal stones.
- Cystine stones comprise approximately 1 per cent of the total.

Pathogenesis

Nephrolithiasis results from super saturation of the urine with crystalloid. There are four possible causes of urinary supersaturation:

- increased urinary excretion of the crystalloid;
- variation of the pH of the urine, resulting in diminished crystalloid solubility;
- deficiency of substances which normally prevent crystallization (e.g. glycosaminoglycans);
- reduced urinary volume.

In an individual patient more than one cause may operate.

Complications

The complications of stone formation give rise to much morbidity and a significant mortality from what is basically a preventable disease in most instances. The main ones are obstruction, infection, local destruction of renal parenchyma and haemorrhage.

Presenting features

- Ureteric colic is characteristic of calculi and consists of excruciating pain which may be described as cramping, sharp or stabbing. The distribution extends from the loin down the line of the ureter to the groin. There is often radiation to the testes in men and to the labia majora in women.
- Loin pain, without ureteric colic or infection.
- Symptoms of urinary tract infection typically associated with infection stones, but which may be the presenting feature in any form of calculi.

- Macroscopic haematuria with or without colic.
- Symptoms of signs of chronic renal failure.
- Loin tenderness, one of the few physical signs.
- Symptoms and signs of acute renal failure, particularly when one kidney has been silently destroyed, and the remaining kidney develops obstruction or acute infection.
- A palpable kidney in the presence of a large staghorn calculus or obstruction.

Diagnosis

This is not difficult, as the history is usually clear, and confirmation simple by appropriate imaging techniques. A plain X-ray of the urinary tract to reveal the presence and size of radio-opaque stones, and an intravenous urogram to demonstrate their relationship to the urinary tract and site of any obstruction, are still the initial imaging investigations in patients with renal calculi. Non-opaque calculi cause negative shadows within the urinary tract on the intravenous urogram. Ultrasound can demonstrate obstruction and the presence of stones and is replacing urography in many centres. CT scanning may reveal non-opaque calculi undetected by conventional techniques. Antegrade pyelography can be performed to demonstrate the level of ureteric obstruction in a non-functioning kidney or to outline non-opaque calculi in the renal pelvis.

Other investigations

The urine must be cultured to exclude infection.

Crystals are commonly detected on urine microscopy. Some, such as crystal calcium and uric acid, may occur in the urine of normal individuals, but in patients with calculi, crystals are often numerous, large or aggregate. Cystine crystals do not occur in normal urine and their presence is diagnostic of cystinuria. Urine pH should always be determined and calcium, urate, cystine and oxalate excretion should be measured. Chemical analysis of the calculus may facilitate the diagnosis of underlying causes. Renal excretory function should be measured, and hypercalcaemia and hyperuricaemia excluded. Obviously any underlying cause of a metabolic abnormality requires investigation in its own right.

Management

Treatment has two aims, to remove or eliminate existing calculi and to prevent recurrence, which is very common.

Medical treatment

If the 24-hour urine volume can be maintained within the range of 2.5–3.5 litres, this simple measure alone will often prevent recurrence.

If this approach is to be effective, the patient must maintain a high night volume and should be encouraged to drink sufficient fluid on retiring to ensure voiding during the night and drink the same volume of fluid after emptying the bladder during the night.

Diet   There is little evidence to suggest that high oxalate absorption contributes to stone formation, except in cases of intestinal oxalosis. Although a purine-free diet has been advocated for the control of uric acid calculi, this regimen is difficult to adhere to and requires life-long compliance. Dietary restrictions are seldom recommended as effective control may be achieved by other methods.

If calcium intake is excessive, a modest reduction may be justified. However calcium restriction increases oxalate absorption from the bowel and is thus of doubtful benefit in prophylaxis.

Idiopathic hypercalciuria   Thiazides increase calcium reabsorption in the distal tubule and correct idiopathic hypercalciuria. A single dose of a thiazide diuretic at night (e.g. bendrofluazide, 5 mg) will enhance noctural urine flow and reduce calcium excretion.

Hyperuricosuria   Hyperuricosuria is associated with the formation of both calcium oxalate and uric acid stones. In many cases, alkalinization of the urine may be prophylactic. Potassium citrate, 40–60 mEq/day is more effective than sodium bicarbonate in preventing recurrence.

Renal tubular acidosis   Potassium citrate, 40–60 mEq/day can be used to reduce urinary calcium excretion and to increase urinary citrate. This regimen will usually reduce or prevent recurrence.

Infection stones   Because these calculi harbour bacteria, their elimination is essential to effective treatment of the infection. Interventional methods facilitate the elimination of most infection stones without open surgery. If intervention is contraindicated, continuous suppressive treatment with an anti-bacterial agent (e.g. amoxycillin,

250–500 mg t.d.s.) is necessary to maintain a sterile urine and thus prevent continued stone growth.

Surgical removal or ultrasound disintegration of infection calculi may fail to eliminate the tiny fragments which lead inevitably to stone recurrence. Citric acid infusion through a percutaneous nephrostomy is therefore recommended as an adjuvant treatment.

Cystine stones may dissolve spontaneously if patients are able to excrete 3 to 5 litres of fluid/day. Penicillamine, 0.25 g–1.5 g/day encourages stone dissolution and prevents recurrence. A urinary pH greater than 8.0 must be achieved before cystine solubility is increased.

Surgical treatment

Although direct surgical removal of stones from the urinary tract is obviously an important and effective procedure, other interventional methods are superceding conventional surgery. These methods are still undergoing modification, and a full appraisal of their pros and cons is not yet possible.

Percutaneous stone removal

The introduction of a percutaneous needle into the renal collecting system under fluoroscopy allows various instruments to be introduced through the dilated tract and used to fragment calculi or to remove them percutaneously; both ultrasonic and laser probes have been used. Fluoroscopy may be used to guide stone retrieval baskets using small tracks (14 F); over 90 per cent of stones less than 7 mm in smallest diameter can be removed by this route.

Although complications, including serious haemorrhage, occur in approximately 20 per cent of patients treated with large calibre tracks (24–35 F), experienced surgeons report complications in only 4 per cent of cases.

Extracorporeal shock wave lithotripsy

In this procedure an ultrasound shock wave is generated and focused on the calculus which is fragmented by repeated treatments. Repeated shock waves, administered over periods of up to 60 minutes, may be necessary. Although the first models were very costly, several second generation machines produced at lower cost are undergoing trials and it is likely that this method will become more widely available.

The new methods afford considerable advantages over the conventional non-interventional approach to calculi under 6 mm in diameter; 4–6 weeks may elapse before the patient passes the stone, during which time recurrent renal colic is common. Given a choice, most patients are likely to favour the immediate relief provided by percutaneous extraction, particularly as the procedure may be performed under local anaesthetic with a minimum of risk and inconvenience.

Obstructive uropathy

Definition

Obstruction occurs when urinary flow is prevented between the renal calyces and the point at which urine is voided from the body.

Pathophysiology

Obstruction below the bladder If bladder pressure is low (despite obstruction) urine flow down the ureter is not prevented and there is no deleterious effect on renal function. If the intravesical pressure is raised throughout the micturition cycle then the effects are as for ureteric obstruction.

Obstruction above the bladder In acute ureteric obstruction, the intraluminal pressure increases and the intrapelvic pressure rises to 50–70 mm Hg. This pressure, transmitted to the collecting ducts and tubules, impairs glomerular filtration. Nonetheless urine formation may continue for some days, even when obstruction is complete, and is due to increased resorption of urine in tubules and collecting ducts. If complete obstruction persists, renal blood flow falls and glomerular filtration ceases within a few days. Initially the kidney swells and the renal pelvis dilates, then the kidney contracts uniformly, and eventually atrophies. In partial ureteric obstruction the renal functional changes depend on the degree of obstruction. Dilation is more gradual. Persistent partial obstruction leads eventually to a very large hydronephrotic kidney with only a thin rim of cortex.

Renal tubular dysfunction Acute partial obstruction can cause a low sodium concentration and a high osmolality, leading to confusion when oliguria is suspected to be due to prerenal causes. If partial obstruction continues, impairment of concentrating mechanisms may cause polyuria and increased sodium loss.

After relief of obstruction, renal blood flow and GFR often recover completely and some recovery of function may occur even in situations which were thought to be irreversible i.e. up to a limit of 8 weeks complete obstruction, after which non-function is almost inevitable. After unilateral obstruction little tubular dysfunction is evident, but after bilateral obstruction serious electrolyte and water loss can occur. Losses of 6–8 litres/24 hours, continuing for several days, are not uncommon. This diuresis may persist despite the development of hypovolaemia.

Causes

The causes of obstructive nephropathy are listed in Table 7.5. The likelihood of any cause in a given patient obviously depends upon age, sex and geography. Obstructive nephropathy is not uncommon. In infants and children, urinary tract obstruction due to congenital anomalies is a relatively common cause of renal failure and in elderly men it is often due to prostatic obstruction. Between the ages of 20 and 60 years the incidence of urinary tract obstruction is higher in women than in men, but over the age of 60, the converse is the case.

Table 7.5   Common causes of obstruction

Intraluminal
Calculi
Bladder or ureteric tumours
Necrotic papillae
Blood clot

Congenital
Pelvic–ureteric junction obstruction
Bladder neck obstruction
Urethral valves
Phimosis

Acquired
Ureteric stricture
Neurogenic bladder
Urethral stricture

Extramural
Prostatic obstruction
Pelvic tumours
Retroperitoneal fibrosis
Trauma including surgery

Presenting features

Upper urinary tract obstruction may be symptomless or cause mild symptoms such as backache and malaise; if infection occurs, malaise, fever, loin pain and symptoms and signs of septicaemia may supervene. Loin pain may be provoked by alcohol, diuretics or excessive fluid intake, which increase urinary volume and cause distension of the collecting system, particularly in pelviureteric junction obstruction.

In bladder outflow obstruction symptoms may be minimal and may be accepted by the patient as normal. Hesitancy, diminished force of the stream, terminal dribbling, and a sense of incomplete bladder emptying are typical. The frequent passage of small volumes of urine may be a prominent symptom–retention with overflow. Acute and complete retention of urine, with severe suprapubic and perineal pain, is a clear clinical picture. Lower urinary tract infection is often associated with bladder outflow obstruction causing frequency, urgency, urge incontinence, dysuria, suprapubic pain, haematuria, and cloudy, smelly urine.

Complete anuria requires exclusion of a diagnosis of complete bilateral obstruction or complete obstruction of a single kidney. The differential diagnosis includes bilateral total renal cortical necrosis, acute anuric glomerulonephritis and bilateral renal arterial occlusion. Polyuria may occur in partial obstruction due to impairment of renal tubular concentrating capacity. Intermittent anuria and polyuria indicate intermittent complete obstruction and are typical of retroperitoneal fibrosis.

Signs

Loin tenderness and/or a palpable enlarged kidney may occur in upper urinary tract obstruction. In acute or chronic retention an enlarged bladder can be felt or percussed. Careful examination of the genitalia, rectum and vagina is essential. The size of the prostate assessed rectally is not always indicative of prostatic obstruction; median lobe enlargement of a normal prostate may give rise to severe obstruction, whereas a grossly enlarged gland may cause little or no obstruction. Additional symptoms and signs due to the underlying cause of the obstruction may also feature in the patients presentation.

Diagnosis

The diagnosis of urinary obstruction is very important since it is eminently treatable and prompt detection and therapy can regain useful renal function. The detection of urinary obstruction is rapid and easy, but a high index of clinical suspicion is vital. Imaging techniques are the keystone to both the diagnosis and the planning of the management of obstruction.

Ultrasound

Ultrasonography has replaced intravenous urography as the initial imaging technique in a patient suspected of having urinary obstruction – it is quick, easy to perform, painless and non-invasive. An experienced operator can by ultrasound readily demonstrate a dilated collecting system including the ureter. Renal stones may also be detected by this technique and renal cortical width can be assessed. Normal ultrasound appearances do not exclude acute obstruction when dilation may be minimal in the early stages. Ultrasound is an excellent way of determining bladder size and of showing intravesical lesions.

Intravenous urography (IVU)   The number of IVUs performed in recent years had diminished due to the advent of other investigative techniques. Nonetheless they are still very important in the diagnosis and assessment of urinary obstruction. Important information is obtained even in the presence of severe renal failure, if a high dose of contrast medium is used in combination with tomography and if films are taken 24 hours after injection. The recent introduction of iso-osmotic contrast media has reduced the toxicity associated with IVUs.

Apart from functional information, an IVU will often demonstrate the anatomical site of obstruction. A delayed appearance of the nephrogram, which eventually becomes denser than that of the unobstructed side and outlines a swollen enlarged kidney, is the first sign indicating obstruction. A negative pyelogram may be seen outlining a distended pelvis. As dye enters the drainage system it will show dilation down to the site of obstruction. In bladder outlet obstruction a distended bladder will be seen which empties poorly after micturition.

CT scanning gives precise anatomical information in a patient with urinary obstruction, particularly if the procedure is enhanced by intravenous contrast media, but is unnecessary for most cases of urinary obstruction. Its uses are when renal failure has led to limited or no excretion of contrast, in assessing tumours of the renal parenchyma and the bladder, when obstruction is due to pelvic or retroperitoneal masses. Retrograde pyelography used to be the standard diagnostic investigation but has now been largely replaced by newer techniques. It involves the risk of general anaesthesia in a patient who may be acutely ill and may introduce infection. It can be useful, however, as an extension of cystoscopy.

Antegrade pyelography has proved a significant advance in diagnosis and management. It is the preferred approach when there is sufficient dilation of the renal pelvis to allow safe placement of a fine catheter. The procedure is performed under local anaesthesia with either image intensifier or ultrasound control. Although significant bleeding is a complication it is uncommon and usually ceases quickly. A perfusion test can be performed through the percutaneous catheter *in situ* in the renal pelvis. Fluid is infused through the catheter at 10 ml/minute and the pressure monitored and compared to bladder pressure monitored simultaneously through a urethral catheter. A pressure gradient of less than 10 mmHg indicates no obstruction and more than 20 mmHg indicates significant obstruction between the two points of measurement.

Cystoscopy, urethrography and urodynamics may be necessary if bladder outlet or urethral obstruction is suspected. Urodynamic studies are essential for diagnosing a neuropathic hypotonic bladder which is radiologically similar to bladder outlet obstruction. If the bladder fails to contract despite the introduction of a large volume of fluid and the intravesical pressure remains low, then a hypotonic bladder is present.

Treatment

Relief of obstruction is clearly the aim of treatment. The details of how this is done obviously vary from case to case, depending upon the causative pathology, and will not be discussed further here. However, certain general principles apply to any patients with obstructive nephropathy.

Defining the cause of obstruction   The investigations described above usually indicate the site of obstruction, and in most instances its cause; the latter may however require laparotomy.

Reversibility of renal function   Before deciding

the definitive treatment, it is necessary to determine how much renal function is recoverable after relief of the obstruction. If the obstructed kidney is severely damaged and likely to contribute little to long-term function after disobstruction then a nephrectomy is indicated, especially if the opposite kidney is unobstructed and normal. There is, however, a much greater tendency in recent years to conserve kidneys and many nephrectomies in the past have been performed when relief of the obstruction lesion would have been preferable. Assessment of recoverability of renal function is most effectively obtained by relief of the obstruction. This can be done temporarily by either percutaneous nephrostomy or through the retrograde insertion of a ureteric catheter. In bladder outlet obstruction, a urinary catheter will achieve temporary drainage. These catheters can be left *in situ* for days or weeks and give a good indication as to the final functional result of definitive surgery.

A guide to individual kidney function is gained from radionuclide scanning. Radionuclide scanning allows for comparative function to be quantitiated, though in the presence of unrelieved obstruction, GFR and renal blood flow may be underestimated.

Post-obstructive diuresis Following relief of obstruction, a huge and obligatory diuresis may occur. Intravenous fluid replacement is essential. Initially the urine should be assumed to be hypotonic and replaced with half normal saline in a volume which equals urine output and insensible losses. Urinary electrolytes should then be determined and intravenous therapy designed to replace losses. Hypokalaemia is particularly likely to develop and, if the diuresis continues, potential loss of other ions should be checked. The diuresis may continue for weeks. After several days the body weight can be allowed to drop cautiously by reducing intravenous replacement, but if renal function deteriorates without affecting urine volume, fluid and electrolyte replacement should be continued until the condition recovers spontaneously.

Careful control of infection is essential at each stage in urinary obstruction management. If infection is suspected at presentation, antibiotics should be started immediately. The antibiotic chosen should give a broad cover against Gram-negative organisms (e.g. an aminoglycoside). If there is no clinical reason to suspect infection, antibiotics should be withheld. However, any invasive procedure (particularly antegrade or retrograde pyelography) should be covered by an appropriate antibiotic. Failure to do this results in a significant incidence of septicaemia in patients who are often already acutely ill.

If drainage tubes are left *in situ* for prolonged periods, urinary cultures will almost certainly become positive; in the absence of fever, malaise and local inflammation antibiotics should be withheld. Repeated courses of antibiotics will not lead to a sterile urine and will only increase the risk of super-infection.

Outcome

Renal function   Four main factors influence the rate at which kidney damage occurs, its extent, and the degree and speed of recovery after relief. These are whether obstruction is partial or complete, the duration of obstruction, whether or not infection occurs, and the site of the obstruction.

Complete obstruction for several weeks will lead to irreversible or only partially reversible kidney damage, but complete obstruction for several months causes total, irreversible destruction. Partial obstruction carries a better prognosis. Bacterial infection commonly occurs with obstruction and stasis, and exacerbates kidney damage. Obstruction at or below the bladder neck may induce hypertrophy and trabeculation of the bladder without a rise in pressure within the upper urinary tract, in which case the kidneys are protected from the effects of back pressure. This is not the case with obstruction at more proximal sites.

Patient survival   this depends upon the severity of the complications of obstruction, and the nature of the underlying disease.

Familial renal disease and tubular disorders

There are many familial disorders with a renal component; involvement of other organs or tissues e.g. eyes or ears, may predominate in the presentation.

Hereditary glomerular disease

Alport's syndrome

The commonest features of Alport's syndrome are persistent or recurring haematuria, which may be preceded by an upper respiratory infection, and proteinuria, which very rarely progesses to the nephrotic syndrome. The renal disease leads to chronic renal failure, usually in adult life. Women are usually less severely affected than men, few of whom survive beyond the age of 40 years without dialysis or transplantation. Nerve deafness has a well-known but variable association with Alport's syndrome and about 15 per cent of patients have abnormalities in the lens. The eye and ear defects may be asymptomatic and renal disease may not necessarily be present. Inheritance is autosomal dominant with a varying degree of penetrance. Twenty per cent of cases are the result of new mutations. There is no single explanation for the variability of the disease presentation, or for the considerable variation between sexes. Antenatal diagnosis is not yet possible. The disease is due to a defect in synthesis of basement membranes, giving a typical appearance on electron microscopy.

Familial recurrent haematuria

Familial recurrent haematuria is dominantly inherited. It is a benign disease without deafness. Although the characteristic ultrastructural lesion of Alport's syndrome is absent, the glomerular basement is abnormally thin.

Congenital nephrotic syndrome, Finnish type

This syndrome is thus known because it occurs in 1/10 000 live births in Finland. The disease starts *in utero* and usually causes premature labour with fetal distress. Other congenital abnormalities such as talipes, wide cranial sutures and a flattened nose occur. Oedema and ascites are present in 25 per cent of affected infants at birth and in all cases by 3 months due to the very heavy proteinuria. The babies fail to thrive and 80 per cent die from persistent infections in the first year of life.

The combination is due to an inborn metabolic error of glomerular basement membrane structure and function. Inheritance is autosomal recessive. Prenatal diagnosis and termination of affected pregnancies are possible because the fetal proteinuria results in high levels of amniotic gamma-fetoprotein in early pregnancy. No specific treatment is available. The nephrotic syndrome responds to symptomatic management, long term survivors have received renal transplants with excellent results.

Congenital nephrotic syndrome, other types

Other types of congenital nephrotic syndrome may be caused by glomerular diseases similar to those found in older children (e.g. focal segmental sclerosis), occurring in families, suggesting a recessive inheritance. Some patients respond to steroid or cytotoxic therapy, but when the disease presents in infancy the prognosis is poor.

Cystic disease

Adult polycystic disease

The presentation is usually around the age of 40, but the disease may occur in childhood. It is a common cause of renal failure in adults. The cause is unknown. The inheritance is autosomal dominant. The gene responsible has not yet been identified, but marker genes have, allowing prenatal diagnosis with some certainty. The cysts are distributed so that renal enlargement is usually unequal. The cysts vary in size, are present in cortex and medulla, and affect all parts of the nephron, including the glomerulus. The liver contains cysts in 50 per cent of patients and about 10 per cent have aneurysms of the cerebral arteries.

Presenting features These include renal pain, stones, haematuria, infection or chronic renal failure. The kidney masses are usually palpable. Proteinuria is common but rarely clinically significant. Diagnosis is confirmed by urography or ultrasonography. The progression is variable, some patients having a normal lifespan, but more commonly, terminal renal failure occurs within 10 years of diagnosis. Liver disease does not develop in the adult form.

Treatment Treatment is that of chronic renal failure. Some patients require supplements for salt loss.

Infantile polycystic disease

Cases range from the newborn baby with huge renal masses to the older child presenting with cystic kidney and liver disease. The cause is unknown, inheritance being recessive.

The kidneys of the newborn are large, spongy and many times the normal weight. The distal tubules and collecting ducts are dilated, but the glomeruli, calyces, pelvis and lower urinary tracts are normal. The liver shows bile duct dilation and proliferation, portal enlargement and fibrosis. Infantile polycystic disease may be diagnosed prenatally using ultrasound.

The baby often looks abnormal with Potter facies (low set ears, a broad flat nose and micrognathos). The large kidneys may obstruct labour. Moderate kidney enlargement and hepatomegaly are found in older children. The progression of hypertension and renal insufficiency is variable; some patients die of hepatic disease.

Treatment   As there is no specific treatment, the management is that of progressive renal failure and, in older children, that of portal hypertension.

Medullary cystic disease/nephronophthisis

These conditions can be regarded as synonymous. In children the disease may progress insidiously and the child presents with chronic renal failure and dwarfism. Hepatic, ophthalmic, neurological and bony abnormalities also occur. Thirst and polyuria are common, but hypertension is rare because of renal wasting of potassium and sodium. Proteinuria is absent. The cause is unknown but two theories have been put forward: a defect in metabolism of Tamm Horsfall protein or an abnormality of tubular handling of potassium. Inheritance is recessive although dominant forms usually occur, particularly in young adults. There is no specific treatment, the appropriate treatment for chronic renal failure should be given. There is no contraindication to dialysis or transplantation.

Medullary sponge kidneys

Although medullary sponge kidneys are mostly sporadic, there are reports of familial cases. They are a developmental abnormality which occurs when the ureteric bud branches and penetrates the metanephros. The papillary medulla contains cavities and cysts connected to tubules. The cut surfaces of the kidney resemble a sponge. Patients present with haematuria, infection or stone formation. Management depends upon that of the last two complications, and, when it occurs, that of chronic renal failure.

Metabolic disorders

Primary hyperoxaluria (oxalosis) is a recessively inherited disorder of two known types:

- *Type I* – the enzyme deficiency results in increased oxalic acid synthesis and excretion with associated increased excretion of precursors (glycollate and glyoxylate);
- *Type II* – there is normal excretion of glycollate but increased L-glyceric aciduria and oxalic acid.

Type I usually presents in the first decade with stones and nephrocalcinosis and continues to renal failure and death by the age of 20 in 80 per cent of cases. Calcium oxalate crystals are distributed widely, especially in the retina, bone marrow, brain and heart.

Type II is a more benign disease with nephrolithiasis being the main complication. Renal failure does not occur.

Diagnosis rests on the clinical features together with a raised oxalic acid excretion. In advanced renal failure oxalate excretion is low but bone marrow trephine biopsy examination allows a diagnosis to be reached. The most beneficial therapy is pyridoxine, which promotes the conversion of glyoxylate to glycine. This must be given when there is reasonable renal function. Phosphate supplements may be required to reduce calcium oxalate formation. Treatment is most effective in the newborn or in transplant recipients. When renal failure supervenes, dialysis and transplantation have been contraindicated because of recurrence of oxalate deposition in the graft. Further experience with pyridoxine therapy may alter this view.

A secondary form of hyperoxaluria occurs after ingestion of oxalate precursors by poisoning (ethylene glycol antifreeze or methoxyflurane), or through excessive absorption in gut disorders (malabsorption, resection).

Vitamin D-dependent rickets

Vitamin D-dependent rickets is a rare, recessively inherited disorder caused by a deficiency of 1-hydroxylase enzyme which converts 25-hydroxycalciferol to 1,25-dihydroxycalciferol in the kidney. The defect causes hypocalcaemia, high parathyroid hormone (PTH) levels, aminoaciduria and phosphaturia. Treatment is with oral vitamin D.

Anatomical abnormalities

Vesico-ureteric reflux

Vesico-ureteric reflux occurs in one-third of children with urinary tract infection and surveys of relatives have demonstrated that it is familial. Inheritance is multifactorial with a 10 per cent chance of a first degree relative being affected.

Ureteric duplication

Ureteric duplication is one of the more common forms of urogenital abnormality with an incidence of 1/200. Renal damage may occur from obstructed ectopic ureters or vesico-ureteric reflux. An autosomal dominant form of inheritance is thought to be responsible.

Other inherited conditions with renal involvement

There are a host of rare inherited disorders with involvement of the kidney, too numerous to detail here. The reader is referred to larger texts.

Renal tubular disorders

These may be inborn metabolic errors which alter transport systems across the tubular epithelium, or acquired due to toxic, immunological or inflammatory mechanisms. The consequences are excretion of substances not present in normal urine, excessive excretion of a component of normal urine or failure to reabsorb a substance. Many tubular disorders are rare. The most common types are described.

Renal tubular acidosis

Abnormalities of renal tubular acidification occur in the disorders known as renal tubular acidosis (RTA). Defects may be quantitative when the number of functioning nephrons is too few to cope with the metabolic acid load, e.g. in chronic renal failure. In such cases individual tubular function is normal. In the proximal and distal types of RTA, individual tubular function is qualitatively abnormal.

Proximal RTA is rare. The primary form presents in infancy with growth failure, vomiting, hypercholoraemic acidosis and alkaline or slightly acid urine. The disorder may also occur at other ages accompanying generalized tubular conditions such as Fanconi syndrome and cystinosis, and following renal transplantation. Excessive parathyroid hormone secretion may also be associated with proximal RTA. The defect is a bicarbonate leak, excessive bicarbonate appearing in the urine at serum bicarbonate levels lower than expected. Causes suggested include carbonic anhydrase deficiency, defects in H^+ secretion or the chloride bicarbonate pump, and hypocalcaemia. These patients excrete normal quantities of acid and can form an acid urine in the presence of severe acidosis. There are no bone changes nor is there nephrocalcinosis. Treatment is the addition of large amounts of alkali, 10 mmol/kg. Thiazide diuretics may decrease these requirements by reducing the extracellular fluid volume and increasing bicarbonate reabsorption. Potassium supplements are required. The prognosis of primary proximal RTA is good and treatment may be reduced or discontinued in later life.

Primary distal RTA (classical RTA) may occur in early life with failure to thrive, polyuria, dehydration and constipation. Some cases are not diagnosed until growth retardation is noted in adolescence. Abnormal distal tubular cell metabolism results in failure of H^+ secretion into tubular fluid in the presence of systemic acidosis. Renal stones, rickets and osteomalacia are common and nephrocalcinosis invariable. Weakness due to potassium deficiency occurs occasionally. Incomplete forms and a recessively inherited acidosis with deafness are described. Diagnosis depends on the clinical findings and demonstrations of a urine pH above 6 with either spontaneous or ammonium chloride-induced acidaemia. Titratable acid and ammonium excretions concentrations are low.

Treatment is with small amounts of alkali, 1–3 mmol/kg/day (1–3 mEq/kg/day) equivalent to daily endogenous production of H^+, and potassium. The dose should be adjusted to keep the urine calcium below 0.05 mmol/kg/day (2 mg/kg/day). If nephrocalcinosis has not developed, the prognosis can be good.

Secondary forms of distal RTA occur in vitamin D poisoning, idiopathic hypercalcaemia, amphotericin nephrotoxicity, and chronic active hepatitis.

The Fanconi syndromes

A number of multiple tubular disorders are cha racterized by glycosuria, phosphaturia, aminoaciduria and tubular acidosis. They are best considered as: Lignac–Fanconi syndrome (cystinosis), idiopathic 'adult' Fanconi syndrome (non-cystinotic Fanconi syndrome), secondary Fanconi syndrome.

Cystinosis

This disease occurs in about 1/40 000 live births. It is usually diagnosed in the first year. Prenatal diagnosis can be made by analysing amniotic fluid cells for cystine.

Cystine crystals are widely deposited in the soft tissues. The proximal tubule is shortened and thickened (swan-neck deformity) but this is not specific. Cystinosis is an autosomal recessive condition. Its pathogenesis is unknown but is thought to be a lysosomal storage disease with impairment of the transport mechanisms responsible for removing cystine from the lysosome.

Failure to thrive in infancy, rickets, polydipsia and polyuria, recurrent vomiting and dehydration are typical symptoms in childhood. Ocular involvement causes photophobia, and later, especially in transplanted patients, hypothyroidism occurs. On investigation a metabolic acidosis with low plasma levels of potassium and phosphate is found. The urine contains glucose, phosphate, amino acids, and there is a concentrating defect. Diagnosis is easily made by demonstrating cystine crystals in the cornea, the bone marrow, or skin, or measuring cystine content of leucocytes.

There is no specific treatment for cystinosis. It progresses to terminal renal failure by puberty. Recently treatment with phosphocystaemine has been introduced. It reduces plasma concentration of cystine, but any long term benefit awaits proof. Symptomatic biochemical abnormalities should be corrected. Dialysis and transplantations have been performed in a large number of cases – cystine reaccumulates in the grafted kidney but has not yet been shown to cause renal failure. Recently, in a small number of cases, dementia has occurred, with eventual death.

Idiopathic 'adult' Fanconi syndrome

This usually presents itself in early adulthood. Recessive and dominant forms occur. There is no cystinosis but intestinal transport defects are found. The presentation is usually with bone pain from osteomalacia, and muscle weakness.

Secondary Fanconi syndromes

These arise from a number of causes such as myeloma, intoxication with heavy metals, and drugs, inborn errors of metabolism such as Wilson's disease or glycogen storage diseases.

Primary tubular concentrating defects

Nephrogenic diabetes insipidus is caused by a block in the antidiuretic hormone-cyclic-AMP pathway affecting water permeability of the distal tubular cell. Inheritance is X-linked and carrier females have a partial defect in concentration.

Secondary tubular concentrating defects

Hypercalcaemia and hypokalaemia impair cyclic-AMP production in the distal tubular cell and water reabsorption. The effects are reversible in the short term but not if structural damage has resulted. Drugs e.g. lithium carbonate and methoxyflurane may cause a similar concentrating defect.

Aminoacidurias

These are primary, with impaired tubular reabsorption but normal blood amino-acid levels (e.g. cystinuria, Hartnup disease), or secondary to hyperaminoacidaemias (phenylketonuria) in which tubular reabsorption is insufficient to deal with the load presented.

Benign renal glycosuria

Benign renal glycosuria affects 1–2 per cent of the population. The diagnosis is made by excluding diabetes mellitus (demonstrating a normal glucose tolerance curve) and other meliturias such as fructosuria. There are two forms of glycosuria: a dominantly inherited form in which tubules cannot reabsorb filtered glucose but the overall Tm glucose is normal, and a low TmG found with other tubular abnormalities e.g. cystinosis. No treatment is required.

Bartter's syndrome

Bartter's syndrome is a recessively inherited condition which usually presents with failure to thrive, a normal blood pressure and polyuria and polydipsia due to failure to conserve salt and water. Hypokalaemia, metabolic acidosis, hyper-reninaemia and aldosteronism and a vasopressin-resistant concentrating defect are biochemical features, and histologically there is hyperplasia of the juxtaglomerular apparatus. The pathogenesis of this heterogeneous condition is unknown: defective tubular sodium handling, angiotensin resistance and excessive prostaglandin synthesis have all been suggested. Symptomatic improvement may occur by correcting the electolyte abnormalities by diet, potassium supplements or spironolactone. Propranolol has been used to suppress renin and prostaglandin synthetase inhibitors e.g. indomethacin or ketoprofen have also been reported as being successful.

Drugs and the kidney

The kidney is the final common pathway for excretion of many drugs and their metabolites, and is exposed to high concentrations of potentially toxic substances. Many drugs therefore can cause renal damage, and their effect is increased in the presence of pre-existing renal disease. It is therefore necessary to consider the damage caused by drugs to the kidneys, and the effect of renal failure on drug prescription.

Renal disease caused by drugs

The main effects of drugs on the kidney are:

- direct nephrotoxicity – acute tubular or interstitial damage and renal papillary necrosis;
- prerenal effects;
- obstructive uropathy;
- allergic or immunological damage;
- vasculitis;
- interstitial nephritis and
- glomerulonephritis.

Up to 20 per cent of cases of acute renal failure are caused by drugs and chemicals, but minor degrees of damage may pass undetected. Chronic damage usually occurs insidiously and the role of drugs may be unrecognized. The clinical features of drug-induced renal diseases are no different to those of spontaneous renal disease apart from the obvious history of exposure to drugs. An accurate drug history must be obtained from any patient with renal disease.

Tubular and interstitial damage

Drugs and their metabolites are selectively taken up and concentrated by the renal tubular cells before excretion. As high intracellular concentrations occur particularly in the renal medulla, direct toxic damage tends to affect the renal tubular cells and renal papillae. Direct nephrotoxicity of this type is usually dose-dependent. Acute tubular necrosis is the lesion usually found due to drug-induced renal failure. Antimicrobial therapy is the commonest cause. Various compounds are implicated in the production of tubular and interstitial damage. Aminoglycosides are excreted unchanged by the kidney. Renal damage is dose-dependent and occurs typically in dehydrated patients and in those with renal failure. Nomograms should be used for calculating the initial dose according to the age, weight and serum creatinine levels of the patient, and subsequent doses should be adjusted according to plasma levels. Potentiation can occur with other nephrotoxic agents.

Cephalosporins produced recently are less nephrotoxic than the originals. But care is needed when used in patients with impaired renal function, especially in combination with aminoglycosides or diuretics.

Colistin and polymyxin B may produce proximal tubular damage even at therapeutic doses. Frusemide may potentiate the nephrotoxicity of aminoglycosides, cephalosporins and polymyxins. Amphotericin is an antifungal agent which causes acute proximal and distal tubular damage, causing renal tubular acidosis, hypokalaemia and nephrocalcinosis. Gold and mercurial compounds produce proximal tubular damage. Both paracetamol and aspirin, in overdosage, may cause renal tubular necrosis.

Acute renal failure may follow contrast radiography, especially in patients with diabetes, jaundice, myeloma, dehydration or pre-existing renal disease. Liver disease prolongs excretion of contrast through the kidneys, resulting in tubular damage. Modern urographic media e.g. diatrizoate and iothalamate are relatively safe, even in renal failure where high doses may be required, but dehydration must be avoided. It is essential that dehydration is avoided in all ill or uraemic patients undergoing contrast radiography, including computerized tomography.

Fluorinated anaesthetic agents such as methoxyflurane cause acute distal tubular damage, resulting in polyuria and hypernatraemia. This effect is less common with enflurane and halothane. Lithium salts can cause nephrogenic diabetes insipidus, unresponsive to vasopressin and aldosterone. Polyuria and dehydration result in renal damage and increasing plasma lithium levels. Both acute and chronic renal failure may occur, with scarring of the interstitium. Lithium salts also cause tubular acidosis, hypocalciuria and membranous nephropathy. Lithium therapy must be monitored by plasma levels and regular tests of renal function.

Demethylchlortetracycline also causes diabetes insipidus. It is used to treat inappropriate antidiuretic hormone secretion, but care must be taken to avoid dehydration and the development of acute renal failure.

Analgesic nephropathy is the commonest form of chronic drug-induced renal damage. It is a major cause of renal failure, accounting for 5–30 per cent of patients with end-stage renal failure in different countries. The importance of recognizing analgesic nephropathy lies in the facts that it is preventable, and discontinuation of analgesics often produces stabilization or improvement in renal function.

Aetiology and pathogenesis

Although phenacetin has borne the brunt of the blame for causing analgesic nephropathy, no analgesic drug can be considered completely safe. In practice, virtually all patients with this condition have taken several drugs over the years, often as mixtures and it is impossible to single out any one as the causative agent. Papillary necrosis can occur following the consumption of 1–2 kg of analgesics, equivalent to six tablets a day for 3–5 years, but many patients have taken more this amount by the time the diagnosis is made.

Presenting features

In the idiopathic form the incidence is higher in women than in men. Apart from features of chronic renal failure, patients are characterized by often being depressed or having other psychiatric disorders, the abuse of purgatives or alcohol, dyspepsia, ischaemic heart disease, recurrent urinary tract infections, and an appearance of premature ageing. Patients may also present with the complications (see below). The long term reason for taking analgesics is often headaches, back pain, or hard to elucidate. In other patients, analgesic nephropathy may arise secondary to a chronic disease accompanied by much pain, e.g. rheumatoid arthritis.

Diagnosis

This depends on a high index of suspicion and an accurate drug history. All patients with renal problems should be questioned about intake of analgesics especially patent remedies for headaches, migraine, backache or rheumatism. Unless the possibility of analgesic abuse is considered, the renal damage may be attributed to chronic pyelonephritis. A sample of urine, sent for estimation of salicylates and paracetamol, will measure analgesic intake within the previous 48 hours.

IVU shows scarred kidneys with absent papillae in many patients due to papillary necrosis.

Complications

Arterial damage causes ischaemic heart disease. Ureteric obstruction may result from the passage of a necrotic papilla or ureteric fibrosis. Transitional cell tumours of the renal pelvis and ureter occur in about 10 per cent of patients.

Treatment

The treatment is to reduce the intake of analgesic, which is often not achieved, either because of the underlying painful condition, or because of the very nature of the abuse.

Allergic or immunological damage

Acute interstitial nephritis is quite common, and may be accompanied by fever and rash. Eosinophilia may be noted in the blood. In most cases, renal function improves when drugs are withdrawn. Interstitial nephritis is seen most commonly with the penicillins, diuretics, and non-steroid anti-inflammatory drugs. It also occurs with rifampicin, sulphonamides, co-trimoxazole, cephalosporins, phenytoin, phenindione and phenazone.

Glomerulonephritis

Many drugs cause glomerular damage associated with the deposition of immunoglobulins and complement i.e. evidence of inflammation and/or immunological damage. It is thought that the drug acts as a hapten or in some other way alters a protein to form an allergen, resulting in the formation of circulating immune complexes. Drugs causing glomerulonephritis are listed in Table 7.4.

Two important forms of drug-induced glomerular disease are discussed in more detail.

Membranous nephropathy

Gold therapy for rheumatoid arthritis may cause membranous nephropathy which may progress to renal failure. Gold treatment must be accompanied by regular urine tests for protein and treatment must be discontinued if proteinuria develops. Penicillamine produces proteinuria in 10–20 per cent of patients, which remits on withdrawal of the drug. Membranous nephropathy has also been described with lithium therapy.

Drug-induced SLE syndrome

The reported incidence with hydralazine varies from 10–20 per cent of patients treated, but renal involvement is rare. The liability to develop hydralazine-associated SLE is genetically linked to the human leucocyte antigen DR4. Procainamide may cause the SLE syndrome in up to 30 per cent of patients on long-term therapy. It occurs both in fast and slow acetylators. Renal involvement is uncommon. Complement levels are generally normal in drug-induced SLE, and antibodies to double-stranded DNA are rare.

Allergic vasculitis is a rare form of renal damage. It may follow thiazide diuretics, penicillamine, and occur as part of drug-induced SLE.

Prerenal damage caused by drugs

Water and electrolyte loss occurs with excessive use of diuretics or laxatives. Lithium carbonate has similar effects, which may be exacerbated by concurrent use of diuretics.

Increased catabolism

Glucocorticoids raise the blood urea by increasing catabolism. Tetracyclines inhibit the incorporation of amino acids into protein, causing a rise in blood urea. In renal failure, tetracycline excretion is delayed, tetracyclines should therefore be avoided in patients with renal impairment, except for doxycycline which has minimal anti-anabolic effects and even in renal failure is eliminated rapidly.

Vascular occlusion

Arteriolar and/or venous occlusion may occur with oestrogen therapy. It is usually reversible but occasionally causes acute renal failure.

Obstructive uropathy

Obstruction to the kidneys may be caused by ureteric fibrosis, calculi blood clots, and/or tubular blockage, all of which can be due to drugs.

Haemorrhage

Anticoagulants or fibrinolytic agents may cause ureteric obstruction by a blood clot within the urinary tract, or by retroperitoneal haemorrhage.

Retroperitoneal fibrosis

Retroperitoneal fibrosis has been attributed to several drugs, including methysergide and methyldopa.

Ureteric fibrosis

Ureteric fibrosis and obstruction due to a sloughed papilla are complications of analgesic nephropathy (see above).

Tubular blockage

Crystalluria Uric acid may be deposited in the renal tubules during the treatment of myeloproliferative disorders with cytotoxic agents. Allopurinol before cytotoxic therapy is started, and a high fluid intake prevent urate deposition.

The early sulphonamides were relatively insoluble and crystallized in acid urine. Modern sulphonamides rarely cause problems, but a high fluid intake must be maintained. Acetazolamide, which is structurally related to sulphonamides, may precipitate in the urine.

Bence–Jones protein can precipitate in the renal tubules of patients with multiple myeloma, especially in the presence of dehydration.

Calcium nephropathy and renal calculi Vitamin D preparations can cause hypercalcaemia and calcium deposition in the kidney. 1-hydroxycholecalciferol is safer than earlier preparations, since its effects are briefer and reversible, but serum calcium levels must be carefully monitored. Renal calculi have been described following excessive consumption of vitamin D, and antacids containing calcium (milk–alkali syndrome). Rarely xanthine nephropathy occurs with allopurinol therapy.

Prescribing in renal failure

Apart from the obvious effect of failure of renal

excretion, renal failure can alter drug metabolism by diminishing protein binding with consequent greater bioavailability of the drug, changing the volume of distribution, and reducing gastro-intestinal absorption.

Prescribing for patients with renal failure therefore requires a knowledge of the metabolism and activity of the drug, its duration of action and method of excretion. The following rules apply:

- choose the drug with minimal nephrotoxic effects;
- use plasma levels to prescribe the dose;
- avoid prolonged courses of toxic drugs;
- avoid nephrotoxic combinations of drugs.

Therapeutic drug levels may be maintained either by reducing doses or by increasing the intervals between doses.

Renal disease in pregnancy

Hypertension and eclampsia

Ten to twenty per cent of pregnancies are complicated by hypertension with accompanying proteinuria. In a normal pregnant women the diastolic blood pressure falls by approximately 15 mmHg, hence the diastolic blood pressure in a normal pregnancy should be below 75 mmHg.

A raised blood pressure is a common complication of renal disease in any patient, and is evident from an early stage in pregnancy; underlying renal disease is found in 50 per cent of women presenting with hypertension or proteinuria during pregnancy. Hypertensive disorders of pregnancy can be divided into two categories – idiopathic hypertension, (pre-eclampsia) and hypertension which derives from underlying renal disease and occurs in both primiparous or multiparous women who develop essential hypertension in pregnancy. Pre-eclampsia seldom recurs after the first pregnancy. When hypertension in pregnancy is a manifestation of latent essential hypertension, or occurs as a complication of renal disease, it usually recurs in all subsequent pregnancies.

Glomerulonephritis and pregnancy

It is important to exclude glomerulonephritis as a cause of proteinuria, hypertension or impaired renal function because patients with this condition constitute a high risk group during pregnancy.

Urine microscopy is the most sensitive method for detecting glomerulonephritis as the presence of increased numbers of glomerular erythrocytes in the urine is a specific indicator of glomerulonephritis. While it is not definite that pregnancy affects the natural history of glomerulonephritis, some patients with lesions which are normally benign, such as membranous glomerulonephritis, may deteriorate sharply during pregnancy.

Urinary tract infection

Bacteriuria (i.e. 10^5 organisms/ml) accompanies pregnancy in 5–10 per cent of women; approximately 30 per cent of untreated patients with bacteriuria will develop acute pyelonephritis. Treatment of bacteriuria with antibacterial agents prevents acute pyelonephritis and it is therefore important to treat bacteriuria promptly. A high proportion of pregnant women with bacteriuria will have underlying renal disease if investigated during the postpartum period.

Reflux nephropathy

This is a common condition, and a large proportion of these patients are at risk of urinary tract infections, and, if there is already elevation of the plasma creatinine then they may undergo an accelerated deterioration to end stage renal failure. Prophylactic antitiotics are indicated during the pregnancy.

Acute renal failure

Acute tubular necrosis may develop during pregnancy as a consequence of either sepsis or haemorrhage. The most common context in which acute tubular necrosis accompanies septicaemia is in septic abortions performed in early pregnancy. The incidence of this complication has fallen to negligible levels in countries where abortion has become accepted. Acute tubular necrosis may accompany haemorrhage or abruptio placentae in late pregnancy, when the much more serious complication of acute cortical necrosis occur. Patients with acute cortical necrosis may recover gradually over 3–6 months to a level at which their own kidneys can sustain adequate function, but for most patients the prognosis is very poor, most requiring maintenance dialysis or transplantation.

Thrombotic microangiopathy is a very uncommon form of acute renal failure similar to the haemolytic uraemic syndrome, and being associated with thrombotic microangiopathy, which usually occurs in the postpartum period. Recovery of renal function is rare in patients with thrombotic microangiopathy, but has occurred following treatment with heparin or plasma exchange.

Renal calculi

Renal calculi are a common form of renal disease and there may be a particular propensity toward this condition during pregnancy. Infection has been implicated as the most likely factor. Infection stones can grow rapidly during pregnancy as can other stones e.g. cystine and uric acid stones.

Pregnancy and impaired renal function

Patients with impaired renal function are at considerable risk of accelerating to end-stage renal failure if they become pregnant. Fertility is diminished in end-stage renal failure, though it may be restored by a successful renal transplant; a small number of women have achieved pregnancy on chronic haemodialysis. Patients with a raised serum creatinine above 200 μmol/litre are generally advised not to become pregnant. In addition, those women with active glomerular disease, e.g. mesangiocapillary glomerulonephritis or lupus glomerulonephritis should avoid pregnancy.

8

Haematology

Anthony Goldstone, Charles Singer, John Gribben

Anaemia

Anaemia is defined as a reduction in the concentration of haemoglobin (Hb) below the normal value for the age and sex of the patient. This results from an inbalance between production and loss of red cells. Relative anaemia is due to an increase in plasma volume with a normal total red cell mass as occurs in pregnancy, splenomegaly, hypoproteinaemia and macroglobulinaemia.

Clinical features

Symptoms and signs are due to the anaemia itself and to the disorder causing the anaemia. The haemoglobin level at which symptoms of anaemia develop depends upon the rate of development of the anaemia and the age and general condition of the patient. Children and young adults tolerate a greater degree of chronic anaemia than older patients because of the inability of the cardiovascular system to compensate efficiently with increasing age. Tiredness, lassitude, fatigue and weakness are the most common and early symptoms of anaemia. The main symptoms of severe anaemia relate to the cardiovascular system and the most common are dyspnoea on exertion and palpitations. With most patients dyspnoea only occurs on exertion but in severe anaemia there may be dyspnoea at rest. Angina, due to myocardial ischaemia, is worsened in anaemia. The haemoglobin should be determined in all patients suffering from angina, since anaemia when present represents a treatable and reversible factor contributing to the myocardial ischaemia.

When the haemoglobin falls below 6 g/dl ECG changes occur in approximately 30 per cent of patients. These include low voltage, depression of the ST segments and flattening or inversion of T

Table 8.1 Aetiological classification of anaemia

Impaired red cell formation
1. *Impaired haemoglobin synthesis*
   - Iron deficiency
   - Impaired iron utilization
   - Impaired haem or globin synthesis
     - thalassaemia
     - sideroblastic anaemia
     - lead poisoning
     - pyridoxine deficiency
     - porphyria
2. *Impaired DNA synthesis*
   - B_{12} deficiency
   - folate deficiency
3. Aplastic anaemia and red cell aplasia
4. Marrow infiltration
5. Metabolic disorders and toxic dyshaemopoiesis

Blood loss

Haemolysis
1. *Congenital red cell disorders*
   - red cell membrane disorders
   - enzyme defects
   - defective haemoglobin synthesis eg. sickle cell anaemia
2. *Immune red cell destruction*
3. *Acquired non immune red cell disorders*
   - paroxysmal nocturnal haemoglobinuria
   - severe burns
   - infections – especially malaria
4. *Hypersplenism*

waves. In the absence of pre-existing heart disease these changes disappear when the anaemia is corrected.

There are two main classifications of anaemia:

- the aetiological classification (Table 8.1) and;
- the morphological classification.

The morphological classification is based on the characteristics of the red cell as determined by examination of the blood film and the blood counters. In order to understand the essential principles of the morphological diagnosis of anaemia it is necessary to understand the 'absolute values' of the red cell. Automated cell counters derive these values from the measured values which are the haemoglobin level, the red cell count and the mean cell volume (MCV). The MCV is a very accurate index when measured on a modern blood counter by electrical impedence (the Coulter method) or by laser scatter of red cells (as in Technicon H1).

The other indices are then defined as follows:

Haematocrit or packed cell volume (PCV) $= \dfrac{MCV \times rbc\ count \times 10^{12}/fl}{1000}$

Mean cell haemoglobin (MCH) $= \dfrac{Hb\ (g/dl) \times 10}{rbc\ count \times 10^{12}/litre}$

Mean cell haemoglobin concentration (MCHC) $= \dfrac{Hb\ (g/dl)}{PCV}$

The most useful index for classifying the anaemias morphologically is the MCV (Table 8.2).

Table 8.2   Classification of anaemias

1. Normocytic anaemias (MCV 76–96fl)
   These are usually also normochromic (MCHC 30–35 %)
   (a) Anaemia of chronic disease where there is impairment of red cell production
   (b) Following haemorrhage or haemolysis
       – there may be a macrocytosis if there is a marked reticulocytosis. The MCV of a reticulocyte is 110fl
   (c) Combined deficiencies e.g. iron and folate.
2. Microcytic anaemia (MCV < 76fl)
   This is usually associated with hypochromia (MCHC < 30 %)
   (a) Iron deficiency
   (b) Thalassaemia
   (c) Sideroblastic anaemia
3. Macrocytic anaemia (MCV > 96fl)
   Most are normochromic
   (a) Megaloblastic erythropoiesis
       Vitamin B_{12} and folic acid deficiency.
   The red cell series will show considerable abnormalities of morphology and there will also be changes in the myeloid and megakaryocytic elements.
4. Normoblastic erythropoiesis
   (a) Due to raised reticulocyte count or following marrow infiltration
   (b) Endocrine disorders – myxoedema and hypopituitarism.

Iron deficiency anaemia occurs when the body content of iron is decreased. In *iron depletion* storage iron is decreased or absent but serum iron and haemoglobin levels are normal. In *iron deficiency* the serum iron and transferrin saturation levels fall and eventually the haemoglobin falls.

Aetiology

Iron deficiency may occur as a result of inadequate iron intake, malabsorption of iron, chronic blood loss, intravascular haemolysis or diversion of iron to fetal and infant erythropoiesis during pregnancy and lactation. In adult males and post-menopausal women the commonest cause is chronic bleeding from the gastrointestinal tract.

Pathogenesis

As the body becomes depleted of iron, changes occur in many tissues. Haemosiderin and ferritin disappear from the marrow and other storage sites. There is a decreased activity of other iron proteins including cytochrome c, cytochrome oxidase, succinic dehydrogenase and myoglobin as well as in other enzymes which do not contain or require iron. This results in disturbances in cellular metabolism in many tissues. Achlorhydria occurs in up to 40 per cent of patients because of a decreased capacity of the stomach to secrete hydrochloric acid. This achlorhydria may be irreversible even after correction of the underlying iron deficiency. Dysfunction in the nervous system may result in paraesthesia. There may be mucosal atrophy of the tongue, stomach and small intestine. In the pharynx, mucosal atrophy may lead to web formation and dysphagia (Plummer–Vinson syndrome).

Clinical features

When anaemia develops slowly there may be remarkable adaptation even if the condition is severe. Fatigue, irritability and headaches are common complaints. Pallor, glossitis, stomatitis and angular cheilitus are common signs. Koilonychia is now rarely encountered. Splenomegaly was primarily reported in early series but is now exceedingly rare in iron deficiency.

Therapy

Once it is established that a patient is iron deficient, replacement therapy should be instituted; it is not justifiable to await the results of investigations to determine the cause of bleeding.

Oral replacement therapy is the preferred form of administration. Indications for parental iron therapy are malabsorption and intolerance to oral iron therapy.

Megaloblastic anaemias

These disorders have in common morphological and functional changes in the cell lines in the marrow which are due to abnormalities in DNA synthesis. Megaloblastic erythrocyte precursors appear larger than the corresponding normoblastic cells with a characteristic open and particulate chromatin in the nucleus. The precise biochemical mechanisms are uncertain but there is impaired conversion of deoxyuridine to deoxythymidine and increased RNA production.

Clinical features

Anaemia may be mild or severe. As it develops insidiously symptoms may be few until anaemia is very severe at which stage congestive heart failure may supervene. Anorexia and glossitis are common. Optic atrophy, peripheral neuropathy, subacute combined degeneration of the cord and dementia may be associated with severe vitamin B_{12} deficiency but have also been described in folate deficiency (Table 8.3).

Laboratory features

The anaemia is macrocytic and the red cell count markedly reduced. Leucopenia with neutrophil 'right shift' results in the characteristic multi-lobed neutrophils. Thrombocytopenia develops as the anaemia becomes more severe.

Treatment

Where possible, the underlying cause should be treated. In vitamin B_{12} deficiency replacement is given by parenteral administration. In folate deficiency 5–15 mg of folate are given orally for about 4 months after B_{12} deficiency has been excluded. Blood transfusion should be avoided since circulatory overload occurs commonly with transfusion. Since the response to therapy is rapid it is seldom necessary to subject the patient to the risks of trans-

Table 8.3 Classification of megaloblastic anaemia

Vitamin B_{12} deficiency
1. *Decreased intake*
    strict vegetarian (vegan)
    impaired absorption
    intrinsic factor deficiency
       autoimmune
       gastrectomy
    malabsorption
       familial
       ileitis, ileal resection, sprue, *coeliac* disease
    competitive parasites
       fish tapeworm
       bacteria in blind loops and diverticuli
    chronic pancreatic disease
2. *Impaired utilization*

Folate deficiency
1. *Decreased intake*
    poor diet
    alcoholism
    haemodialysis
    impaired absorption
    coeliac disease
    intestinal disease
    anticonvulsants, other drugs
2. *Increased requirements*
    pregnancy
    hyperthroidism
    neoplastic disease
3. *Impaired utilization*
    folic acid antagonists e.g. methotrexate, trimethoprim

fusion but this may be necessary when the haemoglobin is less than 5 g/dl or when the patient i debilitated, in heart failure or has severe sepsis.

Inherited defects in haemoglobir synthesis

Thalassaemia

Thalassaemia is not a single disease but a group o disorders resulting from an inherited abnormalit of globin production with defective synthesis o one or more of the globin chains. This pro duces ineffective erythropoiesis, haemolysis and variable degree of anaemia.

Genetic control and synthesis of haemoglobin

Human adult haemoglobulin is a heterogeneous mixture of proteins, the predominant form being HbA with about 2.5 per cent HbA_2. In intrauterine life the predominant form is HbF. They have a similar structure each consisting of two α-like and 2 non-α-like globin chains. Except for early embryonic forms of Hb all the normal human haemoglobins have 2 α chains. In HbA these are combined with β chains ($\alpha_2\beta_2$) in HbA_2 with δ chains (α_2) and in HbF with γ chains ($\alpha_2\gamma_2$). During embryonic development there is an orderly switch from the synthesis of one type of globin chain to another. The switch from γ to β chains is synchronized throughout all fetal organs. There are two α globin chain genes on chromosome 16. The non α genes are on chromosome 11 in a linked, γ, δ, β gene cluster. The defect in thalassaemia is in the DNA sequence but this could be manifest at any of the stages of the protein synthesis and in various forms of thalassaemia defects have been found at all levels. Possibilities include deleted globin genes, partial gene deletions, abnormalities in mRNA processing and point mutations.

Classification

Thalassaemias are classified according to which globin chain (or chains) is synthesized at a reduced rate.

β thalassaemias

In $\beta°$ thalassaemias no β chains are produced. In β^+ thalassaemia there is a partial deficiency of β chain production. Genetically thalassaemia minor or thalassaemia trait refers to the heterozygous state and thalassaemia major to the homozygous state. Clinically these terms refer to the clinical severity with intermedia being used to indicate symptoms of intermediate severity. Thalassaemia can be associated with other structural haemoglobin variants such as HbS and E. HbS interactions are discussed under sickle cell disease. HbE interactions with β thalassaemia behave like β thalassaemia major.

Thalassaemia major

Homozygous $\beta°$ or β^+ produces the clinical picture first described by Cooley in 1925. Affected infants are normal at birth because of normal production of HbF. Anaemia develops during the first few months of life and becomes progressively severe. The infants fail to thrive and have feeding problems. Growth retardation becomes more apparent with age and without regular transfusion death occurs in childhood. If adequate transfusion programmes are possible, few of the complications of the disorder will occur during childhood and the disease will only cause a problem when the effects of iron overloading from ineffective erythropoiesis and from repeated blood transfusion begin to become apparent at the end of the first decade. The first sign of iron overloading is usually absence of the pubertal growth spurt and a failure of menarche. Over the succeeding years a variety of endocrine abnormalities including diabetes mellitus, hypoadrenalism and hypoparathyroidism develop. Towards the end of the second decade cardiac complications arise resulting in death from cardiac siderosis by the end of the third decade.

Present transfusion regimes maintain a high haemoglobin level, suppress abnormal erythropoiesis and permit normal growth. Desferrioxamine is given by slow subcutaneous injection to reduce transfusion siderosis. Splenectomy is indicated if there has been a progresive increase in the frequency of transfusion or the development of pancytopenia attributable to hypersplenism.

β thalassaemia intermedia

Clinically this is defined as an ability to maintain Hb of 7 g/dl with normal growth. It is a heterogeneous group of disorders including homozygotes for mild β^+, homozygotes for β thalassaemia of high fetal haemoglobin type.

The diagnosis is often not made until four or five years of age when intermittent infections precipitate transitory deterioration. Development of splenomegaly may result in subsequent transfusion dependence and may be an indication for splenectomy in some cases.

β thalassaemia minor (thalassaemia trait)

The heterozygous state for β thalassaemia is not usually associated with any clinical disability. Haemoglobin values are usually in the range 9–11 g/dl. The most striking feature is small, poorly haemoglobinized red cells (MCV <80 fl, MCH <26 pg). The HbA_2 level is increased and ranges from 3.5–7 per cent. There is only slight or no increase in HbF. The presence of thalassaemia minor is of no consequence in consideration for general anaethesia.

α thalassaemias

Haemoglobin Bart's Hydrops fetalis syndrome results from a total absence of α chains. No HbA, HbA_2 or HbF is produced. Haemoglobin Bart's results from a tetramer of γ chains. The condition is fatal and is a frequent cause of stillbirth in South-East Asia. Toxaemia during pregnancy is commonly found. Hb Bart's has a high O_2 affinity further contributing to tissue annoxia.

In Haemoglobin H disease with only one functional gene the clinical findings are variable with some patients being as severely affected as in thalassaemia major. It is characterized by the presence of 5–20 per cent HbH (β_4) which is unstable and easily precipitated in the cell, leading to splenomegaly. HbA constitutes the major component.

Thalassaemia traits

These are asymptomatic. They are characterized by Hb Bart's of ≈ 5 per cent at birth. There is a microcytic, hypochromic anaemia with a normal HbA_2 level.

Sickle cell anaemia

Mutations in the gene sequence can cause a variant amino acid to be substituted for the normal component in the amino acid sequence leading to an inherited structural abnormality of the globin chain. In sickle haemoglobin (HbS) valine replaces the normal glutamic acid at position 6 in the β chain. The homozygous state (HbS/S) is referred to as sickle cell anaemia and the heterozygous state (HbA/S) is referred to as sickle cell trait.

The exact reason why this amino acid substitution causes sickling is incompletely understood but the valine residues in the deoxygenated structure become polar and form contacts with adjacent molecules. The molecules polymerize together and are laid down as fibres inside the cell causing it to become rigid.

A large number of inherited and acquired factors influence the pathogenesis of the clinical symptoms, which may vary from the virtually symptomless sickle cell trait to the potentially lethal complications of sickle cell anaemia. A correlation

exists between the concentration of HbS within a cell and its susceptibility to sickling. This is complicated by the high incidence of α thalassaemia within the same populations as the HbS gene since this may ameliorate the clinical severity of HbSS.

The anaemia of sickle cell disease is primarily due to haemolysis. Factors involved in haemolysis include decreased deformability of red cells, increased adherence to vascular endothelium, increased erythrophagocytosis and formation of oxygen radicals by abnormal oxidation. There is formation of 'dense cells' with high Ca^{2+} content which activates Ca^+ dependent K^+ channels particularly K^+ and water loss. The oxygen affinity curve for HbS is markedly right shifted for two reasons. The mean 2, 3 DPG levels are increased but the major component is due to decreased O_2 binding by deoxy HbS polymers so that there is particularly low affinity in the dense cells. There is therefore a relative increase in tissue oxygenation and a resultant decrease in serum erythropoietin.

Geographic distribution

HbS occurs with greatest prevalence in tropical Africa. The heterozygote frequency is approximately 20 per cent but rises to 40 per cent in some areas. Sickle cell trait has a frequency of 8 per cent in the American black population. It occurs to a lesser extent in the Middle East, Greece and in aboriginal tribes in India. It is rarely found in Caucasians except where racial mixture has occurred over the centuries.

The high prevalance of HbS in areas of the world where malaria is endemic suggested the selection advantage with sickle cell trait in this disease. This advantage seems to be restricted to young children with *Plasmodium falciparum*. Although children with sickle cell trait are readily infected, the infected cells are preferentially sickled and destroyed.

Sickle cell trait

Sickle cell trait does not produce any abnormality of the blood counts and is an exceedingly rare cause of morbidity. Red cell survival is relatively normal. Surgical patients with sickle cell trait have been reported to have no greater perioperative mortality than those with normal haemoglobin but it is normal practice to give increased oxygen to these patients as the occasional sickle crisis has been described. The sickle cell screening test is positive. I his test an aliquot of red cells is added to a buffered olution (pH 7.1) containing a reducing agent. HbS s precipitated and the solution becomes cloudy. IbA remains in solution. Haemoglobin electro- horesis demonstrates the presence of HbS in con- entrations of 35–50 per cent.

ickle cell disease

IbSS may be considered the prototype for the roup of sickle cell diseases. The homozygous state S is the most severe of these disorders with HbS/C nd HbS/B⁺ thal being milder and the HbS/E ildest of all. HbS/D is of varying severity depend- g on the specific HbD defect present.

linical features

he fetus and neonate are protected by the high vels of HbF which are maintained during the first ew months of life. The concentration of HbS rises ntil adult levels are present by the sixth month. he high levels of HbF make a sickle screening test nreliable at birth and diagnosis at this stage is by lobin chain electrophoresis. Because of the high vels of HbF presentation does not occur until six onths of age. Screening of all at risk infants ould take place by the age of six months.

rises

any patients are in reasonably good health for uch of the time but may be interrupted perio- ically by a crisis which can have a sudden onset nd occasionally a fatal outcome. Various types of ises arise:

Infarctive (painful) crisis is the most common form of crisis. It results from obstruction of blood vessels by rigid sickled red cells. Pain is the chief clinical manifestation. Infarctive crises may occur in any tissue but particularly in bones, chest and abdomen. Splenic infarctions are so common in childhood that eventually the spleen becomes very small and scarred (autosplenectomy).

Aplastic and megaloblastic crisis where depres- sion in erythropoiesis secondary to infections, particularly of viral origin can cause a catastro- phic fall in Hb because of the very short half-life of red cells in sickle cell disease. A similar picture may be seen in patients who develop folate deficiency.

- *Sequestration crisis* which is a massive pooling of red blood cells may occur in the spleen of infants and young children. As a result the haemoglobin falls catastrophically within a few hours and this is associated with rapid enlarg- ment of the spleen. Such crises are responsible for a large proportion of deaths that occur in the first years of life.
- *In haemolytic crises* the normal haemolysis which occurs in sickle cell disease may be sud- denly increased though this is uncommon.

Laboratory investigations

There is a normochromic, normocytic anaemia with a Hb of 6–11 g/dl. The blood film shows evi- dence of abnormal erythropoiesis and 'sickle cells' may be present. The sickle screening test is positive and haemoglobin electropohoresis shows HbS, no HbA but a varying amount of HbF. Intrauterine diagnosis of the homozygous state can be made from a fetal blood sample and termination of preg- nancy may then be offered. More recently a restric- tion enzyme (MSTII) has been used to identify the specific molecular defect (Val→ Glu 6th amino acid of the β gene) and enables intrauterine diag- nosis by chorionic villus biopsy at ten weeks.

Management

The fundamental point of management is preven- tion of infection, the major precipitating factor in sickle cell crises.

Pneumococcal vaccine is routinely given to children from age two years onwards. Penicillin prophylaxis is given from six months to six years of age. Fever in a child under six years of age with sickle cell disease often indicates life threatening bacterial infection. Such children have a 400-fold increase in pneumococcal septicaemia or meningi- tis. A child in whom sepsis is suspected should be admitted to hospital for treatment. Pneumococcal infections become less frequent after the first decade of life and other pathogens are more commonly encountered. Infections after surgical procedures are a major problem. Osteomye- litis, secondary to salmonella species, staphylo- cocci and enteric organisms are increasing in importance.

Once crisis has occurred there are three essential aspects in the management: adequate hydration, adequate analgesia and identification and treat- ment of any precipitating events.

Hydration is the mainstay of therapy for painful crises. For adult patients 3 to 5 litres/day should be given if the cardiovascular system is stable. Children should receive 100 ml/kg/day. The goal of analgesic therapy is to provide optimal pain relief. Unfortunately this is not often achieved because of lack of understanding of the clinical pharmacology of analgesics and excessive concern about narcotic addiction.

Surgery for patients with sickle cell disease

All patients of African and West Indian descent should have screening for sickle cell haemoglobin on admission to hospital. Screening is also advocated in other groups of non European extraction not only to detect HbS but also other haemoglobinopathies, particularly thalassaemias which may interact with haemoglobin S as previously described. Pre-operative transfusion with packed cells may help to avoid complications in patients with sickle cell disease undergoing surgery. However, simple transfusion can aggravate the clinical state by increasing viscosity (notably in patients with HbSC) and exchange transfusion to obtain a HbA level of 80 per cent is indicated in patients who require pre-operative transfusion. Many experts believe that routine exchange transfusion is not necessary pre-operatively in patients with HbSS. It is our practice to perform a partial exchange transfusion in patients with sickle cell anaemia as preparation for surgery requiring general inhalation anaesthesia, prior to vitrectomy and surgery requiring application of a tourniquet to a limb. Induction of anaesthesia should be rapid and care taken to prevent prolonged hypoxia. The percentage of inspired oxygen should not be less than 50 per cent. Metabolic acidosis should be avoided. Oxygen should be given post-operatively. Chest physiotherapy for sickle cell patients is important post-operatively to prevent development of chest infections.

Special problems in pregnancy and sickle cell disease

Pregnancy carries an increased risk for a woman with sickle cell disease and for her fetus. The risks are not so great as to contraindicate pregnancy in women even with severe sickle cell anaemia. However, the patient should be closely supervised during the pregnancy. Intrauterine growth retardation is not uncommon.

The role of transfusion in pregnancy is controversial. Transfusion is often begun by the third trimester to reduce pre-partum complications. The goal of prophylactic transfusion therapy is to achieve a haemoglobin A level greater than 70 per cent. Where the sickle cell disease accelerates during pregnancy with more painful crises than previously, serious complications or renal capillary necrosis the patient should certainly receive an exchange transfusion. Previous history of such a course should influence the management of further pregnancies.

Delivery

If delivery is uncomplicated local or regional anaesthesia causes no problem. If fetal distress or anatomic considerations prompt caesarian section, general anaesthesia may be necessary. If the patient has not been on chronic transfusion therapy acute exchange transfusion is advisable before operation. Because of the risk of venous pooling some authorities believe that spinal or epidural anaesthesia are contra indicated.

Termination of pregnancy

At less than 13 weeks analgesia rather than anaesthesia is usually all that is required for suction curettage. After this time hypertonic solutions are injected into the uterus and contraction stimulated with prostaglandins. Hypertonic NaCl should not be used as it can cause sickling and therefore hypertonic urea is substituted. Evidence that prostaglandin can induce sickling is not conclusive but prostaglandin F_2 is safe.

Other indications for partial exchange transfusion in sickle cell disease

The following are generally considered to be indications for transfusion:

- life threatening infections;
- acute impending or suspected cerebro-vascular accidents including transient ischaemic attacks;
- acute splenic sequestration crisis;
- acute priapism;
- acute progressive lung disease;
- intractable acute events including painful crises lasting more than 7 days.

Haemolytic anaemia

Hereditary spherocytosis

This is an inherited defect of the membrane cytoskeleton now known to be spectrin deficiency, which causes the red cells to be rounder, more rigid and fragile with increased osmotic fragility.

It is inherited as autosomal dominant with incomplete penetration although in up to 20 per cent neither parent is affected. It affects 1 in 5000 of the population.

Hereditary spherocytes have a diminished life span in the patient with an intact spleen but following splenectomy red cells survival approaches normal.

Clinical features

Symptoms vary in severity. In mild cases there is no anaemia but the anaemia may be moderate or severe in other cases. The spleen is almost always palpable. In the more severe cases jaundice may be present at birth. Because of the increased bilirubin metabolism pigment gallstones are common even in childhood. Depression of the bone marrow as occurs in infections can produce so called 'aplastic crises' particularly in childhood.

Therapy

Splenectomy produces a cessation of haemolysis although the red cell defect persists. Because of the potential gallstones and episodes of aplastic or haemolytic crises, splenectomy is recommended in children and young adults even if the anaemia is mild. Splenectomy should be postponed until the age of 3 years if possible to decrease the risk of infection with pyogenic infections, particularly pneumococcus postsplenectomy.

Hereditary elliptocytosis

This is a rare autosomal dominant condition. It is due to the presence of an abnormal spectrin and produces red blood cells of elliptical shape. It represents a benign condition with no overt haemolysis and therapy is not required in most cases. Where haemolysis is more severe splenectomy is advisable.

Enzyme deficiencies in red cells

The enzyme systems in the red cells are almost exclusively involved in oxygen and carbon dioxide transport. ATP is essential for membrane ion transport and to maintain the bioconcave disc shape of the red cell. ATP is produced by the glycolytic pathway. 2,3 diphosphoglycerate (2,3-DPG) is synthesized by an offshoot of this pathway and modulates haemoglobin oxygen affinity. NADH is also produced by the glycolytic pathway and maintains haem iron in the ferrous state.

Erythrocyte enzyme defects are usually due to the production of an abnormal enzyme rather than the absence of the enzyme protein. Glucose-6-phosphate dehydrogenase deficiency is the only common enzymopathy. Pyruvate kinase deficiency is also relatively commonly encountered. Only these two conditions will be discussed in detail.

Glucose-6-phosphate dehydrogenase deficiency (G6PD)

In this condition, which is inherited as sex-linked, there is a marked decrease in the activity of the enzyme G6PD. The deficiency results from the inheritance of any one of a large number of abnormalities of the structural gene which codes for the amino acid sequence of the enzyme with differences detected in the pathogenesis of the African (A^-) and Mediterranean variants. Eleven per cent of black American males have A^- type G6PD. The frequency of the Mediterranean type variant occurs in the Caucasian population ranging from less than 1 in 10 000 in northern Europe to 50 per cent in Kurdish Jews. G6PD deficiency is also common in areas of China and South East Asia.

Mechanism of haemolysis

G6PD deficient cells have a shortened life span under many circumstances including drug administration and infections. The exact reason is not known.

A large number of drugs have the capacity to precipitate haemolytic reactions in G6PD deficient individuals (Table 8.4).

An episode of drug induced haemolysis usually begins 1 to 3 days after commencement of the drug. Heinz bodies appear in the red cells and the Hb

Table 8.4 Drugs to be avoided in patients with G6PD

Antibacterials
Chloramphenicol
Co-trimoxazole
Furazolidine
Nalidixic acid
Nitrofurantoin
PAS
Sulphonamides
Sulphone e.g. Dapsone

Analgesics and Antirheumatics
Aspirin
Amidopyrine
Phenacetin
Probenecid

Cardiovascular
Procainamide
Quinidine

Antimalarials
Chloroquine
Mepacrine
Pentaquine
Primaquine
Quinacrine
Quinine
Quinocide
Hydroxychloroquine

Miscellaneous
Dimercaprol
Vitamin K aqueous preparations
Doxorubicin

drops rapidly. In severe cases abdominal and back pain occur. In the A⁻ type of G6PD deficiency the haemolytic process is self-limiting since the young red cells produced in response to the haemolysis have near normal G6PD levels. The picture is more severe in the Mediterranean type deficiency.

Haemolysis may follow infections. The anaemia is relatively mild with a drop of haemoglobin of 3–4 g/dl.

Neonatal jaundice may occur in infants with G6PD deficiency and may be sufficiently severe to produce kernicterus. It is rare in the African variety but more common in the Mediterranean and the Far East.

Favism

Favism is potentially one of the most serious clinical consequences of G6PD deficiency. It is more common in children than in adults. The onset of haemolysis may be quite sudden, having been reported within hours of ingestion of fava beans. In severe cases shock may rapidly develop.

Therapy

Individuals with G6PD deficiency should avoid drugs which might induce haemolysis. If haemolysis does occur, good fluid intake should be given to avert renal damage secondary to haemoglobinuria. Infants with neonatal jaundice may require exchange transfusion.

Prognosis

The Hb of affected subjects remains relatively stable except during periods of infection or drug administration. Nearly all patients recover normally from drug or infection induced haemolysis. Favism must be considered a relatively dangerous disease and fatalities are not uncommon. In view of the benign nature of the commonest types of G6PD deficiency screening is not recommended.

Pyrurate kinase (PK) deficiency

This is inherited as an autosomal recessive condition. It is characterized by a moderate to severe haemolytic anaemia. Most patients are of North European origin. There is gross impairment of ATP generation resulting in a shortened red cell life span. The 2,3 DPG levels are raised resulting in a 'shift to the right' in the haemoglobin oxygen dissociation curve. The Hb is usually between 4 and 10 g/dl. Exacerbations occur during infections. Symptoms tend to be less severe because of increased oxygen delivery caused by the shift of the oxygen dissociation curve. Pigment gallstones are common.

Exchange transfusion may be required during the neonatal period. Splenectomy may raise the Hb level and reduce transfusion requirements.

Haemostasis

When vascular endothelium is damaged and subendothelial structures exposed there is activation of a complex sequence of events. There is interaction of platelets and fibrin to produce a blood clot which stops bleeding and acts as a skeleton for repair processes. Five interacting systems contribute to the process:

- The intrinsic coagulation pathway, activated when collagen is exposed.
- The extrinsic coagulation pathway, activated by tissue factor which is a membrane bound glycoprotein.
- The platelets involved in the original haemostatic plug provide platelet phospholipid (platelet factor III), factor V from platelet granules and ADP which activates factors XII and XI in the presence of collagen.
- The fibrinolytic system.
- A system of coagulation and fibrinolysis inhibitors which include antithrombin, α_2 antiplasmin and α_2 macroglobulin. These modulate the serine proteases which are central to the clotting sequences.

Table 8.5   International Committee on Thrombosis and Haemostasis Nomenclature

FVIII/vWF	protein complex
FVIII Act	factor VIII activity as measured by clotting assay techniques
FVIII Ag	factor VIII antigen as measured by immunological techniques
vWF Ag	vWF antigen as measured by immunological techniques
vWF RCo	Ristocetin cofactor activity – the vWF related activity required for the aggregation of human platelets induced by the antibiotic ristocetin.

vWF refers to that part of the FVIII/vWF complex which has vWF RCo and vWF Ag but is devoid of FVIII Act and FVIII Ag. In the older literature vWF Ag was often referred to as factor VIII related antigen (FVIII RAg)

The coagulation system

Coagulation takes place following a complex amplifying system by the conversion of enzyme precursors to serine proteases which act upon their substrate and convert it to a biologically active molecule. Activation of factor X to the serine protease Xa with the generation of thrombin as the common end product of both the intrinsic and extrinsic pathways.

The intrinsic pathway

The enzyme central to this pathway is factor XII. Activated factor XII activates factor XI which in turn converts factor IX to IXa. It is also capable of triggering the kinin pathway, plasminogen activation, activation of factor VII and the conversion of pre-renin to renin.

Identification of plasma proteins involved in contact activation has been based on finding human plasmas deficient in specific plasma proteins. Four proteins are involved in normal contact activation – factor XII, factor XI, prekallikrein and high molecular weight kininogen. The activation of factor X is catalyzed by a complex of factors VIIIa and IXa with phospholipids and Ca^{2+}.

Factor VIII is a complex structure (Table 8.5). Cloning of the factor VIII gene has now conclusively shown that factor VIII is a protein distinct from von Willebrand factor (vWF) but the two factors combine to form a protein complex. The nomenclature has become somewhat confused by changes in the understanding of the molecule.

The Extrinsic pathway

The exposure of blood to a foreign surface activates a membrane-bound glycoprotein – the so called 'tissue factor' which complexes with factor VII to produce active VIIa. This serine protease activates factor X in the presence of phospholipid and calcium ions.

The common pathway

Factor Xa generated via either the intrinsic or extrinsic pathways activates prothrombin (factor II) to produce thrombin, the final proteolytic enzyme of the coagulation process. Proteolytic cleavage of fibrinogen by thrombin produces the fibrin monomer which spontaneously polymerizes to form the insoluble fibrin clot. Thrombin generation from prothrombin is dramatically accelerated by factor V, a glycoprotein co-factor which binds the Xa, prothrombin and Ca^{2+} accelerating thrombin production 10 000–15 000 fold. The fibrin clot is stabilized by activated factor XIII. There are two forms of factor XIII – a plasma enzyme and a smaller enzyme in platelets. Factor XIIIa introduces covalent bonds between fibrin polymers. If cross-linking is defective bleeding may occur.

Hereditary coagulation disorders

These are a rare group of disorders of which haemophilia A, haemophilia B and von Willebrand's disease are clinically the most important. Haemophilia A is the least uncommon of these disorders and occurs in all ethnic groups. Its incidence in the UK is about $100/10^6$ population.

Haemophilia A – factor VIII deficiency

The molecular defect is an absence or low level of plasma factor VIII. It is inherited as an X-linked recessive disorder. The disease is severe if less than 1 per cent of the factor is present, moderately severe at 1–5 per cent and mild if greater than 5 per cent of the factor is present. Haemophilia results from a failure or reduction of synthesis of factor VIII or synthesis of an abnormal variant of factor VIII.

Clinical features

Abnormally prolonged or repeated bleeding occurs characteristically producing haematoma, haemarthroses or other forms of deep tissue bleeding. Primary haemostasis at capillary level is normal so that mucous membrane bleeding is rare and petechiae do not occur. Spontaneous intracranial haemorrhage is rare. The severity of the disease usually parallels the degree of deficiency of factor VIII and usually breeds true within families. The degree of deficiency is almost always constant throughout life in individual patients.

Factor VIII levels are reduced in haemophiliac infants even at birth but they rarely present with bleeding in the neonatal period. Subcutaneous haemotamata develop as the child grows older and begins to crawl. Haemathroses begin as the child starts to walk.

Diagnosis

The full clinical picture of severe haemophilia will readily suggest the diagnosis.. Mild haemophilia should be considered in any male presenting with prolonged posttraumatic bleeding. There is prolongation of the activated partial thromboplastin time. The diagnosis is confirmed by specific measurement of factor VIII levels. The carrier status of the female relatives of affected individuals is determined to assist in genetic counselling.

Successful prenatal diagnosis of haemophilia is now possible and allows a carrier to have a normal son and reduces the number of elective pregnancy terminations.

Treatment

The mainstay of managing bleeding episodes is early treatment with factor VIII concentrates. For spontaneous joint bleeding levels of factor VIII above 20 per cent are usually satisfactory. For major surgery the factor VIII level should be raised to 100 per cent and kept above 60 per cent until healing is completed. For established bleeds 0.5 u/kg per cent rise required of factor VIII are given. If treatment is carried out at home then it can be given at the earliest sign of bleeding. Severe haemophilia can be treated prophylactically by infusion of 25 u/kg factor VIII twice weekly.

Oral antifibrinolytics such as tranexamic acid can assist haemostatis and if given 24 hours before dental extraction may obviate the requirement for factor VIII.

Deamino-D-arginine vasopressin (DDAVP) is a synthetic derivative of vasopressin. When administered intravenously or intranasally it brings about an increase in the level of circulating factor VIII complex in normal individuals, mild haemophiliacs or patients with von Willebrand's disease. The increase in factor VIII seen in some individuals has been sufficiently great to enable surgery to be carried out without bleeding.

Haemophilia B – factor IX deficiency

Haemophilia B is inherited in the same way as haemophilia A and is clinically indistinguishable. The incidence is approximately one-fifth that of haemophilia A. Heat treated factor IX concentrate is the treatment of choice.

von Willebrand's disease (vWD)

After haemophilia this is the next most common inherited bleeding disorder. It is difficult to be sure of the true incidence because of the problems encountered in the diagnosis. It affects both sexes. Various sub-types are now described. It is usually inherited as an autosomal dominant condition. In its usual form mucous membrane bleeding is common while haemarthroses are rare. The bleeding time is prolonged. The vWF Ag is reduced as is the vWF RCo. The different sub-types show differing responses to DDAVP. The patient with vWD who is undergoing major surgery may require factor VIII replacement in much the same way as a haemophiliac although most cases will respond to fresh frozen plasma or DDAVP.

Heparin

The heparins are a group of negatively charged sulphated polysaccharides with an average molecular weight of 15 000. The anti-thrombotic action of heparin requires a plasma co-factor, an α-2 globulin, anti-thrombin III which combines with and inhibits activated clotting factors. Heparin may bind to lysyl residues on anti-thrombin III accelerating inhibitory activity of the anti-thrombin III. Heparin also binds to thrombin and has effects on platelets enhancing primary aggregation directly but perhaps also inhibiting platelet aggregation indirectly by neutralization of the aggregating agent thrombin. Heparin has a multi-site effect on the coagulation cascade and on platelets, affecting many of the laboratory tests of coagulation. The tests involved include the whole blood clotting time, the activated partial thromboplastin time, the prothrombin time and the thrombin time. The reptilase time however is normal and this can be used in determining whether abnormalities of the above tests are due to heparin. None of the above tests are ideal for the control of therapy.

Indications for use

Heparin is used for:

- the prophylaxis of venous thrombosis and pulmonary embolism;
  the treatment of venous thrombosis and pulmonary embolism;
- the treatment of acute arterial occlusion;
- the maintenance of blood fluidity in extracorporeal circulations;
- the treatment of disseminated intravascular coagulation (DIC).

Treatment of venous thrombo-embolism

Patients with popliteal, femoral or iliac vein thrombosis have a high risk of pulmonary embolism and should be treated. Treatment of asymptomatic calf vein thrombosis is controversial but symptomatic calf vein thrombosis is usually treated. Heparin, rather than oral anticoagulants, is usually chosen as initial treatment because of its immediate action and is usually given continuously for 7–10 days. The risk of recurrence of DVT is greatest within the first few weeks after the event and diminishes over the following 6 months. Oral anticoagulant therapy is usually commenced after 7 days of heparin. The heparin is continued for 2 to 3 days after the commencement of oral anticoagulant therapy. Continuous infusion of heparin is preferred to intermittent intravenous injection since it reduces the incidence of significant short term over-anticoagulation with consequent bleeding. Infusion ensures a reasonably constant level of anticoagulant not achieved by intermittent bolus administration because of the short half-life of heparin. For continuous i.v. infusion, heparin is given in a bolus loading dose of 5–10 000 units to an adult and then a continuous maintenance infusion of 25 000–40 000 units/24 hours. The high doses are recommended in acute pulmonary embolism, to neutralize the preformed thrombin and because the high levels of platelet factor IV circulating in this situation tend to neutralize heparin. The dosage is adjusted to keep the PTT or the thrombin time two to three times normal. When monitoring therapy by heparin assay, the heparin level is kept between 0.3 and 0.5 units/ml. Lower doses should be given immediately postoperatively and in patients with liver and renal disease.

The prophylaxis of venous thrombo-embolism

Here low dose heparin is more frequently used and probably inhibits the serine proteases early in the clotting cascade. The high doses of heparin required to neutralize thrombin are not necessary in this context. A number of low dose heparin regimes have been reported to prevent calf, popliteal and femoral venous thrombosis with subsequent pulmonary embolism after elective gynaecological and thoraco-abdominal surgery, but results have been less encouraging after hip surgery and prostate surgery. Low dose heparin is also used in pregnancy for prophylaxis in patients at high risk for DVT. It does not cross the placenta and therefore does not cause bleeding in the fetus. Dosage of subcutaneous heparin before surgery is 5000 units stat and then 5000 units b.d. or t.d.s. starting 12 hours post operatively and continuing for 7 to 14 days. The most important side-effect of heparin is bleeding which is less of a problem at this dosage. Less common complications include osteoporosis, alopecia, hypersensitivity reactions and thrombocytopenia.

Heparin reversal

In many situations heparin does not need to be reversed but stopped as it has such a short half-life. However, overdosage can be immediately neutralized by a strong basic substance such as protamine sulphate, 1 mg of protamine neutralizing 100u of heparin. To neutralize heparin 60 minutes after heparin injection, 50 per cent of the neutralizing dose is given and only 25 per cent at 2 hours after injection. Neutralization is assessed by PTTK or thrombin time immediately after the protamine.

Oral anticoagulants

The number of patients in the UK treated with coumarin drugs has increased several fold in recent years. There has been increased confidence in the recommended therapeutic range and regulation of dosage using the British Comparative thromboplastin. Administration of oral anticoagulants to patients with venous thromboembolism has been accepted practice since the 1940s. Only one prospective randomized trial was reported but was abandoned before completion because of the higher risk in the untreated group. The validity of this study has been constantly challenged but several prospective trials from McMaster University have confirmed that oral anticoagulants are extremely beneficial in preventing recurrence of DVT. The role of warfarin therapy for postmyocardial infarction is more controversial. The initial claims for its efficacy, made in the 1950s, were premature and not made on the basis of sound clinical trials. The use of anticoagulants in this setting cannot be recommended on a large scale at present.

Therapeutic ranges

In order to promote standardization of the prothrombin time for monitoring oral anticoagulants the World Health Organisation developed an International Reference Thromboplastin and recommended that the prothrombin time ratio be expressed according to a uniform system known as the International Normalized Ratio (INR). The INR is the prothrombin time ratio obtained by testing a given sample using the WHO reference thromboplastin.

Haemorrhage

Bleeding remains the major problem without regular laboratory control. Severe haemorrhage is rare in the British System for anticoagulant Control with British Ratios or International Normalized Ratios between 2 and 4. A long-term study from Edinburgh analyzed patients with valvular heart disease and prosthetic valves and showed only 51 haemorrhages in 1199 patient years; 24 were serious haemorrhages with 23 events occurring when the INR was excessively prolonged. Only two events were fatal.

The results of the McMaster clinical studies have established the optimal therapeutic range in patients with venous thromboembolism. In these patients the INR should be in the range of 2.0 to 3.0. In patients with prosthetic heart valves of the mechanical type, current evidence suggests the therapeutic range is 3.0 to 4.5 whereas for patients with valvular heart disease, atrial fibrillation or tissue heart valve replacement a recommended range is 2.0 to 3.0.

Anticoagulants during pregnancy

Special problems arise during pregnancy. The concentration of some blood clotting factors increase while the fibrinolytic mechanism is reduced. These changes promote good haemostasis at delivery but may aggravate tendency to thromboembolism. The risk is greatest in the immediate postpartum period.

Coumarin type drugs are safe and effective for the mother but as they cross the placenta they are a hazard to the fetus. Congenital abnormality, abortion, still birth and perinatal morbidity from fetal haemorrhage are all thought to be increased by the use of oral anticoagulants. Thus they should be avoided in the first weeks of pregnancy or in women seeking to become pregnant. Heparin, which may be given subcutaneously, should be used in early pregnancy in women who require anticoagulation and again at term as finer control of haemostasis during labour is achieved.

Disseminated intravascular coagulation (DIC)

DIC is a pathological disorder arising from activation of the haemostatic system within the circulation in response to injury of some form. This leads to the formation of intravascular fibrin, deposition of platelets and a secondary activation of the fibrinolytic pathway. In the classical case this results in the non-clotting of the blood because of fibrinogen depletion, consumptive thrombocytopenia and the production of fibrin degradation products (FDPs). The clinical hallmark of the disease is haemorrhage, which in some cases may be profuse.

It appears paradoxical that the generation of fibrin within the circulation should produce haemorrhage rather than thrombosis. In practice, the deposition of fibrin within the small vessels is occurring at the same time as defibrination by the fibrinolytic pathway. At autopsy there is seldom any evidence of intravascular fibrin deposition. This illustrates that the body is very efficient at clearing intravascular fibrin from the circulation. The extent to which this fibrin is digested is related to the concentration of fibrinolytic inhibitors in the circulation. The main inhibitors are α-2-antiplasmin, α-2-macroglobulin and α-1-antitrypsin. The relative importance of the various plasminogen activators is less well understood.

Normal haemostasis involves four main components – the blood vessel, platelets, coagulation and fibrinolysis. DIC may be triggered off by injury at any of these levels, although there is usually interaction between these components for established DIC to occur. The main groups of disorders producing DIC are shown in Table 8.6. Frequently two or more factors are in operation at the same time.

Clinical features of DIC

The commonest presenting feature of DIC is haemorrhage which may be profuse. The majority will develop skin haemorrhage. Frank purpura may be an indication of an underlying vasculitis with sensitive fibrin thrombi. In many patients the underlying cause is obvious e.g. septicaemia, but in others clinical suspicion is aroused by features such as excessive bleeding from venepuncture sites.

Clinical evidence of thrombosis is rare and the extent to which microthrombi occur within the circulation is disputed. On the other hand, renal lesions are found in a number of patients and may be due to the deposition of thrombi within the renal microvasculature. In the majority of cases the renal lesions are reversible. In the rare form of acute DIC (thrombotic thrombocytopenic purpura (TTP)), the thrombi occlude the cerebral vasculature leading to multiple neurological lesions of upper motor neurone type. The patient becomes increasingly drowsy often leading to coma and subsequent death.

Laboratory diagnosis of DIC

A few relatively simple tests are sufficient to make the diagnosis of DIC. This can be achieved by performing a clotting screen consisting of a one stage prothrombin time, a partial thromboplastin time, a thrombin time, platelet count, fibrinogen estimation and the estimation of FDPs. An inspection of whole blood allowed to clot in a glass tube gives rapid information during surgery or an obstetric emergency. An abnormal clotting screen which is due to the presence of heparin is distinguished by correction using the Reptilase time. The coagulant venoms can clot fibrinogen in the presence of heparin.

Treatment of DIC

The most important task is to identify and treat the underlying cause. If the precipitating event cannot be reversed rapidly then it is necessary to correct the underlying deficiencies of clotting factors and platelets. Fresh frozen plasma (FFP) can be used both to replace the depleted clotting factors and also as a plasma expander. FFP contains a fibrinogen concentration of approximately 4 g/litre. In the case of severe hypofibrinogenaemia

Table 8.6 Conditions associated with DIC

Acute	Subacute	Chronic
Shock	Disseminated	Liver disease
Septicaemia	malignancy	Myocardial
Acute	Promyelocytic	infarction
intravascular	leukaemia	Neoplasm
haemolysis		Paroxysmal
Acute		nocturnal
pulmonary		haemoglobi-
embolism		nuria
Cardiac arrest		SLE, renal
and		disease,
resuscitation		
Extensive		
trauma		
Major surgery		
Burns		
Placental		
abruption		
Septic abortion		

cryoprecipitate should also be given initially – each bag of cryoprecipitate contains approximately 1 gram of fibrinogen. The beneficial effect of heparin in DIC, if any, has not been demonstrated by controlled trials. It has been the practice to restrict the use of heparin to the relatively rare promyelocytic leukaemia where the onset of DIC may be predicted as soon as anti-leukaemia therapy commences. A recent controlled trial in this setting failed to show any benefit for heparin even in this situation and at the present time the use of heparin in DIC cannot be recommended.

Fibrinolysis

Fibrinolytic drugs have been in clinical use since the late 1950s and their efficacy has been well established in clot lysis. There are three major problems for the practitioner.

- does clinical benefit follow such treatment?
- fear of haemorrhagic complications
- the cost and selection of the best agent

Clinical benefit

Fibrinolytic therapy can be considered for patients with virtually any type or site of clot. Most widespread interest at present is in coronary artery thrombosis associated with acute myocardial infarction. It is now clearly established that early administration of streptokinase can produce reperfusion with improved ventricular function and reduced mortality. The best results are obtained if streptokinase is administered within 4 hours of the onset of symptoms. There is also great debate as to whether these drugs are of benefit in the therapy of deep venous thrombosis or pulmonary embolism. Comparing streptokinase with heparin, thrombolysis is achieved more often with streptokinase but bleeding also occurs more frequently. Similarly, with pulmonary thromboembolism greater resolution of pulmonary emboli with thrombolytic therapy than with heparin has been confirmed by several studies but a benefit in the effect on overall mortality has yet to be established.

Haemorrhagic complications

The major complication remains the risk of bleeding. The risk can be minimized by keeping the course as short as possible, minimizing invasive

Table 8.7 Contraindication to fibrinolytic therapy

- cerebrovascular process
- major surgery, surgical biopsy within 1 week
- postpartum
- recent bleeding, especially from GI tract
- dacron prosthesis
- severe hypertension
- coagulation defect
- diabetic retinopathy

procedures and by excluding those patients with contraindications to therapy (Table 8.7).

Choice of agent

The standard agents are streptokinase and urokinase which have similar half-lives. Streptokinase, but not urokinase, is antigenic but urokinase is more expensive.

The theoretical problem with streptokinase and urokinase is generalised activation of fibrinolysis resulting in defibrination and a generalised bleeding tendency. Acylated plasminogen kinase activated complex (apsac) and tissue plasminogen activator (tPa), which have a more localized effect because of their affinity for intravascular thrombus, have also been studied. Early reports suggest that these agents may produce an even better reduction in mortality but at considerably increased financial costs.

Acute leukaemia

Leukaemia is a malignant proliferation of the blood forming tissues, its two major forms being acute lymphoblastic leukaemia (ALL) and acute myelogenous leukaemia (AML). The term 'acute leukaemia' implies that the cells are morphologically immature.

The precise mechanism of leukaemogenesis is unknown. The leukaemic stem cells divide but fail to differentiate and so accumulate within the bone marrow. Its incidence is 3.5/100 000 and is apparently rising in the Western world.

Clinical features

The presentation of AML and ALL is similar with a sudden onset of the symptoms of marrow failure – lassitude, infection and bleeding. Bone and joint pains may occur particularly in ALL. Lymphadenopathy and hepatosplenomegaly are also more prominent in ALL. Infiltration of other tissues such as skin, gums and perineum usually indicates a monocytic element.

Acute lymphoblastic leukaemia

ALL is most common in children although substantial number of cases occur in adolescence and adults. Patients with ALL can be divided into several immune groups. The most common group are pre-B-cell ALLs which include common form of ALL (cALL). Rarer forms are T cell, null cell and B cell. Patients with the pre-B-cell form of the disease have the best prognosis, particularly in children. Those with T-cell or null phenotype have an intermediate prognosis and those with B-cell ALL have the least favourable prognosis. The presence of a chromosomal abnormality worsens the prognosis particularly in adult ALL. Other factors which have been reported to adversely influence the remission rates include male sex, (associated with testicular relapse), initial presentation with CNS leukaemia, high white blood count on presentation and the presence of a mediastinal mass.

Therapy

Major advances in the treatment of childhood ALL have occurred during the last 20 years. Milestones in the advancement of this treatment have included firstly, the use of multiple chemotherapy regimens and secondly, the introduction of prophylaxis for the CNS. Remission induction therapy of adults with ALL is largely based on the approaches successful in children. Approximately 50 per cent of patients with ALL will achieve remission following therapy with vincristine and prednisolone. Addition of daunorubicin to vincristine and prednisolone will result in remission rates of 70–90 per cent of adults. Several large multi-centre studies are currently underway, notably in West Germany, but at the present time the impact of different schedules of remission induction therapy on remission duration remain uncertain.

CNS Prophylaxis In early studies of childhood ALL up to 50 per cent of patients relapsed in the CNS. CNS prophylaxis is now universally applied. The most commonly used method is 1.8 Gy of cranial irradiation given in 12 fractions, accompanied by up to six doses of intrathecal methotrexate. Although no impact on the survival of adults with ALL has been reported, CNS prophylaxis is still recommended.

Postremission therapy Although it is believed that once remission is induced, consolidation or intensification therapy is effective in adults with ALL, data to support this concept are lacking. Similarly, studies in children with standard risk ALL have failed to demonstrate benefit from consolidation chemotherapy. Considerable data, albeit uncontrolled, do indicate an advantage to consolidation therapy in children with high risk ALL. Since adults with ALL follow a similar course to children with high risk ALL it is reasonable to utilize consolidation chemotherapy in adults. Maintenance chemotherapy in childhood ALL is effective in prolonging remission and decreasing the number of relapses, thereby improving survival. Uncontrolled studies in adults who have received postinduction therapy including consolidation and maintenance appear to have a longer remission. There remains considerable controversy over the intensity and length of postinduction therapy. The most common form of maintenance chemotherapy is methotrexate and 6-mercaptopurine. The use of monoclonal antibodies *in vivo* remains of research interest at the present time.

Relapsed and resistant leukaemia Patients with ALL who relapse are treated by a similar regimen used to achieve the initial remission to attempt second remission. Approximately fifty per cent of adults will achieve a second remission with this approach. Those who relapse while still receiving maintenance chemotherapy have a poorer prognosis than those who relapse after completing maintenance chemotherapy. Those with resistant leukaemia who fail to respond to the induction regimen have a poor prognosis although a minority will subsequently achieve remission using alternative high dose chemotherapy frequently involving high dose methotrexate.

Acute myeloid leukaemia

Prognostic factors

In general terms, excluding the neonatal age group, it is usual to believe the younger the patient the more favourable the outcome. The prognostic significance of a large number of cytogenetic abnormalities that are now being detected in association with AML is an area of considerable interest. Achievement of rapid clinical remission does seem to be associated with a better prognosis. However, at present there remains little evidence that AML is curable by chemotherapy and subsequent relapse seems inevitable, except perhaps in a small proportion of patients.

Therapy

The most commonly used induction regimens consist of daunorubicin, cytosine and 6-thioguanine. The optimal dose and duration of therapy with these agents remains uncertain. Using this approach approximately 70–80 per cent of patients with AML will be expected to achieve remission. The appropriate therapy of patients with AML once they have achieved remission is controversial. However, most people believe that some form of consolidation or early intensification is beneficial. Numerous forms of maintenance chemotherapy have been evaluated but the median remission duration has remained relatively constant despite these major differences. There have been relatively few studies of the use of late intensification therapy in AML and its role remains controversial. In contrast to ALL, CNS involvement in AML occurs in less than 5 per cent of patients. There is no detectable benefit of CNS prophylaxis in this group of patients.

Bone marrow transplantation for acute leukaemia

Allogeneic bone marrow transplantation (BMT) is an effective form of treatment for both acute myeloid leukaemia (AML) and acute lymphatic leukaemia (ALL). It is the treatment of choice for selected patients. The major controversy remains as to which patients should receive BMT early in their disease as opposed to those in whom transplantation should be delayed. When allogeneic BMT was first studied in end-stage leukaemia only ten per cent of patients survived. Studies of transplantation in relapse of leukaemia did however indicate that cure was obtainable in a small proportion of patients. However, BMT also carries a substantial risk of complications causing morbidity and mortality, and these risks must be weighted against the potential benefit of the procedure in the individual patient.

Complications of BMT Allogeneic BMT involves the use of very high dose chemotherapy (usually cyclophosphamide) and total body irradiation to ablate the host bone marrow and any underlying leukaemia. The dose that is administered is limited by the toxicity on normal tissues. It produces mucositis and gastrointestinal toxicity. Life-threatening complications such as pneumonitis and hepatic veno-occlusive disease may occur. Haemorrhagic cystitis is common in patients receiving high dose cyclophosphamide though this is largely prevented by the use of MESNA which binds the toxic metabolites in the urine. The dosage of chemotherapy and irradiation given are potentially carcinogenic and the risk of second malignancies is uncertain at present. Patients have a severe immunodeficiency following BMT and are at high risk of opportunistic infections within the first 6 months. The most important of these is cytomegalovirus which produces an interstitial pneumonitis usually within the first 6 months. Interstitial pneumonitis with pneumocystis carinii was also a not uncommon complication, but the incidence of this has been dramatically reduced by the use of prophylactic 'Septrin' during the first six months post BMT. Following allogeneic BMT the graft may be rejected. This was an uncommon problem following BMT for leukaemia until the introduction of techniques to deplete the graft of donor T lymphocytes using monoclonal antibodies. This has been performed in an attempt to reduce the incidence of graft versus host disease (GVHD). GVHD is due to immunocompetent donor T lymphocytes present in the bone marrow graft reacting aginst the tissues of the immunosuppressed recipient. This manifests itself as skin rash, derangement of liver function and gastrointestinal symptom and remains a major problem in BMT. A number of methods have been used to reduce the incidence of GVHD: prophylactic methotrexate, cyclosporin A or both in combination are widely used. As already stated donor T lymphocyte depletion markedly reduces the incidence but at the price of an increased rejection rate. Transplantation of allogeneic bone marrow also appears to confer a beneficial graft versus leukaemia effect. This has been deduced from analysis of the relapse rate in patients with GVHD of varying severity, and in patients who receive syngenic BMT (from an identical twin) in whom GVHD does not occur and who have twice the relapse rate (40 per cent). At the present time approximately 20–30 per cent of allogeneic bone marrow recipients die of one of these transplant related complications. As a result of the age-related incidence of many of these complications (most notably GVHD), allogeneic BMT is rarely carried out on patients over 40 years of age.

BMT in AML

The results in AML must be compared with recent advances reported with chemotherapy. BMT is clearly superior to alternative forms of treatment for patients with AML in second remission or early relapse. The major controversy centres on whether transplantation should be recommended for patients in first remission. Available data suggests that BMT is superior to postremission chemotherapy for patients under 30 years of age.

BMT in ALL

The majority of children with standard or good risk ALL may achieve prolonged disease free survival with standard chemotherapy. These patients have not been considered for BMT during first remission. Several centres have reported preliminary results of marrow transplantation in patients with poor prognostic features. It is not presently possible to state whether early bone marrow transplantation will improve survival in these patients as analysis is particularly difficult given the recent data of increased survival with intensive chemotherapy.

Autologous bone marrow transplantation (ABMT)

In this procedure the patient's own bone marrow is harvested, after conventional chemotherapy has induced remission of disease, and cryopreserved. The patient then receives high dose chemotherapy and/or radiotherapy at doses which are ablative to the bone marrow. The cryopreserved bone marrow is then returned to the patient allowing reconstitution of haematological elements. Several potential advantages of this mechanism include its availability to patients who do not have an HLA identical sibling, its application to patients of an older age group up to 55-years-old and the decreased morbidity and mortality associated since there is no GVHD. A major concern remains whether residual leukaemia is present in the bone marrow which is cryopreserved and then reinfused to the patient. The rate of relapse of leukaemia is undoubtedly higher in patients receiving autologous versus allogeneic BMT. However, this is offset by the decreased morbidity and mortality associated with the procedure. To date no randomized study has been undertaken of autologous BMT versus conventional chemotherapy although this question should be answered by a study of ABMT in patients with acute myeloid leukaemia in first remission which is shortly to be commenced in the UK.

Bone marrow harvest

What is the risk to the donor in performing bone marrow harvests? In a series reported from Seattle on 1270 harvests from 1160 donors six patients had life-threatening complications. There was one cerebrovascular accident, three had cardiopulmonary problems during the procedure and two developed bacterial infections. Contrary to what might be expected the vast majority of patients do not complain of much pain following the procedure and it is only very rarely that the donor does not leave hospital on the next day. Greater than expected pain is usually due to haematoma at the site of aspiration. General anaesthesia is recommended where possible, but the procedure has been performed under spinal anaesthesia, caudal block and recently the Manchester group have reported the use of marrow harvests under local anaesthesia and intravenous hypnotics.

When feasible an autologous unit of blood is removed from the donor and stored for one week prior to the procedure. This unit is then reinfused during the procedure. Normal banked blood should not be transfused during the procedure to eliminate the risk of contaminating the marrow harvest with viable lymphocytes.

When harvesting from a normal donor an adequate marrow dose can usually be obtained from the posterior iliac crests alone. For this reason the procedure should commence with the patient prone on the table. It may however be necessary to aspirate also from the anterior iliac crests and from the sternum. In the case of autologous bone marrow transplantation, where the donor has received prior chemotherapy, it is the usual practice to harvest first from the posterior iliac crests and then from the anterior crests and finally the sternum to obtain an adequate yield of cells. Intraoperative cell counts to determine the number of cells obtained are now rarely performed.

It has always been anticipated that marrow donations would be associated with a risk of complications arising from the use of general anaesthesia. Of the six life-threatening complications reported from Seattle, three were related to anaesthesia. In the world literature to date there is one fatality reported connected with bone marrow donation.

Supportive care of the neutropenic patient

Previously infection was the most common cause of death in patients with haemotological malignancy. Although morbidity from infectious disease is still a major problem in these patients, therapeutic advances have produced a dramatic decline in the death rate due to infection. Previously the majority of infections were due to gram-negative organisms and *Pseudomonas* was a particular problem. Gram-positive infections are now increasing in number mostly associated with the increased use of long-term indwelling central catheters. These changes have affected the expected outcome as well as the approaches to prevention. Febrile patients with granulocytes less than 0.5×10^9/litre should promptly receive sytemic antibiotics and it is inappropriate to await results of blood cultures before commencing therapy. Typically this involves an aminoglycoside antibiotic and a semi-synthetic penicillin or cephalosporin. There are no convincing data that systemic antibiotics should be given prophylactically and there are several reasons why they should not be given in this way. Once the results of blood cultures are available it may be possible to adjust the antibiotic therapy to tailor the therapy more specifically and avoid the toxicity and cost of broad spectrum regimens. In patients with documented or suspected catheter related sepsis the addition of specific Gram-positive cover using such drugs as vancomycin is indicated. The use of oral non-absorbable antibiotics has been evaluated in several controlled studies to assess the value of 'gut sterilization' with controversial and contradictory results. The addition of anti-fungal agents may be necessary, often empirically. These are usually required following prolonged courses of broad spectrum antibiotics or where there has been no response to fever despite the use of broad spectrum antibiotics. One of the critical decisions to face the clinician treating the patient with haematological malignancy is whether to stop or continue antibacterial therapy in the neutropenic patient. When the patient remains febrile but otherwise clinically well, the discontinuation of antibiotics can be disastrous. It is currently our practice to discontinue antibiotics in the neutropenic patient only when the patient has been afebrile for a period of 5 days.

Viral infections The viral infections most frequently encountered are the herpes virus including *Herpes simplex* and *zoster*. Cytomegalovirus is also a herpes virus which is seen most commonly in the setting of the immunosuppressed patient post transplant. *Herpes simplex* infections will be frequently localized, self-limiting and may differ little from the infections that occur in patients with intact immune defences. However, *Herpes simplex* infections in these patients are often not only more frequent but also more severe. These viral infections have often been associated with a more severe form of mucositis and may produce associated morbidity with increased pain and decreased oral nutritional intake. It is therefore our policy to add parenteral acyclovir therapy to patients at the first sign of any reactivation of *Herpes simplex*. Infections with zoster are also increased in this group of immunocompromized patients. Primary varicella with visceral dissemination and death is not uncommon in children with haematological malignancies. Similarly, atypical generalized zoster is also seen in patients with Hodgkin's or non-Hodgkin's lymphoma, particularly in patients who have had previous radiotherapy. Among immunodeficient adults, however, *Herpes zoster* is the more common viral infection. In patients who have *Herpes zoster*, viral dissemination remains a risk. Parenteral acyclovir therapy is indicated at the first sign of varicella or zoster infections.

Lymphomas

Hodgkin's disease

Hodgkin's disease is a malignant neoplasm arising in a lymph node. It spreads contiguously by the lymphatic channels. The malignant cell is the Reed–Sternberg cell. The origin of this cell has been difficult to determine, but gene rearrangement studies now suggest that it is lymphoid in origin and may be derived from either T or B lymphoid elements. The tumour cells are usually associated with reactive lymphocytes.

It is more common in males and in ages 20–40 years.

Histology

The diagnosis must always be confirmed by biopsy of an affected node. The Reed–Sternberg cell is a large binucleate cell with prominant nucleoli. The histological classification is based on that of Lukes and Butler:

- nodular sclerosis;
- lymphocyte predominant;
- lymphocyte depleted and;
- mixed cellularity.

Paucity of reactive lymphocytes is associated with a poorer prognosis.

Clinical features

Patients present with lymphadenopathy, most frequently involving the cervical nodes. B symptoms are now rigidly defined as weight-loss (more than 10 per cent in six months), fever (over 38°C) and night sweats. Other constitutional symptoms include malaise and pruritus. Alcohol related pain is seen more commonly in textbooks than in patients.

Staging

Accurate staging is very important as it provides a prognostic guide and indicates appropriate therapy.

Ann Arbor staging system
Stage I: single lymph node region
Stage II: two or more lymph node regions on one side of the diaphragm.
Stage III: nodes on both sides of the diaphragm which may include splenic involvement.
Stage IV: diffuse involvement of one or more extralymphatic organs.

Each stage is divided into A or B according to the presence or absence of B symptoms. Staging procedures involve a thorough history and examination including inspection of Waldeyer's ring. Radiological examinations include a chest X-ray, lymphangiogram and computerized axial tomography of chest and abdomen. A bone marrow aspirate and trephine biopsy should be performed. A liver biopsy may be indicated if the liver function tests are abnormal. A staging laparotomy and splenectomy are now only indicated if the result of such a procedure will alter the subsequent management which is usually then restricted to patients with Stage IIA disease who may be restaged as IIIA by the finding of abnormal nodes by multiple nodal biopsy.

Treatment

Radiotherapy is the treatment of choice if the disease is within a treatment field. It is indicated

now in Stage IA and IIA. 40 gy are given in divided doses over a period of 3–4 weeks.

In those patients with B symptoms or in those with advanced (Stage III–IV) disease combination chemotherapy is indicated. The mainstay of treatment is 'MOPP'.

Mustine hydrochloride	6 mg/m^2(Days 1 and 8)
Vincristine (Oncovin)	1.4 mg/m^2(Days 1 and 8)
Procarbazine	100 mg/m^2(Days 1 to 14)
Prednisolone	50 mg/m^2(Days 1 to 14)

Mustine may be replaced by the less toxic chlorambucil without loss of efficacy in treatment.

Chemotherapy is much less well tolerated than radiotherapy. Most men are rendered azospermic and semen should be cryopreserved where possible.

Prognosis

Stages I and II, lymphocyte predominant histology and normal haemoglobin levels are good prognostic features. Stages III and IV, the presence of B symptoms, large mediastinal mass and depleted lymphocyte histology are poor prognostic features. Overall the ten-year survival is about 60 per cent whilst 80–90 per cent of relapses occur in the first two years. There is increasing awareness of the risk of secondary malignancies including acute leukaemia and solid tumours in these patients.

Non Hodgkin's lymphomas (NHL)

These are a heterogeneous group of neoplastic disorders arising from cells of the immune system. Most NHLs originate within lymphoid tissues and are widely disseminated at the time of clinical presentation in nodes, marrow or blood. Later there may be involvement of other organs such as liver, gastrointestinal tract, skin, lung or central nervous system. Staging of the extent of the disease at diagnosis is usually expressed using the Ann Arbor system but is less crucial in NHL than in Hodgkin's disease. It is necessary to distinguish cases of truly localized disease which may be curative by localized radiotherapy.

Histological classification

The classification is far from simple and this is reflected by the large number of histopathological

Table 8.8 International Working Formulation for NHL

Low grade
Small lymphocytic
Follicular, predominantly small cleaved
Follicular mixed small cleaved and large cells

Intermediate grade
Follicular predominantly large cell
Diffuse small cleaved cell
Diffuse mixed small and large cell
Diffuse large cell

High grade
Large cell – immunoblastic
Lymphoblastic
Small non-cleaved cells

Unclassifiable
In about 10 per cent of cases the morphologic pattern does not fit into any of the above groupings.

classification in existence. The most widely used is now the International Working Formulation for NHL (Table 8.8).

Clinical features

Painless lymphadenopathy is the presenting feature in more than two-thirds of patients. Systemic symptoms occur in up to 30 per cent of patients and consist of fever, night sweats, weight loss, fatigue and pruritus. Although marrow involvement is frequent blood counts are usually normal at presentation.

Treatment

Patients with low grade disease should not be treated unless they are symptomatic as there may be long periods of relatively static disease. The optimal therapy for NHL is not defined. Radiotherapy may be curative in those patients with localized disease. It is more commonly used for palliative reduction in tumour mass.

Chemotherapy is employed as single agent therapy with chlorambucil or cyclophosphamide in the low grade histologies or as multi-agent regimes containing adriamycin in the more aggressive forms. CHOP is the most commonly used regime and consists of:

Cyclophosphamide	750 mg/m^2	(Days 1 to 8)
Adriamycin	25 mg/m^2	(Days 1 and 8)
Vincristine	1.4 mg/m^2	(Days 1 and 8)
Prednisolone	160 mg/m^2	(Days 1 to 5)

The lymphoblastic lymphomas are treated as for acute lymphoblastic leukaemia.

Prognosis

Patients with low grade histology have a median survival of approximately seven years. In the higher grades there has been considerable improvement in survival with aggressive therapy. More than 50 per cent of patients now obtain complete remission of disease and more than half of these patients may be cured.

The myelodysplastic syndromes

These are rare conditions which are preleukaemic in nature. They consist of refractory anaemia, refractory anaemia with excess blasts (RAEB), chronic myelomonocytic leukaemia and sideroblastic anaemia. Most patients are over 40 years of age. There is a varying degree of pancytopenia. The frequency of evolution of these syndromes to AML is probably around 20 per cent of patients. There is interest in the use of Interferon therapy in these conditions to prevent progression of disease.

The myeloproliferative disorders

These are a spectrum of neoplastic disorders in which there is proliferation of the myeloid stem cell or its derivatives. The proliferations of the myeloid series are not usually restricted to one cell line and transitions can occur.

Chronic granulocytic leukaemia (CGL)

CGL was the first type of leukaemia to be discovered. The Philadelphia chromosome is present in the granulocytic, erythroid, megakaryocytic and lymphoid cell lines. It results from the translocation of the break point cluster region (bcr) on the long arm of chromosome 22 to the c-abl oncogene region on chromosome 9. The biochemical consequences of the new gene activation has now been investigated in detail but the mechanism whereby this results in neoplastic proliferation is not yet understood.

Clinical features

CGL becomes more common with increasing age. There is a gradual onset of anorexia, weight loss and anaemia. Splenomegaly is almost invariable. The white blood count is raised with the appearance of early myeloid elements in the peripheral blood. The disease runs a chronic course for 18 months to 5 years before transition to an accelerated phase resulting in acute leukaemia, most commonly AML.

Treatment

Treatment remains symptomatic and there is no curative therapy for CGL with the exception of allogeneic bone marrow transplantation. Alkylating agents such as Busulphan will lower the white count and reduce splenomegaly. Such treatment increases the patients' well-being but has no effect on subsequent transformation to the blastic phase. Once blastic change has occurred the disease is often refractory to standard acute leukaemia therapy and there is a dire prognosis. Where possible allogeneic bone marrow transplantation should be performed during the chronic phase.

Polycythaemia rubra vera

This is characterized by excessive production of red cells and an increase in red cell mass in the presence of low levels of erythropoietin. The cause is unknown.

Clinical features

Presentation is usually after the age of 40. The onset is insidious and is often first suspected after a routine full blood count.

The symptoms are related to circulatory disturbances secondary to the increased red cell mass and hyperviscosity which results in vascular distention, impaired blood flow, stasis and ultimately tissue hypoxia. The co-existing thrombocytosis interacts to increase the rate of thrombosis, thromboembolism and haemorrhage to about 40 per cent of patients and these are a common cause of mortality. Central nervous symptoms are most common and are related to the decrease in cerebral blood flow. Headache, dizziness, vertigo, tinnitus and visual disturbances are often present.

Therapy

There are two main approaches to therapy. Phlebo-tomy should be the initial therapy. Phlebotomies of 350–500 ml may be performed every other day until the haematocrit is reduced to the normal range. In the elderly patient smaller volumes may be taken. In emergencies intensive phlebotomy may be accompanied by plasma infusion.

Control of the underlying condition requires myelosuppressive therapy. Radioactive phosphorus (^{32}P) was widely used until recently but its use is now restricted to older patients because of the associated risk of developing of malignant disease (e.g. leukaemia). The alternative use of alkylating agents, most notably chlorambucil has now been shown to carry an increased risk of malignant disease and a recent large series studied by the PRV (USA) study group suggests that hydroxyurea is the treatment of choice.

Prognosis

Untreated, the median survival is 2 years. This rises to 13 years with treatment. Thrombosis and haemorrhage are the major cause of death and 25 per cent progress to acute leukaemia or myelofibrosis.

Secondary polycythaemia

Secondary polycythaemia is an absolute erythrocytosis resulting from enhanced stimulation of red blood cell production. It is secondary to hypoxia in the majority of cases. More rarely it is due to inappropriate erythropoietin production in various renal lesions including hypernephroma tuberculosis and adenoma or to non renal tumours such as cerebellar haemangioblastoma, ovarian tumours, phaeochromocytoma, hepatoma and carcinoma of the bronchus.

The resultant polycythaemia increases the oxygen carrying capacity until whole blood viscosity compromises blood flow and the oxygen carrying capacity begins to fall. Judicious venesection may be indicated if haemotocrits are above 60 per cent.

Blood transfusion

Blood groups were first discovered in 1900 by Karl Landsteiner who described agglutination of the red cells of some individuals when mixed with serum from some but not all other individuals. Classification of the blood groups was based on the realization that a specific antigen – antibody reaction had

Table 8.9   Blood group systems and major antigens

System	Major antigens
ABO	A, B, H
Rhesus	C, c, D, E, e
Lewis	Le^a, Le^b
Kell	K, k, Kp^a, Kp^b, Js^a, Js^b
Duffy	Fy^a, Fy^b
Kidd	Jk^a, Jk^b
Lutheran	Lu^a, Lu^b
MNSs	M, N, S, s
P	P$_1$, P; P^k
Ii	I, i

occurred and over one hundred blood group antigens have now been reported. These are classified into blood group systems, each of which is inherited independently from other systems. The most important systems are listed in Table 8.9.

The red cell membrane

Blood group antigens are situated on the surface of the red cell membrane which consists of a lipid bilayer in which large protein molecules are embedded. Beneath the lipid bilayer is a protein network which maintains the shape of the red cell and provides its deformability. About 10 per cent of the membrane is carbohydrate attached to phospholipids, glycolipids and proteins and situated on the external surface. The carbohydrate residues and the transmembrane proteins exposed on the external surface of the cell provide the antigenic properties of the cells. The high concentration of charged residues on the cell surface produces an ionic cloud when red cells are suspended in saline and the resulting 'zeta potential' is sufficient to keep the cells apart.

The ABO blood group system

The ABO blood group antigens found on red cells are carbohydrate residues synthesized by specific transferases coded for by genes situated on the long arm of chromosome 9 and inherited in an autosomal dominant manner. The A antigen is produced by the addition of N-acetylgalactosamine to an L-fucose residue, the B antigen by the addition instead of D-galactose to the same residue. The product of the O gene, if there is one, has no effect on L-fucose which is produced by another gene labelled H. In the absence of the L-fucose product of the H gene no A or B substance can be produced: this extremely rare situation occurs in the homozygous absence of the H gene, (hh) and has been labelled the 'Bombay' phenotype. These individuals make anti-A, anti-B and anti-H 'natural' antibodies, and compatible blood is difficult to obtain. Blood group A has two main subgroups, A$_1$ and A$_2$ in which the sugar residues are identical, but in A$_1$ the higher density of the residues results in a new antigen called A$_1$. Some individuals in subgroup A$_2$ make anti A$_1$. There are no important subgroups of group B. In the United Kingdom Caucasian population the occurrence of ABO groups is as follows: group O, 47 per cent, group A$_1$ 34 per cent, group A$_2$ 8 per cent, group B 8 per cent, group AB 3 per cent.

Secretors

Approximately 80 per cent of individuals secrete water-soluble substances in saliva that have the same specificity as the A, B or H antigens on their red cells. This is controlled by a secretor gene inherited independently of ABO and H genes. Homozygous (SeSe) and heterozygous (Sese) individuals are secretors; individuals who lack the Se gene (sese) are non-secretors. Water-soluble A, B and H antigens are present in most body fluids of a secretor. The secretor status affects the expression of the Lewis blood group.

Antibodies to the ABO system

Sera taken from individuals over the age of about 6 months almost always contain antibodies to A and B antigens not expressed on their red cells. It is likely that these antibodies are due to exposure to A, B and H antigens widely distributed in nature, in animals, plants and bacteria. These 'naturally occurring antibodies' are commonly IgM though group O individuals may have some IgG anti-A and B. The titre (strength) of the antibodies varies considerably in different sera though in general the strength of anti-A in group B and group O subjects is greater than that of anti-B in group A and group O subjects. They react best at 4°C and are therefore called cold agglutinins. Both IgM and IgG anti-A and anti-B are capable of binding complement causing lysis of the red cells at 37°C.

Immune anti-A and anti-B are the result of direct stimulus with A or B antigens by pregnancy, by transfusion of incompatible blood or plasma or following injection of horse serum, anti-tetanus toxin and some vaccines. These antibodies may also be strongly haemolytic.

Dangerous universal donors

Blood group O has sometimes been referred to as 'Universal donor' blood because group O red cells are not agglutinated by the anti-A and anti-B in the serum of group B and A patients. However, group O donors have anti-A, anti-A_1 and anti-B in their plasma, any of which may agglutinate and lyse the recipient's A or B cells, if present in high titres. Group O blood donations are screened to identify high titre antibodies.

Table 8.10 lists antigens and antibodies in the ABO system.

Table 8.10 Antigens and antibodies in the ABO system

Blood group	Antigens on the red cells	Antibodies in the serum
A_1	(H)A A_1	anti-B
A_2	(H)A	anti-B (2 % anti-A_1)
B	(H)B	anti-A + A_1
A_1B	(H)A A_1B	none
A_2B	(H)A B	none (25 % anti-A_1)
O	H	anti-A + A_1 + B

The Rh blood group system

The importance of this system is due to the ease with which antibodies are produced when Rh-D positive blood is transfused to an Rh-D negative person. In addition, because they are usually IgG, these antibodies can result in haemolytic disease of th newborn.

The Rh blood group system is controlled by three very closely linked genes carried on chromosome 1, each of which has a number of alleles. The commonest Rh genotypes in the United Kingdom are shown in Table 8.11. When Rh groups are reported on patients 'Rh positive' means D antigen positive (DD or Dd) and 'Rh negative' means D negative (dd). However, only CDE negative donor blood (cde/cde) is labelled 'Rh negative'. From Table 8.10 it may be seen that only 15 per cent of the UK population is Rh-D negative. In practice the D antigen is most important due to its greater potential to evoke an immune response. It seems likely that there is no d antigen and inheritance of the d gene results in merely the absence of D. The

Table 8.11 Commonest Rh genotypes in the UK

Genotype	Short Notation	Approximate incidence (%)
CDe/cde	R^1r	31
CDe/CDe	R^1R^1	16
cde/cde	rr	15
CDe/cDE	R^1R^2	13
cDE/cde	R^2r	13
cDE/cDE	R^2R^2	3

antigens C^w and D^U may be regarded as weak forms of the C and D antigens respectively.

The Rh antigens are well developed at birth and are not known to be present on cells other than red cells.

Antibodies to the Rh system

Naturally occurring antibodies are rare, weak and not of clinical importance. The commonest immune antibody was anti-D though due to anti-D prophylaxis this is no longer true. About 20–30 per cent of sera containing anti-D also contain anti-C activity. This is not a separable antibody and is termed anti-G. The next most common antibodies formed are anti-c and anti-E.

All the antibodies of the Rh system have caused haemolytic transfusion reactions and haemolytic disease of the newborn. These antibodies are almost invariably IgG (apart from a small proportion of 'naturally occurring' IgG anti-E) and do not agglutinate saline-suspended Rh-positive red cells but can be detected using a colloid medium (e.g. bovine albumin) which reduces the zeta potential or by the indirect antiglobulin test. In the indirect antiglobulin test, incubation of donor red cells with patient serum at 37°C is followed by addition of anti-human globulin which causes cross linking of antibody-coated red cells and visible agglutination.

Haemolytic disease of the newborn (HDN)

HDN is caused by sensitization of the mother to a blood group antigen borne by her fetus. Most blood groups can be involved but the most severe cases have been caused by differences in the Rh system, most notably when the mother is Rh-D negative (dd) while the fetus is Rh-D positive (Dd or DD). The pathogenesis depends on an IgG antibody response permitting placental passage of antibody. Hence it does not occur with naturally occurring IgM anti-A or anti-B antibodies and is uncommon in a first pregnancy (unless the mother has been sensitized by an incompatible transfusion). In this latter case sensitization usually occurs during delivery when sufficient fetal red cells cross the placenta and enter the maternal circulation to immunize the mother. The IgG antibodies formed as a result will cross the placenta in a subsequent pregnancy and result in haemolysis of the fetal red cells if they too bear the appropriate antigen. High levels of antibody early in pregnancy or a rising titre of antibody in the maternal serum is an ominous sign and is an indication for careful monitoring of the fetus by ultrasound and amniocentesis. Subsequent pregnancies are characteristically progressively more severely affected, with a progression from neonatal jaundice (with the potential complication of kernicterus) and anaemia (direct antiglobulin test positive) to intrauterine death from cardiac failure and ascites (hydrops fetalis).

Treatment of a neonate with HDN consists of exchange transfusion with fresh group O red cells compatible with any antibody present in the maternal serum and matched against maternal and neonate's sera. Severity is best indicated by the haemoglobin level in cord blood and the bilirubin level and nucleated cells in the infant's blood. Intrauterine transfusion with fresh group O cells compatible with maternal serum by intraperitoneal or umbilical vein cannulation can reverse hydrops and maintain fetal survival until delivery at 32–34 weeks.

HDN due to anti-D has been dramatically reduced by the injection of 500 i.u. IgG anti-D intravenously to all Rh-D negative women within 72 hours of delivery of a Rh-D positive infant. This is believed to result in the rapid destruction of any fetal cells in the circulation thus preventing an immune response. Because feto–maternal haemorrhage can occur at other times in pregnancy 250 i.u. i.v. anti-D is also given to Rh-D negative women for threatened abortions, abortions, ectopic pregnancies and amniocentesis before the 20th week and 500 i.u. i.v. anti-D is given for antepartum haemorrhage, external cephalic version and stillbirth after the 20th week.

Rh-D is still the commonest antigen implicated in severe haemolytic disease of the newborn. Less commonly HDN may be due to other rhesus antigens (c, E, e) or antigens of other blood group systems e.g. ABO Kell or Duffy.

Other blood group systems of note

Lewis

Occasional severe haemolytic transfusion reactions. Poorly developed antigens at birth are therefore not a cause of HDN.

P

Very rarely associated with severe transfusion reactions. Donath–Landsteiner antibody found in paroxysmal cold haemoglobinuria has anti-P specificity.

Ii

Anti-I associated with chronic cold haemagglutinin disease and *M. pneumoniae* infection. Anti-i is found briefly after infectious monucleosis and may cause haemolysis. These are cold antibodies and of no clinical importance.

Kell

Immune anti-K is the most common and clinically important antibody outside the ABO and Rh systems. Ninety one per cent in the UK are Kell negative (kk) and may produce this antibody following transfusion or pregnancy. Kell antibodies can cause severe haemolytic transfusion reactions and severe HDN.

Duffy

Anti Fy[a] is rare but occasionally occurs following transfusion usually in patients with other antibodies already. It may cause transfusion reactions and HDN.

Kidd

Antibodies are rare but can occur following transfusion or pregnancy and can cause severe delayed haemolytic transfusion reactions and HDN.

Practical blood transfusion serology

A recipient's ABO blood group is first determined by testing his red cells with known sera and his serum with known red cells. The D-group is also determined using at least two known anti-D sera. An antibody screen may then be performed to exclude the presence of antibodies to other Rhesus system antigens and to other systems. This is performed by testing recipient serum against group 0 red cells from two to three individuals, who between them carry all important red cell antigens. A number of techniques are used to ensure that the screen is capable of detecting all significant antibodies (saline room temperature, enzyme 37°C and indirect antiglobulin tests). In the event of a positive result, the antibody is identified using an extended panel of group O cells. The presence of an antibody may delay the provision of compatible blood.

When blood is to be transfused, the cross-match is carried out as the final test of compatibility. Recipient serum and cells from each donor unit to be transfused are incubated together at 37°C using a number of techniques. Donor units giving a positive result are rejected. Recently, however the absolute necessity of the cross-match to exclude significant incompatibility has been questioned.

In the presence of a negative antibody screen, some centres now carry out no further matching for many elective surgical procedures for which blood is not regularly transfused. Such procedures, where formerly blood was routinely matched but rarely transfused, include cholecystectomy, hiatus hernia repair and abdominal hysterectomy. If blood is required, a 30 minute cross-match is carried out using modern transfusion techniques or in an emergency, group specific blood is immediately available.

The question of antibody screen or cross-match is as yet unresolved. The 'group, screen and save' policy reduces wastage of donor units that are otherwise repeatedly cross-matched for a series of patients but never used. However, the cross-match safeguards against the presence of antibody to a rare antigen absent on the screening cells but present on donor cells.

Transfusion of red cells

Red cell concentrates

The introduction of 'optimal additive solutions' has permitted increased yield of plasma for fractionation and improved the shelf-life and flow characteristics of red cell concentrates. The maximum amount of plasma is removed from a freshly collected donation leaving a haematocrit of about 90 per cent and 100 ml of a solution of saline, adenine, glucose and mannitol (SAG-M or ADSOL) is added. This provides adenine, glucose and mannitol for red cell metabolism and reduces the haematocrit to 60 per cent. These preparations

have a shelf-life of 35 days at 4°C. Adenine provides better ATP synthesis during storage though 2,3 DPG levels still deteriorate rapidly resulting in increased oxygen affinity and a left shift in the oxygen curve. Complete restoration of 2,3 DPG levels to normal takes up to 24 hours after transfusion.

The simple transfer of a unit of blood from donor to recipient is not only wasteful but also constitutes a needless exposure of the recipient to potentially harmful or immunogenic elements. Red cell concentrates are the products of choice for nearly all routine transfusions. These products permit replacement of oxygen-carrying capacity without unnecessary volume expansion and liberate the other blood components for use for other patients. When necessary, red cell concentrates may be transfused in combination with colloid or electrolyte solutions as indicated. The only clear indication for transfusion of whole blood is continuing massive haemorrhage when both red cells and volume need to be replaced.

The routine ordering of blood for surgery on the basis of the patient's haemoglobin level must be challenged. Many factors, including of course the plasma volume, affect the patient's haemoglobin level. The need for red cell transfusion must be assessed for each patient in a much more serious way than hitherto and the potential risks to the patient of any transfusion must be taken into account. In addition, there are advantages during the surgery of having reduced haemoglobin levels because reduction of blood viscocity improves blood flow.

Leucocyte poor red cells

The transfusion of leucocyte poor red cells is indicated in patients who have developed non-haemolytic febrile transfusion reactions due to anti-leucocyte antibodies. These usually only develop in patients who have had multiple transfusions. A number of techniques have been used to reduce the leucocyte content of transfused blood. Filtration of blood through specially designed wool or nylon filters seems to be as effective as the use of multiply washed reconstituted frozen red cells.

Autologous blood transfusion

The use of autologous blood has the advantages of absolute compatibility and the absence of risk of disease transmission. The emergence of HIV as a transfusion risk has increased interest in this technique. However, it is only feasible for elective procedures and even then the unpredictability of requirements and the lack of facilities both for donation and storage make it impractical at the present time in the UK. The unpredictability of requirements is clearly the major obstacle. If additional blood is transfused, it may be argued that the infective or sensitization risks are reduced, but clearly much of the advantage (except conservation of homologous blood stocks) is lost.

Blood can be collected and stored either in liquid or frozen state and then reinfused into patients during elective procedures. In recent years a number of centres in the USA have provided facilities for the collection and storage of autologous blood. An objection frequently raised is the fitness of the patient to donate blood preoperatively. However, centres in which the autologous transfusion is routine, frequently carry out venesection on elderly patients and those with compromized cardiovascular status. Indeed, it can be argued that any patient fit enough to undergo elective surgery is medically fit to donate blood preoperatively. However, no more than 450 ml should be taken at a single donation and donations should be no more frequent than every 4 days. The haemoglobin should be 11 g/dl or greater and iron supplements are advisable. Finally, at least 72 hours should elapse between the last donation and major surgery. The major risk is of reinfusion of the wrong blood to the wrong patient. In general, unused autologous units are not reassigned for homologous use. But if they are, all criteria for donor selection must be fulfilled. Autologous transfusion is clearly very useful for the rare patient for whom compatible blood is hard to find. An alternative source of autologous red cells for transfusion is blood shed at an operative site. This can be retrieved by specially designed equipment (e.g. Haemonetics 'Cell Saver') which anticoagulates, filters, washes, packs and concentrates the red cells to a haematocrit of 50 per cent. The cells are prepared in a standard transfusion pack and have a shelf-life of 24 hours.

Whilst the provision of facilities for collection and liquid storage of red cells for autologous transfusion may be a reasonable approach to the anxieties of patients concerning the risks of blood transfusion, it seems unlikely that the storage of frozen red cells will be of any value for emergency use in view of the problems of storage, the delays inherent in thawing and washing and the delivery of the cells to the site at which the emergency occurs. The provision of blood from a specific donor e.g. spouse, parent or sib, is not believed to be appropriate as there is no reason to believe that even if it is compatible (a point often forgotten by the anxious patient or relative), the unit of blood would not be any less of an infective risk than that of a screened anonymous donor.

Cryopreserved red cells

Standard packed red cells may be preserved for several years in the frozen state if mixed with glycerol and frozen under carefully controlled conditions. The cryopreservant glycerol prevents cellular damage from ice crystal formation. When required, the frozen cells are rapidly thawed and serially washed in saline solutions. The process of thawing and washing takes about 1 hour and the cells have a shelf-life of 12 hours. As a result their use is limited. They are useful for preserving stocks of rare blood groups. Frozen-thawed red cells are also depleted of leucocytes but this is more economically achieved by filtration.

Red cell substitutes

The problems associated with the supply, storage, compatibility and potential hazards of donated blood encouraged research into the development of blood substitutes. No current substitute meets all the necessary requirements but some compounds have achieved clinical use in Japan and the USA. Perfluorocarbon emulsions have been used clinically but require inspiration of hyperbaric oxygen and are difficult to store and reconstitute. In addition, sensitivity has been reported and test doses are recommended. Modified haemoglobin solutions are not at such an advanced stage of development but are easier to store, achieve a greater oxygen delivery to tissues and on preliminary studies appear non-toxic. In addition, they are compatible with aqueous solutions, require no cross-match and are free of the risk of hepatitis.

Platelet transfusion

Platelet concentrates are prepared from donor blood by centrifugation within 6 hours of collection and contain 5×10^{10} platelets in 50–70 ml of plasma. Usually six packs are transfused with the intent of raising the platelet count by 40–60×10^9/litre. An alternative source of platelets for transfusion is by plateletphoresis using a cell separator: a single donor pack obtained in this way should contain at least 3.5×10^{11} platelets in about 250 ml plasma. Single donor packs are usually used in patients who have become refractory to random donor platelets as a result of HLA antigen sensitization from previous transfusions. Patients with aplastic anaemia for whom marrow transplantation is planned may receive single donor platelets to reduce the possibility of sensitization but these should not come from potential bone marrow donors.

Platelet transfusion is indicated in patients with major bleeding who have a quantitative or qualitative platelet defect. In addition, prophylactic platelet transfusion is often indicated in patients with a platelet count less than 20×10^9/litre and a product defect i.e. leukaemia or aplasia. No crossmatch is required but ABO compatible platelets are probably more effective and due to red cell contamination 'Rh-positive platelets' should not be given to Rh-negative female patients. Chill-fever reactions following platelet transfusion are associated with allo-immunization and failure to obtain a platelet increment. Such patients may respond to HLA-matched platelets. The likelihood of controlling haemorrhage is directly related to the post-transfusion increment. Although patients with alloantibodies, sepsis, splenomegaly or DIC may not have a post-transfusion increment, they should, nevertheless, receive platelet concentrates if they have thrombocytopenic bleeding.

When surgical procedures are planned in thrombocytopenic patients, a full assessment of the platelet count and the coagulation system must be made. A patient with a low platelet count may well have clotting factor abnormality in addition, particularly in the case of disseminated intravascular coagulation (DIC). Such patients may require platelet and clotting factor transfusion immediately before and during surgery. Close liaison should be made with the haemotologists *well in advance* (if possible) of the procedure. Platelets should be stored before use at room temperature and not in the 4°C refrigerator or the deep freeze. Anaesthetists must be extremely cautious and well informed of the storage temperatures appropriate for blood products before use.

Granulocyte transfusion

These are indicated as an adjunct to established anti-infective therapy for infections in neutropenic patients. There is no evidence that prophylactic granulocyte transfusions are of value. Indeed the risks of hypersensitivity, allo-immunization and cytomegalovirus infection make prophylactic granulocyte transfusion unacceptable. Granulocytes are obtained by leucapheresis on a cell separator and the larger numbers obtained from patients with chronic granulocytic leukaemia may result in better clinical responses.

Table 8.12 Plasma components and their important clinical indications

Product	Unit value (ml)	Clotting factors	Non-icterogenic	Storage (°C)	Indications
Plasma protein fraction† (PPF/SPPS)	400	No	Yes	2–25	Oligaemic shock, burns plasma exchange
Salt poor albumin‡	100	No	Yes	2–25	Liver disease, nephrotic syndrome
Fresh frozen plasma (FFP)	200	All	No	−30	Haemostatic disorders, von Willebrand's disease, haemophilia B
Cryoprecipitate	30	VIII fibrinogen fibronectin	No	−30	Haemophilia A, acquired haemostatic disorders
Factor VIII concentrate	15	VIII	No	+4	Haemophilia A
Factor IX concentrate	20	II, IX, X	No	+4	Haemophilia B, reversal of warfarinization

Key
†Protein content 4.5 g/100 ml, sodium content 3.1 mmol/g protein
‡Protein content 20 g/100 ml, sodium content 0.65 mmol/g protein

Plasma components and fractions

The plasma removed from units of donated blood is processed in a number of ways to provide blood components and fractions in high demand. The major products and their important clinical indications are summarized in Table 8.12.

Albumin products

These preparations are heated to 60°C for 10 hours and are free of infective risk from hepatitis and HIV. Plasma protein fraction (PPF) is a useful volume replacement fluid during major haemorrhage and its oncotic effect is more prolonged than electrolyte solutions which can result in pulmonary oedema. PPF is preferable to synthetic plasma substitutes such as urea-linked gelatin and dextran 70 whose only advantage is cost and availability and which may be associated with anaphylactic reactions and disturbances of haemostasis. PPF is also useful for replacement of protein loss after severe burns though this is best deferred for 24 hours whilst capillary integrity is poor. PPF or salt poor albumin infusions are indicated in reversible hypoproteinaemic states such as acute nephrosis and acute hepatocellular failure. The use of albumin preparations in chronic hypoproteinaemic state is more controversial as repeated infusions are extremely expensive. Anaphylactic and febrile reactions may occur with these products as with any other blood product. PPF contains no clotting factors and potentially worsens some situations in which there is already a bleeding tendency. Each anaesthetist must be aware of the difference between PPF and FFP (fresh frozen plasma) which does contain clotting factors.

Fresh frozen plasma

This product is prepared by careful separation of blood cooled immediately after venesection and has a shelf-life of 3–6 months at −30°C. It is useful in the treatment of conditions where replacement of several coagulation factors is required e.g. following massive transfusion of stored blood, liver disease or disseminated intravascular coagulation (DIC). In addition, it may be used to reverse the effects of oral anticoagulants in patients undergoing elective surgery. By supplying all the vitamin K dependent factors (II, VII, IX and X), it provides a rapid yet short lived correction of haemostasis which is useful in patients who must resume anti-coagulation promptly after surgery. An injection of vitamin K would take some 24 hours to be effective and frequently causes subsequent resistance to warfarin. FFP is also useful in the treatment of von Willebrand's disease, mild Factor IX deficiency (Haemophilia B) and other rare congenital deficiencies. FFP should be ABO compatible with the recipient and Rh-D compatibility is especially important for Rh-D negative females. It should be thawed quickly and infused immediately and rapidly. The infective risk is low because of donor screening but no sterilization process is possible with this product.

Cryoprecipitate

This product is prepared by thawing frozen single donor plasma and is then stored at or below −30°C. It has high concentrations of factor VIII and appreciable quantities of fibrinogen and fibronectin. Due to their single donor origin the amount of factor VIII in each pack varies widely but for the same reason the infective risk has been lower than that associated with pooled factor VIII concentrate. The concentrates should be thawed rapidly and used immediately – six to ten packs are usually transfused at a time. The major use of this product is in mild to moderate haemophilia A. However, in acquired haemostatic disorders where fibrinogen is low e.g. liver disease and some cases of DIC, infusion of cryoprecipitate along with FFP is often helpful, since it supplies additional factor VIII and fibrinogen in large quantities in a relatively small volume. Sometimes in overwhelming DIC, cryoprecipitate can be very helpful in providing a great deal of clotting factors in a minimal volume. In addition, cryoprecipitate may reverse the acquired platelet defect associated with uraemia.

Factor concentrates

The factor VIII rich cryoprecipitate and factor IX rich supernatant fluid can be subjected to further purification but at the expense of further losses. Pooling of the products of many donations is carried out to achieve standardization of the preparation. The potential infectivity of the product is dependent on the screening of donors and the sterilization of the product: filtration to remove bacteria, some viruses and fungal spores and since 1985, heat treatment at 80°C for 72 hours to eliminate HIV. Unfortunately, the sterilization process results in a further loss in potency and does not eliminate non A non B hepatitis.

Factor VIII concentrate is widely used in the treatment of haemophilia A. Its ease of storage and administration has resulted in the development of home treatment and revolutionized the treatment and lifestyle of severely affected patients. However, the problems associated with pooling donations from healthy carriers of viral disease are now well recognized. The screening of donors and heat sterilization should prevent a repetition of the HIV-AIDS episode but the development of recombinant factor VIII should supercede this form of therapy.

Factor IX concentrates are clearly most useful in the management of haemophilia B (Christmas disease). The preparative process results in appreciable concentrations of factors II, VII and X also. Hence this product can also be used to reverse warfarinization. In addition activation of some of the factor X during the preparative process makes it a useful therapy for patients with haemophilia A no longer responsive to factor VIII concentrates due to anti factor VIII antibodies. The problems of pooling and infection also apply to factor IX concentrates, and this preparation is also now heat treated.

Immunoglobulin preparations

A number of immunoglobulin preparations for subcutaneous or intramuscular administration are prepared from unselected healthy donors (human normal immunoglobulin; HNI) or from individuals with a high titre of antibodies of particular specificity (tetanus, hepatitis B, rabies, cytomegalovirus, herpes simplex, measles, mumps, rubella, vaccinia and herpes zoster). HNI is used in the treatment of general immune deficiency states and also to provide passive prophylaxis against hepatitis A as a high level of antibody to this virus is present in the normal donor population. Specific immunoglobulins are used to provide passive prophylaxis against these diseases following accidental or suspected exposure. The specific immunoglobulins are scarce and should be used with discretion e.g. in immunosuppressed patients. The chemical fractionation process used to prepare immunoglobulins itself results in stabilization and heat treatment is not required to eliminate the infective risk.

Anti-D immunoglobulin is required for passive prophylaxis of all Rh-D negative mothers, and is obtained from Rh-D negative volunteers deliberately immunized with Rh-D positive red cells. An alternative source in the form of monoclonal antibodies produced from a human cell line has been developed.

An immunoglobulin preparation suitable for intravenous infusion has been evaluated recently. It has been shown to be beneficial in the treatment of refractory immune thrombocytopenia (ITP) with at least a transient elevation of the platelet count in all patients. Its cost prohibits prolonged courses of treatment but it is useful for the preparation of thrombocytopenic patients for surgery. The mechanism of action appears to be reticuloendothelial system blockade. The same preparation has been shown to improve the neutrophil count in immune neutropenia and to reduce infective episodes in chronically immunosuppressed patients.

Antithrombin III concentrates

Deficiency of this circulating inhibitor of thrombin and other activated factors results in the development of recurrent venous thromboses. Inheritance is autosomal dominant and thrombotic events, often in unusual sites, usually occur in response to a challenge e.g. trauma, pregnancy or surgery. Affected individuals are usually maintained on long-term warfarin anticoagulation, but several antithrombin III concentrates are now available for prophylactic therapy in circumstances associated with a severe challenge e.g. elective surgery, labour.

Complications and hazards of blood transfusion

Febrile reactions

A non-haemolytic febrile transfusion reaction occurs in about 5–10 per cent of transfused patients, and these have various causes including antibodies to leucocyte or platelet antigens and sensitivity reactions to foreign proteins. Mild reactions can be prevented by an injection of chlorpheniramine (Piriton) at the beginning of the transfusion. Rarely severe reactions with chest pain and hypotension may occur and are an indication for termination of the transfusion as they are difficult to distinguish clinically from haemolytic transfusion reactions. In some sensitive patients, filtered blood can be used to prevent reactions to leucocyte antigens.

Haemolytic transfusion reactions

The severity of the reaction to incompatible transfusion is dependent on the antibodies and blood group antigens involved. If haemolysis is predominantly intravascular as in ABO incompatible transfusion, an immediate severe reaction commonly occurs, with rapidly developing fever, dyspnoea, intense headache, a feeling of constriction in the chest and often intense pain in the lumbar region. Hypotension and circulatory collapse may follow, as may disseminated intravascular coagulation, renal failure and finally jaundice. A transfusion of 100 ml or more has usually been given before the appearance of symptoms. In predominantly extravascular destruction, as with IgG antibodies, the reaction is less severe with chills and later jaundice. The cross-match procedure is designed to detect the antibodies responsible for most of these reactions: when reactions occur they are usually due to mislabelling of submitted blood samples or misidentification of patients. Transfusion of outdated blood or blood haemolysed by freezing, heating or infection can produce a similar haemolytic reaction. In the unconscious or anaesthetized patient these signs are easy to miss, unexplained hypotension and oozing from surgical wounds may be the only clues to a haemolytic reaction.

A delayed transfusion reaction may occur due to the development of significant levels of IgG antibody after the transfusion. The rising level of antibody leads to extravascular haemolysis a few days after the transfusion with unexplained jaundice and anaemia.

When a haemolytic transfusion reaction is suspected, the transfusion must be stopped immediately and saline or plasma infused as necessary. Artifical plasma expanders are contraindicated. The patient and blood pack identifications should be checked and the samples listed in Table 8.13 should be taken. These tests should confirm the presence of haemolysis. Subsequent management is determined by the severity with early support of renal function and replacement of labile coagulation factors important in the most severe cases.

Circulatory overload

The risks of cardiac failure and pulmonary oedema in elderly patients is reduced by the use of red cell concentrates rather than whole blood. Judicious use of diuretics is also helpful in such patients receiving transfusion.

Table 8.13 Response to suspected haemolytic transfusion reaction

- Stop transfusion. Replace with saline/plasma.
- Check patient and blood pack identification.
- Take the following samples:
  1. haemoglobin + platelet count
  2. heparinized blood for plasma haemoglobin, bilirubin, U + E, haptoglobin + methaemalbumin
  3. coagulation screen
  4. fibrinogen + FDP's
  5. clotted blood for direct antiglobulin test, blood group checking + antibody screen + cross-matching more blood if necessary.
- Return all blood packs + infusion sets to Blood Bank for investigation of donor blood group and antibody screen.
- Save the next specimen of urine to test for haemoglobin and microscopy.

Infection

Infected blood

Careful precautions are taken to prevent significant bacterial contamination of blood during collection. Blood that subsequently undergoes manipulation involving a breach of the closed pack system (e.g. filtered red cells) has a shelf-life of only 12 hours. No units should be left out of cold storage for longer than 30 minutes. The initial reaction to transfusion of contaminated blood may be indistinguishable from a severe haemolytic reaction. The diagnosis is confirmed by microscopy and culture.

Disease transmission

The diseases which may follow transfusion are listed in Table 8.14. Risks are reduced by using only normal healthy adults as donors. Donors who have been vaccinated with live virus within 3 months or jaundiced in the preceding year are deferred. So should donors who have recently travelled in a malarial area. All donations are tested for hepatitis B virus surface antigen (HBsAg), syphilis and antibodies to human immunodeficiency virus (HIV). The risk of disease transmission by blood must be borne in mind when labelling specimens for laboratory analysis. The relative infectivity of these agents is indicated by the incidence of disease following needle-prick injury etc.

Table 8.14   Disease transmitted by transfusion of blood or blood products

Viral infections	Bacterial infections	Parasitic infections
Hepatitis B	Syphilis	Malaria
Hepatitis A	Brucellosis	Chaga's disease
Non A, non B hepatitis	Rickettsial infection	Toxoplasmosis
Cytomegalovirus		Kala-azar
Epstein–Barr virus		African trypanosomiasis
Parvovirus		
Human immuno- deficiency virus (HIV)		

Hepatitis

Screening of all blood donors for HBsAg has dramatically reduced the incidence of post-transfusion hepatitis due to hepatitis B virus. This was previously the most important cause of transfusion associated infection. Total elimination has unfortunately not occurred as undetectable levels of antigen may occur after acute infection or in a few chronic carriers. The HBsAg is usually produced in large quantities during active infection and provides a useful and reliable marker of infective blood by radio-immunoassay or passive haemagglutination. During the evolution of the disease the HBsAg and other virus particles: core antigen (HBcAg) and the e antigen are initially found in the blood. As the infection is terminated, the corresponding antibodies take their place. About 5 per cent of infected individuals become chronic carriers and approximately 1 in 500 new blood donors are positive. Positive donors are further investigated by testing for HBcAg, HBeAg and antibodies to these particles. The presence of HBeAg suggests high infectivity because it is associated with the presence of the whole virus (Dane particle), whilst the presence of anti-HBe is associated with the convalescent state, chronic hepatitis or persistant carrier status.

Positive donors are excluded from further donation and their antigen and antibody status is monitored. Those who develop antibodies may be useful for the production of specific immuno-globulins.

Hepatitis A is an uncommon cause of post-transfusion hepatitis. It is generally a milder disease with a shorter incubation time and differentiation is easy by antibody studies.

Most cases of post-transfusion hepatitis are now thought to be due to the so called non-A, non-B virus or group of viruses. This condition has a variable incubation period of 2 weeks to 4 months and is not exclusively a transfusion-associated infection: indeed the majority of cases do not follow transfusion. Most patients do not become jaundiced, and most cases are subclinical with transient elevation of transaminases (transaminitis). The reported incidence following transfusion has ranged from 4–18 per cent according to the socio-economic background of donors and recipients. Some cases of non A, non B posttransfusion hepatitis progress to chronic hepatitis and cirrhosis. This agent(s) is presumed to be responsible for the high incidence of hepatitis in haemophiliacs following treatment with factor VIII concentrate. Clearly the pooled nature of this product is responsible for the higher risk among these individuals. Prevention is solely by exclusion of donors with a history of jaundice or hepatitis since the causative virus(es) is unknown. Exclusion of donors on the basis of raised hepatic transaminases is deemed impractical by most authorities.

Cytomegalovirus (CMV)

The transmission of CMV by transfusion is of little consequence to most recipients. Subclinical infections probably occur in about 16 per cent of immunocompetent transfusion recipients. Transmission of the infection is due to transfusion of virus-containing leucocytes from a seropositive donor. The prevalance of CMV antibody in donors varies with age, sex and social class and there is a steady seroconversion in any CMV-negative donor panel. Immunosuppressed CMV negative individuals and premature neonates are at risk of post-transfusion CMV and some centres have established panels of seronegative donors for such patients. The infection rate in transplant recipients may be reduced by passive immunisation with CMV-immune globulin.

HIV – AIDS

The transmission of human immunodeficiency virus (HIV) and the subsequent development of acquired immunodeficiency syndrome (AIDS) following transfusion of blood and blood products from an infected donor is well recognized. The major group of recipients to experience this complication are haemophiliacs due to contamination of large pools of Factor VIII concentrate by a few infected donations. However, it is clear that a number of cases of infection have occurred as a result of transfusions of a single unit of blood from an infected donor. The response to this hazard has been the elimination of donations from individuals in high risk groups, i.e. homosexuals, bisexuals, intravenous drug abusers and the sexual partners of these individuals. In addition, since late 1985 all blood donations have been screened for the presence of antibody to HIV-1. An assay suitable for the routine detection of viral antigens is not yet available (an assay to detect viral nucleic acid may be a future possibility) and although HIV-1 virus isolation has been reported from antibody negative subjects, assays for antibody to HIV-1 are currently the only practical screening test for infective blood.

The speed with which useful tests have been developed has been impressive and has been due to collaboration between commercial organizations and major research groups. Two main types of antibody tests exist and have been designed to achieve the optimum balance of specificity and sensitivity i.e. to limit false positives without missing false negatives. One is an 'enzyme-linked anti-globulin test' using viral antigen absorbed onto a solid phase (e.g. petri dish) to 'fix' any antibody in the donor serum which is then detected by an enzyme labelled antibody to human immuno-globulin. This test is liable to give false positives if the donor's serum contains HLA antibodies as HLA antigens are absorbed into the virus coat during tissue culture. The second assay is a 'competitive assay' which again uses solid phase absorbed viral antigen but is more specific as antibody in the donor serum must compete for binding with enzyme labelled specific anti-HIV-1. A positive test must be confirmed by a further technique and this is usually carried out by a Western blot assay. Positive blood donations must not be used and the donors must be counselled. The presence of antibody to HIV-1 is an indication of previous exposure to the virus which then may become latent in the host's CD4 lymphocytes. At the time of writing, it is estimated that 25–50 per cent of people infected with HIV-1 will develop AIDS. In a screening programme carried out recently by the National Blood Transfusion Service in the UK only 4 of more than 3 million donations were found to be positive in individuals who denied being in a high risk group. Thus the risk of infection follow-ing blood transfusion is extremely low, and screening of donors is reducing it even further. However, it seems prudent not to use unscreened 'emergency donors' and special donor panels for neonatal units and cell separator units must be screened if they are to be safe.

The discovery of another virus (HIV-2) in West Africa which is associated with an AIDS-like disease and is antigenically distinct from HIV-1 i.e. does not cross-react with anti-HIV-1 antibodies, presents a new problem as screening donors for antibodies to HIV-1 will not detect individuals infected with this agent. This virus has been detected in Europe among individuals of West African origin but whether it represents an infective hazard on the scale of HIV-1 is not yet clear. Interestingly, the virus appears more closely related to a simian immunodeficiency virus (SIV) which causes an AIDS-like disease in monkeys, suggesting that the theory that these viruses originate from simian hosts in Africa may well be correct. It is possible that the development of a screening test for viral DNA may detect both viruses as there is some homology in the more conserved genes of HIV-1 and HIV-2.

The risk of transfusion-associated HIV-1 infection has been greatest following transfusion of blood products pooled from many thousands of donations, most notably factor VIII concentrate. A further approach introduced to reduce the risk of infection is that these products are now heat-treated to 80°C for 72 hours. This eliminates HIV but unfortunately not non A or non B hepatitis.

The risk to health-workers appears to be extremely low. Only a small proportion of cases of 'needle-stick' injuries have resulted in sero-conversion which suggests that the agent is of low infectivity compared to hepatitis B virus. Nevertheless, all venepunctures, blood sample submissions, and manipulations involving body fluids should be performed with an awareness that the fluid concerned is a potentially lethal health hazard.

Complications from massive transfusion

Transfusion of large volumes of stored red cells as occurs routinely during cardiac surgery or unpredictably in patients with uncontrolled haemorrhage requires special additional measures. Even whole blood becomes progressively depleted of coagulation factors and platelets on storage at 4°C. This is clearly much more certain when these components have been removed and replaced by optimal additive solutions. Thus transfusion with large volumes of stored red cells results in dilution of circulating platelets and coagulation factors (most notably the labile factors V and VIII) in addition to the loss of these components with continuing haemorrhage. Hence replacement of these components with platelet concentrates and fresh frozen plasma should be considered in any patient who rapidly receives 6 to 10 units of red cells. The requirement for each of these components should be monitored by performing a platelet count and coagulation screen. An ongoing requirement for transfusion requires careful monitoring. This is preferable to a rule of thumb approach such as giving 1 unit of platelets and 1 unit of FFP with every 4 units of red cells after the first 6 units.

Metabolic effects are complex as the acidity of stored blood may cause an acidosis whereas the citrate anticoagulant may cause an alkalosis. Rarely does significant hyperkalaemia occur due to leakage from stored cells. The infused citrate may produce a fall in ionized calcium resulting in tetany and occasionally in arrhythmias. This is avoided by the intravenous administration of 10 ml 10 % calcium gluconate with every 1 litre of red cells infused rapidly. When large volumes of cold blood are transfused it is easy to 'chill' a patient and this can also result in arrhythmias. The use of regularly serviced blood warmers is advisable under these circumstances.

A fall in the concentration of 2,3 DPG in stored red cells results in a high oxygen affinity. In theory, this will impair oxygen delivery to the tissues, however it has proved difficult to demonstrate a detrimental effect from transfusion of 2,3 DPG depleted cells. Whilst it is probably prudent to use relatively fresh blood if massive transfusions are to be given, this often proves difficult in practice.

Finally, it must be emphasized that the emergence of HIV has ensured that, at last, blood transfusion is being taken seriously by doctors as a procedure not without risk. All anaesthetists must ensure that they have a basic grasp of the significance of transfusing blood and its derivatives to the unsuspecting or unconscious patient.

Further reading

Boral, L.I. (1979). A guideline for anticipated blood usage during elective surgical procedures. *American Journal of Clinical Pathology* **71**, 680–84.

Collins, J.A. (1983). Pertinent recent developments in blood bank. *Surgical Clinics of North America* **63**, 483–95.

Kay, L.A. and Huehns, E.R. (1985). *Clinical Blood Transfusion*. Pitman Publishing, London.

Mollison, P.L. (1983). *Blood Transfusion in Clinical Medicine*. Seventh Edition. Blackwell Scientific Publications, Oxford.

Petricciani, J.C., Gust, I.D., Hopp, P.A. and Krijnen. (1987). *AIDS: The Safety of Blood and Blood Products*. John Wiley, London.

Race, R.R. and Sanger, R. (1975). *Blood Groups in Man*. Sixth Edition. Blackwell Scientific Publications, Oxford.

Singer, C.R.J. and Goldstone, A.H. (1985). Recent advances in blood transfusion and blood products I and II. In: *Anaesthesia Review 3*, pp. 156–82. Edited by Kaufman, L. Churchill Livingstone, Edinburgh.

9

Gastrointestinal and Liver Disorders

Ian McNeil

Introduction

Gastroenterology has been transformed in the past 10–15 years with the development of the fibreoptic endoscope, which has enabled direct visual examination of the upper and lower gastrointestinal tract to become a routine procedure. Pancreatic and biliary structure can be examined endoscopically to facilitate diagnosis. Therapeutic endoscopy has become generally available with respect to the management of oesophageal strictures and varices, and in particular to biliary tract disease, contributing greatly to the quality of life and life expectancy of many patients. Polypectomy in the colon has become the treatment of choice for small and medium size polyps: the effects of this on the incidence and prognosis of colonic cancer may become apparent.

The pharmacology of some gastrointestinal disorders has also advanced rapidly. This is particularly true of peptic ulcer disease where a variety of effective agents are available and more are being developed. These new modes of therapy have had a profound effect on the need for gastric surgery. Advances in the knowledge of the physiology and pathophysiology of the gastrointestinal tract offers hope of further improvements in therapy.

Nevertheless, the increasing prevalence of some diseases (e.g. colonic carcinoma) invites particular concern. Prevention may be progressively more important in this and the other 'Diseases of Western Civilization' that involve the gastroenterologist. The introduction of a cheap hepatitis B vaccine world-wide may have profound effects for the health of people in the Third World.

The oesophagus

The cardinal symptoms of oesophageal disease are pain and dysphagia. The commonest pain is heartburn; others include spasm, that can produce symptoms almost inseparable from ischaemic cardiac pain, and impact pain (odynophagia).

Reflux oesophagitis

After a heavy meal there is often gastro-oesophageal reflux associated with burning retrosternal discomfort; however, in a substantial minority of the population symptoms occur frequently and with much less provocation.

Squamous epithelium is sensitive to the reflux of gastric acid and pepsin, resulting in inflammation oesophagitis. Oesophagitis can also occur after a total gastrectomy: bile and trypsin are likely to be further corrosive agents.

The presence of acid in the oesophagus has several determinants. The resting tone of the lower oesophageal sphincter and the effect of abdominal pressure in keeping the intra-abdominal oesophagus closed will generally prevent reflux. The efficacy of peristalsis will moderate how rapidly refluxed acid is cleared into the stomach. Reflux depends on derangement in the anatomical barrier and physiological and pharmacological effects on the lower oesophageal sphincter. Sphincter tone is reduced by chocolate, fatty foods and smoking and by anticholinergic drugs, particularly atropine, and raised by gastrin and metoclopramide. With a sliding hiatus hernia, some anatomical reasons for preventing reflux are lost. However, lower oesophageal sphincter tone can still prevent reflux in hese patients and this is well demonstrated clinically by a poor correlation between the presence of a hiatus hernia and reflux oesophagitis. Acid clearance by peristalsis can be reduced in a variety of diseases, including achalasia.

In reflux oesophagitis the typical symptom is heartburn, often with acid regurgitation to the throat and mouth, which is worse lying down or bending forward. The pain lacks the periodicity of peptic ulceration, symptoms often being present daily for many years; meals may promote a bout of symptoms.

Diagnosis is principally based on the history. Severe oesophagitis may produce chronic, or rarely acute, blood loss. Barium swallow and meal, particularly in the head-down position may demonstrate reflux. Endoscopy will show both reflux and friable red mucosa which can be confirmed histologically as oesophagitis. A Bernstein test may be performed, or the more recent alternative, placing a pH electrode in the lumen of the lower oesophagus and recording luminal pH and symptoms over 24-hour periods.

Treatment

Medical management includes general measures such as weight reduction, avoiding tight clothing, attention to posture and elevating the head of the bed. Careful selection of meals is helpful and surprisingly infrequently advised. Antacids are effective in most patients and taken when symptoms arise, especially immediately after meals and on going to bed. Current preparations often include an alginate that promotes the formation of an antacid raft over the gastric contents, so that the antacid raft is likely to be refluxed rather than acid.

A course of H_2 receptor antagonist may be necessary if symptoms are severe, allowing antacids to become effective again. Often the H_2 receptor antagonists are used only at night. Finally, metoclopramide promotes gastric emptying, increases acid clearance from the oesophagus and increases lower oesophageal sphincter tone. Surgery is rarely indicated for oesophagitis except when it is associated with hiatus hernia.

Hiatus hernia

A hiatus hernia is a common finding during both barium examinations and endoscopy and generally is of the sliding type.

Symptoms are generally due to associated complications, particularly gastro-oesophageal reflux. A sensation of fullness or early satiety occurs. Prior to the wide-spread introduction of endoscopy, hiatus hernia was often considered the source of occult gastrointestinal blood loss. Endoscopy has recognized the relative infrequency of this complication by finding previously unidentified ulcers, oesophagitis etc., as the source of blood loss.

A particular complication of paraoesophageal or rolling hiatus hernia is gastric torsion producing strangulation or volvulus. This will present as severe chest and epigastric pain and may be readily mistaken for cardiac pain.

Diagnosis is based on history, by finding a retrocardiac fluid level on chest X-ray or by barium swallow and meal. Early investigations should be made as these complications are an indication for early surgical intervention.

In general, treatment of hiatus hernia depends upon symptoms. Sliding hiatus hernia per se requires no treatment and many physicians would not mention its presence to a patient. Reflux oesophagitis should be treated as above. Surgery is indicated in under 5 per cent of patients. Indications include potential torsion or volvulus, persisting symptoms despite careful prolonged medical management of reflux oesophagitis and perhaps troublesome peptic stricture of the oesophagus. Typically some form of hernia reduction with fundoplication and repair of the hiatus is undertaken. More recently a silastic ring has been placed round the lower oesophagus. This, called the Angelchick prosthesis, seems to prevent reflux effectively and improve oesophagitis in selected patients. Its exact mechanism of action is unclear.

Peptic stricture

Recurrent peptic ulceration with subsequent fibrosis will eventually produce a stricture which usually occurs at the junction of squamous and columnar epithelium. The development of stricture will produce slowly progressive dysphagia (Table 9.1).

Barium swallow is the investigation of choice. Subsequently endoscopy should be carried out; this allows biopsy and cytology specimens to be taken before dilatation.

Currently most benign strictures are dilated under diazepam sedation. Perforation is an occasional complication but fortunately this usually

Table 9.1 A comparison of malignant and benign oesophageal strictures

	Malignant	Benign
Symptoms	Little or no indigestion	Long history of heartburn
	Sudden start to dysphagia that progresses rapidly, Weight loss, Odynophagia	Dysphagia of gradual onset that may vary in severity
Radiology	Irregular long stricture with shouldering	Smooth narrowing often short
Endoscopy	Normal oesophagus, often pushed up over pale, friable masses of tumour	Smooth stricture, often with inflammation

responds to conservative management. Surgery for strictures is rarely indicated, particularly now endoscopic dilatation is widely available and is a relatively uncomplicated procedure for even the frailest elderly patient.

Barrett's oesophagus

In this rare condition the lower oesophagus is lined with columnar (gastric) and not squamous epithelium. This may be a congenital anomaly or progressive replacement of damaged squamous epithelium by relatively acid-resistant columnar epithelium. Clinically the patient suffers from heartburn and later dysphagia. Investigations may show a high stricture with an oesophageal ulcer, typically occurring in the gastric type mucosa. Endoscopy will reveal the change in mucosa from squamous to columnar. Treatment is the same as for reflux oesophagitis and peptic stricture but in the presence of an ulcer, H_2 receptor antagonists should be given in full dose for at least 6 weeks. It is believed that adenocarcinoma occurs more frequently in patients with Barrett's oesophagus and this is considered an indication for endoscopic follow-up.

Carcinoma of the oesophagus

Primary carcinoma of the oesophagus is usually of the squamous type. The lower oesophagus can be involved by adenocarcinoma arising in the fundus which produces symptoms of dysphagia similar to squamous carcinoma.

The aetiology of oesophageal carcinoma is unknown. Smoking and alcohol abuse are associated with the disease. There is a striking geographical variation with the incidence in areas of Asia and Africa being up to 50 times greater than that in Britain: dietary carcinogens must also play a role. Other risk factors include hereditary tylosis, the Plummer–Vinson syndrome, achalasia and Barrett's oesophagus.

Men are affected twice as frequently as women with most lesions being in the middle and lower thirds of the oesophagus. Dysphagia is the principal symptom (*see* Table 9.1). Inhalation of oesophageal contents or bleeding are less common presenting complaints. Physical signs include lymph node enlargement in the neck or evidence of recurrent laryngeal nerve palsy. Lesions of the upper third of the oesophagus are divided more equally between women and men and in some are associated with the Plummer–Vinson syndrome.

The diagnosis is generally made by barium swallow followed by endoscopy with biopsy and brush cytology. Assessment of spread in order to plan treatment includes abdominal ultrasound for liver metastases and thoracic CT scanning to determine local involvement.

Treatment depends upon the extent of the carcinoma at presentation. Although curative surgery is ideal, the illness has already passed beyond this stage in many patients, and treatment can only be palliative. Nutritional support is particularly important for carcinoma of the oesophagus in view of the rapid weight loss. Opportunities for passing a small bore enteral feeding tube or commencing total parenteral nutrition should be taken whenever possible so that the patient is in optimal condition for whatever mode of treatment is planned.

Extensive surgery may be required for carcinoma of the lower and middle third of oesophagus as the tumour tends to spread longitudinally. The stomach is mobilized and anastomosis made to the remaining oesophagus in the chest or neck. Colonic or jejunal transposition is rarely required.

Palliation will depend on the techniques available locally and on the site and extent of the tumour. More than one method may be combined to achieve better results. In some series radiotherapy has proved as effective as 'curative surgery', and is the treatment of choice for upper third tumours. In the early stages however, there is often considerable swelling of the tumour and placing a naso-jejunal fine-bore feeding tube before treatment enables nutrition to continue. Surgical palliation of lower and middle third carcinomas is similar to curative excisions. The blind ends of the involved length are oversewn but no attempt is made to excise the malignancy.

Celestin tubes can be placed through the oesophageal carcinoma. This is usually done endoscopically after dilatation but can also be done under anaesthesia when an exploratory laparotomy has shown the tumour to be widespread. Other endoscopic techniques that are being evaluated involve tumour destruction by laser or diathermy to provide a lumen for swallowing.

The prognosis is poor. Overall survival is under 10 per cent at 5 years. Surgery has a high mortality – 10–20 per cent – and only improves 5-year survival by 10–20 per cent.

Achalasia

Though uncommon this is the most frequently encountered disorder of oesophageal motility. The cause is not known but the illness is primarily a denervation of the smooth musculature of the lower two-thirds of the gullet. The result is failure of relaxation of the lower oesophageal sphincter with impaired peristalsis above. Oesophageal manometry shows pressure in the lower sphincter to be increased two to three-fold, with only partial relaxation at best following a swallow. The response of the lower sphincter to gastrin is exaggerated and cholinergic drugs produce a great increase in pressure with uncoordinated or absent relaxation and even pain. Manometry of the lower third of the oesophagus shows failure of peristalsis and tertiary contractions.

Achalasia occurs at all ages. The characteristic symptom is dysphagia. Liquids may be as troublesome as solids, with several years intermittent difficulty, often exaggerated by stress. Gradually the dysphagia worsens and becomes permanent. Pain from oesophageal spasm can occur at any stage. Weight loss occurs late in the disease. The oesophagus becomes dilated leading to regurgitation of undigested food without acid or bile. Inhalation may occur leading to bouts of coughing especially at night time and resulting ultimately in pulmonary fibrosis.

The diagnosis is usually made radiologically. A dilated oesophagus may show on chest X-ray, and barium studies will show a widened oesophagus containing food, poor peristalsis and a smoothly tapering sphincter which opens irregularly. The indication for endoscopy is concern about invasion of the lower sphincter by a carcinoma of the stomach. Oesophageal manometry remains the ultimate diagnostic method and may be needed in the early case, particularly if chest pain is a troublesome feature.

Medical treatment is unhelpful. Though various nitrates and nifedipine will lower sphincter pressure experimentally they tend to be of little practical value. Dilatation, as practised for a stricture, is of short-term benefit only. Forcible pneumatic rupture of the lower oesophageal sphincter is one approach that can be repeated as necessary. The alternative is surgical division of the muscle coat down to the mucosa over the sphincter zone (Heller's cardiomyotomy). Cardiomyotomy is frequently complicated by reflux and peptic stricturing so the operation is generally combined with an anti-reflux procedure.

The dysphagia is relieved in about 80 per cent of patients by either method. However, muscular tone never returns and each patient should be advised about eating late at night so that pulmonary spillage does not occur. The incidence of carcinoma is increased, and typically occurs in a dilated oesophagus, so dysphagia develops long after any prospect of curative treatment.

Diffuse oesophageal spasm

This motor abnormality of unknown aetiology presents with chest pain and intermittent episodes of dysphagia. Non-propulsive contractions that may be abnormally powerful occur spontaneously, often diffusely through the lower two-thirds of the oesophagus or are brought on by swallowing.

Difficulty occurs in separating this condition from cardiac anginal pain, particularly when the pain starts at times other than meals. The pain lasts up to an hour, may radiate to the arms or neck and be relieved by glyceryl trinitrate. Dysphagia is very inconstant and often worse in stressful situations. Radiology may be normal but the typical appearance is of an irregularly contracting 'corkscrew' oesophagus. Manometry again provides the diagnosis, particularly in those patients with normal radiology.

Careful explanation and reassurance is the first stage in treatment. Any tendency to reflux oesophagitis should be treated vigorously. Glyceryl trinitrate (GTN) or nifedipine may be tried and are beneficial in some patients. Balloon dilatation of the affected lengths of the oesophagus is employed for moderate to severe cases, and in a few patients myotomy has been tried.

Other oesophageal conditions

Diverticula

Oesophageal diverticula are generally of no consequence.

Plummer–Vinson syndrome

The concurrence of an upper oesophageal web with iron deficiency anaemia produces intermittent dysphagia. Treatment consists of rupturing the web at endoscopy.

Scleroderma

Scleroderma affects the oesophagus producing firstly a loss of peristalsis as the muscle coat is replaced by fibrous tissue and secondly, the loss of lower sphincter tone. Reflux with subsequent stricturing is frequent and troublesome. Dysphagia is very common both before and after a stricture develops. The barium swallow is diagnostic. Treatment is aimed at preventing damaging reflux oesophagitis.

Monilia

This is the commonest oesophageal infection, producing dysphagia, pain and anorexia with tell-tale signs of monilia in the pharynx of debilitated patients. Severe disease with ulceration and haemorrhage may occur. Treatment is usually with nystatin.

Chemical injury and stricture

Accidental consumption of strong caustic solutions is the classic cause. Recently, attention has been paid to early treatment of caustic injury with milk, demulcents and then mild antacids in an attempt to reduce stricturing. Patients with an established stricture have often learnt to dilate them at home, but present from time to time at hospital with bolus obstruction. This can be relieved endoscopically. Oesophageal ulceration can result from pharmaceutical agents including emepronium bromide for urinary problems, tetracycline as well as aspirin and non-steroidal anti-inflammatory agents.

Perforation

Spontaneous rupture in vomiting bouts (Boerhaave's syndrome) occurs but the increase in diagnostic and particularly therapeutic endoscopy has resulted in iatrogenic performations becoming commoner. Chest pain is the most important feature and diagnosis may be aided by fever or signs of a pneumothorax. Abnormal appearances on a chest X-ray include air in the pleural cavity, mediastinum, or the upper abdomen. Early diagnosis and treatment are vital. Conservative treatment involves broad spectrum anti-biotics with total parenteral nutrition. Nasogastric drainage is less important. Early surgery is probably equally effective. The importance of early diagnosis is shown by recent series demonstrating no mortality if treatment was started within 24 hours but this was increased to 50 per cent when treatment was delayed.

Stomach and duodenum

Many recent advances have been made in gastric physiology. Firstly, gastric emptying can now be examined by a series of techniques enabling physiological controls to be explored. Contractions of the stomach are regular and pass into and through the pylorus, particularly after eating. Nausea and vomiting are associated with impaired contractions and also some reflux through the pylorus from duodenum to stomach. This reverse reflux is known to occur at other times and bile is felt to be one of the ulcerogenic factors and may contribute to oesophagitis.

A series of important causes of delayed gastric emptying have now been clearly established including pain, particularly from abdominal inflammation, and immobilization as well as a variety of metabolic and electrolyte disturbances which are complicated by gastric retention and even acute dilatation. Finally a variety of drugs reduce gastric emptying including opioids, atropine and ganglion-blockers. Patients with diabetes are prone to develop gastroparesis. Some anti-emetics, e.g. metoclopramide and domperidone, increase gastric emptying and use is being assessed in this complication of diabetes.

Secondly, gastric secretory physiology is better

understood. The mechanisms involved include neural control via acetyl-choline, gastrin release in both cephalic and gastric phases of secretion, as well as histamine. Hydrogen ion is secreted by an ATPase whose isolation has opened up a new pharmalogical area and omeprazole has been developed as a specific inhibitor of the H^+/K^+ ATPase.

How the mucosa protects itself against acid has also been better characterized. Secretion of bicarbonate by the mucosal surface of stomach and duodenum has been measured. The ability of mucus to limit hydrogen ion diffusion enables the mucus-bicarbonate layer to reduce exposure of the gastric surface to damaging low pH. The maintenance of the mucus-bicarbonate layer depends on several factors including prostaglandins which are also able to speed mucosal healing of breeches in the columnar cell layer, these various actions being known as cytoprotection.

Peptic ulceration

Peptic ulceration is declining in incidence in the UK. Although the aetiology is unknown, peptic ulceration is related to a break-down of the balance between acid and pepsin production and mucosal protection or resistance. Acid secretion rates in duodenal ulcers are normal or high, but in gastric ulcer low or normal. Duodenal ulceration may represent an increased acid output overcoming a normal mucosal resistance, whereas in gastric ulcers the major component may be breakdown of mucosal resistance in the presence of normal or reduced acid production.

Factors that are known to contribute to peptic ulcer include male sex, family history and diet, with dietary fibre and milk being protective. Smoking seems to be a risk factor for developing duodenal ulceration though it is well recognized as being an inhibitory factor in the healing of peptic ulcers. The relationship to drugs is more complex. Corticosteroids have still not been proven to be ulcerogenic. However, non-steroidal anti-inflammatory agents seem to be related to gastric ulceration, possibly because they alter prostaglandin metabolism. Alcohol seems to be damaging in the short term but there is no evidence in the long term that it is harmful. Many patients with chronic obstructive airways disease have ulcers or have had operations for peptic ulcers. Furthermore they tend to have recurrent or poorly healing gastric ulcers, though this may relate to continued smoking rather than the patient's obstructive airways disease.

In duodenal ulcer the pain is felt in the epigastrium and related to meals, typically between 30 and 120 minutes after meals. The pain is frequently relieved by milk, antacids or a further meal. Awakening with pain in the early hours of the morning is an important symptom. Radiation to the right upper quadrant or the back occurs. In common with gastric ulceration there is usually a periodicity in symptoms, with episodes every few months which last for perhaps 2–3 months before settling. The frequency of recurrences varies greatly from patient to patient. Physical signs are remarkably few, some people having a little tenderness in the epigastrium or right upper quandrant of the abdomen.

In gastric ulceration, the patient is often elderly rather than the young man with a duodenal ulcer. Again the pain is related to meals: however it tends to occur during a meal or soon after a meal. Vomiting is a more frequent symptom which may produce pain relief. Anorexia is more common and weight loss much more frequent. Examination may reveal epigastric tenderness.

Investigations should include a blood count for anaemia. However the investigation of choice lies between a double contrast barium meal and endoscopy. The choice of investigation is less important in duodenal ulceration though endoscopy is probably more accurate, particularly if the duodenal bulb is scarred and distorted by past ulceration. In gastric ulceration, the question of malignancy is important. Malignant gastric ulcers may produce similar symptoms to benign lesions and under these circumstances it is most important for endoscopy to be carried out. Only by doing biopsies and brush cytology at endoscopy is there any chance of finding early gastric cancer which is discussed below.

The relationship between benign gastric ulceration and subsequent development of gastric carcinoma is not completely clear.

The aims of treatment are firstly to relieve the patient's symptoms, secondly to heal the ulcer and thirdly to try and break the cycle of remission and relapse. Some general measures that are employed include diet. There is no evidence that special diets are of any particular benefit other than providing a degree of symptomatic relief. However stopping smoking is important as smoking hinders ulcer healing. Finally, it is important to check that no remedial factor is present, particularly in relation to non-steroidal anti-inflammatory drugs.

Various agents have been used in the treatment of peptic ulcer (Table 9.2). Antacids are usually a

Table 9.2   Treatments for peptic ulceration

Antacids	May be curative in high and medium doses. Important for symptomatic relief	
H₂ receptor antagonists	Cimetidine Ranitidine Famotidine Nizatidine	Divided or single night time dose
Surface acting agents	Sucralfate	Anti-pepsin and binding to exposed surfaces
	Bismuth chelate	May inhibit *Campylobacter pylori*
Anticholinergic agents	Pirenzepine	Side-effects of glaucoma, urinary retention etc encountered
Liquorice derivatives	Carbenoxolone	For gastric ulceration. Mineralocorticoid side-effects very common

mixture of magnesium and aluminium salts but occasionally indications exist for these salts to be given separately. Calcium antacids are available, frequently over the chemist's counter but they are not to be recommended as calcium elevates gastrin levels and therefore promotes increased gastric secretion.

Specific ulcer healing drugs are now available with various modes of action. Four histamine H₂ receptor antagonists are currently available while others are being developed. Cimetidine is now being used so frequently world-wide that its side-effects are well established, including alterations in liver function tests and hepatic drug metabolism, and gynaecomastia. Ranitidine seems to have slightly fewer side-effects.

The next category is the surface acting agents which comprise sucralfate and tri-potassium dicitrato bismuthate. Side-effects do occur, particularly after the bismuthate with black tongue and black stools being features. The fourth category is anti-cholinergic agents. Pirenzepine seems currently to be the most effective because it is moderately specific for gastric muscarinic receptors.

Two new groups of anti-ulcer agents are currently undergoing clinical trials. A series of sub-stituted prostaglandins is now available derived from prostaglandin E₁ or E₂. Ulcer healing tends to occur at higher doses than cytoprotective effects and is related to inhibition of acid secretion. Diarrhoea is likely to be a troublesome side-effect. Omeprazole, the H⁺/K⁺ ATPase inhibitor is also at the trial stage. It is a very potent inhibitor of acid secretion in the recommended doses and will produce almost absolute inhibition of gastric acid secretion.

For treatment of active duodenal ulceration there is a wide choice. Pirenzepine, one of the surface acting agents or an H₂ receptor antagonist will heal about 80 per cent of ulcers in 4 weeks, compared with 40–50 per cent healing over the same period with placebo treatment. The natural history of duodenal ulcer is one of a slowly settling lesion over a few weeks with spontaneous healing. About 20 per cent do not heal in the initial period with the first chosen agent. As this is mostly likely to have been an H₂ receptor antagonist, the options are to increase the dose or change the treatment to one of the surface acting agents. There seems to be a progressive healing of duodenal ulcers under either option.

Gastric ulcers tend to be more difficult to treat. It is likely that prolonged treatment with H₂ receptor antagonist will slowly heal gastric ulcers, but the results are much less absolute than they are for duodenal ulcers. The other agents are probably also effective, including carbonoxolone. Many physicians find that they need to treat people with gastric ulcers for several months and may change the treatment two or three times in this period.

With effective treatment for duodenal ulceration it was soon realized that a proportion of healed ulcers quickly relapsed when treatment was stopped. Maintenance treatment for these patients was developed, particularly as asymptomatic recurrence could be found at follow-up endoscopy. Currently maintenance treatment would be used in patients whose ulcer has quickly recurred after treatment or who have only short periods between recurrences. Low dose nocturnal H₂ receptor antagonists are usually used. In recent trials bismuth chelate (DeNol) reduced the recurrence rate when compared with H₂ receptor antagonists.

The indications for surgery are changing and include firstly failed medical treatment. The development of a complication of peptic ulceration is a very frequent indication for surgery and these are discussed below. A further indication is the difficult gastric ulcer, a category that embraces

Table 9.3   Consequences of gastric surgery

Recurrent ulceration
Postvagotomy diarrhoea (with steatorrhea)
Bilious vomiting
Anaemia (iron and B_{12} deficiency)
Osteomalacia
Dumping
Early satiety and vomiting
Weight loss

the poorly healing gastric ulcer and also those patients in whom fear or concern about malignancy exists. Since the introduction of the more effective forms of treatment of peptic ulceration, the numbers of patients coming to operation have fallen. A wider range of operation is employed including highly selective vagotomy, now the operation of choice for uncomplicated duodenal ulceration in many centres. Vagotomy and pyloroplasty is also frequently performed. However for gastric ulceration the preferred treatment is partial gastrectomy.

Peptic ulcer surgery is associated with a series of adverse effects (Table 9.3). Recurrent ulcer occurs in up to 10 per cent of patients after operations for duodenal ulcer but much less frequently following gastric ulceration. Diarrhoea, although generally mild, and steatorrhoea occur frequently after vagotomy. Bilious vomiting can be a difficult problem in patients who have had a gastroentrostomy or pyloroplasty. Reconstructive surgery for this complication may be necessary.

Dumping, which is an unpleasant sensation of sweating, dizziness, faintness and perhaps sleepiness after a meal may be followed by vomiting. Dumping can be helped by taking small meals, not drinking at the same time as eating and resting for a period after a meal. Dumping tends to settle gradually in most patients, though rarely some form of reconstruction is required.

Complications of peptic ulceration

Perforation   The typical symptoms of perforation usually arise from an anterior duodenal ulcer, and consist of the sudden onset of upper abdominal pain which spreads throughout the abdomen, with the signs of rigidity, tenderness and absent bowel sounds. Prior to perforation there may have been an increase in peptic ulcer symptoms, though pain-free ulcers are known to perforate. There seems to be a recent increase in perforation of gastric ulcers which may be related to non-steroidal anti-inflammatory drug consumption. Perforation is confirmed by the X-ray finding of a pneumoperitoneum. The pain may restrict breathing leading to pulmonary collapse.

Patients should be adequately resuscitated prior to operation: surgical closure or repair of the perforation and peritoneal toilet remains the mainstay of treatment. Medical treatment consisting of nasogastric suction, antibiotics and intravenous fluids and feeding, has been used in some centres and also in those unfit for surgery.

Penetration   Erosion of an ulcer outside the gastrointestinal wall with involvement of adjacent tissues is the retroperitoneal equivalent of perforation. Symptoms include radiation of pain to the back and loss of the typical periodicity of ulcer pain after food. Development of resistance to treatment which the patient previously found a relief, such as antacids, should lead to suspicion of penetration. The pancreas is commonly invaded, though omentum and liver, can also be involved. Treatment is usually surgical as the complication is considered to be a failure of medical treatment. The diagnosis may be difficult to confirm without surgery.

Pyloric stenosis   This complication is less frequently encountered than perforation or haemorrhage. Peptic ulceration or, less frequently, carcinoma of the stomach are the usual causes. In peptic disease there is often a long history of relapse and remission of the ulcer and then vomiting, anorexia and weight loss may occur. Stenosis is generally caused by duodenal ulceration and rarely by antropyloric gastric ulceration. Physical examination shows a dehydrated patient with some evidence of malnutrition. A succussion splash and occasionally visible peristalsis may be present.

Metabolic changes can be profound. Dehydration will be manifest by a raised blood urea. Hypokalaemia, hypochloraemia and alkalosis are frequent and eventually hyponatraemia may also occur. Anaemia and hypoproteinaemia occur in 25 per cent of patients with this complication.

A barium meal shows a large food and fluid filled stomach. Passage of barium into the duodenum is impaired or absent. Endoscopy may be hazardous as gastric contents may be regurgitated and inhaled. However after a period of nasogastric wash-out endoscopy can be performed to ensure that there is no malignant involvement of the pylorus.

Treatment is essentially surgical after correcting the electrolyte and possibly nutritional disturbances. Commonly a patient will have been started on an intravenous H_2 receptor antagonist at diagnosis. Endoscopic balloon dilatation is being considered as an alternative to surgery.

Acute upper gastrointestinal haemorrhage This section will discuss the causes and management of this common problem, of which peptic ulceration is only the commonest of many causes. Upper gastrointestinal bleeding remains a major cause of hospital admissions with a seasonal variation, being most commonly encountered in Spring and Autumn. Overall mortality has not fallen and remains at about 10 per cent. This is felt to reflect the increasingly aged population that presents with this complaint and the fact that many patients have another illness that impairs their recovery. Several recent studies have shown an increased consumption of non-steroidal anti-inflammatory drugs in patients with haematemesis or melaena when compared with a matched control population.

The commonest cause of acute upper gastrointestinal bleeding remains peptic ulceration, which accounts for over 50 per cent of the total. Other lesions which account for about 5–10 per cent include oesophagitis with oesophageal ulcer and the Mallory–Weiss tear. Varices probably contribute under 5 per cent in the UK but there is a considerable geographical variation in their frequency. Malignancy of the stomach (and rarely of the oesophagus) contributes about 3 per cent.

Making a diagnosis from the history is notoriously difficult. Physical examination may show features of chronic liver disease or gastric malignancy. However, the history may enable some prognostic features to be evaluated. There is evidence that vomiting coffee grounds without fresh blood or passing melaena without vomiting fresh or altered blood are associated with an improved prognosis. Adverse prognostic features of importance include clinical anaemia, hypotension with systolic BP under 100 mmHg, tachycardia over 100/min as well as being aged over 60. The general fitness of the patient is a major influence on the outcome.

Endoscopy has become the investigation of choice for determining the source of bleeding as it will generally enable the bleeding lesion to be identified. Endoscopy will also ascertain whether bleeding is continuing, and provide an opportunity for endoscopic treatment. Skilled endoscopists should perform these examinations and most gastroenterologists feel that the endoscopy should take place within 24 hours of admission.

A major problem is recognizing the sub-group of patients who are likely to re-bleed. As well as a history of vomiting red blood or vomiting blood with the passage of melaena, there are several endoscopic signs that are associated with an increased likelihood of re-bleeding. About 20–25 per cent of all admissions are likely to bleed again, but this can be raised to 50 or even 75 per cent when the following have been found at endoscopy: the presence of a vessel in the ulcer base, the visible vessel, and a firmly adherent clot over the ulcer which cannot be dislodged. Bleeding throughout the examination is associated with an increase in operative intervention.

A barium meal as a diagnostic examination is becoming less common as particularly skilled radiology is needed, especially for diagnosis of erosions and similar small lesions. Separation of bleeding from non-bleeding lesions is also difficult radiologically.

In management, the prime aspect is still the proper assessment and resuscitation of the patient. Correction of blood volume by transfusion after the necessary assessment using central venous measuring and haemoglobin is one of the first responsibilities. Assessment of any complicating illness and the effects of bleeding, for instance renal failure, are also necessary. When the patient is fit enough, endoscopy is the next step in management.

In patients with peptic ulceration, treatment consists of drugs, endoscopic therapy and surgery. H_2-receptor antagonists have not been shown to be beneficial in any trial, but when all the trials are combined there is a trend in favour of clinical benefit. Other treatments tried have been tranexamic acid and somatostatin, the former showing a favourable trend. Therapeutic endoscopy involves the application of heat or electricity to the bleeding ulcer and beneficial results have been obtained in several trials of laser therapy. Diathermy electrodes and the heater-probe for coagulation are alternative ways of preventing rebleeding via the endoscope.

Decisions about the appropriate moment for surgery are difficult to make. Recent studies have given conflicting results for both aggressive and conservative approaches. Continued or renewed bleeding are firm indications for surgery. The difficulty lies in how best to manage a patient over 60-years-old with a single major haemorrhage. The aggressive approach which requires early surgery in these patients has produced good results in some centres though not in others. An important aspect is close medical-surgical cooperation to maintain a low mortality rate in these difficult patients.

Treatment of other lesions varies. Oesophageal varices will be discussed under portal hypertension. Oesophagitis should be treated medically and very rarely requires any surgical intervention. Similarly a Mallory–Weiss tear very rarely requires surgery, but a course of H_2 receptor antagonists is commonly prescribed. Gastric carcinoma, if found, will need assessment and surgical treatment (*see* below). Erosive gastritis fortunately settles in nearly all patients with antacids and H_2 receptor antagonists as surgery often involves a total gastrectomy – a not inconsiderable risk.

Zollinger–Ellison syndrome

This syndrome consists of the association of hypergastrinaemia with acid hypersecretion, i.e. the level of gastrin is inappropriate and maintained even when acid is being produced in large amounts. The principal cause of the syndrome is a gastrin producing tumour of the pancreas which may be multifocal or malignant. Other causes include antral G-cell hyperplasia – a normal source of gastrin but no longer under physiological control.

Clinical suspicion is the most important factor behind diagnosis, such as the association of peptic ulceration with diarrhoea, ulcers in unusual places, recurrent ulceration after surgery and unexplained watery diarrhoea and dyspepsia in patients who have familial multiple endocrine adenomatosis. Investigation involves the measurement of a fasting gastrin level followed by a secretin stimulation test of gastrin output where indicated. Gastric acid secretion tests have been shown to provide little additional diagnostic benefit.

H_2 receptor antagonists, often in supranormal doses, will suppress the acid hypersecretion. However, not infrequently, the treatment fails and the patient requires surgery after a few years. The operation of first choice for most patients is a total gastrectomy with pancreatic exploration. In only a minority is a surgically curable lesion of the pancreas found. However malignant, or metastatic disease, is often slowly progressive and compatible with survival of over 20 years.

Gastritis – erosive gastritis

Abnormal and inflamed gastric mucosa is frequently seen at endoscopy and confirmed histologically. The relevance and pathological significance of gastritis has not been clarified but certain types are well recognized. Multiple gastric erosions, erosive gastritis, are seen after aspirin ingestion and may produce an acute upper gastrointestinal bleed. Bile damages the gastric mucosa and inflammation around the stoma after partial gastrectomy is regularly found. Bile may also play a part in the increased 'stump cancer' found after gastric surgery. Atrophic gastritis, associated with pernicious anaemia, is commonly seen in the elderly. The association of gastritis with *Campylobacter pylori* infection is being assessed as a treatable cause of gastritis and gastric symptoms.

Gastric carcinoma

The incidence of this tumour is declining as is the incidence of peptic ulceration, yet it remains the fourth commonest carcinoma in England and Wales. In Japan the incidence is two to three times higher and much effort has been put into its early detection, leading to the clear categorization of early gastric cancer which is of much better prognosis.

The aetiology of gastric carcinoma is not known. There is a small genetic factor and major environmental influences. Nitroso compounds formed from nitrates in the diet are considered a likely carcinogen. Other pre-disposing conditions to carcinoma are gastric polyposis and a previous partial gastrectomy.

Early gastric cancer is defined as a carcinoma involving only the mucosa and sub-mucosa but not the muscle coats or serosal surface. Mass screening in Japan has allowed classification of the early lesion and enhanced its recognition both on double contrast barium meal and on endoscopy. The early lesion may remain localized for a prolonged period but is thought to become an advanced carcinoma eventually. The importance of diagnosis lies in its prognosis: at 5-years 95 per cent survive in Japan. The lesion is being recognized in Europe and seems to behave similarly.

Advanced gastric cancer can present as a malignant ulcer, as a polypoidal and fungating mass or as diffuse involvement of the whole stomach with little or no mucosal abnormality – linitis plastica. Both local spread, and widespread metastases to liver and distant lymph nodes are common.

Symptoms experienced by patients vary a great deal, and may be particularly insidious. Anorexia and weight loss are frequent and abdominal pain that may be either deep and boring, epigastric, and worsened by food is common. Flatulence, a sensation of fullness and vomiting after meals occur not infrequently. The symptoms may be similar to those of a benign gastric ulcer. Presentation with either haematemesis or the development of a microcytic anaemia is uncommon. The presence of physical signs indicates a lesion past cure. Metastasis may be manifest as hepatomegaly, ascites or left supraclavicular lymph node enlargement (Troisier's node). A palpable mass usually indicates a large tumour with local involvement.

Diagnosis is made by either barium meal or endoscopy. Linitis plastica is better detected by barium meal but endoscopy has the advantage of obtaining tissue for histological and cytological examination. Either radiology or endoscopy will provide information about the extent of the disease within the stomach preoperatively.

Treatment is surgical. Involvement of the pylorus with gastric outlet obstruction is common and best relieved or prevented by gastroenterostomy. Resection occasionally is curative but commonly palliative. Chemotherapy and radiotherapy have proven to be of little benefit.

The outlook is poor with 5-year survival of under 10 per cent, a figure that has not changed for 40 years. This underlines the importance of detecting early gastric cancer whenever possible. A high index of suspicion is needed so that dyspeptic middle aged patients are appropriately investigated early. Apparent healing of small ulcerating lesions is well recognized and so a trial of treatment, particularly without diagnosis, is not indicated.

Other gastric conditions

Leiomyoma

These tumours of the muscle layer are generally benign. Commonly asymptomatic and of no consequence, bleeding is the principal manifestation. The tumours that are large and bleed ulcerate at their apex. A leiomyoma appears as a smooth mass bulging into the stomach with gastric folds displaced by the mass and often a central ulcer. Treatment is by resection.

Ménétrièr's disease

This rare disease is characterized by giant gastric folds with a typical histological appearance. Symptoms include pain, vomiting, the consequences of hypoproteinaemia or bleeding. Diagnosis is best made by a full thickness biopsy. Treatment is usually partial resection to control the patient's symptoms and reduce the surface from which protein exudation occurs.

Non ulcer dyspepsia

Originally a radiological diagnosis, endoscopy has shown that some of these patients have ulcers etc., that have been missed. Nonetheless the management of a patient with typical dyspeptic symptoms and normal investigations remains a considerable problem. Treatment with antacids and even formal courses of ulcer treatment may be needed as well as repeat endoscopy, particularly during bouts of symptoms. The relation to *Campylobacter pylori* infection of the stomach is being assessed.

Hereditary haemorrhagic telangiectasia (Osler–Weber–Rendu disease)

This familial condition presents as bleeding from the nose, pharynx or the upper gastrointestinal tract. Telangiectasia are found on lips, tongue and mucosal surfaces as well as the hands and in the lungs and liver. Treatment is with transfusions and iron therapy; oestrogens have been shown to reduce the rate of blood loss but are only appropriate in female patients. A direct approach to the lesions can be undertaken surgically. The laser, heat and cautery have been recently studied in an attempt to reduce or stop the blood loss.

Gastric lymphoma

Lymphomas of the stomach are increasingly being recognized. They may present as benign or malignant ulcers but are characterized histologically. Before involvement of other organs occurs with the lymphoma, gastrectomy may be curative and can be supported by chemotherapy or radiotherapy. Close follow-up to prevent recurrence of the lymphoma in the stomach is needed in these patients.

Small intestine – absorption and malabsorption

The process of digestion and absorption occurs in a series of stages which have been well described in texts of physiology.

Table 9.4 lists the features produced by failure to absorb the many nutrients, and outlines the clinical tests employed for detecting malabsorption. Carbohydrate and fat together provide the bulk of energy supply and so their malabsorption produces weight loss. The established tests for carbohydrate malabsorption have been recently complemented by the newer tests of permeability. One or several non-metabolizable sugars are given orally and the amounts appearing in the urine measured over a predetermined time period. The absolute amounts and ratios of the sugars is determined and used to measure permeability. The xylose test is a long established test of permeability using a single sugar. Hydrogen breath tests are also used to measure carbohydrate absorption – for example, a lactose-hydrogen test used in alactasia.

The investigation of people with established or potential malabsorption employs various other tests. These include disease specific tests which are discussed with the diseases and some non-specific tests. A barium meal and follow through is commonly undertaken. In malabsorption, dilatation of the intestine with dilution and clumping of the barium occurs. A specific diagnosis, particularly Crohn's disease, can also be made on a barium meal follow through. Plain abdominal X-ray may be helpful and abdominal ultrasound may also provide evidence for hepatic, biliary or pancreatic disease that is responsible for malabsorption.

The principal causes of malabsorption are listed in Table 9.5 using a classification established to emphasize the mechanisms behind malabsorption. Clearly some diseases produce malabsorption by more than one mechanism. Crohn's disease is the typical example, and may produce malabsorption through mucosal damage, bacterial overgrowth, and previous intestinal resections. The most frequent causes of malabsorption that are clinically significant are coeliac disease, Crohn's disease, pancreatic insufficiency and bacterial overgrowth. The malabsorption associated with gastric surgery is generally mild.

Table 9.4 Investigations and consequences of nutrient malabsorption

Nutrient	Consequence of malabsorption	Investigations to demonstrate malabsorption
Carbohydrate	Diarrhoea, weight loss	Glucose tolerance test, lactose tolerance test, xylose test, breath hydrogen study, permeability of non-metabolizable sugars
Protein	Wasting, oedema	Plasma albumin
Fat	Steatorrhoea, weight loss	3($-$5) day faecal fat on a normal fat intake, radiolabelled fat absorption study
Calcium, magnesium	Tetany, osteomalacia	Plasma levels
Sodium, water	Diarrhoea, hypotension	Plasma levels
Potassium	Hypokalaemia	Plasma levels
Iron	Anaemia	Blood level, ferritin
Fat soluble:		
Vitamin A	Night blindness, skin changes	Blood level
Vitamin D	Osteomalacia, myopathy	Blood level, plasma calcium, phosphate
Vitamin K	Clotting disorder, bruising	Clotting screen
Water soluble:		
Vitamin B_{12}	Pernicious anaemia: sub-acute combined degeneration	Plasma level, Schilling test
Folate	Macrocytic anaemia, metal changes	Plasma or red cell level
Vitamin C	Anaemia, scurvy	
Bile salts	Fat malabsorption, diarrhoea	^{14}C glycocholate breath test, sehcat test

Table 9.5   Causes of malabsorption

Anatomical/ postoperative changes	Postgastrectomy Crohn's disease Intestinal resection
Specific mucosal enzyme defects	Alactasia A β-lipoproteinaemia
Mucosal disease	Coeliac disease Tropical sprue Whipple's disease Crohn's disease Lymphoma
Bacterial contamination	Blind loops Fistulae Diverticula Scleroderma Diabetes mellitus Crohn's disease (Tropical sprue)
Maldigestion	Pancreatic insufficiency Bile salt deficiency Zollinger–Ellison syndrome
Abnormal motility	Scleroderma Diabetes mellitus
Others	Radiotherapy Addison's disease Thyrotoxicosis Parasites (giardia and roundworms) Drugs e.g. neomycin, colchicine Tuberculosis Ischaemia

Presentations of malabsorption are many and typical consequences of malabsorption are shown in Table 9.4. Anaemia which may prove to be multifactorial is one of the most frequent consequences. Diarrhoea, weight loss, and a rather poorly localized abdominal discomfort are also common. As well as finding evidence for specific deficiencies, patients with malabsorption are often pale with distended abdomens. Treatment frequently involves attention to the nutrition of the patient as well as specific measures directed at the cause.

Coeliac disease

Coeliac disease occurs when a susceptible person is exposed to gluten, a protein of wheat, and barley, oats and rye, that induces a hyperplastic response immunologically with alteration in the small intes-

tinal architecture. Coeliac disease has an increased incidence in families, being related to HLA-B8 and HLA-DW3. Its incidence geographically varies considerably, being particularly high in Western Ireland.

The mucosal lesion of coeliac disease is 'villous atrophy'. The villous pattern of the small intestine is lost, the villi being replaced by thickened mucosa with a dense cellular infiltrate. The crypts are hyperplastic extending further towards the surface epithelium. The epithelium is abnormal with disruption of the brush-border and glycocalyx, and numerous lymphocytes are found between epithelial cells. These changes are most pronounced in the proximal jejunum becoming less severe distally into the ileum, where absorptive function will also be better. The histological features are typical but not necessarily diagnostic of coeliac disease.

The clinical features are essentially those of malabsorption as outlined above. Children are commonly investigated for failure to grow or to develop. Adults may give a history of many years duration or provide evidence for malabsorption as a child with anaemia, delayed puberty or relative small stature being features. Physical examination generally shows no specific findings though clubbing is occasionally encountered.

The diagnosis of coeliac disease is based upon the demonstration of malabsorption in the presence of total or partial villous atrophy, both of these improving after exclusion of gluten from the diet. Thus two jejunal biopsies are needed as a minimum to provide a diagnosis.

The basis of treatment is the gluten free diet. Patients, and their relatives if necessary, need to have the diagnosis and treatment carefully explained with regular review by a physician and a dietitian. Specific nutrient deficiency should also be corrected. The Coeliac Society is a valuable self-help group. Although symptomatic response may be swift, recovery of the mucosa may take a prolonged period, particularly in adults. A third or fourth biopsy over periods of 12 months or longer may be needed to demonstrate improvement of the jejunal histology.

Some patients fail to respond to a gluten free diet. This may be due to failure to comply with the diet. It may be necessary to allow a longer period on the diet before reassessing the patient. Concomitant pancreatic disease may require pancreatic supplements, or alactasia may be unmasked. Steroids are occasionally given for non-responsive coeliac disease.

A wide variety of complications of coeliac disease have been described. Intestinal complications include ulceration and stricturing which present as bleeding, diarrhoea and pain, with obstruction later and have a high mortality. Of equal severity is the increased incidence of malignant disease. Both carcinoma of the gastrointestinal tract and small intestinal lymphoma, typified as malignant histiocytosis of the intestine are more frequent.

Dermatitis herpetiformis

Dermatitis herpetiformis is an uncommon skin disease with an itching, blistering rash. Nearly all patients have an enteropathy with the histological appearances of coeliac disease. Dapsone is an effective treatment of the rash but does not alter the intestinal lesions. A gluten free diet however will improve the intestinal lesion and allow the dapsone to be reduced in dose or withdrawn completely.

Tropical sprue

This disease occurs in people who visit the tropics and who then develop an illness with features of malabsorption. Currently the disease is thought to start with an episode of travellers diarrhoea. An abnormal small intestinal flora then develops. Mucosal damage occurs and nutritional deficiency, particularly of folate and vitamin B_{12}, delays or limits the ability of the mucosa to recover.

Tropical sprue is confined principally to India, South-East Asia and some areas of the Caribbean. Both visitors and the indigenous population can suffer the disease with a well described delay in some patients between exposure and development of the disease in a temperate climate.

Most patients have diarrhoea, anorexia, and abdominal swelling with often an acute episode of diarrhoea initially. The illness is typified by episodes of remission and relapse. Progressive weight loss and nutritional deficiencies occur. Physical examination shows a thin person who may be anaemic with a distended abdomen and increased bowel sounds. Investigations show evidence of malabsorption including a megaloblastic anaemia due to B_{12} or folate deficiency. Jejunal biopsy may show changes with reduction in villous height and an increase in inflammatory cells as with any other disease such as giardiasis. Jejunal aspiration and cultures should be undertaken at the same time as jejunal biopsy.

Diagnosis is based on the findings of malabsorption with an appropriate history. Treatment consists of correction of the nutritional deficiencies and administering vitamin B_{12}, folate and antibiotics. Tetracycline is usually given for up to 6 months in the first instance.

Alactasia

The progressive diminution of the enzyme lactase in the small intestinal brush border with adult life is very common world-wide. Many patients do not have symptoms but mild diarrhoea is a presenting feature, often at a time of dietary change. Diagnosis can be confirmed by a lactose tolerance test, a lactose breath hydrogen study or lactase levels in a jejunal biopsy specimen.

The illness can be a trap for the unwary. Clinical suspicion and a trial treatment of a lactose free diet is often all that is needed to make a diagnosis.

Whipple's disease

Though rare this illness is a multisystem disorder with deposition of a glycoprotein in macrophages, shown by electron microscopy to be masses of bacteria. The cause has not been further defined. Men in middle age are usually the sufferers with weight loss, diarrhoea, and polyarthropathy. Fever is present in over half the cases as well as lymphadenopathy, pigmentation and evidence of nervous system involvement. Diagnosis is established by jejunal biopsy when the architecture is grossly distorted by numerous macrophages filled with PAS positive material. Treatment is with antibiotics. Two weeks penicillin and streptomycin are given, then tetracycline for an initial period of 1 year. Clinical responses are often very rapid though changes in histology may take a considerable or indefinite time to become manifest. Careful follow-up is needed as relapse occurs, requiring further courses of antibiotics.

Bacterial contamination of the small intestine

The healthy small intestine contains relatively few microorganisms. If intestinal function is impaired, bacterial overgrowth can occur with subsequent malabsorption. This can result from surgical blind loops, diverticula, strictures with dilated segments as well as from motility disorders such as systemic sclerosis and contamination with faecal organisms in gastrocolic or jejunocolic fistulae. A mixed anaerobic flora usually develops.

The effects of the overgrowth include the deconjugation of bile salts resulting in impaired fat absorption and bile-salt induced diarrhoea. Intraluminal carbohydrate is metabolized. Fats are metabolized to hydroxy-fatty acids which produce diarrhoea. Vitamin B_{12} deficiency can arise.

Diagnosis is based on clinical suspicion in the presence of a suitable anatomical cause demonstrated radiologically. A ^{14}C-glycocholate breath test or a hydrogen breath test help make the diagnosis. Jejunal aspiration is the best method of confirming the diagnosis. Surgical correction of some lesions is possible. Most patients however need antibiotics. Tetracycline and metronidazole are commonly used and after initial success given as courses whenever symptoms recur. Some patients need cycles of antibiotics to remain well.

Miscellaneous disorders

Tumours

Small intestinal tumours are rare. Benign tumours, such as leiomyomas may present as occult bleeding and may prove very difficult to diagnose. Carcinoma is rarely encountered, though its frequency is increased in Crohn's disease and coeliac disease.

Lymphoma

Primary lymphoma may arise from the small intestine presenting with bleeding, perforation or the features of obstruction. Mediterranean lymphoma and alpha chain disease are more diffuse small intestinal lymphomas with malabsorption, fever and finger clubbing being presenting features. Diagnosis of the lesion is made by radiology and biopsy. Treatment is by resection with supplementary chemotherapy and radiotherapy. Isolated primary lymphomas may respond to this.

Ischaemia

Chronic ischaemia is uncommon and clinical features relate poorly to angiographic findings. Abdominal pain after meals, diarrhoea and weight loss are typical symptoms. No findings are specific. Diagnosis is often delayed with the patients being considered to have a functional illness after a prolonged period of unrewarding investigation. Sur-

gical correction of the arterial stenoses may improve the patient's condition. Acute ischaemia due to superior mesenteric artery occlusion producing an acute abdomen is a surgical emergency with high mortality and morbidity.

Large intestine

The role of the colon beyond the preparation and storage of faeces has been poorly recognized and remains improperly understood. The colon has the capability of compensating to a considerable degree for small intestinal failure. It is likely that bacteria may alter components of the diet to produce carcinogens.

Colonic disease shows wide geographical variations. Carcinoma and diverticular disease are typical illnesses of Western civilizations. Sigmoid volvulus on the other hand is a Third World problem.

Carcinoma and adenomatous polyps

Colonic carcinoma is the commonest or second commonest malignancy in the Western world and its incidence is still increasing. It is also of importance because surgical cure is possible at an appropriate stage and because a substantial proportion are distributed within easy reach of a sigmoidoscope.

The aetiology is unknown. Environmental factors are most important, as shown by the way population groups who migrate from low to high incidence areas develop the high incidence of their new home. Certain conditions predispose to colonic cancer though they contribute relatively few cases examples of which are familial polyposis coli, inflammatory bowel disease and familial colonic cancer. It is now widely considered that adenomatous polyps are premalignant, because the distribution of polyps in the large bowel is the same as carcinoma, and with increasing size polyps have an increasing likelihood of containing malignant foci – for polyps less than 1 cm in diameter under 2 per cent are malignant but in polyps over 2 cm 46 per cent prove to be malignant. Also, the age at which patients present with adenomatous polyps is about 4 years younger than that at which carcinoma presents. Finally, colons with a carcinoma commonly contain one or more adenomatous polyps.

Clinical presentation of colonic carcinoma

depends on position in the colon. Right colonic tumours present with iron-deficiency anaemia, weight loss, dyspeptic abdominal pain or as a mass. Obstruction is uncommon. Left colonic tumours produce alteration in bowel habit, rectal bleeding or obstruction. Rectal carcinoma typically produces tenesmus with rectal bleeding. Physical findings of carcinoma include the presence of a mass or evidence of obstruction, as well as metastasis, particularly to the liver. Many polyps are found coincidentally; sometimes they can produce bleeding or colicky pain. Large left-sided villous adenomas may produce watery mucus in sufficient quantities to become diarrhoea.

Diagnosis depends upon the sequence of rectal examination, sigmoidoscopy and barium enema being carried out in all patients with suggestive symptoms. If there is doubt colonoscopy may be necessary to establish the true diagnosis.

Treatment of colonic carcinoma is surgical, the operation being determined by site of the lesion and the presence or absence of metastases. At present, polyps are generally treated colonoscopically. The finding of a polyp on any examination of the bowel should be followed by colonoscopy of the whole colon, any polyps found can be excised for histology. Other lesions, such as carcinoma, may also be found. Colonoscopy should be repeated at a 6–12 monthly interval initially as people who have had a polyp are likely to have others. Some large villous adenomas of the rectum need an endoanal excision under anaesthesia to effectively remove them.

Prognosis of colonic carcinoma depends on the extent of the disease. Overall survival for 5 years is about 40 per cent, but carcinoma localized to the bowel wall has a 65 per cent 5-year survival, of whom most have been cured of the disease. Full thickness involvement of the bowel wall, however, with involvement of lymph nodes is of much poorer prognosis with a 15 per cent 5-year survival.

Diverticular disease

Diverticular disease is a common problem with an incidence that increases with age, about 40 per cent of people over 60 years having diverticula present. The aetiology is not known.

The diverticula develop most commonly in the sigmoid colon. It is believed that increasing segmentation, perhaps related to low fibre intakes, produces very high luminal pressures and gradually outpouchings of mucosa appear at the weakest points, where blood vessels pass through from serosa to mucosa. This accounts for the prominent muscle hypertrophy which is found and for the pressures recorded in patients with diverticular disease.

Symptoms are difficult to attribute to diverticular disease being similar to the irritable bowel syndrome. However, change in bowel habit with rectal bleeding does occur raising the possibility of carcinoma. In uncomplicated diverticular disease, a palpable and slightly tender left iliac fossa colon may be present.

Diagnosis is generally confirmed by barium enema. If rectal bleeding has occurred it is often necessary to proceed to colonoscopy because views of the sigmoid colon may not be adequate on a barium study to exclude carcinoma.

Treatment is by explanation of the changes and a high fibre diet. Sometimes a smooth muscle relaxant helps. Complications include acute diverticulitis. In this, a diverticulum becomes obstructed and an abscess develops. Symptoms of abdominal pain, vomiting, fever and constipation result. Pus may spread locally to produce a pericolic abscess and a tender left iliac fossa mass will be palpable. The abscess can subsequently extend into the peritoneal cavity or the bladder as a colovesical fistula. Treatment of acute diverticulitis is with intravenous fluids, antibiotics and analgesia (pethidine being preferred to morphine). If the abscess does not resolve then surgery to excise the inflamed length of sigmoid colon is required. Peritonitis and colovesical fistula are indications for surgery.

Ischaemia

Large intestinal ischaemia is more common than small intestinal, occurring in the elderly. The splenic flexure and descending colon are most commonly involved. Typically the illness is short-lived and confined to the mucosa, producing left-sided abdominal pain with bloody diarrhoea. The area is tender without evidence of peritonitis. Plain abdominal X-ray will show an abnormal bowel outline at the splenic flexure. If needed, a barium enema shows 'thumb printing' in the area involved. Treatment is conservative.

A few patients develop full thickness ischaemia – gangrene of the colon. Peritonitis rapidly develops and early surgery is needed, though despite successful excision mortality is high.

Irritable bowel syndrome

A definition of irritable bowel syndrome is particularly difficult to present. It is basically a pooling of those patients with abdominal pain, distension and with change in bowel habit, who also have no other demonstrable illness – the majority of patients attending a gastrointestinal outpatient clinic.

A variety of abnormalities have been described including altered motility and altered sensitivity to both luminal distension and bile acids. The irritable bowel syndrome can also present as a consequence of a previous gastrointestinal problem, acute gastroenteritis being a typical example.

There are three major groups of symptoms which are worse with stress. The most common presentation is with colicky lower abdominal pain and an abnormal bowel habit often associated with meals. Commonly defaecation will alter the pain making it better or worse. The change in bowel habit is very variable. Diarrhoea may occur on some days, constipation on others as well as days with the passage of a normal stool. Mucus may be passed with pellety or rabbity stools and a sensation of incomplete rectal evacuation is common. Rectal bleeding should not occur.

The second presentation is that of upper abdominal pain which may be postprandial. The pain is generally poorly localized and poorly defined, rarely occurring at night. Nausea is frequent but vomiting uncommon. Patients have often been extensively investigated for peptic ulceration or gall bladder disease, and it is not infrequent to find that they have had cholecystectomy without relief of symptoms. A final group of patients have painless diarrhoea, typically occurring first thing in the morning but never at night. Weight loss is uncommon.

Most patients are young adults though any age may present with the irritable bowel syndrome. Physical examination including rectal examination and sigmoidoscopy is normal. Investigations are also normal. In the young these generally consist of blood count, ESR and plasma biochemistry. In the elderly a barium enema is an important investigation to exclude carcinoma.

Difficult though it may be, a positive diagnosis of the irritable bowel syndrome should be made where possible. This assists in the care of the patient in that a cohesive approach is possible from the outset. The first aspect of management is careful explanation and reassurance. As constipation plays a part in many if not most patients, a high fibre diet is recommended. Symptomatic treatment is also employed, including antispasmodics, antacids and anti-diarrhoeal agents. Food allergy has been proposed as the cause of the irritable bowel syndrome but evidence for this is unconvincing. A few patients however benefit from avoiding some foodstuffs, such as cereal products. Tranquillisers or antidepressants are also of benefit in patients who are anxious or depressed, a not infrequent finding.

Infectious diarrhoea

A wide variety of organisms produce acute infectious diarrhoea. The principal symptoms are well known but nausea and vomiting, malaise, headache and fever are important aspects of the early part of most illnesses. In most instances the illness is self-limiting and its source and infecting organism are rarely identified. Treatment consists of rest and an adequate oral fluid intake. Intravenous fluids are occasionally indicated if hypotension is present or if vomiting prevents adequate oral rehydration. Advances in gastrointestinal physiology have led to the use of oral rehydration preparations that have been of profound benefit world-wide. There is evidence that antibiotics and anti-diarrhoeal preparations tend to prolong the illness, if not the symptoms, and particularly to prolong the carrier state with a slowed clearance of the infecting organism from the patient's gastrointestinal tract.

Specific infections and their distinctive features include:

Staphylococcus aureus and Clostridium perfringens

These produce a heat stable enterotoxin. The incubation period after eating contaminated food is 30 minutes–5 hours. Vomiting is a prominent feature of the illness. The toxins can occasionally produce circulatory collapse requiring hospital admission.

E. coli

Enterotoxigenic *E. coli* are important in producing illnesses with watery diarrhoea world-wide although some may produce a more haemorrhagic colitis. Oral rehydration therapy is the most important aspect of management, antibiotics generally having no place.

Salmonella infections

A vast number of salmonella organisms have been identified as causing food poisoning, being particularly associated with mass catering and processed foods. Multiple drug resistance is becoming a problem in management of invasive salmonella infections that produce illnesses similar to typhoid fever (*see* below). For *Salmonella gastroenteritis*, antibiotics are not indicated. Occupational health assessment and evidence of clearance of infection are important parts of the management of these patients.

Typhoid and paratyphoid fevers

The early features of typhoid are those of any systemic infection. After a 10-day incubation period there is a gradual onset of headache, fever and cough. Constipation at this stage is common. The pulse is typically disproportionately slow in relation to the fever and the abdomen may feel doughy and slightly tender. The spleen may be palpable and, in a minority of patients, rose spots can be found over the abdomen. Though the illness is initially systemic the second phase of the illness includes many serious abdominal problems. Massive haemorrhage and small intestinal perforation are two particular gastrointestinal complications with a high mortality. Onset of diarrhoea and passage of organisms occurs at this stage of the illness. Metastatic abscesses may develop anywhere. Diagnosis depends on finding the organism in blood cultures taken in the first week, or in stool in the second and third weeks. The Widal test may show changing titres after 10–14 days of overt illness. Treatment is with parenteral chloramphenicol or ampicillin initially. Stool and urine specimens should be followed till six negative specimens consecutively have been obtained.

Shigella

Shigella infections produce predominantly a colitis with bloody diarrhoea and abdominal pains. Infections acquired in the UK are generally due to *Shigella sonnei* and are milder than those due to *S. flexneri* or *S. shigae* from abroad. Diagnosis is by stool culture. As an exception to the rule, antibiotics have a role and tend to speed systemic recovery. Co-trimoxazole is the treatment of choice. Reiter's syndrome may complicate some shigella infections.

Campylobacter

Campylobacter species are being increasingly recognized as a major cause of diarrhoea and vomiting in the UK and elsewhere in the world. After a 3–5 day incubation period, abdominal pain is a prominent early symptom followed by diarrhoea that is frequently bloody. Systemic features vary considerably and if severe are an indication for antibiotic treatment, usually erythromycin.

Pseudomembranous colitis

Though known from the period before antibiotics, pseudomembranous colitis is generally seen in relation to antibiotics, particularly if the patients are at increased vulnerability through a recent operation or severe illness. Pseudomembranous colitis has been described as complicating most, if not all, antibiotics. Lincomycin and clindamycin have the highest incidence in relation to the number of courses prescribed. The illness usually commences several days after the course of antibiotics has been started. Diarrhoea is of very variable severity with the passage of mucus but very rarely blood. In severe episodes fever, prostration, hypotension and abdominal pain may occur. Sigmoidoscopy may be normal or demonstrate plaques of the pseudomembrane with distinctive histology.

The illness is likely to be a super-infection by *Clostridium difficile* when the normal flora has been disturbed by antibiotics. Diagnosis is based on finding the enterotoxin and the organism in the stools. Treatment is by oral vancomycin and supportive measures as needed. Metronidazole is an alternative therapeutic agent.

Amoebic dysentery

Amoebic infections occur principally in warmer climates. The severity of the disease depends upon the equilibrium between host and parasite. Immuno-suppression and corticosteroids impair the host response whereas the enzyme composition of the parasite, the zymodene, and the ability to produce histiolytic enzymes enhance the illness produced by the parasite.

Infection occurs after cysts have been swallowed and then developed into active amoebae. In many people the infection produces few or no symptoms and is mostly present in the right colon. Invasive amoebic disease produces amoebic colitis, with bloody diarrhoea, fever and weight loss. There may be colonic tenderness. Sigmoidoscopy can show ulcers that appear deep and discrete. Histologically these ulcers are flask shaped without a prominent leucocytic response. Scrapings taken at sigmoidoscopy from ulcers show active amoebae with ingested red cells. Active amoebae may also be seen in rapidly examined faecal specimens.

Invasive amoebiasis can be complicated by perforation, haemorrhage or an amoeboma. This is a mass of inflammatory tissue with secondary bacterial infection. It may be mistaken for carcinoma or Crohn's disease, both clinically and radiologically. Abscess formation may occur away from the colon, most frequently in the liver which is described below.

Diagnosis of amoebic disease depends on finding the cysts or active organisms in the stools and on positive antibody titres. In the symptom-free disease only cysts will be found. Active colitis will have few cysts but active amoebae should be present. Serology is usually positive. Liver abscess is generally associated with positive serology as well as the appearance of an abscess on ultrasound and other imaging procedures.

Treatment of amoebic colitis is with metronidazole for a 5-day course. Patients with colitis and asymptomatic carriers should then be treated with Diloxanide furoate 500 mg t.d.s. for a further 10-day period, to clear asymptomatic infection and stop passage of cysts. Liver abscesses are treated with metronidazole.

Familial polyposis coli

In this autosomal dominant condition, during early teenage years there is the gradual development of numerous adenomatous polyps in the colon and rectum. If left untreated malignant change occurs. Current treatment consists of colectomy, usually in the late teens, with either ileostomy or ileorectal anastomosis. The latter has considerable advantages for social reasons, as well as having a lower incidence of infertility in men. However, the risk of malignant change in the rectal stump persists and follow-up with fulguration and removal of all polyps is required lifelong. Distinction between familial polyposis coli and other intestinal polyp conditions, particularly Gardner's syndrome, is becoming less. In Gardner's syndrome polyps are also found in other parts of the gastrointestinal tract, with skin lesions, and multiple osteomas that appear in adolescence producing distortion of the facial skeleton.

Pneumatosis coli

This uncommon condition is characterized by gas filled cysts in the wall of the colon. The origin is unknown though current theories relate the cysts to anaerobic bacterial infection. The condition is associated with mechanical obstruction of the gastrointestinal tract and with chronic lung disease.

The symptoms are of change in bowel habit with mucus and blood, and cysts rarely rupture to produce a pneumoperitoneum. The cysts can be seen on sigmoidoscopy, biopsy and barium enema. Treatment, determined by symptoms, consists of a continuous increase in inspired oxygen concentration by nasal cannulae. Blood gases are carefully monitored in view of the fact that patients also have chronic respiratory disease.

Inflammatory bowel disease

An understanding of inflammatory bowel disease has been slowly gained over the past century. After separation from infectious diarrhoeas the inter-war years saw the recognition of Crohn's disease and its gradual distinction from ulcerative proctocolitis followed. More recently, whether these are separate diseases or opposite ends of a spectrum of a single disease has been questioned. In this section the two diseases will be discussed separately as they can be separated clinically in 95 per cent of patients.

Ulcerative colitis

Ulcerative colitis is most frequently a disease of white Westerners, but occurs occasionally in the Third World. The incidence in the UK and Scandinavia seems to be static. Immigrants, particularly those to the UK, do develop the illness though it is not known if the incidence matches that of the indigenous population – one person in 1400. There is an increased familial incidence, with both ulcerative colitis and Crohn's disease. The aetiology of ulcerative colitis is not known. A wide variety of immunological abnormalities have been recognized, which may be primary or secondary. If primary it is possible that they are the consequences of exposure to an infectious agent or to various dietary antigens. A psychosomatic aetiology is very unlikely though psychosomatic events seem to precipitate some relapses.

Symptoms vary with extent of the disease and

severity of the attack. Though the illness may start at any age, its peak incidence is in young adult life. Symptoms of the passage of blood per rectum, and diarrhoea usually gradually worsen. The most severely ill are those patients with involvement of all the colon, total colitis, in an acute attack. They will have frequent diarrhoea with blood and mucus, and the systemic features of fever, malaise and weight loss. Diarrhoea may occur up to 20 or 30 times daily and at night. Generalized abdominal pain is common and it may worsen prior to defaecation. These patients are often thin, anaemic and febrile, and may show signs of iron deficiency. A tachycardia of over 100 beats/minute is common. Dehydration can occur. Abdominal examination may be normal or show diffuse tenderness and some distention.

Milder attacks can occur in patients with extensive disease or in patients with colitis limited to the left colon. The diarrhoea is less severe, e.g. 3–5 stools day, and anaemia rare. Abnormal physical signs including fever are less likely to occur. The least extensive disease, proctitis, very rarely produces constitutional symptoms. Patients with proctitis pass blood and mucus with tenesmus and urgency, yet no alteration in the frequency of defaecation. A wide variety of events has been recognized as precipitating attacks in people with established ulcerative proctocolitis, including stress, upper respiratory tract infections and particularly gastrointestinal infections. Patients who have ulcerative colitis are less likely to be smokers than the general population.

Diagnosis is based on finding clinical, histological and radiological evidence of ulcerative colitis in the rectum and to a variable extent proximally. True ulcerative colitis not involving the rectum is very rare if it exists at all. The most important first investigation is sigmoidoscopy and biopsy. Though the rectal mucosa may return to normal in remission, the changes in a mild attack include a granular and friable mucosa with abnormal vessels. Moderately active disease shows more pronounced mucosal inflammation with mucopus. In severe attacks spontaneous bleeding may result in a rectum filled with mucopus and blood. Ulcerations may be seen.

The histological features of ulcerative colitis are inflammation generally limited to the mucosa with surface ulceration. The glands may be irregular or absent, generally empty of mucus and show crypt abscesses. In very severe disease, extensive areas of the bowel may show loss of the entire mucosa.

Other investigations include stool culture to exclude infectious diarrhoea, blood count for anaemia and liver function tests for albumin.

After sigmoidoscopy and biopsy, radiology would be the next investigation. Plain abdominal X-rays may show an empty colon with irregular walls due to oedematous mucosal islands surrounded by ulcerated bowel in an acute attack. A barium enema may be dangerous in patients with a severe acute attack. In proctitis, it is often normal. Generally a granular or ulcerated outline of the bowel wall can be followed from the rectum proximally, to delineate the extent of the disease. Patients who have had a severe attack often show pseudopolyps, smooth strictures and an abnormal ileum due to reflux ileitis. Leucocytes, labelled with indium[111], have been shown to localize in inflamed intestine, an alternative way of assessing the extent of the disease.

Colonoscopy has an important role to play in ulcerative colitis. It can be helpful in establishing the diagnosis and the extent of the disease, as well as the follow-up of that sub-group with an increased incidence of carcinoma.

Complications of ulcerative colitis include those involving the intestine and the extraintestinal manifestations. Colonic complications of a severe attack are principally toxic megacolon and perforation. In toxic megacolon the colon is greatly dilated and aperistaltic. Codeine phosphate and other opioid antidiarrhoeal agents may exacerbate or precipitate the condition. Patients with acute attacks of colitis are best followed by serial abdominal X-rays where colonic diameter can be measured. Steroid treatment may mask any physical signs. Toxic megacolon is an indication for urgent surgery, as perforation frequently ensues. Even if an episode of toxic megacolon has responded to medical treatment, the patients seem to never completely settle and come to a colectomy during the same admission. Perforation most often occurs in toxic megacolon. Signs of perforation, such as increased pulse rate, temperature, abdominal pain and rigidity, may be suppressed by concurrent steroid treatment. Thus perforation is a further reason for daily abdominal X-rays. Treatment is surgical. As emergency colectomy carries an appreciably higher mortality than early elective colectomy surgical treatment should be undertaken before the colon perforates. Both toxic megacolon and perforation seem to be decreasing in frequency, possibly due to increasing recognition of the hazards of the use of codeine phosphate.

Massive haemorrhages are a rare but dangerous complication of an acute attack. Treatment is by resuscitation followed by colectomy. Rectovaginal fistula, ischiorectal abscess and fissure *in ano* also occur. Their presence should lead to suspicion of the diagnosis. Fibrous strictures occur in the involved intestine. Initially soft and disrupted by sigmoidoscopy or colonoscopy they later progress to smooth strictures. Fortunately they rarely need any treatment but need to be examined to ensure that they are not malignant.

Ulcerative colitis is a premalignant condition, an important problem late in the course of the disease. The groups most at risk are well recognized, but the likelihood of developing cancer is a matter of debate. Patients at an increased frequency of malignancy, have total colitis and duration of disease of 15–20 years before the start of the increased occurrence of malignancy. Thereafter the possibility of developing a carcinoma progressively increases such that, after having the illness for about 25 years, approximately 8 per cent of patients have developed carcinoma. Carcinoma is often associated with the development of severe dysplasia of the mucosa in other parts of the colon, which can be found on routine biopsies. This aspect of the management of ulcerative colitis has become the major indication for colonoscopy, repeated every 1–2 years in patients with total colitis over 10 years in duration. Some centres perform colectomy for persistent severe dysplasia and find small carcinomas in a high proportion of the colons of these patients.

A wide variety of extraintestinal manifestations have been recognized in ulcerative colitis and Crohn's disease. Arthritis, or pain in a joint is common. Large joints are typically involved and the arthropathy may migrate from joint to joint, particularly in the lower limbs. The colitis is usually active when joint disease occurs and treatment of the bowel is beneficial to the joints. Ankylosing spondylitis is twenty times more common in ulcerative colitics than in the rest of the population. Sacroiliitis is very frequent – perhaps 15 per cent of colitics have it. Clubbing is also seen in inflammatory bowel disease. Skin lesions include pyoderma gangrenosum, erythema nodosum and vasculitis. Pyoderma gangrenosum is characterized by necrosis of the skin exposing the underlying tissues and is rarely seen in Crohn's disease. Pyoderma gangrenosum is poorly related to activity of colitis, and treated with high dose corticosteroids. Vasculitis is much less common and may, like all the other extra intestinal complications, be a manifestation of immune complex deposition. Ulcers of mucous membranes, generally oral ulcers, are seen.

The ocular complications of inflammatory bowel disease, uveitis and episcleritis, are less common than the arthritis and skin manifestations. There are several hepatic complications in ulcerative colitis. Abnormal liver function tests are relatively common. Chronic active hepatitis is rare. Specific hepatobiliary problems related to ulcerative colitis are sclerosing cholangitis and carcinoma of the bile duct. Chronic fibrosis in the biliary tree produces a series of strictures with dilated segments in sclerosing cholangitis and the symptoms are jaundice, itching and weight loss. Infection and biliary stones occur. Treatment of sclerosing cholangitis is difficult and principally aimed at preventing infection. Carcinoma of the bile duct is perhaps four times more frequent in ulcerative colitis. Pulmonary function tests may be abnormal, especially involving a reduction in lung transfer factor while fibrosing alveolitis has been reported. Pleuropericarditis has also been described in inflammatory bowel disease.

Management of ulcerative colitis depends on the current state of the illness and its extent. In a severe attack admission to hospital with careful observation of girth, pulse, temperature and plain abdominal X-rays are necessary. An intensive course of medical treatment is begun with usually a 5-day limit. The treatment consists of high-dose prednisolone – 60 mg or more daily – intravenous fluids, blood and possibly intravenous nutrition. Many patients settle rapidly but those who have not settled at 5 days are carefully reviewed with a view to early colectomy. Some patients are continued on this regime for longer periods but the incidence of surgery is very high. If the patients have settled they are changed to treatment employed for a moderately severe attack consisting of prednisolone, 40 mg daily by mouth, the introduction of oral sulphasalazine 2–6 g a day and steroid enemas. With recovering health the patient is discharged from hospital and the steroid dose reduced in outpatients. Mild attacks of colitis can be treated by sulphasalazine 4 g daily, and local steroids, either prednisolone enemas, hydrocortisone foam or suppositories. An attack of proctitis is usually treated with local therapy. Local steroids are used as well as sulphasalazine which can be administered locally or more usually orally.

Maintenance treatment is an important aspect of

the management of patients with ulcerative colitis. In patients in remission continuing oral corticosteroids confers no benefit in general, though a small group of patients require a small dose of corticosteroids to prevent relapse. Most patients are able to discontinue steroids completely but take oral sulphasalazine which has been demonstrated to maintain remission. The usual maintenance dose is 2 grams daily.

Thus the drugs usually employed in ulcerative colitis are corticosteroids and sulphasalazine. Corticosteroids have the expected side-effects. They may mask perforation in people with a severe acute attack. Given locally they produce minimal side-effects. Sulphasalazine is poorly absorbed but broken down by the intestinal microflora, mostly in the colon, to sulphapyridine which is the carrier molecule and 5-aminosalicylic acid which is the active part. Sulphasalazine has been shown to be of benefit in the mild acute attack though it is not as effective as corticosteroids. Its principal role is in remission to prevent further relapse. Side-effects are common. These include nausea, vomiting and dyspepsia which can be helped by enteric coated tablets. Rashes, headache, disorientation and haemolytic anaemia also occur. Dyspnoea and X-ray changes of interstitial infiltration, and changes compatible with bronchiectasis have been reported. Reversible oligospermia is an important cause of reduced fertility in men. As many of the side-effects are thought to be related to the sulphapyridine attention has now been paid to preparing tablets or compounds of 5-aminosalicylic acid that do not break down until they reach the terminal ileum or colon. Mesalazine or 5-aminosalicylic acid is likely to be as effective as sulphasalazine and probably has fewer side-effects. Other medications used in ulcerative colitis include codeine phosphate, and loperamide to control diarrhoea. Many people with proctitis and left-sided disease develop functional right-sided constipation which produces symptoms of bloating, abdominal distension and discomfort. Isogel and other fibre supplements are useful ways of managing this difficulty.

Over the past few years the importance of follow-up and early treatment of a relapse has been emphasized and it is possible that this has reduced the number of admissions, the length of admission and possibly the number of perforations in patients with ulcerative colitis.

Surgical treatment has an important place in the management of patients with ulcerative colitis.

There are both urgent indications and early elective indications. Proctocolectomy with a terminal ileostomy has been the standard operation but in emergencies and now in the younger patient colectomy, temporary ileostomy and a mucus fistula for the rectum has become the operation of choice, because this reduces mortality and allows a second more careful approach to the rectal stump. In the young patient, various alternative approaches such as an ileorectal anastomosis or the formation of a pelvic pouch with ileoanal anastomosis can be undertaken. Indications for emergency surgery include perforation, toxic megacolon and haemorrhage. The failure of a severe attack to settle on medical management requires early elective surgery. Similarly early elective operations are carried out for carcinoma, severe dysplasia and much more infrequently for severe extraintestinal manifestations of the disease.

Crohn's disease

Crohn's disease, a chronic intestinal inflammatory illness, differs from ulcerative colitis in that any part of the gastrointestinal tract may be involved, its histology is different and also the disease is often discontinuous.

The incidence of Crohn's disease is still increasing, this being more than reclassification of ulcerative colitis. The disease is commonest in whites and has a bimodal age distribution. Most patients have the onset of the disease in early adult life but there is also a gradually increasing incidence in the elderly. The cause is unknown but current views still support the concept of an infectious agent though 20 years' research have not convincingly demonstrated any responsible agent. In common with ulcerative colitis a variety of immunological abnormalities have been described though their role in aetiology is speculative.

The clinical features of Crohn's disease vary both from the parts of the gastrointestinal tract involved and from the severity of the disease. In the small intestine active disease, which frequently involves the distal ileum with perhaps a small cap of caecum and large intestine, usually produces abdominal pain and diarrhoea. The pain felt may be related to inflammation of overlying peritoneum or to the colic produced by obstruction in a thickened oedematous length of intestine. The diarrhoea usually consists of three to four watery stools a day passed without blood or mucus. Steatorrhoea may be apparent. Weight loss, fever and anaemia are frequent in active disease. Inactive disease, due to

Table 9.6 A comparison of ulcerative colitis and Crohn's colitis

	Ulcerative colitis	Crohn's colitis
Clinical:		
Bleeding	Usually present	Uncommon
Urgency, tenesmus	Usually present	Uncommon
Anal disease	Rare	Frequent
Sigmoidoscopy:		
Inflammation present	Always, with friable mucosa and mucopus	Variable, nil to total rectal involvement
Radiology:		
Continuity	Continuous from rectum proximally	Typically discontinuous
Right colonic disease	In total colitis	Common
Ulceration	Often mild – granular, appearance – or if severe widespread undermining	Deep – 'rose thorn' or 'collar stud' or linear producing cobblestone appearance. Aphthous sometimes seen
Strictures, fistulae	Rare	Common
Pseudopolyps	Common	Rare
Histology:		
Dept of involvement	Mucosa and submucosa	Full thickness
Granulomas	Rare	Common
Fissures	Rare	Common
Discontinuity of involvement	Not seen on small biopsies	Common

damage in previous attacks, or an excision of the small intestine, results in diarrhoea in many patients. Healed lesions may lead to fibrous strictures that produce the symptoms of intestinal obstruction intermittently. Colonic disease may be very similar to ulcerative colitis and features that differentiate the two are given in Table 9.6.

Anal disease is a common feature of Crohn's disease, though rectal involvement at the same time is uncommon. The features of anal disease are oedematous discoloured skin tags, fissures and fistulae. Cavitating ulcers occur and can lead to ischiorectal abscess formation. When florid the appearances are easily recognizable, though more subtle changes may be present for some years before a diagnosis of Crohn's disease is made, often after previous local treatment. Crohn's disease of other regions of the gastrointestinal tract is well known. Oral ulceration is found with typical histology. The disease has also been described in the oesophagus and occurs in the stomach and duodenum resulting in peptic ulceration and obstruction. Widespread small intestinal involvement may be found as opposed to terminal ileal disease. In many, several skip lesions can be demonstrated with generally severe symptoms of malabsorption as well as obstruction.

Physical examination also varies. Clubbing, anaemia, oral aphthous and fissuring Crohn's ulcers may be found. A tender right iliac fossa mass suggests ileal disease. Signs of intestinal obstruction may be present. The perianal area should be carefully examined.

Routine investigations include blood count for anaemia and liver function tests to demonstrate a low albumin due to malabsorption or protein losing enteropathy. Hepatic enzymes may be deranged in acute episodes. Vitamin B_{12} levels may be low in terminal ileal disease. Histological features of Crohn's disease are most important in making the diagnosis (Table 9.6). Granuloma can be seen at any level and even in the draining lymph nodes. Ulceration varies from discrete superficial aphthous ulcers to fissures extending deep into the muscle layers. Sheet ulceration can also occur in Crohn's disease. The discontinuity of Crohn's disease can be recognized microscopically with inflammatory involvement of some glands while adjacent ones are normal. The histological features may be apparent on biopsies throughout the gastrointestinal tract including an apparently normal rectum.

Radiology is extremely valuable in making the diagnosis requiring barium enema and follow through (Table 9.6). Typical features include firstly discontinuous involvement of the intestine producing skip lesions, in both small and large bowel. The discontinuity may produce involvement of one wall of the colon only. Secondly, there may be stricturing. Frequently a length of ileum is seen with a long narrow stricture of the lumen – the String sign. Ulceration in Crohn's disease tends to be deep, producing 'rose thorn' ulcers or linear fissures and areas where linear ulceration breaks the mucosa up to produce a cobblestone appearance. Aphthous ulcers of the intestinal wall may also be seen. Fistulae commonly are found passing from an area of Crohn's disease to adjacent intestine.

Endoscopy is principally of value in helping make a diagnosis in difficult cases and establishing the extent of the disease. It can be used to obtain specimens for histology from abnormal areas on X-ray and to examine anastomoses for evidence of recurrence which can be difficult to determine on X-ray.

The separation of complications from primary disease is particularly difficult in Crohn's disease. Malabsorption for example, has many causes which include bacterial overgrowth, bypassing of intestine by fistulae, bile acid depletion due to terminal ileal disease as well as widespread mucosal involvement. Enterocutaneous fistulae occur, often soon after laparotomy and can produce particular management problems. Fistulae to bladder, vagina, and urethra are also found. Carcinoma of the large and small bowels are increased but for colonic disease the incidence of carcinoma is much less than in ulcerative colitis.

More specific complications related to Crohn's disease include stone formation. In ileal disease, malabsorption of bile acids predisposes to gallstone formation. The associated steatorrhoea produces hyperoxaluria, one of several mechanisms that lead to the well recognized increased incidence of renal stones. Many of the extraintestinal complications of ulcerative colitis are found in patients with Crohn's disease particularly in colonic Crohn's disease. These include arthritis and spinal disease, erythema nodosum and ocular problems. Metastatic Crohn's disease, is occasionally encountered.

Treatment of Crohn's disease is complex, and as the majority of patients come to surgery at some stage, it is often shared between physician and surgeon. The natural history of the disease is one of recurrence and remission, with gradual spontaneous settling of recurrences. Medical management depends on steroids, sulphasalazine and nutrition in the first instance. A series of trials have shown that oral corticosteroids induce remission in Crohn's disease of both the large and the small intestine. Prednisolone, 40–60 mg daily, is a standard starting dose and the steroid dosage is gradually reduced as the disease settles. Steroids, in common with all other forms of treatment, have not been shown to benefit patients already in remission, but clinically one frequently encounters patients who require steroids to remain well after an acute attack. Sulphasalazine has also been shown to benefit active disease but it is not so effective as corticosteroids, with which it is frequently combined. In distinction to ulcerative colitis no benefit as a maintenance treatment has been demonstrated for sulphasalazine.

Nutrition in patients with Crohn's disease is most important. Indeed some authorities contend that it is the most important aspect in promoting remission. Correction of obvious nutritional deficits and prophylactic vitamin B_{12} for ileal disease or resection are necessary. Patients with severe small intestinal Crohn's disease and functional intestinal failure require total parenteral nutrition which may be started in hospital and continued at home. Once nutrition has improved the patient's body weight and general health, surgical correction of the various intestinal abnormalities can be undertaken. Other dietary approaches, such as high fibre diets, have been tried without particular benefit, except for one small study which showed an elemental diet to be as effective as corticosteroids in inducing remission.

More controversial drugs include azathioprine, 6-mercaptopurine and metronidazole. Azathioprine acts by reducing steroids in those requiring large doses. It has been used in people with enterocutaneous fistula though it has been difficult to show if it is beneficial. 6-mercaptopurine presumably acts in a similar manner. Metronidazole has also been used in long trials of treatment but results are controversial.

As the disease settles the doses of steroids and sulphasalazine are reduced and if possible stopped, though a proportion of patients prove to need maintenance steroids. In these patients azathioprine can be used if steroids were needed at over 10 mg daily or were producing side-effects.

Cooperation between physician and surgeon has led to a clearer understanding of the place of surgery. Surgical intervention is rarely undertaken for active disease but for complications of Crohn's disease. Intestinal obstruction, commonly due to fibrous stenosis as opposed to active disease, is one of the commonest indications. Resections are kept to a minimum. In small intestinal disease with many strictures, stricturoplasty rather than excision or bypass is being considered, and may prove the operation of choice. Abscess formation, which may be anywhere in the abdomen, and fistulae are important indications. Abscesses are carefully drained hoping not to create a fistula. Fistulae need to be excised *en bloc* with the associated active disease. Haemorrhage or perforation occur very rarely and are treated surgically. In Crohn's colitis symptoms are often so continuous and severe that colectomy with ileostomy or ileorectal anastomosis but not the formation of small intestinal pouches becomes the treatment of choice. Some patients have chronic ill health and require surgery for this indication alone. The recurrence rate after 'curative surgery' which means that all macroscopic disease had been resected, is about 3 per cent per annum. Recurrence frequently occurs at and just proximal to an anastomosis.

Inflammatory bowel disease in pregnancy

Many patients with ulcerative colitis and Crohn's disease are young women. In ulcerative colitis their fertility seems to be normal though in patients who have active Crohn's disease and possibly those with chronic ulcerative colitis, fertility is reduced. In men sulphasalazine produces reversible oligospermia and this may be a cause of infertility. Treatment with mesalazine instead of sulphasalazine allows restoration of a normal sperm count a few months after stopping the sulphasalazine.

Patients with ulcerative colitis in remission who become pregnant generally have no ill effects during pregnancy and the standard medicines do not seem to produce problems with the fetus. However, in active disease the spontaneous abortion rate is high. The picture in Crohn's disease for pregnant patients is less clearly understood but it seems likely that inactive disease is unlikely to complicate the pregnancy. Authors of papers discussing this topic uniformly stress the importance of using medical treatment to maintain the health of the mother. It is most important to reassure patients who are pregnant that they should attend if symptoms occur and that the medicines – steroids and sulphasalazine – particularly if used locally, will not be deleterious to their pregnancy. The incidence of relapse in either disease does not seem to be particularly increased in pregnancy but may occur in the puerperium.

Inflammatory bowel disease in childhood

Inflammatory bowel disease presents particular problems in childhood. Firstly diagnosis may be delayed even longer than it is in adults. Treatment is the same as in adults but special attention should be shown to nutrition. Secondly, growth retardation is produced by active disease, particularly Crohn's disease and by the steroids used for treatment. To overcome this various strategies have been used. Surgical intervention has been used as a carefully considered treatment to allow a growth spurt once active disease has been excised. Other centres use steroids in various ways including short sharp courses or alternate day doses so that growth retardation is minimized.

Ileostomies

Life with an ileostomy has been described as an improvement on the chronic diarrhoea of ulcerative colitis. However, at present the number of operations for chronic disease seems to be falling, the more important indications for surgery being a complication or a fulminant acute attack. For these patients it is important to stress that an ileostomy will be no handicap. Patients with an ileostomy should return to normal diet, normal work and normal social lives. Notwithstanding, ileostomists are prone to an increased incidence of renal stones and gallstones. In hot weather, and with gastroenteritis they are vulnerable to salt and water depletion because their ileostomy imposes an obligatory loss of 50–100 mmol of sodium each day with 500–1000 ml of water.

Young patients who have established ulcerative colitis, after a careful histological review, are considered for the formation of a pelvic pouch and ileo-anal anastomosis. If this functions normally the ileostomy can be closed. These pouches however are difficult to construct and prone to various complications: experience of their use is being gained slowly. Colostomies are rarely performed for inflammatory bowel disease.

Not unnaturally the physical aspects of appliances for both people with ileostomies and colostomies becomes most important once they have regained health. Access to a stoma therapist, usually a nurse, is particularly valuable.

The pancreas

The pancreas lies on the posterior wall of the abdomen, and develops from separate outgrowths from the intestine, the dorsal and ventral pancreatic buds. Each has its own duct but the two buds fuse to form a single gland. This fusion occasionally fails leading to a congenital anomaly which may be an annular pancreas or an isolated ventral pancreas. The head of the pancreas lies in the duodenal loop, the body is posterior to the stomach and lies anterior to the spine at T_{12}–L_1 while the tail extends into the splenic hilum. Splenic vessels are intimately related to the pancreas and may be damaged in pancreatic disease as may the portal vein lying behind the head of the pancreas. Microscopically the pancreas consists of acini of exocrine tissue draining into the ductal system and of the Islets of Langerhans.

Exocrine secretions, amylase, lipase and peptidases, are released in an inactive form within a bicarbonate-rich pancreatic juice. Secretion is controlled by the vagus, secretin, cholecystokinin-pancreozymin and vaso-active intestinal polypeptide (VIP), and probably inhibited by pancreatic polypeptide. The endocrine pancreas produces insulin and glucagon which are concerned in carbohydrate metabolism. Other hormones produced include somatostatin which is a powerful inhibitor of many hormones.

Synthetic analogues of somatostatin are being assessed, and they are of benefit in patients with vipomas, glucagonomas, and the carcinoid syndrome. Acromegalics lose their headache and have lower growth hormone levels. In gastroenterology, synthetic somatostatin improves dumping, but is of little or no benefit in acute gastrointestinal bleeding.

Acute pancreatitis

This is a major cause of abdominal pain where a self-perpetuating inflammation involves the gland and surrounding tissues.

The two principal aetiological agents are gallstones and alcohol. Infrequent causes include trauma, viral infections such as mumps, hyperparathyroidism, hyperlipidaemia and drugs such as steroids and thiazides. Even rarer is familial acute pancreatitis, and many other diseases have been linked in case reports.

Over 95 per cent of patients with acute pancreatitis have pain, typically felt in the epigastrium or the right and left hypochondria. The severity varies greatly from mild to excruciating and the pain may radiate round the abdomen into the back. Examination in the initial phase of the illness may reveal only mild tenderness with slight guarding. Fever and intestinal ileus may develop and vomiting may be severe. Discolouration of the flanks (Grey–Turner's sign) or around the umbilicus (Cullen's sign) is seen in some severe cases. Shock with hypotension and peripheral circulatory failure is evidence of a severe attack, when hypoxia and respiratory failure can occur.

The diagnosis is usually made by measuring serum amylase although lipase estimations are an alternative. Plasma calcium often falls. Radiology should include chest X-ray and plain abdominal view. The former may show evidence of pleural effusions, and the latter dilated loops of a generalized ileus or an ileus localized to viscera around the pancreas. Abdominal ultrasound and CT scanning will show an inflamed abnormal gland as well as gallstones if they are the precipitating factor. Pseudocysts are a common complication. Indeed with these newer imaging techniques small cysts within the gland have been found to be a very frequent accompaniment of episodes of acute pancreatitis. Barium studies and pancreatic radioisotope scans are rarely used now.

Complications in the initial period include shock, respiratory failure with accompanying cyanosis and disseminated intravascular coagulopathy. Hypocalcaemia may be so severe as to produce tetany. Local complications that take a few days to develop include pseudocysts, fistulae and abscess formation. Diabetes is usually transient. Swelling of the pancreas can cause mild obstructive jaundice.

The management of the illness depends on the severity of the disease. Two-thirds of patients have a mild attack with a mortality of 1–2 per cent. Those factors associated with a severe attack are shown in Table 9.7; three or more indicate a severe attack. The persistence of an elevated urea after adequate fluid replacement is more important than an elevated value on presentation.

A mild attack is treated with analegsia, intravenous fluids and 'nil by mouth' regime. A nasogastric tube is unnecessary unless vomiting is persistent. Although the attack usually subsides within 2–3 days, the cause must always be sought.

Table 9.7 Factors that indicate severe pancreatitis

WCC over 15×10^9/litre
Glucose over 10 mmol/litre
Urea over 16 mmol/litre
Calcium under 2.0 mmol/litre
Albumin under 32 g/litre
Lactate dehydrogenase over 600 u/litre
Arterial PaO_2 under 7.5 kPa

Considerable attention, however, must be devoted to patients with severe attacks. Treatment consists of adequate analgesia and rapid fluid replacement with saline and proteins; central venous pressure monitoring is usually necessary. 'Nil by mouth' regime is started while acid secretion is suppressed by an H_2 receptor antagonist. Peritoneal lavage (similar to peritoneal dialysis) may benefit selected patients. Oxygen will be needed continuously with some patients progressively deteriorating and needing ventilating. Clinical deterioration suggests abscess formation or a necrotic pancreas and ultrasound and CT scan should be undertaken urgently. Under these circumstances laparotomy is indicated.

Pseudocysts are recognized by persistent pain and a failure of the amylase level to return to normal. With conservative care these present no further problems, but those in the lesser sac often require surgical treatment and this is undertaken when the cyst becomes well encapsulated after a few weeks. Fistulae usually close spontaneously.

Chronic pancreatitis

Chronic pancreatitis is a disease where continued inflammation gradually destroys the gland, replacing functioning tissue by fibrous tissue.

Alcohol consumption is the major cause of chronic pancreatitis. Other, rare causes of chronic pancreatitis include hypercalcaemia and tropical calcific pancreatitis probably caused by severe protein-calorie malnutrition. Gallstones are believed to be responsible for a small proportion of cases, as are hypercalcaemia and familial causes. Pancreas divisum, or the isolated ventral pancreas, may also produce chronic pancreatitis when the dorsal part of the gland, draining through the duct of Santorini, develops a stenosis close to the duodenum.

The most important clinical features of chronic pancreatitis are abdominal pain, weight loss and diabetes mellitus. Pain occurs in 75–90 per cent of patients and varies from epigastric discomfort to severe constant gnawing abdominal and back pain requiring opiate analgesia. Leaning forward helps: patients with severe pain often have a pronounced stoop. 'Binge' drinking may exacerbate the pain, as may food. Weight loss occurs in all patients and is probably due to a combination of pain, fear of eating and malabsorption. Steatorrhoea, the most important manifestation of pancreatic malabsorption may not appear till many years after the onset of the disease. Frank diabetes mellitus eventually develops in about one-third of patients with one-third more having abnormal glucose tolerance.

Clinical signs are few. Evidence of weight loss might be present. Upper abdominal tenderness may be the only abdominal sign.

The investigations employed in chronic pancreatitis define structural changes or functional changes. Pancreatic calcification is diagnostic but relatively uncommon in the UK. Ultrasound or a CT scan may show an enlarged gland with diffuse textural changes and even scattered pinpoint calcifications, as well as cyst formation. Endoscopic retrograde cholangiopancreatography (ERCP) is particularly valuable being able to demonstrate more precise changes including dilatation of the duct system, strictures and intraductal stones. ERCP will help separate pancreatic carcinoma from chronic pancreatitis and in assessing which patient should have surgery. Tests of pancreatic function in chronic pancreatitis involve a variety of indirect and direct tests (Table 9.8).

The pancreolauryl test measures the efficacy of a lipolytic enzyme and the PABA test a proteolytic enzyme. The principle for each of these screening tests is that a non-absorbed marker is hydrolysed by a pancreatic enzyme to an absorbed marker, fluorescein or PABA, which is measured in the urine. Direct tests involve placing a tube in the duodenum and measuring pancreatic juice production,

Table 9.8 Tests of pancreatic function

Indirect	Direct
Faecal fat collection	Pancreozymin-secretin
Radiolabelled fat	test
absorption study	Lundt test meal
Stool examination for fat	
and meat fibres	
Pancreolauryl test	
PABA test	
Glucose tolerance test	

stimulated either by pancreozymin and secretin or by the liquid meal used in the Lundt test.

Medical treatment consists of pain relief, trying to limit progress of the disease, and treatment of pancreatic insufficiency and diabetes. Pain relief can be particularly difficult. Opiate analgesics are required in many patients and subsequent addiction is common. The addition of a tricyclic antidepressant or a non-steroidal anti-inflammatory drug may improve the results. Attempts to alter the progress of the disease include abstinence from alcohol and the treatment of precipitating events such as hypercalcaemia or gallstones. Pancreatic insufficiency is relatively straightforward to treat. A low fat, adequate calorie diet is allied to oral enzyme replacement. A variety of high potency enzyme preparations are now available and their dosage is adjusted using faecal fat estimations as markers of adequacy. H_2 receptor antagonists reduce gastric acid degradation of these enzymes and increase their potency. Diabetes on the other hand requires insulin and careful control of the diet, malabsorption making control of the diabetes particularly difficult.

Several techniques to limit the disease or its effects have been tried recently but are of limited value including complete destruction of the exocrine pancreas by injection of acrylic polymers endoscopically and trials of washing out protein plugs at endoscopy. Coeliac plexus block provides pain relief in many patients, but is generally effective for only a few months and repeat attempts are much less successful: carcinoma is a more appropriate indication for this technique.

Surgery is principally undertaken for intractable pain. If ERCP has demonstrated strictures with disease limited to the tail then excision of this part of the pancreas may be very successful. Other approaches include total pancreatectomy, 95 per cent pancreatectomy leaving the residual 5 per cent alongside the duodenal loop or a Puestow procedure.

Complications of chronic pancreatitis include obstructive jaundice. Fibrosis and oedema in the head of the pancreas produce a long stricture of the lower common bile duct. A bypass procedure or an endoscopic prosthesis will relieve the jaundice in patients who do not settle spontaneously. Similarly fibrosis and oedema can produce stenosis of the duodenum or transverse colon necessitating surgical correction. Fluid with high enzyme levels may accumulate in the pleural cavity, pericardium or peritoneum. Thrombosis of the splenic vein is potentially very troublesome. Mild splenomegaly is the usual consequence but about 15 per cent of patients develop gastric or gastro-oesophageal varices that bleed, and are particularly difficult to diagnose and manage. Pseudocysts also occur in chronic pancreatitis.

Chronic pancreatitis tends to be an illness that slowly progresses until little gland remains. At this stage the pain is much less though malabsorption and diabetes will not change. Mortality in these patients is related to surgery, diabetes and the effects of alcohol.

Carcinoma of the pancreas

This malignancy is increasing in the population yet its outlook remains abysmal. Periampullary carcinoma has a better prognosis and is considered separately. Pancreatic carcinoma is now the fifth most common carcinoma. Men are affected twice as often as women and the incidence increases with age. Smoking, heavy drinking, diabetes mellitus and a high dietary fat intake are associated with the disease. Most carcinomas arise in ductal epithelium; the distribution being about 70 per cent in the head, 20 per cent in the body and 10 per cent in the tail. The first symptoms are often vague and poorly localized; abdominal discomfort and malaise are typical. This delays presentation and diagnosis. Thereafter two groups of symptoms predominate; jaundice with weight loss, or pain. If the body or the tail is the site of the disease, deep boring pain, radiating to the back and relieved by leaning forwards, occurs. Weight loss is usual but jaundice rarely occurs. These symptoms are similar to those of chronic pancreatitis. Jaundice and pain occur in carcinoma arising in the head. A few patients present with diabetes or acute pancreatitis. Depression is common in patients with carcinoma of the pancreas.

Examination of the jaundiced patient demonstrates a palpable gall bladder (Courvoisier's law) in a little less than 50 per cent. Hepatomegaly or a palpable mass may be found. Migratory thrombophlebitis is a rare feature of the disease. Diagnosis in the patient with obstructive jaundice involves blood liver function tests followed by an ultrasound. A dilated common bile duct should be seen and a mass in the head may be visible. Absence of gallstones helps. Subsequently ERCP is the investigation of choice to demonstrate the site and nature of the blockage of the bile ducts, and show if an ampullary or peri-ampullary carcinoma is present which can be biopsied. In carcinoma of the body and tail, separation from chronic pancreatitis may be difficult. Ultrasound and CT scan may delineate a lesion and guided aspiration cytology provide diagnostic material. ERCP will show a stricture but may not always clearly demonstrate this to be a carcinoma.

The treatment is almost wholly aimed at relief of symptoms. Jaundice can be relieved surgically by a cholecyst-jejunostomy with or without gastro-jejunostomy or endoscopically by placing a drainage tube across the strictured length of the bile duct (stenting). Survival time is similar for these two techniques. Percutaneous stenting is an alternative approach. Surgical resection of a tumour may be a valuable way of relieving pain, particularly in cases of carcinoma of the body and tail, but attempts at curative surgery in general do not provide worthwhile improvements in survival times. Radiotherapy and chemotherapy are not of great benefit, increasing survival time for perhaps a few weeks only.

The prognosis is very bad. Over 50 per cent of patients die within 9 months; 5-year survival is well under 5 per cent. Not surprisingly some centres do not believe that 'curative' surgery has a place. A few long survivors after bypass are reported but in many, if not all, no histological confirmation of the diagnosis had been made.

Periampullary and ampullary carcinoma present early with obstructive jaundice. Investigation shows dilated bile ducts and pancreatic ducts and the carcinoma may often be seen at endoscopy. Diagnosis is usually obtained at ERCP. A stent may be placed to improve the patient's jaundice as he is prepared for operation. The treatment of choice is a Whipple procedure, pancreaticoduo-denectomy. Though this is associated with a high operative mortality, the 5-year survival is 30–50 per cent, a worthwhile approach for this group of tumours.

Cystic fibrosis

This illness with an autosomal recessive inheritance is now being increasingly encountered as the patients' survival increases. Most patients have suffered in childhood from frequent respiratory infections and have malabsorption, the diagnosis being originally confirmed by a sweat test. Respiratory disease is a major aspect of the illness with severe infections leading to bronchiestasis and to cor pulmonale, needing appropriate antibiotics, physiotherapy and bronchodilators. Most patients also have pancreatic malabsorption treated with pancreatic supplements, H_2 receptor antagonist, and a diet that is adequate nutritionally, produces no side-effects and no barrier to growth.

Problems being encountered in adolescence and young adulthood include small bowel obstruction which usually settles on conservative treatment. A variety of hepatic problems include fibrosis, cirrhosis, gallstones and even variceal bleeding.

Endocrine tumours

Pancreatic tissue is the origin of a variety of endocrine tumours. Insulinoma with hypoglycaemia is the commonest. The Zollinger–Ellison syndrome is the consequence of a gastrin secreting tumour. Glucagonomas have been described producing mild diabetes and a particular migratory rash mostly seen on the peripheries. Vasoactive intestinal polypeptide (VIP) secretion produces the pancreatic cholera syndrome.

Anaesthesia and gastrointestinal disease

Patients undergoing abdominal surgery may present with additional problems associated with gastrointestinal disorders. Continuous suction via a nasogastric tube may lead to fluid and electrolyte loss resulting in alkalosis and hypokalaemia. Malnutrition may be elicited from the history and a clinical examination may reveal loose skin folds and muscle wasting. If the weight loss does not exceed 10 per cent of the ideal body weight, then routine nutritional support is probably unnecessary. However, a severely catabolic patient who has lost weight and is likely to have continuing absorptive difficulties postoperatively should benefit from intravenous alimentation. Patients who are malnourished may have fatty infiltration of the liver, cardiac failure due to thiamine deficiency and anaemia of multifactorial origin. Prolonged diarrhoea or vomiting are likely to lead to electrolyte disturbances and hypokalaemia. In the malnourished patients there are increased risks of infection as well as interference with temperature control. Post-operative complications increase 5-fold if the serum albumin < 3.2 g/dl.

Anaesthetic agents may interfere with gastrointestinal function. Relaxation of oesophageal sphincters may lead to regurgitation of gastric contents which may be inhaled unless considerable precautions are taken. Gastric emptying is impaired by opiates, atropine-like drugs, pain and immobilization. Beta adrenergic receptor blocking agents may reduce the lumen of the bowel while drugs and techniques, which reduce the blood flow especially to the mucosa of bowel, can impair the integrity of intestinal anastomoses.

Biliary disease

Gallstones

Bile contains three principal constituents whose balance is important in gallstone formation. These are cholesterol, bile salts (also known as bile acids) and phospholipids, principally lecithin. The bile salts maintain the other two components in watery solution. As the relative proportion of bile salts falls and that of cholesterol particularly rises, the bile becomes supersaturated and cholesterol may precipitate out. Bile in this state is described as lithogenic. Cholesterol concentrations are raised by obesity, excess fat in the diet and oestrogens. Precipitation of cholesterol, where recognized, seems to centre on mucus, gall bladder polyps and precipitated bilirubinate following infection. Most gallstones are mixed stones composed of cholesterol (major component), calcium salts and bilirubin. Pure cholesterol stones and pure bilirubin stones occur less frequently.

Gallstones are very common in Western populations. Up to 30 per cent of elderly women have them, the incidence in men being lower. Increasing age and obesity are important predisposing factors. Bilirubin stones are most commonly encountered in patients with a haemolytic anaemia or haemoglobinopathy. Most gallstones are silent, the person eventually dying of other disease unaware of their presence and having had no symptoms. For reasons that are at present unknown, a variety of manifestations can develop (Fig. 9.1).

Chronic cholecystitis is one of the commonest. The wall of the gall bladder becomes inflamed and gradually thickens. Symptoms include flatulent dyspepsia, nausea and pain. Flatulent dyspepsia is associated with belching, fatty food intolerance and often heartburn. The pain is generally in the epigastrium, right hypochondrium or even in the lower chest and is often vaguely localized. This pain can be rather chronic, though other patients may have biliary colic for a few hours which is thought to be due to recurrent but transient obstruction by stones to flow of bile in the gall bladder. The only abnormal physical sign may be mild tenderness over the gall bladder. A change of bowel habit is common: this is likely to be the result of dietary change.

Acute cholecystitis occurs when the gall bladder becomes truly obstructed. Nausea and vomiting and severe right hypochondrial pain which may radiate to the back between the scapulae are the usual symptoms. There is tenderness and guarding in the right hypochondrium and Murphy's sign is generally positive. The patient is usually febrile and ill.

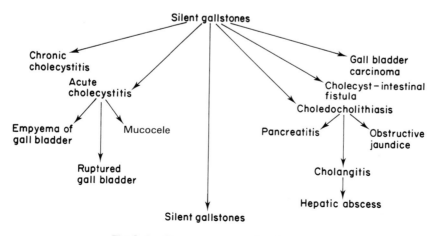

Fig 9.1   Consequences of gallstones.

Routine haematology and biochemistry in chronic cholecystitis are usually normal but may show a leucocytosis and mildly abnormal liver function tests in acute cholecystitis. Abdominal ultrasound is the most useful initial investigation. In chronic cholecystitis a contracted, thick walled gall bladder with stones should be visible. In acute cholecystitis ultrasound will allow early confirmation of the presence of gall bladder disease. Oral cholecystography, however, has been the commonest investigation for gall bladder disease. Though dependent on near normal liver function it is a valuable method of demonstrating gallstones and shows whether there is good filling of the gall bladder with bile. Nonetheless, gall bladders fail to opacify both for intrinsic reasons (disease) as well as extrinsic (failure to swallow contrast tablets, malabsorption, poor liver function, etc.). Cholecystography has been used at an interval of 6–8 weeks after acute cholecystitis to attempt to demonstrate the gall bladder. Radioisotope scanning with HIDA is a useful initial investigation in acute cholecystitis when the gall bladder fails to fill. It probably produces slightly more accurate results than ultrasound or the other imaging techniques. ERCP has relatively little to offer in cholecystitis.

Treatment is mostly by cholecystectomy, though medical dissolution of gallstones for chronic cholecystitis is employed. In chronic cholecystitis the operation is elective. An operative cholangiogram is becoming a routine feature of all cholecystectomies. In acute cholecystitis initial management involves intravenous fluids, analgesia and antibiotics. Morphine may cause spasm of the sphincter of Oddi and intensify the pain, producing symptoms not dissimilar from that of myocardial infarction. (Morphine is also better avoided in patients who had a cholecystectomy, as it may also produce pain by a similar mechanism.) Cholecystectomy is now being undertaken more frequently as an early operation – within days of onset of the disease rather than waiting the time-honoured 2–3 months. This delay may allow further episodes to occur.

Medical management is by gallstone dissolution therapy. Patients must be carefully selected. Non-opaque stones, preferably under 2 cm in diameter, in a functioning gall bladder are necessary. Chenodeoxycholic acid, ursodeoxycholic acid or a combination are given as a night-time dose for periods up to 18 months to dissolve the stones. There are side-effects of liver dysfunction and diarrhoea from taking chenodeoxycholic acid but ursodeoxycholic acid has relatively fewer side-effects. Unfortunately, after stopping treatment the stones recur in many if not most patients, sometimes within months. It has been put forward that a radical change to a high fibre diet may reduce the lithogenic nature of the bile in these patients.

The complications of cholecystitis include cholecyst-intestinal fistula. A gallstone, usually large, erodes through the gall bladder into adjacent small intestine. This passage is usually asymptomatic but gallstone ileus may result when a large stone reaches a narrower segment such as the ileum. On plain abdominal X-ray a stone may be seen in the right iliac fossa and gas in the biliary tree. Following acute cholecystitis several events may occur. Continuing obstruction with sterile gall bladder contents may result in the gradual accumulation of mucus from the lumen to produce a mucocele. This should be excised. If the bile is infected continued obstruction results in an empyema of the gall bladder. Pain and fever persist with continued tenderness and guarding in the right upper quadrant of the abdomen. Emergency cholecystectomy is needed. Gall bladders occasionally perforate in acute cholecystitis to produce a biliary peritonitis. Early surgery with peritoneal lavage is needed for this complication, which if left carries a high mortality.

Acalculous cholecystitis occurs in about 10 per cent of acute cholecystitis, and is a complication encountered in patients in the intensive care unit. No stones are seen on ultrasound or cholecystogram. Initial treatment may require percutaneous gall bladder drainage and antibiotics. Most patients have a cholecystectomy eventually for persisting symptoms and in many an abnormal mucosa with Rokitansky–Aschoff sinuses or cholesterol deposits is found.

Not all patients lose their symptoms after cholecystectomy. In this difficult group explanations include misdiagnosis such as silent stones and the irritable bowel syndrome, retained stones in the common bile duct or cystic duct remnant and the post-cholecystectomy syndrome. This last is poorly defined and includes stenosis of the sphincter of Oddi and tonic bile duct pain.

Choledocholithiasis

Stones in the common bile duct can arise from the gall bladder and pass the cystic duct or originate *de novo* in the common bile duct or the hepatic biliary tree. About 15 per cent of patients with gall bladder stones also have them in the common bile duct.

Typical symptoms consist of biliary colic, jaundice, ascending cholangitis and pancreatitis. Biliary colic is a severe colic, arising from the epigastrium and right hypochondrium which radiates to the back in the region of the tips of the scapulae. Obstructive jaundice, with or without colic, is an important aspect of stones in the bile duct. It can mimic a pancreatic neoplasm in the elderly with quite marked weight loss and can also produce intermittent jaundice. Ascending cholangitis occurs when infections arise in the biliary tree. Poor or absent drainage of bile is a requisite feature. As well as stones other causes include neoplasm and stricture of the bile duct. The symptoms are those of Charcot's triad – pain, rigors and jaundice.

Physical findings in biliary colic are typically minimal. A little tenderness may be present in the right hypochondrium. Jaundice may be transient. In ascending cholangitis the features of severe infection are present – prostration, high fever and hypotension. Jaundice rapidly worsens and the liver becomes quite tender.

Diagnosis and treatment of the conditions vary. Biliary colic needs analgesia before investigations can be begun. The first investigation, an ultrasound may show a dilated duct containing one or several stones. In obstructive jaundice treatment follows diagnosis. The steps in the sequence of investigation are usually ultrasound followed by ERCP or percutaneous transhepatic cholangiography. CT scanning may play a small role in reaching a diagnosis. Vitamin K should be given to correct clotting abnormalities in prolonged jaundice.

Ascending cholangitis however needs urgent treatment. After blood cultures have been obtained, antibiotics should be started as soon as possible. Amoxycillin or cefuroxime with metronidazole would be a suitable combination. Vitamin K may be needed. Investigation should be delayed till the patient is starting to recover if possible. Ultrasound and other imaging procedures should be used to fully outline the duct system. A cause for blockage should be extensively sought in all patients who have episodes of ascending cholangitis.

Definitive treatment is either surgical or endoscopic. Operative clearance of the bile duct has been an operation used for many years. However, it has a considerably higher mortality than cholecystectomy and in many patients an indwelling T-tube is needed. Endoscopic treatment by sphincterectomy and the clearing of the bile duct with a balloon or Dormia basket has been developed. Overall mortality is lower than exploration of the bile duct; morbidity is reasonable.

Patients who have been treated early generally have a good outcome from their treatment. However untreated stones in the common bile duct, particularly in the presence of obstructive jaundice, are complicated by episodes of ascending cholangitis and the development of secondary biliary cirrhosis.

Carcinoma of the gall bladder

This relatively rare malignancy nearly always arises in gall bladders containing gallstones. The incidence is highest in women in the 70–80 year age group. The ways the tumour presents include:

- unexpected operative finding;
- similar to chronic cholecystitis;
- abdominal mass;
- obstructive jaundice.

Treatment is surgical but in many patients the tumour has spread before diagnosis is made. The prognosis is poor.

Carcinoma of the extra-hepatic duct

These tumours are about as frequent as carcinoma of the gall bladder. Painless jaundice is the usual presentation. Physical signs are generally unhelpful. At ultrasound the level of blockage producing the obstructive jaundice may be found. If the block seems to be low, near the duodenum, then ERCP would be the next investigation; if high many patients would next have a plasma thromboplastin component (PTC) as their investigation of choice. Carcinoma of the bile ducts is a tumour that often grows slowly and may be amenable to surgery. Unfortunately cure is uncommon though reasonably long survival may result. In some patients non-operative treatment is undertaken. This involves placing drainage tubes across the tumour either using the endoscope or a percutaneous route.

Cholangio carcinoma of the intra-hepatic biliary tree behaves in a very similar manner to hepatoma.

Benign biliary stricture

Cholecystectomy is the usual cause of benign biliary strictures. They present with jaundice or ascending cholangitis. Full visualization is needed using endoscopic and percutaneous routes to plan treatment. Surgery with high anastomosis to jejunum is an excellent treatment but is particularly dependent upon the skill of the surgeon. In unskilled hands a 10–15 per cent mortality is recognized. Secondary biliary cirrhosis is a common complication of biliary strictures.

Clonorchis sinensis infestation

Clonorchis sinensis, a worm which principally inhabits the biliary tree is contracted from eating raw fish and is usually found in people from China, Japan and South East Asia. Abdominal pain and recurrent cholangitis are the symptoms encountered. After diagnosis clearance of the worm should be attempted using hexachloroparaxylol, or chloroquine. Multiple biliary strictures may result from infestation.

The liver

The liver is the most important organ of metabolism. The physiology and function of the liver are of particular value in assessing liver function clinically and in determining the consequences of liver disease.

Metabolic processes dependent on the liver are many (Table 9.9). The liver is one of the most important regulators of body protein, amino acid and carbohydrate metabolism. Most urea is excreted in the kidney but approximately one-fifth is degraded in association with the intestinal wall to produce ammonia which is subsequently converted to amino acid and urea after passing to the liver in portal blood. Synthesis of many other proteins occurs in the liver including important proteins such as most of the clotting factors (except Factor VIII), many carrier proteins and non-gamma globulins.

Lipid metabolism by the liver is of two types. Cholesterol is synthesized and much is then secreted in the bile as cholesterol, or as bile acids after being further metabolized. Triglycerides are also synthesized and released into the circulation by the liver. Bilirubin is taken up from albumin in the circulation, transported by carrier proteins to the glucuronidases. The bilirubin diglucuronide formed is water soluble and secreted into the bile cannaliculus.

Drug metabolism by the liver is of great significance. A variety of processes occurs. The

Table 9.9 Some metabolic functions of the liver and the consequences of liver disease

	Function	Effect of disease
Carbohydrate metabolism	Glycogen synthesis	Hypoglycaemia
	Glycogenolysis	Diabetes mellitus
	Gluconeogenesis	
	Lactic acid metabolism	
Protein metabolism	Albumin synthesis	Low albumin-oedema
	Clotting factor synthesis	Impaired clotting
	Urea synthesis	Impaired ammonia metabolism – encephalopathy
	Amino acid deamination	
	Ammonia incorporation	
Lipid metabolism	Triglyceride synthesis	Impaired biliary lipid production
	Cholesterol synthesis	Fatty liver
	Bile acid synthesis	
Drug metabolism	Oxidation Conjugation	Increased sensitivity especially of liver

cytochrome P450 system principally oxidize aliphatic and aromatic groups in the drug molecule: the effect is usually to reduce the pharmacological activity of the drug, but a few drugs (e.g. imipramine) are transformed to active metabolites. The second major action is to conjugate the drug with glucuronic acid or other water soluble molecules. This leaves the drug soluble and so excretable in urine or bile.

In liver disease, particularly when severe, many or all of these functions can be disturbed (*see* Table 9.9).

Liver function tests

Liver function tests measures several aspects of both function and damage. For example bilirubin assesses in part secretion by the liver; albumin and clotting factors assess synthesis while the enzymes demonstrate damage to the liver cells. The general liver function tests are described here and other ways of assessing liver function follow.

Bilirubin

Bilirubin is measured as a total and then as a conjugated or water soluble glucuronide.

Jaundice as shown by Table 9.10 has many causes. Prehepatic and some hepatic causes are associated with an elevated unconjugated bilirubin, whereas posthepatic lesions produce almost entirely conjugated bilirubin in the serum and urine.

Table 9.10 Causes of jaundice and hyperbilirubinaemia

Haemolytic disease
Septicaemia
Severe infection (e.g. pneumonia)

Gilbert's disease and other hereditary
    hyperbilirubinaemias
Hepatitis (viral, autoimmune, alcoholic)
Intrahepatic cholestasis
Decompensated cirrhosis
Intrahepatic tumours

Gallstones
Pancreatitis
Carcinoma of bile ducts
Carcinoma of pancreas
Bile duct stricture
Biliary atresia
Ascending cholangitis

Albumin-prothrombin time

These are measures of synthetic activity in liver. Though albumin levels may fall for many reason, if the prothrombin time is also prolonged this suggests diminished hepatic synthetic activity. Abnormal clotting may be produced by malabsorption and biliary obstruction too.

Alkaline phosphatase

In the liver this enzyme is localized to the region of the bile cannaliculus. Obstruction to the biliary tree produces marked elevations though alkaline phosphatase may be elevated in hepatocellular damage. However, the liver is not the only source; alkaline phosphatase can be elevated in bone disease and pregnancy (from the placenta). Additional enzymes that act as markers of a hepatic source for an elevated alkaline phosphatase are 5'nucleotidase or gammaglutamyl transferase.

Alanine transaminase-aspartate transaminase

These enzymes are released from damaged hepatocytes. Aspartate transaminase is produced by damage to many other tissues including heart, skeletal muscle and kidney, so is much less specific as a marker of liver disease. Alcoholics may have higher aspartate than alanine transaminases, a reversal of the usual pattern.

Gamma-glutamyl transferase

This enzyme is a non-specific marker, elevation being due to a mixture of cell damage and enzyme induction. It is useful in confirming the liver as a source of elevated alkaline phosphatase and is commonly used as an indicator of heavy alcohol consumption.

Interpretation of liver function tests

Though some patterns of abnormality of liver function tests are well recognized the interpretation of others is particularly difficult. All depend on a clinical assessment to give them a real value. The well recognized patterns are:

- *Cholestasic* – elevated bilirubin, markedly elevated alkaline phosphatase with near normal albumin and transaminases. The prothrombin time may be prolonged by vitamin K malabsorption.
- *Hepatitic* – elevated bilirubin, markedly elevated transaminases, low albumin and prothrombin time with a normal or mildly abnormal alkaline phosphatase.

When assessing other patterns particular note needs to be made of the patient's diagnosis and treatment. Many severe illnesses produce abnormal levels of transaminases and lower plasma albumin. Numerous drugs cause liver damage – often clinically unimportant on first appearance but sufficient to elevate the plasma enzymes. These changes may indicate potentially severe side-effects from a drug and would be an indication to change treatment.

Other investigations

Imaging

A variety of techniques have been used to examine the liver. Currently ultrasound is the first investigation. Cysts, metastases, abscesses, liver texture (e.g.

for cirrhosis) and the state of the biliary tree and blood vessels can be assessed. Subsequently CT scanning would be the next investigation in many centres. Additional information such as the relative amount of fat can be added to the findings of an ultrasound scan.

Radioisotope scans are being less frequently used. A variety of techniques are in use including Tc^{99} sulphur-colloid for liver size, presence of intra-hepatic lesions and evidence of reticulo-endothelial dysfunction. Hepatocellular carcinoma can be detected with a gallium scan.

Advanced liver disease may make angiography necessary. Coeliac and superior mesenteric arterio-graphy outlines the hepatic artery and later the portal vein. Splenoportography involves punc-turing the spleen and injecting contrast medium to outline the splenic and portal veins. Splenic pulp pressure can be measured simultaneously. Digital subtraction angiography (DSA) may replace these techniques as amounts of contrast needed are lower and the quality of the images obtained is better.

As previously discussed the biliary tree can be outlined by ERCP or transhepatic chol-angiography.

Liver biopsy

Percutaneous biopsy using one of several needles and techniques is widely used to make a diagnosis in chronic liver disease. The procedure has a mor-tality of under 0.1 per cent. Patients at greater risk include those with advanced liver disease and poor coagulation. Complications include haemorrhage and, to a much lesser extent, biliary leakage and damage to lung, kidney and intestine.

Alternative techniques include laparoscopic con-trol of the biopsy needle for examination of specific lesions. Transjugular biopsy is employed in patients with poor coagulation.

Measurement of blood flow, pressure and metabolism

Hepatic blood flow can be measured using the clearance of indocyanin green. Steady state or single bolus approaches are used. Portal vein pressure, an important measurement in cirrhosis, can be assessed by direct puncture, or a more indirect measurement, wedged hepatic vein pressure. Liver function can be measured by several other techniques. Bromsulphothalein reten-tion times are used as a comparison between diffe-rent patients. C^{14} aminopyrine breath test is used as an alternative approach to measuring overall liver function. These two last tests tend to be used more as research tools.

Physical signs in liver disease

Signs of liver disease can be found in the limbs, skin and over the head as well as the abdomen. They are listed in Table 9.11. Several disease-specific signs may be present and are described as appropriate to the disease.

Table 9.11 Physical signs in liver disease

Hands	Palmar erythema	Finger clubbing
	Leuconychia	Dupuytren's contracture
Skin	Jaundice	Bruising
	Spider naevi	Pigmentation
	Scratch marks	Xanthomata
	Gynaecomastia	
Face	Parotid enlargement	Paper money skin
	Fetor hepaticus	
Abdomen	Hepatomegaly	Splenomegaly
	Ascites	Testicular atrophy
	Dilated veins	Hepatic rubs and bruits
Limbs	Oedema	Muscle wasting

Liver disease

Viral hepatitis

Though many viruses cause hepatitis, the illness has common clinical features. The severity of the attack can vary from an asymptomatic illness through the easily recognized icteric illness which is typical of the disease, to fulminant hepatic necrosis.

In a typical attack, after an incubation period that varies with the causative virus, a prodromal period is the first indication of the illness. Symp-toms are non-specific and include anorexia, malaise, and mild fever. Patients frequently lose their taste for cigarettes or alcohol. After a few days these symptoms fade and jaundice develops. Urine darkens and stools become pale. Signs may be apparent with tender hepatomegaly and occa-sionally splenomegaly. This icteric phase usually lasts a few weeks with slow recovery. Tiredness and mild ill health are a not uncommon part of con-valescence from acute hepatitis.

Anicteric and asymptomatic episodes of viral

hepatitis appear to be relatively common; many people having antibodies but no history of illness. In a fulminant attack, at the opposite end of the spectrum, the liver damage becomes progressively more severe. Evidence of organ failure develops with bruising, ascites and encephalopathy. Some patients pass from an icteric phase to an episode of cholestasis. There is a gradual change in their liver function tests to the high bilirubin and alkaline phosphatase of cholestasis as their transaminases, markers of the acute attack, are falling.

In the prodromal phase transaminases are elevated. These rise further in the icteric phase of the illness with rising bilirubin, mostly conjugated. Alkaline phosphatase will be only slightly elevated. The blood count will be normal, only rarely showing haemolytic or aplastic anaemia. Urine tests reveal bilirubin. Evidence of a specific viral cause should be sought. Liver biopsy is very rarely needed in the acute illness, though occasionally needed in the cholestatic attack.

Treatment of an attack after diagnosis is principally supportive and symptomatic. In the icteric phase, bed rest is helpful while fat and alcohol should be avoided. Advice about preventing the spread of the virus should be given to the patient and his family. Most patients do not need admitting to hospital for a typical attack of viral hepatitis. Steroids are of no proven benefit in the acute illness but are sometimes used in a cholestatic episode following the acute attack when they produce a rapid clinical improvement.

Hepatitis A (infectious hepatitis)

This small RNA-containing enterovirus is acquired by the faecal-oral route. It is a common cause of illness in the tropics and wherever hygiene is poor, 95 per cent of these populations having had the illness compared to 20–50 per cent in the Western world, where the highest incidence occurs in the Winter. The incubation period is short, 2–4 weeks. Young people are most commonly afflicted and usually the illness is mild. The virus appears in the faeces and urine in the second half of the incubation period and in most patients the onset of the clinical illness heralds a rapid decline in infectivity.

Diagnosis is made by history with appropriate liver function tests and a rising titre of IgM antibodies to hepatitis A. The presence of IgG anti-hepatitis A antibody indicates a past infection only. Sequelae are few. Chronic hepatitis rarely develops and then only the chronic persistent type.

Prophylactic immune serum globulin can be used to provide passive protection to travellers to high risk areas. A vaccine is being developed.

Hepatitis B (serum hepatitis)

This is the most important viral hepatitis world-wide, because of its prevalence, severity and sequelae.

Hepatitis B has an incomplete strand of DNA and a structure like the earth's with surface and core. Various viral proteins are distributed through the particle and act as antigens for the immune response and as markers for detecting the presence of hepatitis B (Fig. 9.2).

Hepatitis B is acquired by parenteral routes. Contaminated needles, blood products, oral and sexual contact are the usual means. The incidence varies greatly world-wide, being particularly low in the United Kingdom where about 5 per cent of people have been exposed but very high in South Africa and South East Asia where 90 per cent or more of the population have antibodies or are carriers.

The incubation period is from 2–6 months. In the prodromal period features akin to serum sickness are found such as urticaria, joint pains and proteinuria. The acute illness is generally more prolonged and more severe than hepatitis A with about a 3 per cent fatality.

Diagnosis depends on detecting markers of hepatitis B, including both antigens and antibodies. The

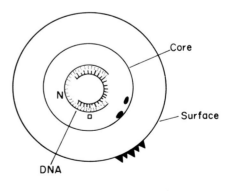

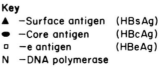

Key
▲ — Surface antigen (HBsAg)
● — Core antigen (HBcAg)
□ — e antigen (HBeAg)
N — DNA polymerase

Fig 9.2 The hepatitis B viral particle.

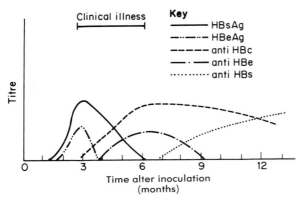

Fig 9.3 Distribution of serum markers in acute hepatitis B.

Table 9.12 Interpretation of serology in hepatitis B

• HBsAg +ve HBeAg +ve Anti HBc −ve	Incubation period	Highly infectious
• HBsAg +ve HBeAg +ve Anti HBc +ve	Clinical illness or chronic carrier	Highly infectious
• HBsAg +ve Anti HBe +ve Anti HBc +ve	Resolving clinical illness or chronic carrier	Slightly infectious
• HBsAg −ve Anti HBs −ve Anti HBe +ve	Convalescent phase	Not infectious
• Anti HBs +ve	Previous infection and immune	Not infectious

pattern of these markers in an acute illness that resolves completely is shown in Fig. 9.3. Titres and timing of the e antigen (HBeAg) and DNA polymerase are identical and are of identical significance. At the start of the icteric phase of the illness anticore antibody (anti HBc) appears, initially as an IgM antibody, subsequently as IgG. About 10 per cent of people become chronic carriers of the virus. The serology in these circumstances shows persisting HBsAg after the clinical illness: if they have persisting HBeAg these patients are highly infectious but if they develop anti HBe they are only minimally infectious. The interpretation of the serology of hepatitis B is shown in Table 9.12.

Treatment is supportive. The illness can be prevented. High titre immunoglobulin for hepatitis B has been available for several years. It is used after accidental inoculation, usually needle-stick injuries in hospitals. It is most effective if given within 48 hours of exposure. Hepatitis B vaccines are also available. One uses highly purified surface antigen protein after a complex preparation that inactivates all known viruses, including HIV. Three doses are given with intervals of 2 and 6 months. It is effective and indicated for people at increased risk of exposure to hepatitis, such as sexual contacts of carriers and newborn children of mothers who are carriers as well as medical personnel. The children of mothers who are both HBsAg and HBeAg positive should be protected by immune globulin at birth followed by a course of vaccine. Recombinant DNA vaccines are now appearing. They will be of benefit world-wide in preventing the disease and its sequelae if they

become sufficiently cheap.

The sequelae of hepatitis B infection are many (Fig. 9.4). All are associated with becoming a carrier of the virus, indicating persisting viral replication many months (at least 6) after an acute illness. Chronic persistent hepatitis is the commonest of these sequelae, occurring in 7–10 per cent of patients after acute hepatitis B. Patients either feel well, or suffer from malaise and fatigue easily. Hepatomegaly and rarely splenomegaly may be present. The diagnosis is suggested by persisting elevation of transaminases. An interval of at least 6 months after acute hepatitis, or evidence of equally prolonged abnormalities of transaminases in the absence of acute hepatitis should precede liver biopsy. The diagnostic features on biopsy are persistence of inflammation in the portal tract without involvement of the parenchyma of the liver. No treatment is indicated. The illness gradually improves, symptomatically and on biochemical testing. Clearance of the virus occurs with cure of the illness eventually.

Chronic active hepatitis follows about 3 per cent of acute attacks. This is a more serious illness that is discussed below. Cirrhosis may result from prolonged chronic active hepatitis or be the presenting feature of the illness. Though HBsAg is positive this is often at low titres and associated with anti-HBe.

Hepatoma, or hepatocellular carcinoma, is an important consequence of hepatitis B infection. The clinical features are discussed later. It is believed that in carriers of hepatitis B the viral genome becomes incorporated into the human DNA. This event, which can occur at any stage, is

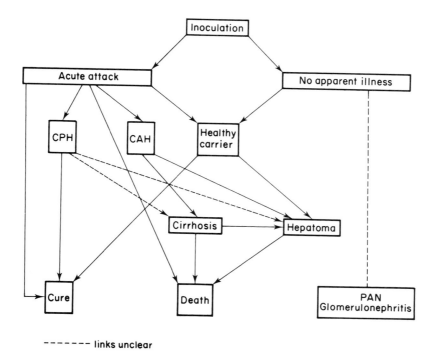

Fig 9.4   Sequence of hepatitis B infection.

associated with cessation of the production of surface antigen and viral particles. The interval to development of hepatocellular carcinoma is not known.

Many associated immunological consequences of the hepatitis B carrier state are known. Polyarteritis nodosa and the manifestations of glomerulonephritis are two of the most important. Other manifestations include vasculitis, arthritis and haemolytic anaemia.

Delta agent hepatitis is an uncommon complication of hepatitis B. The delta agent is an incomplete virus that can only replicate in the presence of the hepatitis B virus. It produces severe, often fatal, attacks of hepatitis and is generally spread parenterally. Delta agent infections can occur during an initial acute hepatitis B illness or produce an episode of hepatitis in a chronic carrier.

Non A-non B hepatitis

The virus or viruses responsible for this clinical picture have yet to be identified. The commonest presentation is an episode of hepatitis 6–12 weeks after parenteral transmission, i.e. intermediate between hepatitis A and hepatitis B. The severity of

the attack is similar to the range encountered in hepatitis B. Persistently abnormal liver function tests are common with rises and falls for up to 12 months. It is believed that at least 20 per cent of patients develop chronic liver disease and cirrhosis which may require steroid therapy. This type of hepatitis is now the commonest posttransfusion hepatitis, though sporadic cases are equally commonly encountered.

A short incubation period hepatitis has also been described. Again this has not been identified further.

Other viral hepatitis

Yellow fever is transmitted by mosquitoes from a monkey reservoir. Though infection is most frequently followed by an unapparent illness, occasional severe outbreaks do occur. Fever, vomiting and jaundice are presenting features, with pain occurring later in the course of the illness. Prognosis is poorer if nervous system or renal involvement occurs or if there is a bleeding diathesis. Immunity can be achieved using an attenutated viral vaccine.

The Epstein–Barr virus produces a hepatitis. In

infectious mononucleosis abnormal liver function tests are common but a clinical hepatitis rare.

Cytomegalovirus and herpes simplex virus cause hepatitis, particularly in immune compromised patients. Other viruses producing hepatitis include Lassa fever, Marburg virus and Ebola virus.

Chronic immune liver disease

Chronic active hepatitis

This progressive liver disease characterized histologically by inflammation in the portal tract and surrounding liver parenchyma has several causes (Table 9.13). Autoimmunity plays an important part in several of them. In the UK the two most common are autoimmune and hepatitis B associated chronic active hepatitis.

Table 9.13 Causes of chronic active hepatitis

Autoimmune (Lupoid)
Hepatitis B associated
Non A-non B hepatitis associated
Haemochromatosis
Wilson's disease
$\alpha1$ anti-trypsin deficiency
Alcohol
Drugs: Methyl dopa,
      isoniazid,
      oxyphenisatin

The autoimmune or lupoid hepatitis occurs most commonly in women, usually premenopausally and often under the age of 30. Symptoms include lassitude, anorexia and weight loss. Jaundice is a common feature at presentation. Signs include palmar erythema, acne and spider naevi. Tender hepatomegaly is the rule. Splenomegaly and fluid retention shown by ascites and oedema occur later in the course of the disease. Many other systems show manifestations of the autoimmune disease process, with diabetes, thyroid disease, glomerulo-nephritis, fibrosing alveolitis and renal tubular acidosis being well recognized.

Liver function tests show an elevated bilirubin and transaminases, the alkaline phosphatase elevation being modest. Plasma albumin is low. Both ESR and IgG are elevated. Tests for hepatitis B are negative. Nearly all patients have a positive test for smooth muscle antibody (SMA). Antimito-chondrial antibody (AMA) is detectable in 30 per cent of patients, rheumatoid factor in 20 per cent and LE cells in a few patients. There is a strong

association with HLA B8, DW3, and A1.

Diagnosis requires appropriate histology. Though portal tracts are inflamed as in chronic persistent hepatitis, the inflammation is not confined by the edge of the portal tract but spreads over to involve the adjacent liver parenchyma. Tentacles of inflammatory cells can be seen surrounding hepatocytes, some of which are ballooned and swollen – piecemeal necrosis. Inflammation, and subsequently fibrosis, join adjacent portal tracts to produce bridging necrosis. Cirrhosis may be seen. In active disease piecemeal necrosis spreading out from any fibrous tissue can be seen.

Treatment is of particular benefit in this liver disease. Corticosteroids are used, initially at a high dose, to correct the liver function tests. The dose of steroids is then reduced, being followed by liver function tests. Repeat biopsy will show an improvement to normal or to the appearances of chronic persistent hepatitis. If particularly high doses of steroids are needed to maintain remission azathioprine can be added and the dose then reduced. Duration of treatment is not known. Some studies have stopped steroids after a period of remission with normal liver function tests and histology but a substantial proportion of the patients subsequently relapse. Untreated the disease progresses to cirrhosis that eventually decompensates.

Hepatitis B chronic active hepatitis represents an immunological response to hepatocytes containing the hepatitis B virus. This type of chronic hepatitis is more common in men and occurs in a slightly older age group. Though symptoms of lassitude and jaundice can occur the finding of abnormal liver function tests is a very common presentation. The autoimmune diseases described above are much less common, though glomerulonephritis and arteritis can be encountered. Liver function tests show elevated transaminases but rarely an elevated bilirubin. These abnormalities vary to-and-fro through the course of the illness.

Diagnosis is based on abnormal liver function tests, evidence of continuing presence of hepatitis B and a liver biopsy. The histological features are the same, with evidence of hepatitis B in hepatocytes. Steroids are of no proven benefit. Immuno-suppression may delay conversion from HBeAg positive to anti-HBe. Antiviral therapy is of some benefit in HBeAg positive patients when, after a period of increased activity, viral replication can be suppressed and the activity of the liver disease will settle.

The other causes of chronic active hepatitis are rarities. However, they are well worth considering when this diagnosis has been made as some of them are treatable.

Primary biliary cirrhosis

Primary biliary cirrhosis is a chronic destructive disease of small intrahepatic bile ducts, and is believed to be immunologically mediated. Cirrhosis is a late stage of the disease.

Primary biliary cirrhosis occurs eight times more frequently in women, especially those aged over 40. The aetiology is unknown though recent studies have found some geographical linkage of cases and the possibility of environmental factors has been raised. The clinical features of the disease can be considered as early symptomatic, advanced symptomatic and asymptomatic. The symptoms early in the disease are principally itching and referral to a dermatologist may occur first. Jaundice is present in a minority of patients at this stage. Signs at this stage of the illness consist of scratch marks, hepatomegaly, and in one-third of patients a palpable spleen. Advancing disease leads to a more easily recognized presentation. Jaundice, pale stools and dark urine now accompany the pruritis. Physical examination reveals a pigmented patient often with xanthelasma: hepatosplenomegaly is present. Further progression is likely to lead to development of features of decompensated cirrhosis including ascites, portal hypertension and encephalopathy. Associated diseases include rheumatoid arthritis, scleroderma, renal tubular acidosis and the sicca syndrome of dry eyes and dry mouth.

Asymptomatic patients are being discovered in increasing numbers. They are diagnosed by liver biopsy following the finding of persistent abnormal liver function tests or hepatomegaly.

Diagnosis commences with finding evidence of cholestasis on the liver function tests. Alkaline phosphatase is generally five or more times elevated. The bilirubin may be normal initially and elevated in more advanced disease. A mild elevation of transaminases may occur. The ESR is increased and IgM is also at a high level. The specific autoimmune manifestation is the antimitochondrial antibody (AMA), positive in over 90 per cent of patients. Histology provides the diagnosis. Stage 1 lesions are pathognomonic – medium sized bile ducts are damaged, surrounded by inflammatory cells and granulomata. Sub-

sequently there is loss of medium size bile ducts from portal tracts, proliferating ductules and periportal invasion by inflammatory cells. The final stage is cirrhosis. If there is any doubt about the diagnosis ERCP should be undertaken to confirm that the extrahepatic biliary tree is normal.

The natural history of the symptomatic patient is slowly progressive deterioration. Bilirubin levels may be stable for prolonged periods. Mean survival in these patients is about 7 years. Towards the end, bilirubin slowly rises, and problems, particularly from portal hypertension and bleeding oesophageal varices may arise. The prognosis of the asymptomatic patient is unknown: some progress to symptomatic disease, others remain unchanged for many years.

Treatment is supportive. Steroids and azathioprine have not been found to be useful. Penicillamine has been shown to reduce the copper overload that occurs with prolonged cholestasis but is relatively toxic, of limited benefit and now little used. Pruritus is treated with cholestyramine, antihistamines or occasionally phenobarbitone, if topical treatment does not work. Because progressive cholestasis leads to shortages of fat soluble vitamins, monthly injections of vitamin D, vitamin K and vitamin A should be given. These help prevent the development of bone disease which is common and which appears to be a mixture of osteoporosis and osteomalacia.

Primary biliary cirrhosis is an indication for liver transplantation, which is at present undertaken when an advanced stage of the disease has been reached.

Inborn errors of metabolism

Gilbert's syndrome

This common condition presents difficulties only when it has not been recognized. The unconjugated bilirubin level is elevated and there is a defect in hepatic uptake and conjugation of bilirubin. Up to 5 per cent of people are affected, the syndrome running in families and usually presenting in young adult life. There are generally no symptoms but a small minority of patients have malaise and other non-specific features. Liver function tests show the elevated unconjugated bilirubin as the only change. Diagnosis theoretically requires a liver biopsy to demonstrate normal liver tissue. This is rarely carried out, and usually preceded by provocation tests such as a 48-hour fast or intravenous nicotinic acid which both elevate the bilirubin. It is most important to tell patients the diagnosis and its implications so that they are not repeatedly investigated or have their treatment denied or altered because their liver function tests are abnormal. Gilbert's syndrome is completely benign.

Other congenital hyperbilirubinaemias

This group of illnesses is much less common than Gilbert's syndrome. The Crigler–Najjar syndromes are a pair of rare unconjugated hyperbilirubinaemias that present in infancy. The basic defect is absence or virtual absence of bilirubin glucuronyl transferase. Type 1 presents in the first days of life with jaundice and kernicterus rapidly ensues. No effective treatment exists. Type 2 is less rare than Type 1 and presents as jaundice in the first year of life. Kernicterus is a rare complication and phenobarbitone produces a marked reduction in the bilirubin. The prognosis is good.

The Dubin–Johnson syndrome is the commoner of the two conjugated hyperbilirubinaemias, which have impaired biliary excretion of bilirubin as the defect. Jaundice is the usual symptom and physical finding. Bilirubin levels are generally less than 80 μmol/litre and other liver function tests are normal. Oral cholecystography fails to demonstrate the gall bladder in these patients. Liver biopsy produces a black core of liver tissue which is virtually diagnostic. No treatment is needed. Rotor's syndrome also presenting in childhood or early adult life is very similar clinically and on liver function tests. Oral cholecystography however is not impaired and liver colour is normal on biopsy. Urinary coproporphyrins are elevated. Again the outlook is good without treatment being required.

Wilson's disease

Though rare this inherited abnormality of copper metabolism is treatable in the early course of the disease. Recessively inherited, the defect is an impaired excretion of copper into bile. Copper deposition follows in liver and brain to produce hepatolenticular degeneration.

The clinical features depend upon the age of presentation for the most part. The severity of liver damage varies greatly – patients with more rapidly progressive liver disease will tend to present under 14 years of age with hepatic features, those with slower hepatic deterioration will more often pre-

sent with nervous system features in their late teens. Hepatic presentations include a hepatitis-like illness, chronic active hepatitis and one of the complications of cirrhosis.

Neuropsychiatric features include development of tremor, dysarthria and abnormal movements. Some intellectual impairment may occur. Psychiatric illness commonly is present in addition to the extrapyramidal features. Other associated illnesses include renal tubular acidosis, renal stones, haemolysis as well as bone and joint problems. In these patients the Kaiser–Fleischer ring is virtually diagnostic and present in over 80 per cent. Other signs include hepatomegaly and the nervous system features.

Diagnosis depends on clinical suspicion of this disease in young patients with hepatic or nervous system problems. Investigations should demonstrate a reduced blood copper and caeruloplasmin levels and elevated 24-hour urinary copper excretion. Liver biopsy should be carried out and part of the specimen analyzed for copper content. Once diagnosed, patients' siblings should have blood and urinary copper estimations carried out.

Wilson's disease is treated with oral penicillamine. This is usually fairly well tolerated up to 1.5 or 2 g daily. Improvement is shown by loss of the Kaiser–Fleischer ring and improvement in the nervous system and hepatic features. Despite the possibility of side-effects, drug dosage should be continued indefinitely at a dose low enough to maintain urinary copper losses. Alternative treatment includes the use of BAL. For patients diagnosed early in the disease, the outlook is excellent and good results can be obtained in many patients with advanced disease also.

Haemochromatosis

This chronic condition arises from the deposition of excess iron in the body tissues. In idiopathic haemochromatosis the intestine inappropriately absorbs more than the 1–2 mg of iron required daily by adults. Total body stores increase from 5 g to between 30 and 50 g. Secondary haemochromatosis produces a clinically identical illness, and arises in people who are regularly transfused (e.g. thalassaemia major) or who have high oral iron intakes, either therapeutically or dietary.

Clinical features reflect the organs into which iron is deposited, the liver, skin, pancreas, heart, pituitary and testes. Typical symptoms are of lassitude, fatigue and the development of mild diabetes mellitus. Men are very much more commonly affected as women are protected for many years by menstruation. Impotence is a common problem, though it is also a feature of both diabetes and cirrhosis. Physical signs include pigmentation of a brown-grey colour to the skin, hepatomegaly and testicular atrophy. In some patients cardiac involvement produces heart failure or cardiac arrhythmias.

Diagnosis is made by demonstrating iron overload. Liver function tests show non-specific changes. Serum iron is elevated, and ferritin is generally very high. Liver tissue should be stained for iron and iron should be estimated quantitatively whenever possible. Primary haemochromatosis can be separated from the iron overload problems found in some alcoholic cirrhotics by venesection as anaemia develops in the latter.

Regular venesection is the treatment of choice. Weekly removal of 500 ml of blood should be carried out until the evidence for iron overload (serum iron, ferritin, liver biopsy) has returned to normal. Hepatomegaly, diabetes mellitus, and heart disease generally improve. Unfortunately other features respond unpredictably to this form of treatment. Once brought under control, monthly venesection is usually adequate to maintain health in people with primary haemochromatosis. It is most important to screen relatives as they may be detected earlier in the course of the disease before some of the untreatable features have developed. Hepatoma or the consequences of portal hypertension are a major cause of death.

Other inherited hepatic disease

As the liver contains large amounts of glycogen it is vulnerable to damage in the glycogen storage diseases. Most of this group of diseases produce hepatomegaly, some with hypoglycaemia. Galactosaemia results in a macronodular cirrhosis which has become the cause of death in many of the longer survivors. α1-antitrypsin deficiency produces an illness that starts with jaundice in infancy. The development of cirrhosis will become clinically apparent by early adulthood.

Hepatic malignancy

Hepatoma

Hepatoma or hepatocellular carcinoma is the commonest primary malignancy of the liver. It is infrequent in the UK but in parts of Asia and Africa is one of the commonest of all malignant diseases. About 80 per cent of hepatomas arise in a cirrhotic liver. World-wide, persistent carriage of hepatitis B with incorporation of the viral DNA into the hepatic nuclear material is the commonest cause. In the UK it is not known how important this mechanism is. The association with alcoholic cirrhosis is the commonest cause in the UK, though hepatoma will develop in other causes of cirrhosis, such as haemochromatosis.

Symptoms and signs are generally those of rapidly deteriorating hepatic function in a patient known to have cirrhosis. Increasing fatigue, weight loss, fever, right upper quadrant pain and swelling are common. Rupture of hepatocellular carcinoma occurs from time-to-time producing peritonitis and shock. In non-cirrhotic patients symptoms are similar or may be reminiscent of gallstones. Examination demonstrates hepatomegaly, perhaps with a distinct mass. A bruit or rub may be audible.

Liver function tests show a rising alkaline phosphatase. Serum alpha-fetoprotein is elevated in 70–90 per cent of patients. Ascitic fluid can be aspirated and is often bloodstained, with a high protein content and occasionally cytology is positive. Ultrasound, CT scan and isotope liver scans frequently demonstrate the hepatoma. However, because the carcinomata arise in a cirrhotic liver, confusion with large regeneration nodules can occur. Liver biopsy will confirm the diagnosis.

Treatment has little to offer the majority of patients. Surgical resection is attempted in the minority of patients with a single lobe of the liver involved, no metastases to bone or lung and, most importantly, a non-cirrhotic liver on biopsy. Transplantation of the liver has been used as treatment but distant recurrent disease is the rule. Chemotherapy with adriamycin may produce a temporary remission in some patients. Some help for the rare metabolic effects of hypercalcaemia, hypoglycaemia or polycythaemia can be given.

The prognosis is poor. The overwhelming majority of these tumours have infiltrated most of the liver at presentation and survival for 6 months occurs in less than 50 per cent. A few have slow-growing tumours with much longer survival.

Intrahepatic cholangiocarcinoma behaves in a similar manner to hepatoma but on a slower time scale and with a higher frequency of presentations due to jaundice. Drainage of obstructed biliary segments provides some palliation in addition to the treatment described above.

Secondary tumours

The liver is one of the most frequent sites for metastasis. In patients with established malignant disease, a progressive elevation of the alkaline phosphatase may pre-date the symptoms of right upper quadrant pain or heaviness, dyspepsia, weight loss and a loss of well being. Jaundice is unusual initially. Patients with symptoms usually have irregular hepatomegaly when examined. Investigations used to demonstrate metastases include ultrasound and isotope liver scan on which deposits may be seen. Liver biopsy which can be ultrasound or CT guided may be needed when there is no known primary site or doubt about the diagnosis.

Though occasional patients have a single resectable metastasis, treatment is symptomatic for most. Chemotherapy, sometimes given via the hepatic artery, or embolization of the tumour may reduce the size of painful metastatic masses.

The liver in infectious disease

Pyogenic liver abscess

Bacterial abscesses of the liver are commonly due to Gram-negative organisms, though anaerobic infections are being recognized with increasing frequency. Abscesses may follow portal pyaemia secondary to an intra-abdominal collection of pus or ascending cholangitis, though most occur spontaneously. Clinically the infections present with high fever, rigors, jaundice and right upper quadrant abdominal pain. Tender hepatomegaly may exist with a rub or a right pleural effusion. Under these circumstances the diagnosis is relatively straightforward. However persisting fever may occur with few other features that localize the problem to the liver and so liver abscess must also be considered when patients have a pyrexia of unknown origin.

Liver function tests show an elevated alkaline phosphatase, possibly elevated transaminases and bilirubin – the derangements seen with an intra-hepatic mass. Blood cultures may be positive and a leucocytosis found. Isotope scanning and ultrasonography have made diagnosis much easier. Current treatment involves aspiration of as much pus as possible, usually carried out after ultrasound guided placement of the aspiration needle. A prolonged (3–4 weeks) course of microbiologically appropriate antibiotics is employed. Multiple small abscesses require antibiotics only, aspiration of one or two of them providing pus for microbiology.

Amoebic liver abscess

The clinical features of this condition are fever and right hypochondrial pain, with a tender enlarged liver. The history of travel is almost invariable, though the interval between exposure to *Entamoeba histolytica* and the development of an abscess may be long. Colitis rarely occurs at the same time.

Diagnosis is based on demonstrating an abscess, in the same way as a pyogenic abscess, and also confirming amoebic disease by antibody tests and stool specimens. When aspirated chocolate-brown pus is obtained. As the abscess may be complicated by rupture into pleura, lung or peritoneal cavity, or even secondary infection, treatment should be started immediately. Metronidazole, 400 mg t.d.s., is the standard approach as for amoebic colitis.

Hydatid disease

Hydatid cysts arise when man becomes the intermediate host to the dog tapeworm, *Echinococcus granulosus*, instead of the sheep. Mediterranean countries, Australia, New Zealand and South America are the regions from which patients are most likely to originate. Though the liver is the commonest site they have also been found in the brain, lungs and bones. The illness is frequently symptom-free and found when another disease is being investigated or when hepatomegaly has been found. Right upper quandrant discomfort or the effect of a cyst rupturing into peritoneum or the biliary tree may cause the illness to present. The contents of hydatid cysts are potent allergens and rupture or needling may produce anaphylactic shock. The structure of the cysts with walls of fibrous tissue, chitinous endocyst, then germinal layer and the presence of daughter cysts, make hydatid disease easily recognizable on ultrasonography and CT scanning. Calcified cysts are also seen on abdominal X-rays.

It is often difficult to decide whether to treat an individual patient. Symptomatic disease is generally treated by surgery. Great care is taken to prevent spillage of cysts and their contents as seeding may occur or anaphylactic shock result. Albendazole is reasonably effective in treating hydatid disease medically and may be valuable prior to operation.

Schistosomiasis

This major problem world-wide is still spreading in the wake of irrigation projects, etc. The cercariae of *Schistosoma mansoni* and *S. japonica* are found in fresh water and penetrate the skin. After migrating to the portal system they involve the intestine initially, producing numerous eggs in the intestinal lumen. Subsequently the adult worms end up in the portal system of the liver where they excite a fibrous reaction. The result is portal hypertension and hepatic fibrosis (pipe-stem fibrosis). Hepatosplenomegaly is usual. Ova may be present in the stool and liver biopsy may also show ova embedded in the portal fibrosis. Portal hypertension can be treated as described below, as the hepatic parenchyma is usually not prejudiced and so shunt surgery is often well tolerated by these patients. Praziquantel is the treatment of choice to kill the trematodes, though oxamniquine is also used.

Other bacterial infections

Septicaemia and pneumococcal pneumonia are often complicated by mild jaundice and abnormal liver function tests. Leptospirosis is rare, producing a bacterial hepatitis with jaundice and bleeding due to hepatic disease and disseminated coagulopathy. Renal failure occurs. Penicillin at the start of the illness may be effective, otherwise treatment is supportive.

In miliary tuberculosis the liver is usually involved. Caseating granulomata will be found on biopsy – this approach can also help in determining causes of pyrexia of unknown origin and occasionally in assisting the diagnosis of active TB at other sites. Similarly syphilis can involve the liver producing hepatitis in the secondary stage and gumma in the tertiary.

Cirrhosis

Cirrhosis is a chronic disease where liver cells necrose with accompanying inflammation. The liver then consists of areas of regeneration (nodules) surrounded by bands of fibrous tissue which replaces the necrotic cells and occasional areas of necrotic liver cells (seen on macro and microscopic examination).

The size of the nodules and the general appearance of the liver has been used in the past to classify the cirrhosis using terms such as macronocular and micronodular, Laënnec's, portal or postnecrotic.

Table 9.14 Causes of cirrhosis

Alcohol
Viral hepatitis – B
non A   non B
Chronic active hepatitis
Primary biliary cirrhosis
Secondary biliary cirrhosis
Drugs – methyl dopa, isoniazid
Wilson's disease
Haemochromatosis
$\alpha 1$ anti-trypsin deficiency
Galactosaemia
Congestive cardiac failure
Budd–Chiari syndrome
Veno-occlusive disease
Jejeuno-ileal bypass
Cryptogenic

However, most causes can produce a mixture of these appearances in different individuals or even in different parts of the same liver. Cirrhosis is best classified by cause (Table 9.14). Most are self-explanatory and a few are treatable. Cryptogenic cirrhosis probably represents the endstage of an autoimmune process, and is found mostly in women.

Cirrhosis which is uncomplicated may be discovered by chance as at this stage of the illness. Symptoms of weakness, lethargy and slight ill health may be absent. Liver palms, a palpable liver and a slight fever may be the accompanying physical signs. At this stage – compensated cirrhosis – liver function tests may be normal. Diagnosis is made by liver biopsy. The outlook for compensated cirrhosis is relatively good.

Decompensated cirrhosis, that is when complications develop, has a much worse prognosis. In alcoholic cirrhosis, 1-year survival for compensated cirrhotics is about 80 per cent and 5-year survival about 50 per cent, but when complications develop survival is reduced to 20–40 per cent at 1 year and 0–30 per cent at 5 years.

Child's classification of liver function was introduced so that prognosis after portosystemic shunt surgery could be assessed. It is basically a division of liver function into good, moderate and poor and the classification applies to outcome after the development of many of the complications (Table 9.15). The complications of cirrhosis can be loosely divided into those related to portal hypertension and those related to liver cell failure. However, there is considerable interdependence between the

Table 9.15 Child's classification

| | | Liver function | |
	Good	Moderate	Poor
Bilirubin (μmol/l)	< 35	35–50	> 50
Albumin (g/l)	> 35	35–30	< 30
Encephalopathy	None	Minimal	Advanced
Ascites	None	Easily controlled	Poorly controlled
Nutrition	Excellent	Good	Poor

various complications in their aetiology and treatment.

Portal hypertension

The pressure in the portal vein is normally slightly higher (3–5 mm Hg) than the pressure of the inferior vena cava. Portal hypertension results from obstruction to outflow as well as an increase of the inflow of blood from the systemic circulation. Obstruction to flow can be considered as hepatic, prehepatic (lesions of the portal vein) and posthepatic (lesions or high pressure in hepatic veins). In portal hypertension the effects of increased pressure result in an enlarged spleen, as well as collateral vessels that develop to provide alternative connections between the portal system and the systemic circulation. The important sites for these are:

- submucosally in the oesophagus draining the left gastric vein into the azygos venous system;
- in the posterior abdominal wall to the renal veins, etc.;
- in the haemorrhoidal plexus and;
- through the remnant of the umbilical vein to the anterior abdominal wall.

Physical signs in patients with portal hypertension include a palpable spleen and dilated abdominal wall veins which radiate and flow away from the umbilicus. A caput medusae may be present in a few patients. Continuous venous hums are sometimes heard in the umbilical vein and its connections. Features of portal hypertension can be investigated in a variety of ways. Imaging can be attempted using ultrasound or CT scan for splenic size, portal venous size and thrombosis of the portal vein. A barium swallow or endoscopy can demonstrate oesophageal varices. Angiographic evaluation of portal hypertension can be under-

taken with an estimate of portal pressure being made. Alternative ways of measuring the pressure in the portal system are to measure wedged hepatic vein pressure, or the more recently developed method for measuring tension in oesophageal varices. In patients who have had a haematemesis or are suspected of having slowly bleeding varices, endoscopy is the investigation of choice.

Bleeding oesophageal varices provide the most important clinical manifestation of portal hypertension alone. Bleeding from haemorrhoidal plexus communications is of virtually no clinical importance in the adult. The severity of variceal bleeding varies greatly from rapid exsanguination to very slow oozing producing melaena or encephalopathy. Haematemesis is typically pain free. It is not known why varices rupture and the incidence of bleeding is not related to progressive increases in portal pressure once a threshold pressure of about 15 mm Hg has been passed. Hypotension and the other features of haemorrhagic shock are common in bleeding oesophageal varices.

A major bleed may produce a deterioration in liver function, almost certainly because of reduced hepatic perfusion. Thus, following bleeding oesophageal varices jaundice is common and encephalopathy occurs frequently.

The management of bleeding oesophageal varices can be considered as an immediate phase and as a long-term phase. In the immediate phase, the first priority is resuscitation. Transfusion will correct the blood loss but if the prothrombin time is particularly prolonged fresh frozen plasma should be administered. Large amounts of intravenous saline are likely to be only of temporary benefit in many, if not most patients, as the saline will tend to increase ascites and peripheral oedema without expanding blood volume. Hypoglycaemia should be considered and treated appropriately. As soon as is feasible endoscopy should be undertaken. As long as the patient is not bleeding briskly emergency sclerotherapy can be performed. Lactulose and neomycin should be used for encephalopathy and ranitidine and antacid may be needed for control of oozing from erosive gastritis which can be found in these patients. Nasogastric tubes should not, in general, be passed for bleeding oesophageal varices. They may, however, have a place to play if encephalopathy becomes the major problem in management.

If the patient is no longer bleeding further immediate therapy is not needed. However, continued or renewed bleeding within 24–48 hours is particularly common and there are several ways of trying to combat this, the choice depending on what is *available* and the skill of the staff looking after the patient. Vasopressin is frequently employed, though arguments still continue about how effective it is. Vasopressin is best given as a continuous infusion at 0.4–0.8 units/kg/hour for up to 24 hours. Colic and diarrhoea are the rule if adequate dosage is employed but angina can also occur. A synthetic vasopressin analogue is available (trilysylvasopressin), that is given in bolus form with perhaps fewer side-effects. Vasopressin is effective in about 50 per cent of patients but re-bleeding occurs often.

A Sengstaken tube is an alternative way of controlling active bleeding if it is due to a varix. The use of Sengstaken tubes requires a level of skill and experience in both medical and nursing staff, as their misuse can be particularly hazardous. The tube, preferably 4 lumen, is introduced through the mouth, or the nose, and passed so that the gastric balloon is in the stomach. This balloon is then inflated with about 500 ml (check the balloon first) and pulled gently back to the cardia. The tube can be fixed in place using tape or a weight of 250–500 g so that the balloon is occluding blood flow from the stomach to the oesophagus at the cardia. If fresh blood is still being aspirated at the oesophageal aspiration port then the oesophageal balloon should be inflated, the pressure being maintained at 30–40 mmHg. It is a wise precaution to check the position of the gastric balloon radiologically after it has been inflated. If bleeding ceases the oesophageal balloon can be cautiously deflated and must be deflated at 24 hours as oesophageal necrosis may occur. *Tamponade* is effective in the short-term in patients with bleeding varices and may allow time for sclerotherapy or surgery to be considered and the patient resuscitated in other ways. Alternative therapeutic regimens for lowering portal pressure are currently under evaluation. Trinitrine and beta blockers have been used with

benefit, the aim being to reduce cardiac output and hence portal arterial inflow.

Continued bleeding after sclerotherapy, balloon tamponade and vasopressin requires surgery. Assuming the patient is able to withstand the operation, the simplest techniques which provide a few weeks before varices recur should be undertaken. A typical approach would be oesophageal transection directly or using the stapling gun. One or two centres world-wide perform emergency portosystemic shunts which are discussed below.

The mortality of acute variceal bleeding is substantial. About 30 per cent of patients die during the single admission to hospital, often from other features of poor liver function; the mortality increases as liver function and reserve deteriorate.

Long-term treatment of oesophageal varices has the aim of reducing portal pressure to normal or of obliterating the vulnerable varices. The past few years have seen a major change in this aspect of treatment. The traditional method of controlling oesophageal varices has been a portosystemic shunt. A variety of shunts have been used including portocaval anastomosis, mesocaval shunt and the distal splenorenal shunt. All shunt surgery is complicated by encephalopathy and by a progressive atrophy of the liver with resulting liver failure. Shunt surgery has been shown not to be beneficial as a prophylactic measure and therefore is reserved for people with bleeding varices.

The rise of sclerotherapy has virtually replaced shunt surgery. The technique involves injection of visible varices endoscopically. The frequency of bleeding and the incidence of fatal bleeding are reduced. However in common with shunt surgery, there is little evidence that life expectancy is improved.

Portal hypertension can also be managed with beta blockers. Propranolol has been shown to lower portal pressure and to reduce the chance of varices bleeding. Further studies of pharmacological methods of controlling portal hypertension are underway.

Portal hypertension due to portal vein thrombosis or schistosomiasis is often associated with good liver function. Portosystemic shunts are well tolerated by these patients and so are of value in preventing further oesophageal bleeding. A rare variant of portal hypertension is that complicating splenic vein thrombosis. Splenomegaly with gastric varices may result, diagnosis is difficult and splenectomy is the treatment of choice.

Splenomegaly is frequently found when portal

pressure is elevated. Hypersplenism can occur and is one of the explanations for the anaemia or thrombocytopenia seen in chronic liver disease.

Fluid retention

In patients with chronic liver disease fluid retention presents as ascites and peripheral oedema. The mechanisms involved are complex but secondary hyperaldosteronism, hypoalbuminaemia, portal hypertension, inappropriate antidiuretic hormone and alterations in renal blood flow are involved.

The clinical features include abdominal distension and discomfort, shortness of breath and swelling of the ankles. Large quantities of ascites are easily detected, but small amounts may require careful assessment of shifting dullness. Hernias fill and become prominent, and pleural effusions may be present.

Investigations include chest X-ray and liver function tests, particularly for plasma albumin. Because total body sodium and water are greatly increased but not necessarily equally, plasma electrolytes may show hyponatraemia as well as the hypokalaemia which reflects low total body potassium in secondary hyperaldosteronism. Small amounts of ascites can be detected by ultrasound or CT scan. A diagnostic aspiration should be carried out and fluid sent for culture, white cell count and cytology. In the ascites of chronic liver disease the first line of treatment is salt restriction (Table 9.16). In a proportion of patients this will be sufficient to start a diuresis when the patient is on bed rest. Spironolactone is the first diuretic of choice for most physicians. It tends to prevent hypokalaemia developing or worsening at doses that can be increased to 400 mg daily. Spironolactone produces gynaecomastia in men. The response of the patient is best measured by daily weight change and by urinary electrolytes. Weight loss of 0.5 kg daily in the absence of peripheral oedema is satisfactory, greater falls producing hypovolaemia leading to impaired renal and hepatic function.

A thiazide or loop diuretic can be added to the

Table 9.16   Sequential treatment of ascites

Low sodium diet (20–40 mmols/day)
Potassium sparing diuretic (spironolactone or
  amiloride)
Thiazide or loop diuretics
Fluid restriction
Leveen shunt

regime if the diuresis obtained is poor. Sodium restriction should be maintained. Care should also be taken not to promote hypovolaemia with hypotension, or hypokalaemia.

The problems arising during treatment are firstly hyponatraemia. Plasma sodium is often below the normal range in patients with cirrhosis but a falling sodium or values below 125 mmol/l are indications for fluid restriction. Renal failure can arise during even relatively mild treatment and should be detected early by following blood urea and creatinine levels. Diuretics should be reduced or stopped depending on the severity of the progressive renal dysfunction or the progressing hyponatraemia.

Resistant ascites not responding to maximal doses of diuretics and confirmed sodium restriction can be treated by re-infusion. Extracorporeal ultrafiltration removes some water and electrolytes and then returns the protein concentrate intravenously. An alternative is the use of the peritoneovenous shunt, or Leveen shunt which drains ascitic fluid subcutaneously into a vein, with a one-way valve to prevent reflux. These shunts are followed by a diuresis and a surprising improvement in many patients. Disseminated intravascular coagulopathy always occurs but is generally clinically insignificant.

Lastly it is now realized that peritonitis develops in patients with ascites. In this condition, spontaneous bacterial peritonitis, there is an infection with a single organism, which is usually also present in the blood-stream. The commonest organisms are *E. coli* or *Pneumococcus*: anaerobes are very rare. The symptoms range from general deterioration in an afebrile patient to pain, ileus and pyrexia. Diagnosis is made by finding a high white cell count in the ascitic fluid and by growing the organism in either ascitic fluid or blood. Treatment starts after the raised white cell count has been discovered with broad spectrum antibiotics. Mortality is high – up to 65 per cent.

Encephalopathy

Hepatic encephalopathy is a syndrome of progressive deterioration in cerebral function in patients with liver disease. Starting with drowsiness and slight confusion, progressive severity is indicated by asterixis and more mechanical behaviour, with coma following that may deepen to complete loss of response to painful stimuli.

Table 9.17 Precipitating events for encephalopathy

Gastrointestinal bleeding
Infection
Hypokalaemia
Constipation
High protein diet
Sedative drugs – especially opiates
Diuretics
Renal failure
Drainage of ascites
Therapeutic portacaval shunts
Operations

The mechanisms are complex and poorly understood. However, the toxins seem to be intestinal metabolites, mostly from protein in the large intestine, that have not been detoxified by the liver. This may be because the liver is functioning inadequately or because blood is shunted from portal to systemic circulations inside and away from the liver. The events that precipitate encephalopathy are listed in Table 9.17.

Clinical features are drowsiness, personality change and confusion initially. An hepatic flap can be demonstrated. The patient will be unable to copy a drawing (classically a star) or consecutively join a series of numbers scattered over a page (trail test). Hepatic fetor is normally present. Occasionally nervous system signs are focal. Chronic encephalopathy occurs with psychiatric manifestations, Parkinsonism or permanent focal signs.

Arterial ammonia levels and the EEG change in proportion to the severity of the encephalopathy and can be used to assess an episode. Diagnosis is essentially clinical.

Management consists of identifying and treating the precipitating events. Dietary protein is stopped and adequate calories are given as carbohydrate. The GI tract is cleared of protein with purges of magnesium sulphate and with enemas. Two more specific measures include the administration of neomycin by mouth and lactulose. Chronic encephalopathy can be treated by low protein diet, lactulose (aiming for two bowel actions daily) but not neomycin. Colonic exclusion and bromocriptine have also been used in a few patients with chronic encephalopathy.

Hepatorenal syndromes

A group of complications of advanced liver disease with progressive renal dysfunction are known as the hepatorenal syndromes. In operations for jaundice renal failure has been an important cause of mortality: its management is discussed below.

Infection and disseminated intravascular coagulopathy predispose to renal tubular necrosis. Vigorous diuresis can bring about renal failure but this can often be relieved by reducing the treatment and waiting for renal function to recover – it probably represents hypovolaemia.

Spontaneous progressive renal failure is the typical hepatorenal syndrome. Patients usually have advanced cirrhosis and often superadded alcoholic hepatitis. Ascites is usually present. Plasma creatinine progressively rises and urea follows. This syndrome is frequently accompanied by deteriorating encephalopathy, ascites may worsen and bleeding may occur.

Treatment is for any precipitating factor and then giving adequate salt-poor plasma protein. Dialysis is of benefit in a few patients, most not being suitable.

Infections

Many infections occur more commonly in cirrhotics than in the non-cirrhotic population. These include subacute bacterial endocarditis, pneumonia and spontaneous bacterial peritonitis. As in the elderly the general manifestations of an infection may not be manifest. Septicaemia occurs often.

Hepatic failure

Rapid decompensation in established liver disease can lead to a rapidly progressive hepatic failure. Typical precipitating events include gastrointestinal bleeding, fluid and electrolyte disturbance, infection, drugs and surgery. Encephalopathy, deepening jaundice and increasingly resistant ascites occur. Renal function deteriorates. There is a deterioration in prothrombin time and an increased amount of bruising and bleeding. Oesophageal varices are likely to bleed.

The outlook is particularly poor and each element should be treated individually.

Other features

Hypogonadism and feminization occur in males with cirrhosis. The mechanisms are inadequately understood. As loss of libido is the major complaint there is often little hope of providing effective treatment.

Pulmonary complications of cirrhosis are found. Oxygen desaturation to levels 60–70 per cent of normal occurs. This is of little clinical effect in most patients though shortness of breath, cyanosis and alterations in chest X-rays have been found. There are abnormal arteriovenous anastomoses, and functional ventilation–perfusion defects that account for these findings. Ascites and pleural effusions may exacerbate this condition. Pulmonary infections and inhalation are more common in patients with cirrhosis.

Alcohol

As will be seen from Table 9.18 a wide range of direct effects of alcohol are recognized. Added to these are the complications of acute intoxication such as inhalation of vomit, fractured ribs and radial nerve (drunkard's) palsy.

Table 9.18 Alcohol-induced disease

Nervous system	Acute alcoholic intoxication
	Withdrawal syndrome – delirium tremens
	Epileptic fits
	Wernicke–Korsakoff syndrome
	Peripheral neuropathy
	Retrobulbar neuritis
	Cerebellar and cerebral atrophy
	Psychiatric disease
Cardiovascular system	Cardiomyopathy
	Hyperlipidaemia
Gastrointestinal tract	Fatty liver
	Alcoholic hepatitis
	Alcoholic cirrhosis
	Pancreatitis – acute and chronic
	Parotid enlargement
	Gastritis
	Mallory–Weiss tear
	Malabsorption
	Diarrhoea
	Carcinoma of tongue, pharynx, oesophagus
Obstetric	Fetal alcohol syndrome
Musculoskeletal system	Gout
	Myopathy
	Dupuytren's contractures
Haematology	Macrocytic anaemia
	Zieve's syndrome

Gastrointestinal disease is a common consequence of alcohol abuse. Both acute and chronic pancreatitis are well recognized consequences and are described above. Gastritis is frequent. This may present as early morning retching, dyspepsia and nausea, much of which may be relieved by a drink. Alcohol is an infrequent cause of malabsorption. Diarrhoea is a common event and is multifactorial. Parotid enlargement and Dupuytren's contractures probably reflect alcohol intake rather than liver disease in most patients showing these signs.

Chronic alcoholic abuse can be difficult to detect. Careful history taking, may be revealing and physical examination may show malnutrition, or loss of concern about appearance. An inappropriately high plasma ethanol is helpful. Other helpful blood tests include an elevated mean corpuscular volume (MCV) and gamma-glutamyl transferase. Treatment generally requires prolonged psychiatric and social support with disulfiram in some patients. The relapse rate is high.

Alcoholic liver disease

The incidence of cirrhosis is proportional to national alcohol consumption. Though less common in the UK than elsewhere the amount of alcohol consumed and the frequency of alcoholic liver disease are both rising for men and women. It has been well demonstrated that women do not need to drink as much as men in absolute amounts or in duration to develop alcoholic cirrhosis.

Fatty liver

This early stage in alcoholic liver disease is reversible and is the commonest form of damage due to alcohol. Fatty liver can be found after a single 'binge' and can usually be found in the liver which has hepatitis or cirrhosis.

The only sign of consequence is hepatomegaly which may be tender. History taking may reveal evidence of alcohol abuse such as retching and nausea, right upper quadrant pain or diarrhoea.

Liver function tests may show mildly elevated transaminases with an elevated gamma-glutamyl transferase. A macrocytosis may be present. Treatment is by abstinence from alcohol.

Fatty liver is a feature of other problems including diabetes mellitus, morbid obesity, inflammatory bowel disease and heart failure.

Alcoholic hepatitis

This lesion is less frequent than fatty change and more serious as a proportion of patients progress to cirrhosis. Alcoholic hepatitis develops after several years heavy drinking.

The histological changes are of hepatic inflammation with ballooned hepatocytes being surrounded by inflammatory cells. Mallory's hyaline is seen in cells in the centre of the lobule. Though other causes are recognized, Mallory's hyaline is virtually restricted to alcoholic hepatitis in the UK. Centrilobular fibrosis may also be found.

Typical symptoms are of fever, jaundice and right upper quadrant pain. The liver is large and tender, with cutaneous stigmata of liver disease present. Severe cholestasis may occur and the diagnosis is easily mistaken for an acute biliary stone problem. At its most severe alcoholic hepatitis is accompanied by ascites and encephalopathy with liver cell failure.

Investigations show a leucocytosis and a mild anaemia. Liver function tests show an elevated bilirubin and the various enzymes are usually abnormal. Typically AST is higher than ALT. Liver biopsy may be necessary to confirm the diagnosis.

Treatment is by avoiding further alcohol and adequate nutrition. Corticosteroids have been used but no convincing evidence for their benefit exists. The course of the illness can be complicated by the development of cholestasis after entering hospital and stopping drinking, and by Zieve's syndrome, features of which include alcoholic hepatitis with gross hyperlipidaemia and haemolysis. Alcoholic hepatitis takes 3–6 months to settle and may result in cirrhosis.

Patients with evidence of liver failure have a mortality of 50–80 per cent.

Cirrhosis

Alcohol is the commonest cause of cirrhosis in the UK and, with viral hepatitis, one of the two commonest causes world-wide. The role of malnutrition in addition to alcohol is still being assessed.

People with HLA-B8 seem to be more susceptible and Dupuytren's contractures, gynaecomastia, testicular atrophy and parotid enlargement are commonly found in alcoholic cirrhosis.

Alcohol and anaesthesia

Though alcohol was a major anaesthetic in Nelson's ships it has also long been recognized as a hazard in the development of modern anaesthesia.

The problems in anaesthetizing patients who are chronic alcoholics include resistance to anaesthetic drugs with alterations in their distribution and metabolism. The requirements for halothane are increased but for suxamethonium, for example, decreased. Hypoglycaemia may occur.

Other potential problems include hypokalaemia, and clinically inapparent water and salt loading, which with a cardiomyopathy that is sensitive to anaesthetic agents are liable to produce serious circulatory problems.

Alcohol withdrawal states can be troublesome. An early postoperative fit or the development of delirium tremens while recovering from an anaesthetic can be hard to recognize. Progressive hypokalaemia, hypophosphataemia or hypomagnesaemia are features of the severe alcohol withdrawal syndrome and may compound perioperative and postoperative care in alcoholics.

Anaesthetic agents may be required in smaller amounts in the intoxicated patient requiring emergency surgery. There are the added problems of the full stomach which may require to be emptied prior to induction. Anaesthetic agents may be potentiated in the presence of high blood alcohol level and postoperative ventilation may be necessary. Techniques involving local anaesthesia may be considered but the patient may prove uncooperative.

Drugs and the liver

The importance of the liver in metabolism of drugs and the sensitivity of the liver to some have important consequences in hepatology.

Role of the liver in drug metabolism

In the pharmacological sequence from administration to elimination, some aspects of liver function are important in drug metabolism. Protein binding, mostly to albumin, is a principal carrier system around the body. Albumin levels will play a part in determining loading doses and in the availability of drugs which are effective in their non-bound state. For most drugs hepatic metabolism is a prerequisite to excretion. The endoplasmic reticulum is the major site with microsomal metabolism taking

Table 9.19 The effects of liver disease on drug metabolism

Drug	Effects	Alteration in dosage	Comments
Paracetamol	Little or none	None	Only altered in overdose
Aspirin	Little or none	None	Contraindicated because of bleeding
Morphine	Increased cerebral susceptibility	Reduce	
Pethidine	Prolonged half-life	Greatly reduce	Avoid
Thiopentone	Prolonged half-life Lowered protein-binding	Reduce	
Phenobarbitone	Prolonged half-life	Perhaps reduce	Mostly renal excretion unchanged
Phenytoin	Unbound fraction increased	Reduce	Toxicity more likely
Benzodiazepines (Diazepam)	Unbound fraction increased Increased cerebral susceptibility	Reduce	
Phenothiazines	Increased cerebral susceptibility	Reduce	
Prednisolone	Altered protein binding Prolonged half-life	Reduce	
Sulphonylureas	Reduced protein binding Possibly prolonged half-life	Reduce	Hypoglycaemia easily induced
Biguanides		Avoid	High risk of lactic acidosis
Digoxin	None	None	
Propranolol	Reduced first-pass metabolism Long half-life	Reduce	
Lignocaine	Prolonged half-life	Avoid	
Warfarin	Increased sensitivity	Reduce	Use with great care if genuinely indicated
Thiazide/loop diurietics	Increased sensitivity	Reduce	See section on fluid retention
Penicillins	Reduced metabolism		Generally only important if renal failure also present. Avoid talampicillin (liver metabolism) and nafcillin (biliary excretion)
Chloramphenicol	Reduced conjugation	Avoid	
Trimethoprim	Altered absorption Prolonged half-life	Use with care	Also co-trimoxazole
Gentamicin	None	None	Dose determined by renal function
Erythromycin	? prolonged half-life	Use with care	
Clindamycin/lincomycin	Prolonged half-life	Avoid	
Fusidic acid	Impaired biliary excretion	Reduce	
Rifampicin	Increased incidence of liver damage	Avoid	
Isoniazid	None	None	Maybe hepatotoxic
Ethambutol	None	None	
Pyrazinamide	Not known	Avoid	Hepatotoxic
Theophylline	Prolonged half-life	Reduce	

place there. Metabolic pathways include the cyto-chrome P450 system. Alternative pathways include flavin enzymes and various esterases. The next stage in drug metabolism is to render a drug soluble and excretable by glucuronide synthesis or a similar mechanism. Finally, some drugs are excreted in the bile.

In established liver disease these mechanisms are altered and the effects vary from drug to drug. The effects of liver disease with respect to the use of important drugs is shown in Table 9.19.

Drug-induced liver damage

Hepatic complications, in common with other systems that suffer drug complications, may be dose related and predictable or idiosyncratic and upredictable. The principal reactions are choles-tasis or a hepatitis, though rarer events, such as granuloma formation or chronic liver disease, do occur. Clinically, there is often some overlap between cholestasis and hepatitis in the reaction to many if not most drugs.

Cholestasis results from obstruction to cana-licular flow, with bile plugs and inflammatory change that are probably secondary to intracel-lular damage. Jaundice and pruritis are the usual symptoms. The liver is enlarged. Liver function tests are typical of cholestasis. After withdrawal of the drug, symptoms resolve in a few weeks in most patients, though 9–12 months may be needed in a small minority before normal liver function returns.

Hepatitic reactions are equally poorly under-stood. For many drugs, the liver metabolizes the drug to produce a toxic metabolite. Immune res-ponses may be a further manner in which hepatic damage occurs. Thus fast acetylators, those who have enzyme system induction (cytochrome P450) and those who are particularly well nourished may be more vulnerable. Re-exposure to an hepatotoxic drug often produces a severe recurrence.

The features of the two common drug responses are described in more detail below and Table 9.20 lists drugs and their hepatotoxicity. Several environmental and industrial agents are hepa-totoxic. These include fungi (e.g. the death cap), carbon tetrachloride, phosphorous and tannic acid.

Chlorpromazine produces an idiosyncratic cho-lestasis. It occurs in about 1 per cent of patients taking the preparation. Anorexia and vomiting can precede the jaundice, which can last many weeks after stopping chlorpromazine. Liver biopsy shows the features of cholestasis and an eosinophillic infiltration may be present in some patients. A blood eosinophilia may also be found. Treatment is supportive and by removing the offending cause.

Paracetamol overdose in contradistinction to chlorpromazine produces a dose-dependent hepa-titic reaction. Around 10–15 g is the minimum required. There may be a little nausea initially but, after 24–72 hours, vomiting, jaundice and tender hepatomegaly develop. Aminotransferases are ele-vated on the first day and worsen with gradual pro-longation of prothrombin time. Massive fatal hepatic necrosis can occur and is treated like viral hepatitis. It is now realized that paracetamol levels in the early hours can be a predictor of which patients are likely to develop hepatic complications and a nomogram for this exists. Specific treatment, either oral methionine or intravenous acetylcy-steine, is given as soon as possible to provide alternative sulphydril groups for binding the toxic metabolites. Liver necrosis is not succeeded by chronic liver disease, recovery being full in those who survive.

Anaesthesia and liver disease

Drug metabolism

The effect of liver disease on drug metabolism depends upon the severity of the liver disease. In advanced disease, care in the choice of agents and their doses will need to be exercised. These are con-sidered in detail in the standard anaesthetic textbooks, but a few general points are listed.

Opiates should be given in reduced dose, and if they have to be prescribed regularly, it should be at prolonged intervals until the patient's tolerance is understood. Similarly other sedatives, including phenothiazines, may need to be given with caution.

The duration of action of barbiturates is likely to be prolonged and recovery delayed after thiopen-tone or methohexitone. Drugs such as etomidate and propofol may be preferred, although the former reduces plasma cortisol levels.

Pseudocholinesterase levels are often low lead-ing to prolonged action of suxamethonium. Resis-tance to curare is said to occur but the use of atracurium, which is destroyed by non-enzymatic means, helps to avoid potential problems. Moni-toring of neuromuscular blockers is also advisable.

Table 9.20 Drug induced hepatotoxicity

Drug	Reaction	Comment
Paracetamol	Hepatitis	In overdose – *see* text
Aspirin	Hepatitis	In high doses
Indomethacin	Hepatitis	Rare
Halothane	Hepatitis	Discussed below
Carbamazepine	Cholestasis	Rare
Sodium valproate	Hepatitis	May be severe
Phenytoin	Hepatitis	Rare
Phenothiazines	Cholestasis	*See* text
Benzodiazepines	Cholestasis	Rare
Monoamine oxidase inhibition	Hepatitis	Occurs in 1–2 % – up to 20 % may be fatal
Tricyclic antidepressants	Cholestasis (hepatitis uncommon)	Rare: mildly abnormal LFT common
Methyltestosterone	Cholestasis	Dose dependent
Oestrogens	Cholestasis (hepatic tumour, peliosis hepatis)	Patients will have cholestasis in pregnancy often
Sulphonylureas	Cholestasis (rarely granulomas)	Mostly chlorpropramide – may mimic pancreatic carcinoma
Methyl dopa	Hepatitis (chronic active hepatitis rare)	
Penicillin	Hepatitis (granulomas)	Rare features of hypersensitivity
Chloramphenicol	Hepatitis	Uncommon side effects
Erythromycin	Cholestasis	With *estolate* ester, not other esters
Tetracycline	Fatty change and necrosis	Usually in treatment in late pregnancy. Associated renal and pancreatic damage
Sulphonamides	Hepatitis (granulomas)	Uncommon
Rifampicin	Hepatitis: hyperbilirubinaemia	1–4 % patients: mostly at higher doses: many respond to lower dose without stopping drug
Isoniazid	Hepatitis	Transient elevation of transaminases that settle. Common in early stages of treatment: hepatitis may be exacerbated by contemporary rifampicin use
Pyrazinamide	Hepatitis	Commonest side effect and reason for limited use of drug
Azathioprine	Mixed hepatitis/cholestasis	Uncommon
6-mercaptoprine	Hepatitis	More common than when using azathioprine: drug not advised in liver disease
Methotrexate	Fatty change, portal fibrosis, cirrhosis	Low incidence in first 2 years then greatly increased
Iron salts	Hepatitis	Following overdose (mostly children)

Although lignocaine metabolism may be impaired in liver disease and its use is potentially hazardous, the amount used in clinical practice does not usually present any major hazard.

Obstructive jaundice

Surgery in patients with severe obstructive jaundice has been long recognized as leading to renal failure.

Attention to detail in the preoperative and operative period has greatly reduced this complication.

Preoperatively, adequate clotting should be achieved with vitamin K. Hypovolaemia should be prevented with the administration of adequate intravenous fluids. It is advisable to insert a catheter preoperatively especially in patients with severe jaundice. Urine output should preferably be assessed preoperatively. Mannitol is used to maintain a good urine output, aiming for approximately 1 ml/kg/hour. In the mildly jaundiced patient mannitol will be needed if the urine output is below this value despite adequate hydration. In the severely jaundiced patient however mannitol (5–10 per cent) should be started preoperatively and continued until 24 hours postoperatively.

Antibiotics should be given and a wide choice is available. An obstructed bile duct is commonly infected and its manipulation likely to lead to bacteraemia in the absence of adequate antibiotic cover.

During the operation hypotension, and particularly hypovolaemia should be avoided and urine volume maintained with mannitol as appropriate. Fresh frozen plasma may be used to assist the abnormal clotting.

Hepatitis

Operations during acute hepatitis, that is moderately severe or worse, have an increased morbidity and an increased mortality. Any elective surgery should be delayed till 1–4 months (from various authorities) after the return of the liver function tests to normal.

A past history of hepatitis or jaundice will raise the possibility of a hepatitis B carrier state and should be checked preoperatively where practical and appropriate precautions taken when doubt remains.

Chronic liver disease

Two particular aspects of anaesthesia are of concern in chronic liver disease. First, hepatic blood flow may be reduced. If this occurs hepatic function deteriorates and in the postoperative period mortality is increased. Hypotensive anaesthesia should not be used in any cirrhotic patient, even those with well compensated disease. Liver blood flow is reduced by hypoxia, hypercarbia, intermittent positive pressure ventilation and inappropriate traction on abdominal viscera and vessels.

The second major problem is postoperative recovery. This may be delayed and assessment of encephalopathy can be particularly difficult in the early postoperative period. Maintained ventilatory support and minimal sedation will allow the picture to become clearer and appropriate measures to be

used wherever possible.

Slow 5 % dextrose is the intravenous fluid of choice if plasma sodium concentrations are normal. Purified protein fraction and fresh blood may be needed as well as platelet infusion. Intravenous saline is likely to lead to salt and water retention and may allow hypoglycaemia to develop.

Halothane

Halothane hepatitis is an uncommon and potentially fatal result of general anaesthesia. There is evidence that an immune basis for the complication exists.

In essence, a hepatitis occurs generally in patients who have had several anaesthetics with halothane, often with several exposures within a month. A mild fever may be apparent 1–2 weeks after an anaesthetic, though this may not be noticed as other reasons for fever could be present or the patient already be at home. Subsequently fever, jaundice and liver cell dysfunction occur at a shorter interval after the anaesthetic.

The mortality in patients who develop jaundice is high – about 30–40 per cent and is increased by the number of previous anaesthetics using halothane. Further anaesthetics should avoid halothane and the patient warned about this. In the events of liver failure standard management is all that can be employed.

Postoperative jaundices

Postoperative jaundice may be attributed to the anaesthetic agents used. However, many causes for postoperative jaundice are recognized, apart from halothane hepatitis and are listed in Table 9.21.

Table 9.21 Causes of postoperative jaundice

Halothane hepatotoxicity
Haemolysis of transfused blood
Resorption of a haematoma
Postoperative intrahepatic cholestasis
Heart failure
Decompensation of chronic liver disease
Bile duct obstruction due to stone, injury or
  pancreatitis
Non-A- non-B hepatitis

10
Rheumatic Disorders

Allan Binder and David Isenberg

Introduction

Rheumatic disorders are numerous and their course is highly variable. While many soft tissue or localized lesions are of no importance in anaesthetic practice, diseases which affect the cervical spine, the temperomandibular and crico-arytenoid joints, the mouth and nasopharynx may result in difficulty and increased risk during intubation, maintenance and recovery from general anaesthesia. Furthermore, constitutional illness and specific organ involvement is common in many of the autoimmune rheumatic diseases and may further complicate anaesthetic management. The medication used to treat these diseases may also be important. This review will concentrate on the clinical features and laboratory abnormalities of those

Table 10.1 Rheumatic disease classification relevant to the anaesthetist

The autoimmune rheumatic diseases
  Rheumatoid arthritis
  Juvenile chronic arthritis
  Systemic lupus erythematosus
  Sjogren's syndrome
  Polymyositis and dermatomyositis
  Scleroderma (and variants)
  The vasculitides
The spondarthropathies
  Ankylosing spondylitis
  Reiter's disease and reactive arthropathies
  Enteropathic arthritis
  Psoriatic arthritis
  Behçet's syndrome
Crystal arthropathies
  Gout
  'Pseudo' gout
Miscellaneous conditions affecting the cervical spine
  Osteoarthritis, osteoporosis, Paget's disease

rheumatic conditions relevant to the anaesthetist with suggestions about the general approach for the anaesthetist and the potential 'pitfalls' of each disease.

The classification of diseases to be considered is shown in Table 10.1.

The autoimmune rheumatic diseases

Rheumatoid arthritis (RA)

Rheumatoid arthritis is a systemic disease with emphasis on joint inflammation. The prevalence is 2–3 per cent of the population, with females being affected three times as often as males and onset occuring at any age. Any synovial joint may be affected by rheumatoid arthritis though the most commonly involved joints are the wrists, metacarpophalangeal and proximal interphalangeal joints in the hands, the knees and the small joints in the feet. IgM rheumatoid factor as detected by the standard Latex test is present in 70 per cent of cases, especially in those with severe disease. Normochromic, normocytic anaemia and a reciprocal rise in the erythrocyte sedimentation rate are associated with active disease.

The arthritis is classically symmetrical and erosive. The most important joints involved in anaesthetic practice are the cervical spine, temporomandibular and crico-arytenoid joints. Cervical spine disease is common and may not cause symptoms even in the presence of radiological instability. In long-standing RA, approximately one-third of patients have radiological instability and 2–5 per cent of these have clinical myelopathy (Marks and Sharp, 1981; Stevens, et al., 1971). With aggressive disease, subluxation may occur within 2 years of the onset of the disease (Windfi-

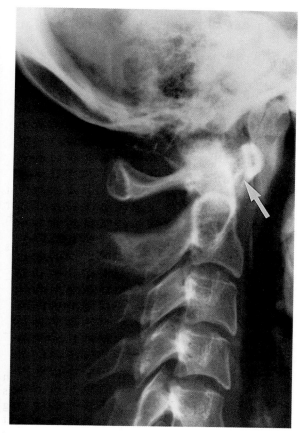

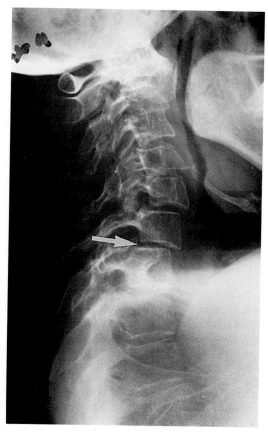

Fig 10.1   Plain X-ray of the cervical spine in a patient with rheumatoid arthritis showing atlanto-axial sub-luxation and a gap of over 6 mm between the dens and arch of the atlas.

Fig 10.2   Lower cervical instability is demonstrated.

eld *et al.*, 1981). Instability is most common at the atlanto-axial joint (Fig. 10.1), but any level may be involved (Boyle, 1971) (Fig. 10.2). Patients with disease of the cervical spine usually present with neck pain radiating to the occiput, but paraesthesia and variable degrees of limb weakness may develop. Some association has been noted between cervical subluxation and sero-positivity and seve-rity of the disease, and there is a suggestion that systemic corticosteroid therapy may accelerate the spinal disease. Cervical spine instability constitutes a serious risk especially if unrecognised, as myelo-pathy may follow intubation (Gardner and Holmes, 1961).

Temporomandibular joint (TMJ) involvement can limit mouth opening and also complicate intubation, especially when restriction in cervical spine movement is also present. In a study of 65 RA patients, 55 per cent had symptoms of TMJ arth-ritis and 86 per cent radiological abnormality of these joints (Ericson and Lundberg, 1967). Although TMJ arthritis may complicate anaes-thesia, deterioration of TMJ function rarely follows the surgery (Taylor *et al.*, 1968). Crico-aryteroid joint (CAJ) arthritis can be difficult to recognize (Bienesstock *et al.*, 1963), but may be found in 30 per cent of RA patients (Lofgren and Montgomery, 1962). Presenting symptoms can be hoarseness, an abnormal sensation in the throat, dysphagia, night stridor or dyspnoea. On occasion acute CAJ inflammation may develop, especially following anaesthesia, with immobilization of the vocal cords in the midline and resultant inspiratory stridor requiring emergency tracheostomy. Less severe CAJ disease has been associated with aspiration of pharyngeal contents at night or following anaesthesia.

Constitutional symptoms such as malaise, weight loss and tiredness can be prominent or even overshadow the joint symptoms. Anaemia, inadequate nutrition and increased susceptibility to infection may also occur. The anaemia, in particular may need to be corrected by transfusion prior to surgery.

Extra-articular features may also develop, especially in seropositive disease. Pulmonary involvement can be of several types. Progressive dyspnoea is usually due to fibrosing alveolitis with an increasing restrictive defect on pulmonary function tests. Pulmonary nodules on chest X-ray resemble rheumatoid nodules in the subcutaneous tissues. The nodules are especially prominent in association with pneumoconiosis (Caplan's syndrome), but result in little respiratory difficulty. Pleuritic chest pain and small or even massive pleural effusions are recognized features of the disease. Cardiac complications can also be diverse. Pericarditis has been found in 50 per cent of RA cases at autopsy (Bonfiglio and Atwater 1969; Lebowitz, 1963) and 31 per cent investigated by echocardiography (MacDonald et al. 1977), but it is often not recognized clinically nor does it create clinical problems other than occasional cases of constrictive pericarditis (Thadani et al., 1975). Myocarditis can develop, but is rarely clinically significant (Leibowitz, 1963) and conduction defects are uncommon. Vasculitis is usually confined to nailfold lesions, but severe lower limb ulceration and systemic vasculitis may occur. Renal function generally shows a mild non-specific deterioration during the course of the disease (Burry, 1972). Serious renal failure may occur, usually due to amyloidosis or related to anti-rheumatic therapy or other unrelated causes.

Sjogren's syndrome complicates about 20 per cent of RA cases. It causes marked dryness of the mouth, which often results in a poor dental state and is discussed later in this chapter.

Felty's syndrome

Felty's syndrome describes seropositive RA in association with splenomegaly and leucopenia. Severe articular and extraarticular features of RA are usual and an increased susceptibility to infection may be found.

The most common drugs used to treat RA are non-steroidal anti-inflammatory drugs (NSAIDs), gold salts, D-penicillamine and sulphasalazine, but systemic corticosteroid and cytotoxic agents are also sometimes required.

Anaesthetic management

Pre-anaesthetic evaluation must include assessment of the range of neck movement, mouth opening and the state of the oral mucosa. The notes of a patient at risk of cervical instability must be clearly marked to indicate the problem and a collar fitted around the patient's neck, pre-operatively, to alert all theatre staff. If CAJ arthritis is suspected, indirect laryngoscopy or fibroscopic examination of the cords must be performed, as pre-operative tracheostomy is occasionally necessary. Plain X-rays of the cervical spine in flexion and extension and special through-mouth views of the odontoid peg are mandatory, whether neck symptoms are present or not. Chest X-ray (CXR) and resting electrocardiography (ECG) are sufficient for routine cardiopulmonary assessment, but if abnormalities are suspected, pulmonary function tests (PFT), blood gas analysis, 24-hour Holter monitor and echocardiographic assessments may be required. Anaemia may be a prominent feature of active RA and may be exacerbated by drug related gastrointestinal bleeding. Anaemia may also be due to marrow suppression caused by one of the drugs used to treat the RA. If the haemoglobin concentration is less than 10 g, transfusion of whole blood or packed cells should be performed before surgery.

Great care is required when moving the patient from bed to trolley to operating table and back again. As joint involvement is widespread, special care is necessary in positioning the patient and protecting the skin which is often thin in association with the chronic illness or steroid therapy. There is also a danger of pressure sores developing during lengthy surgery especially if sacral nodules are present.

Intubation may be difficult and care is necessary to avoid hyperextension or extreme flexion of the neck. Awake or fibreoptic intubation may be advisable and consideration should be given to the use of regional anaesthesia where general anaesthesia is considered too hazardous.

Postoperative extubation must be deferred until the patient is able to maintain an independent airway, and observation continued to ensure that acute CAJ arthritis does not intervene. Unusual sensitivity to narcotic analgesics has been reported in RA (Gardner and Holmes, 1961), especially in the presence of respiratory complications.

Juvenile chronic arthritis (JCA)

Juvenile chronic arthritis can begin at any age before 16 years, but onset is especially common from 1–3 years and during adolescence. The IgM rheumatoid factor is usually absent in children with rheumatoid disease. Three distinct sub-groups of JCA have been recognized on the basis of the mode of onset.

Polyarticular onset JCA

Polyarticular onset JCA is found in 40 per cent of patients who present with five or more affected joints in the first 6 months. The symmetrical poly-arthropathy is similar to adult RA, but children complain less of pain and morning stiffness. Cervical spine involvement is early and severe with complete loss of movement and occasionally acute torticollis. Early atlanto-axial or lower cervical spine instability may be aggravated by bony fusion at other levels. Abnormalities of vertebral body growth and secondary disc degeneration contribute to the cervical spine disease. Involvement of the hypophyseal joints of the thoraco-lumbar region are usually not recognized but scoliosis is 30 times more common in JCA (Svantesson et al., 1981). Temporomandibular joint arthritis in childhood (Larheim et al., 1981; Larheim et al., 1981) leads to failure in the normal development of the TMJ growth centre and hence micrognathia. The most severe changes are those associated with early onset of the disease, but lesser degrees of mandibular abnormality may occur with onset up to 12 years of age. Deficient bite, pain and ankylosis of the TMJ may occur. Crico-arytenoid joint arthritis is uncommon in JCA (Jacobs and Hui, 1977). Constitutional illness may be severe, but systemic complications such as pericarditis and uveitis are rare. After adolescence, seropositive disease (juvenile rheumatoid arthritis) becomes more common and cervical instability, similar to adult RA, is more usual.

Pauciarticular onset

Pauci-articular onset JCA is found in 50 per cent of patients, who present with four or fewer affected joints in the first 6 months. While knees, ankles and wrists are the most often affected, any joint including the cervical spine can be involved.

Chronic uveitis is the only common systemic feature and is most likely in patients who have a positive antinuclear antibody in their blood. One-third of patients progress to polyarticular disease.

Systemic onset JCA (Still's disease)

Systemic-onset JCA (Still's disease) makes up the remaining 10 per cent of cases. Constitutional illness is severe, with high spiking fevers and erythematous morbilliform macular rash on the face, trunk and proximal extremities. Objective arthritis is often mild and can be delayed for several years. Although systemic features are common, they can be insidious and escape recognition. Pericarditis has been reported to be clinically evident in 7 per cent of patients, but has been found at autopsy in 45 per cent of cases (Lietman and Bywaters, 1963). Constrictive pericarditis may also develop (Scharf et al., 1976). Myocarditis, endocarditis, pulmonary fibrosis, neurological abnormalities and renal glomerular disease has been reported (Wortmann et al., 1980). Severe growth retardation is characteristic of systemic onset and severe polyarticular disease, but may also result from corticosteroid therapy used to treat the systemic disease.

Anaesthetic management

The preoperative assessment of patients is dependent on the type of disease. Early onset polyarticular disease is associated with severe cervical spine ankylosis, TMJ and mandibular abnormality; intubation may be impossible (D'Arcy et al., 1976; Hodgkinson, 1981; Roelofse and Shipton, 1983; Smith, 1985). Awake intubation is unacceptable in childhood and ketamine anaesthesia is preferable (D'Arcy et al., 1976). Fibreoptically-guided tracheal intubation via a rhinoscope is a useful alternative procedure (Smith, 1985). Seropositive polyarticular disease found in the older age groups is associated with atlanto-axial and lower cervical instability which is similar to, but sometimes more severe than adult RA. Careful radiological assessment is mandatory in all cases. Patients with systemic onset JCA or polyarticular disease with systemic features also need detailed cardiopulmonary, biochemical and haematological assessment.

Postoperative observation must be prolonged and extubation delayed until laryngeal reflexes have returned (Smith, 1985). With ketamine anaesthesia, a quiet dark environment in the postoperative period is necessary to prevent hallucinations which are especially common in the older children.

Systemic lupus erythematosis (SLE)

SLE is a multisystem autoimmune disease characterized by a broad spectrum of clinical features and serological abnormalities. High titres of antibodies to double-stranded DNA are found in many lupus patients during disease exacerbations. Females outnumber males by 9:1 and while onset can occur at any age, it is most common from 15–35 years.

Constitutional illness is often severe during active disease, with fever, malaise, lymphadenopathy, mouth ulcers and weight loss being prominent features. Over 90 per cent of patients have arthralgia or a symmetrical arthritis involving the hands, wrists, knees and other joints. While the distribution of affected joints is similar to RA and deformity may develop, synovitis is less marked and erosions rarely develop. Cervical spine instability and TMJ and CAJ arthritis are much less common than is RA. A characteristic photo-sensitive 'butterfly' rash may develop on the face and changes in pigmentation, cutaneous vasculitis and hair loss may occur. Approximately 25 per cent of all patients develop Sjogren's syndrome and 5 per cent myositis.

However, in SLE the most important factor in anaesthetic practice relates to the presence and severity of organ involvement. Raynaud's phenomenon is found in 50 per cent of cases and may precede other manifestations of the disease by many years. Cutaneous and systemic vasculitis may occur. Cardiac involvement is common and 15 per cent of patients develop pericarditis often in association with an effusion (Chia et al., 1981). Myocarditis, coronary arteritis and endocarditis occur. Pleuropulmonary features are even more frequent and over 40 per cent of patients develop pleuritic chest pain at some time. Pleural effusions also occur. Interstitial lung disease is common, with acute pneumonitis being found in 5–15 per cent of patients (Matthay et al., 1975) and fibrosing alveolitis following in many cases. A decrease in diffusion capacity in pulmonary function tests often precedes dyspnoea or radiological changes.

Haematological abnormalities are diverse and include normochromic normocytic anaemia, haemolytic anaemia, leucopenia, thrombocytopenia and cryoglobulinaemia. Coagulation defects also occur and a lupus anticoagulant has

been identified and often associated with antiphospholipid antibodies which have been linked with spontaneous abortion, cerebral disease, thrombocytopenia and, paradoxically, a thrombotic tendency which may become manifest following surgery (Shaulian et al., 1981). Renal damage develops in at least 50 per cent of cases and may present with proteinuria, systemic hypertension or progressive renal failure. Psychiatric and neurological features can be found and drug hypersensitivity and susceptibility to infection are important secondary effects.

The clinical course of SLE is usually prolonged and is characterized by relapses and remissions lasting months or years. Corticosteroid and cytotoxic drugs are often used in the treatment of the systemic features of the disease.

Drug-induced SLE

Hydrallazine, procainamide, isoniazid, chlorpromazine and oral anticoagulants have been reported to induce a syndrome similar to SLE in some patients after prolonged use. Arthralgia, arthritis, pleuropulmonary and cardiac features are common but vasospastic phenomena, neurological features and renal disease are rare. The disease is usually mild and remits after stopping the drug. Nevertheless, pericardial tamponade can develop spontaneously (Ghose, 1975) or during surgery (Goldberg et al., 1980).

Anaesthetic management

In severe SLE, the preparation of patients for anaesthesia can be difficult in view of the constitutional symptoms and complex cardiopulmonary, renal and haematological abnormalities. Chest X-ray, ECG, echocardiography and pulmonary function tests are usually necessary whilst blood gas estimation and 24-hour Holter monitor may be required. With renal disease, where electrolytes and plasma protein levels must be checked, creatinine clearance and 24-hour urine protein measurements may also be important to define the severity of the renal lesion. Full haematological assessment is also mandatory and must include platelet count and coagulation studies. The presence of a cryoglobulin and the lupus anticoagulant may also affect anaesthetic practice. Rarely, the lupus anticoagulant has been found to be associated with excessive operative haemorrhage, especially when hypoprothrombinaemia and/or thrombocytopenia is also present. In these patients, fresh frozen plasma and platelet packs should be available before surgery is undertaken (Shaulian *et al.*, 1981). As renal disease is a prominent feature of SLE and drug hypersensitivity a recognized risk, especial care must be taken with the drugs and dosage during anaesthesia of these patients. Control of ambient temperature and blood pressure in the perioperative period is also important, especially in patients with severe vasospastic symptoms. Many lupus patients will be on regular corticosteroids and intravenous schedules providing approximately twice the oral maintenance dose are usually required. To reduce the risk of infection it is advisable to stop other immunosuppressive drugs prior to surgery.

Sjogren's syndrome

Sjogren's syndrome is a chronic autoimmune disorder characterized by keratoconjunctivitis sicca (dry eyes) and xerostomia (dry mouth). Lacrimal and salivary gland hypertropy may be accompanying features. Sjogren's syndrome can be a primary problem or secondary to another auto-immune rheumatic disease notably RA, or SLE. Less frequently, scleroderma, polyarteritis nodosa or dermatomyositis are complicated by the sicca syndrome. Patients with Sjogren's syndrome are over forty times more likely to develop a lymphoma (Kassan *et al.*, 1977).

Xerostomia causes chronic lip ulceration, angular stomatitis and ulceration and atrophy of the oral mucosa and tongue. Dental caries and candida infection may follow. The inflammatory process can involve the nasal mucosa and extend to the lungs with development of chronic bronchitis, recurrent pneumonia or interstitial fibrosis (Strimlan and Rosenow, 1976). Gastrointestinal involvement can lead to dysphagia. Labial gland biopsy is usually diagnostic.

Renal tubular defects, immune-complex glomerulonephritis and hypertension may develop (Talal *et al.*, 1968) and vasospastic phenomena and vasculitis are common. Non-organ specific auto-antibodies are frequently found.

Anaesthetic management

The major anaesthetic problem is associated with the difficulty in intubation of patients with severe xerostomia. Other problems are associated with the pulmonary and renal complications of Sjogren's syndrome and to the underlying autoimmune rheumatic disease.

Polymyositis (PM) and dermatomyositis (DM)

This idiopathic, auto-immune syndrome may only affect the skeletal muscle (PM), or also involve the skin (DM). Symptoms usually begin between 20 and 60 years of age and may occur alone or in association with features of the other auto-immune rheumatic diseases. These disorders are commoner in women (3:1) except for those cases occurring in patients over the age of 50 in association with underlying malignancies (Barnes and Mawr, 1976), where men are twice as likely to have the myositis.

The characteristic features are proximal muscle weakness with or without the classical violaceous rash on the eyelids, knuckles, chest and extensor surfaces of the forearms and shins. The creatine kinase is raised (up to 100 times the upper limit of normal) in 80 per cent of the patients. Severely affected patients may also develop respiratory distress due to respiratory muscle involvement (Hepper *et al.*, 1964). Impairment of proximal pharyngeal muscle function also increases the risk of aspiration pneumonia, especially following anaesthesia (Eisele, 1981; Metheney, 1978).

Fibrosing alveolitis has been reported (Hepper *et al.*, 1964; Schwartz *et al.*, 1976), but where treatment has included cytotoxic agents, the aetiology of the lung fibrosis is uncertain. Symptomatic cardiac involvement is relatively uncommon, but dysrhythmias, congestive cardiac failure and sudden death has been reported as a result of myocardial fibrosis (Hill and Barrows, 1968). Furthermore, ECG evidence of pericarditis, myocardial dysfunction, conduction defects or arrhythmias has been reported in 30–50 per cent of patients kept under prolonged review (De Vere and Bradley, 1975; Bohan *et al.*, 1977). Myositis is treated with corticosteroids and/or cytotoxic agents.

Anaesthetic management

Patients with myositis may be seriously ill with profound muscle weakness and features of lung or cardiac involvement. Occasionally there may also be an underlying malignancy. A full and detailed cardiopulmonary work-up is necessary in preoperative assessment as abnormalities are common. The creatine kinase level in the blood may also help in estimating the severity of the myositis. As swallowing may be poor due to laryngeal muscle weakness, care must be taken to avoid aspiration of gastric contents. Head-up induction, nasogastric suction or pretreatment with H$_2$-receptor antagonists or antacids may be helpful (Eisele, 1981). General anaesthesia is also preferable to regional blocks as the airway can be controlled with greater certainty. This is especially important as the respiratory muscle can be weak, and controlled ventilation may be necessary during the anaesthetic and continued into the postoperative period. There has also been a suggestion of increased sensitivity to muscle relaxants and they should be used with care (Eisele, 1981). A myasthenic effect seen in a few patients with PM given muscle relaxants may have been related to underlying malignancy. A test dose may obviate serious problems. Airway protection should be continued until full recovery to reduce the risks of aspiration pneumonia.

Scleroderma and its variants

Scleroderma

Scleroderma (systemic sclerosis) is a multisystem disorder characterized by obliterative microvascular and proliferative fibrotic changes which affect the skin and many organs. The disease is more common in females with onset usually from 30–50 years.

Skin involvement is the hallmark of the disease, but is insignificant in 5 per cent of cases. In the early stages, the hands and feet show transient puffiness and non-pitting oedema on waking. With disease progression, swelling becomes persistent and then gradually subsides to be replaced by fibrotic material which limits joint movement. Similar changes often affect the face to give the characteristic pinched nose and tight mouth. Severe skin involvement can limit TMJ and cervical spine movement and reduce chest wall expansion (Bohan et al., 1977). With or with treatment, partial or even complete resolution of the skin changes can occur – usually after many years (Weisman and Calcaterra, 1978). Raynaud's phenomenon is usually prominent and may cause or exacerbate digital ulceration or gangrene.

Oesophageal fibrosis and hypomotility affects 90 per cent of patients, (Orrigner et al. 1976), but many do not admit to dysphagia or other symptoms. Severe oesophageal involvement increases the risk of aspiration, especially following anaesthesia. Malabsorption and chronic diarrhoea may result from fibrotic extension to the small bowel. In some cases a 'blind-loop syndrome' may develop due to secondary overgrowth of organisms.

Cardiac involvement has been found in 80 per cent of cases but is often asymptomatic (Clements et al., 1981; Ferri et al., 1985). In a study of 52 patients, only 19 per cent had symptoms (Clements et al., 1981). Myocardial fibrosis can result in cardiac failure, arrhythmias or conduction defects (Ferri et al., 1985). Ischaemic changes and angina may occur in the absence of coronary occlusion and is believed to be due to small vessel disease (Bulkley et al., 1976). Pericarditis and pericardial effusions may occur and are often silent.

Pulmonary disease may be of several types. Pulmonary fibrosis is the most characteristic lesion which causes a progressive reduction in lung compliance and vital capacity (Schneider et al., 1982). Gas transfer impairment can result in pulmonary hypertension (Steckel et al., 1975). Pleuritic chest pain, pleural effusions and chest wall fibrosis may also occur.

Renal disease is uncommon, but is associated with a very poor prognosis (LeRoy and Fleischmann, 1978). Whilst fulminant renal failure and malignant hypertension may occur, proteinuria, haematuria, hypertension and slowly progressive deterioration in renal function are more common. Proximal myopathy, arthritis and neurological abnormalities may also occur. D-penicillamine, colchicine and corticosteroids are often prescribed, but are of dubious value.

CREST syndrome

The CREST syndrome refers to a combination of Calcinosis, Raynaud's phenomenon, Oesophageal hypomotility, Sclerodactyly and Telangectasia. Cardiac and renal complications are less common, and it was originally thought that this syndrome had a better prognosis than scleroderma, but this may not be correct as the visceral lesions do occur and the prognosis is not very different in the two conditions.

Diffuse eosinophilic fasciitis

Diffuse eosinophilic fasciitis occurs in young males who present with induration and fibrosis of the skin of the extremities and trunk but sparing the fingers and not associated with vasospastic features. The inflammatory changes affect the subcutaneous tissue and fascia and often have a prominent eosinophilic infiltrate. Visceral lesions do not develop (Kanard, 1977).

Anaesthetic management

Detailed pre-anaesthetic evaluation is important and full cardiopulmonary and renal investigations must be undertaken as suggested for SLE. Mouth opening and neck range must also be assessed. With serious limitation of mouth opening, blind awake intubation or fibre-optically assisted intubation via the nasal route may be advisable (Thompson and Conklin, 1983). If the oral route is used, severe perioral lacerations or bleeding from telangiectasia may follow difficult intubation (Davidson–Lamb and Finalyson, 1977). Furthermore, carious teeth which are associated with poor mouth opening may also be a source of infection. It may be necessary to remove these before intubation can be attempted, but the patient should be warned that the fitting of dentures to replace the missing teeth may prove impossible.

Vasospastic phenomena are an important aspect of scleroderma and vasodilation must be anticipated following induction of anaesthesia (Eisele, 1981). Plasma expanders or blood may be required to maintain the blood pressure. With renal disease, care must be taken with drugs used and dosage given. With cardiac involvement, particular sensitivity to digitalis has been found.

Venous access may be difficult in scleroderma patients and intravenous induction of anaesthesia may provoke a painful cyanotic reaction similar to Raynaud's phenomenon in the fingers (Davidson-Lamb and Finlayson, 1977). Where no large veins can be found, gaseous induction is preferable (Smith and Shribman, 1984). The measurement of blood pressure can also be difficult and even misleading in patients with Raynaud's phenomenon (Eisele, 1981). Nevertheless, arterial cannulation must be avoided due to the risk of arterial thrombosis. The maintenance of ambient temperature in the perioperative period is especially important in this disease.

Patients with severe oesophageal dysfunction require special care in protecting the lungs, and gaseous induction may be unsafe (Davidson-Lamb and Finlayson, 1977; Smith and Shribman, 1984). A rapid sequence induction is not practicable because of the difficulty in intubation and pretreatment with H_2 receptor antagonists or antacids, emptying the gastric contents, or head-up induction are alternative approaches (Smith and Shribman, 1984).

Regional anaesthesia may be considered preferable especially in patients with serous pulmonary complications (Eisele, 1981; Neill, 1980; Thompson and Conklin, 1983). Local anaesthetic agents can result in prolonged but reversible sensory blockage (Eisele and Reitan, 1971; Lewis, 1974; Neill, 1980), which is useful as analgesia (Eisele, and Reitan, 1971; Neill 1980) but can be associated with prolonged vasospastic change (Sweeney, 1984).

Vasculitic syndromes

Vasculitis is a pathological process characterized by inflammation and necrosis of arteries of any size. The process may also involve veins. Vasculitis can occur as part of an auto-immune rheumatic disease such as RA, SLE, myositis or scleroderma, but there is a group of diseases where it is the predominant feature. Corticosteroid and cytotoxic agents are often used in therapy.

The more common vasculitic syndromes will be considered:

Polyarteritis nodosa (PAN)

Polyarteritis nodosa (PAN) is a systemic illness with the emphasis on damage affecting the small and medium-sized vessels, and frequent involvement of the skin, joints, kidneys and peripheral nerves. However, any organ can be affected. The disease is more common in males and can begin at any age. The presentation and course of this disease is variable. Constitutional symptoms such as fever, malaise and weight loss are often prominent.

The cutaneous lesions are vasculitic, with tender nodules along involved vessels, purpura, livido reticularis and digital ischaemia and gangrene. Peripheral neuropathy or mononeuritis multiplex develop in 50–70 per cent of cases and involves both upper and lower limbs, with progressive sensory and motor deficit (Frohnert and Sheps, 1967). Clinical renal abnormality also develops in 70 per cent of cases (Wainwright and Davson, 1950) with proteinuria, systemic hypertension and progressive renal failure. Cardiac damage is common at autopsy, but less often clinically evident. Congestive cardiac failure may follow hypertension or coronary insufficiency and myocardial infarction may be silent (Holsinger et al., 1962). Critical ischaemia and progressive distal gangrene affects upper and lower limbs. Lung involvement is not a prominent feature in PAN, but is found in other vasculitic syndromes.

Allergic angiitis and granulomatosis (Churg–Strauss vasculitis)

This is a variant of PAN is which lung disease is prominent, often antedating the vasculitic abnormalities. Respiratory features such as asthma, bronchitis and pneumonitis occur. Peripheral blood eosinophilia and extravascular granulomata may also be present in association with the features of cutaneous and systemic vasculitis.

Giant cell arteriitis and polymyalgia rheumatica

There is increasing acceptance that polymyalgia rheumatica (PMR) and giant cell arteritis (GCA also called temporal, cranial or granulomatous arteritis) form a spectrum of disease which affects middle-aged and elderly patients. Polymyalgia rheumatica causes morning stiffness and aching in the muscles of the shoulder and hip girdles, in association with malaise, weight loss and predominantly axial joint pain. Giant cell arteritis has the myalgic symptoms of PMR together with evidence of arteritis which may be confined to the cranial branches of the aortic arch vessels or can be more widespread. Temporal headache, scalp tenderness and transient or permanent visual loss may occur and tender non-pulsatile temporal arteries may be found. As medium and large-sized arteries can be affected in other sites, bruits over large vessels, limb gangrene, myocardial infarction and aortic dissection may occur.

Wegener's granulomatosis (WG)

Wegener's granulomatosis (WG) is characterized by necrotizing granulomatous and vasculitic lesions involving the respiratory tract, kidney and other organs. The commonest early manifestation is giant cell granulomata affecting the upper respiratory tract and causing nasal ulceration and destruction, chronic sinusitis and by contiguous spread, orbit involvement. Fever, weight loss and malaise are usually prominent. Widespread vasculitic lesions of small arteries and veins also develop. The granulomatous and vasculitic lesions may spread to the lower respiratory tract and cough, haemoptysis and dyspnoea appear. Up to 85 per cent of patients also develop renal lesions with proteinuria, haematuria and renal insufficiency but rarely hypertension (Fauci and Wolff, 1973).

Lethal midline granuloma (LMG)

Lethal midline granuloma (LMG) is a rare, but invariably fatal condition, which begins with granulomatous lesions in the upper respiratory tract with progressive destruction of bone, cartilage and skin. The lesions can replace the midface, oropharynx and nasopharynx to cause airway obstruction. Nutritional difficulty can lead to cachexia and death usually within a year. Vasculitis does not occur.

Anaesthetic management

The constitutional illness and widespread systemic disease necessitate careful pre-anaesthetic evaluation in these patients. Detailed cardiac, pulmonary and renal assessments are necessary and hypertension must be controlled before anaesthesia. In WG and LMG, the severity and extent of upper airway obstruction must be defined by clinical, radiographic and histological means and the anaesthetic approach planned accordingly. In severely affected patients or emergency situations, pre-operative tracheostomy may be the only safe method of establishing an airway (Eisele, 1981). Severe and widespread consolidation due to infection, secondary to the upper airway obstruction often complicates advanced disease.

Acute pharyngeal oedema has been described in systemic vasculitis associated with PAN and GCA and may complicate intubation (Martin, 1969). Tongue infarction in GCA may have a similar effect. Acute blindness may be precipitated by general anaesthesia in patients with active GCA and non-urgent surgery should be deferred until control of the vasculitis has been achieved (McGowan, 1967).

Table 10.2 summarizes the pre-anaesthetic assessment required in patients with the autoimmune rheumatic diseases.

Spondarthropathies

The seronegative spondarthropaties are a group of disorders characterized by a propensity to involve the axial skeleton, an absence from the serum of IgM rheumatoid factor and a strong association with the histocompatibility antigen HLA-B27. The group is composed of ankylosing spondylitis, Reiter's disease and reactive arthritis, psoriatic arthritis, Behçet's syndrome and the arthropathies associated with ulcerative colitis, Crohn's disease and Whipple's disease.

Table 10.2 Summary of pre-anaesthetic assessment in patients with autoimmune rheumatic diseases

	Rheumatoid arthritis	Poly/pauci onset juvenile chronic arthritis	Systemic onset juvenile chronic arthritis	Systemic lupus erythematosis	Sjogren's syndrome	Myositis	Scleroderma	Polyarteritis nodosa	Giant cell arteritis	Wegener's granulomatosis	Ankylosing sponylitis (AS)	Sero-negative spondarthropathy (without AS)	Behçet's syndrome
Assess neck range	m	m	m	m	m	m	m	–	–	–	m	m	occ
Assess mouth opening	m	m	occ	occ	m	–	m	–	–	m	m	m	–
Assess mouth, teeth and pharynx	m	–	occ	m	m	–	m	occ	m	m	–	m	m
Assess chest expansion	occ	–	–	–	–	m	m	–	–	–	m	–	–
X-ray cervical spine	m	m	m	m	m	–	m	–	–	–	m	m	occ
Indirect laryngoscopy	occ	occ	–	occ	occ	occ	occ	–	–	m	occ	–	m
Pulmonary function tests	occ	occ	m	m	m	m	m	m	occ	m	m	occ	occ
Blood gases	occ	occ	occ	occ	occ	m	m	m	occ	m	m	occ	occ
24-hour Holter monitor	occ	occ	m	occ	occ	occ	occ	occ	–	occ	occ	–	occ
Echocardiography	occ	occ	m	m	occ	m	m	m	occ	occ	occ	m	occ
Coagulation screen	occ	–	–	m	occ	–	–	–	–	–	–	–	occ
24-hour proteinuria and creatinine clearance	occ	occ	occ	occ	occ	–	occ	m	occ	m	occ	–	occ

Key
m = most important
occ = test occasionally required

All require full blood count, sedimentation rate, creatinine, chest X-ray, resting electrocardiography and urine test for protein.

Ankylosing spondylitis (AS)

Ankylosing spondylitis is an inflammatory arthropathy usually diagnosed in males under the age of 40 years. The previously reported male to female ratio of 10:1 is, however, probably an overestimate as females often have a milder form of the disease. The primary sites of involvement are the sacroiliac joints and spine, but up to 35 per cent of patients have some peripheral joint involvement. Furthermore, early morning stiffness, constitutional illness and extra-articular features may also occur.

The spinal disease usually manifests with low backache due to lumbar spine and sacroiliac joint involvement. Thoracic and cervical spine disease invariably follow, although the rate of progression and severity are highly variable. Only a small proportion of patients develop complete spinal ankylosis. The degree of cervical spine disease is most important to the anaesthetist, as patients with severe and advanced disease who have complete ankylosis present major difficulties in intubation and maintenance of the airway during anaesthesia. Furthermore, vertebral fracture and instability may be missed on radiological assessment and even when asymptomatic may progress to myelopathy with a poor prognosis for recovery (Murray and Persellin, 1981). Thoracic spine ankylosis and costovertebral joint involvement can seriously impair chest expansion. Respiration is normally well maintained by diaphragmatic movement, but in the presence of other respiratory disease, the pulmonary reserve may be seriously reduced and respiratory failure may ensue spontaneously or following anaesthesia (Radford et al., 1977). Lumbar spine involvement may lead to canal stenosis and makes placement of a spinal or epidural needle difficult or impossible (Sinclair and Mason, 1984). Sacroiliitis is invariably bilateral in AS and when unilateral involvement persists, especially in drug addicts, septic arthritis of the sacroiliac joints must be excluded (Gomar et al., 1984).

The peripheral joint involvement is asymmetrical with a predilection for involvement of the hips, knees, shoulders and ankles. Temporomandibular joint arthritis is found in 10 per cent of cases, but with prolonged follow-up the incidence has been reported at 30–40 per cent (Resnick, 1974), with many cases progressing to ankylosis. Crico-arytenoid joint involvement is less common than in RA (Bienenstock and Lanyi, 1977).

The constitutional features such as fatigue, weight loss and morning stiffness are similar to RA and anaemia and rise in ESR also occur. Iritis has been reported in 20–25 per cent of patients and may lead to blindness (Horvath and Fajnor, 1968). Upper lobe pulmonary fibrosis is a well recognized respiratory complication of long standing AS and usually presents with cough, haemoptysis and progressive dyspnoea. Chest wall rigidity and recurrent pulmonary infections may further compromise the respiratory status. Cardiovascular involvement has been reported in 3.5–10 per cent of patients under prolonged follow-up (Calin, 1985). Aortitis and aortic incompetence are the most common features but defects in cardiac conduction, cardiomegaly, mitral valve disease and pericarditis may occur. Cardiac disease may remain unrecognized or may dominate the picture. A study of AS patients kept under review for 13 years showed death from cardiovascular disease to be double that in controls (Calin, 1985). Neurological changes may also occur (Thomas et al., 1974) and amyloidosis (Jayson et al., 1971) may complicate long-standing disease. Nonsteroidal anti-inflammatory drugs are the only agents commonly used in therapy.

Reiter's syndrome and reactive arthritis

Both terms apply to the same non-infective arthropathy which may follow venereal contact or a trivial dysenteric or streptococcal infection. The post-venereal form has been associated with *Chlamydia* and *Mycoplasma* and the post-dysenteric form with *Shigella, Salmonella, Campylobacter* and *Yersinia* infections. In many cases no organism is found. The term 'reactive' is used as the synovial fluid from affected joints is invariably sterile. The peripheral arthropathy is asymmetrical with particular involvement of the large lower limb joints. Classical ankylosing spondylitis develops in some cases. Mucocutaneous features such as urethritis, prostatitis, conjunctivitis, mouth ulcers, circinate balanitis and keratodermia blennorrhagica may occur. Serious uveitis has also been reported. The peripheral arthropathy and mucocutaneous features often show relapses and remissions.

Enteropathic arthritis

Ulcerative colitis (UC) and Crohn's disease (CD) may be associated with a non-deforming peripheral arthropathy which is asymmetrical and often migratory. This arthritis has been reported in 20 per cent of patients with CD (Haslock and Wright, 1973) and 9–11.5 per cent with UC (Greenstein et al., 1976; Wright and Watkinson, 1965) with the highest frequency where disease is confined to the colon. With UC but not CD a clear association has been found between exacerbations of colitis and the peripheral arthritis. Ankylosing spondylitis has been found in both UC and CD with an incidence of 4 per cent in each case. The spinal disease may precede bowel symptoms by several years but once established follows a course similar to the idiopathic forms of AS.

Psoriatic arthritis

An inflammatory arthropathy has been reported in 2.6–7 per cent of psoriatic patients (Baker, 1966), but the frequency is difficult to ascertain as the skin lesions may be insignificant and in some cases may precede the arthritis by many years. There is no consistent association between the activity of the arthritis and skin disease. The arthritis can take several forms. Distal interphalangeal joint changes may predominate or the disease may resemble RA. Mono- or oligoarthritis or a severely deforming mutilans form may occur and 5 per cent of patients develop AS. Constitutional illness and extra-articular features are uncommon.

Behçet's syndrome

Behçet's syndrome is a multisystem disorder characterized by recurrent oral and genital ulceration, arthritis and some other features including uveitis. Aphthous ulceration occurs in crops and usually precedes other symptoms by many years. Oral ulcers can involve the lips, tongue and buccal mucosa and can extend to involve the pharynx and gastrointestinal tract (Griffin et al., 1982). The ulcers are very painful and cause serious disability. With pharyngeal involvement, hoarseness and serious dysphagia may follow. The mucosal atrophy which follows long-standing disease may complicate anaesthetic intubation (Turner, 1972). Uveitis is common and results in blindness in many cases after an average of 3.6 years (Colvard et al.,

1977). The peripheral arthropathy rarely causes permanent damage and AS is uncommon (Dubost et al., 1985). However, erythema nodosum, superficial thrombophlebitis, arterial and venous thromboses, meningoencephalitis, pericarditis, pulmonary vascular disease and mild nephritis may occasionally complicate the anaesthetic management. Corticosteroid and cytotoxic agents are used to treat the serious systemic features of the disease.

Anaesthetic management

Ankylosing spondylitis requires careful pre-anaesthetic evaluation of the cervical spine, TMJ and CAJ. Measurement of chest expansion, pulmonary function tests and CXR are mandatory and blood gas estimation may be necessary in severely affected patients. As cardiac lesions may remain unrecognized (Bromley and Hirsch, 1984; Tucker et al., 1982), ECG, 24-hour Holter monitor and echocardiography may be required in long standing disease. With aortic or mitral valve disease, antibiotic cover should be provided following surgery. A temporary cardiac pacemaker (Bergfeldt, 1983) is occasionally necessary before surgery can be carried out.

With severe limitation of neck range or mouth opening, blind intubation may be dangerous or impossible (Hill, 1980). Awake intubation (Sinclair and Mason, 1984) and fibre-optic laryngoscopic (Lloyd, 1984) methods of intubation have been advocated, although tracheostomy may rarely be necessary. Caudal anaesthesia via the sacral hiatus has also been described for major surgical procedures, even when the epidural and spinal routes are blocked (Deboard et al., 1981). However, the latter method does not guarantee the airway and is therefore not a satisfactory alternative to general anaesthesia in most cases.

During anaesthesia, assisted ventilation is often necessary in view of the reduced chest expansion. Careful postoperative observation and early chest physiotherapy are also important to prevent chest infection.

Where AS develops in association with the other seronegative conditions, the anaesthetic management is the same as with the idiopathic form. Ankylosing spondylitis associated with inflammatory bowel disease (UC and CD), superimposed osteoporosis or osteomalacia may increase the risks of compression fracture of the cervical spine during anaesthesia. Without AS, cervical spine involvement only occurs in the mutilans form of psoriatic arthritis.

Mucosal lesions are common in Reiter's syndrome, but do not influence anaesthetic practice. However, the oro-pharyngeal ulceration associated with Behçet's syndrome can seriously complicate intubation and ketamine or regional anaesthesia may be safer alternatives (Turner, 1972).

Anaemia, hypoalbuminaemia and nutritional deficiencies are associated with inflammatory bowel disease and may influence anaesthetic practice. Widespread psoriasis may also increase the risks of infection. Behçet's syndrome may have serious systemic features which may also be important.

Table 10.2 summarizes the pre-anaesthetic assessment required in patients with spondarthropathies.

Crystal arthropathies

Gout

Gout is an arthropathy resulting from urate crystal deposition in and around joints in association with hyperuricaemia. While the arthropathy does not complicate anaesthesia in its own right, it is associated with obesity, diabetes mellitus, hyperlipidaemia, hypertension, atherosclerosis, renal stones and chronic renal failure which can all increase the risk of general anaesthesia. The stress associated with surgery can also precipitate acute gout in predisposed individuals.

'Pseudo' gout

Calcium pyrophosphate deposition disease 'pseudo' gout may also be precipitated by stress such as surgery and may need to be differentiated from gout and septic arthritis.

Anaesthetic management

Whilst the anaesthetist should be aware of these conditions, as they may flare following surgery, no special precautions need to be taken other than checking the serum urate preoperatively. It should be noted that stopping allopurinol therapy suddenly may be followed by an attack of acute gout.

Miscellaneous conditions affecting the cervical spine

Any condition affecting the cervical spine can complicate anaesthetic intubation. Cervical spondylosis is the commonest cause of neck pain and results from progressive degenerative changes in the intervertebral discs with similar changes in the apophyseal and neurocentral joints. In the early stages, symptoms are often absent and there is a poor correlation between clinical and radiological features. With progression of the disease, cervical spine movement is reduced and subluxation and osteophyte formation can cause neurological abnormalities. In patients with advanced disease, intubation may be difficult and myelopathy may follow. Diffuse idiopathic skeletal hyperostosis (Forestier's disease) is a variant of degenerative disc disease where exuberant flowing ossification of the intervertebral ligaments causes immobility of the spine, but with preservation of the disc spaces on X-ray. Large osteophytes can also protrude anteriorly into the oesophagus causing dysphagia. Paget's disease, osteoporosis, osteomyelitis and primary and secondary tumours can also involve the cervical spine with a risk of inducing myelopathy during anaesthetic intubation. All patients who complain of neck pain or neurological abnormalities suggestive of cervical myelopathy or radiculopathy require preoperative radiological assessment of the cervical spine.

Anti-rheumatic drugs and anaesthesia

Simple analgesic and non-steroidal anti-inflammatory agents (NSAIDs) are the most frequently prescribed agents for musculo-skeletal disorders. However, other more potent agents are also required to treat the connective tissue disorders. Gold compounds, D-penicillamine, antimalarial agents and sulphasalazine are used to control RA and JCA. The antimalarial agents are also used in SLE and D-penicillamine in scleroderma. The drugs with the possible exception of sulphasalazine are ineffective in the seronegative spondarthropathies. Corticosteroid and cytotoxic agents are occasionally used in RA especially for extra-articular manifestations or where the joint disease cannot be controlled by other agents. They are however frequently required in the treatment of systemic JCA, Behçet's uveitis, SLE, DM/PM, and the vasculitides. The only drugs to be discussed are those with possible relevance to anaesthesia.

Non-steroidal anti-inflammatory drugs (NSAID)

The NSAID's reduce platelet aggregation and some, for example aspirin, also prolong the prothrombin time. Haemostasis during anaesthesia may therefore be mildly impaired and this may persist for 1–2 weeks after stopping therapy. All these agents inhibit prostaglandin synthesis by local and systemic effects and with mucosal irritation may result in bleeding. Iron-deficiency anaemia may therefore complicate the anaemia of chronic disease.

Hepatotoxicity has been reported with some of the newer agents as well as aspirin. The NSAID's have several effects on renal function. Inhibition of renal prostaglandin synthesis can cause salt and water retention and result in oedema and systemic hypertension. A further effect is to block the action of diuretics, to further complicate the management of congestive cardiac failure and hypertension. Acute allergic interstitial nephritis, analgesic nephropathy and acute renal failure have been reported with NSAID use. This is a particular problem in the elderly when NSAIDs are used in combination with loop diuretic.

Corticosteroid therapy

Prolonged corticosteroid therapy is associated with osteoporosis, deficient wound healing and reduced resistance to infection. However, the suppression of the hypothalmo-pituitary-adrenal (HPA) axis is the most important side-effect and may persist for up to a year after therapy has terminated. Cortisol levels do not indicate whether HPA suppression has occurred and other functional tests of the HPA axis are complicated and often unreliable. Steroid cover should therefore be given to those patients on steroid therapy and those who received this in the previous year. Intravenous hydrocortisone should be given before starting the surgery with tapering doses over the next 2–15 days. With uncomplicated surgical procedures, steroid cover should be withdrawn or returned to maintenance levels within 2 weeks.

Second line drugs used in RA

Gold salts and D-penicillamine have been shown to have many *in vivo* and *in vitro* immunological effects, but the significance of these effects is unclear. They do not seem to increase the risks of infection. However, renal damage and bone marrow suppression may occur with these agents and obstructive pulmonary disease and myasthenia gravis have occasionally complicated penicillamine therapy.

Cytotoxic immuno-suppressive agents

Azathioprine, methotrexate, cyclophosphamide, chlorambucil and, more recently, cyclosporin A have been used in the treatment of the autoimmune rheumatic diseases. They all act as immuno-suppressive agents and are therefore associated with an increased risk of infection especially when prescribed in combination. Marrow suppression is common, and hepatic, and renal dysfunction may occur. Pulmonary fibrosis has also been reported with cyclophosphamide. The oncogenic potential is a further cause for concern.

Conclusions

Patients with auto-immune rheumatic diseases suffer chronic ill health with severe constitutional symptoms during periods of disease activity. Major mechanical problems may complicate intubation of anaesthesia and maintenance of the airway. Furthermore attempts at intubation in the presence of cervical spine instability can exacerbate or even induced myelopathy. Serious organ damage is also common with possible involvement of the respiratory, cardiovascular, renal and haemopoietic systems. The rheumatic diseases therefore present major challenges to the anaesthetist.

References

Baker, H. (1966). Epidemiological aspects of psoriasis and arthritis. *British Journal of Dermatology*, **78**, 249–61.

Barnes, B.E. and Mawr, B. (1976). Dermatomyositis and malignancy. A review of the literature. *Annals of Internal Medicine*, **84**, 68–76.

Bergfeldt, L. (1983). HLA B27-associated rheumatic diseases with severe cardiac bradyarrhythmias. Clinical features and prevalence in 223 men with permanent pacemakers. *American Journal of Medicine*, **75**, 210–5.

Bienenstock, H., Ehrlich, G.E. and Freyberg, R.H. (1963). Rheumatoid arthritis of the cricoaryteroid joint: a clinicopathological study. *Arthritis and Rheumatism*, **6**, 48–63.

Bienenstock, H. and Lanyi, V.F. (1977). Cricoaryteroid arthritis in a patient with ankylosing spondylitis. *Archives of Otolaryngology*, **103**, 738–9.

Bohan, A., Peter, J.B. Bowman, R.L. and Pearson, C.M. (1977). A computer-assisted analysis of 153 patients with polymyositis and dermatomyositis. *Medicine* (Baltimore), **56**, 255–86.

Bonfiglio, T. and Atwater, E.C. (1969). Heart disease in patients with seropositive rheumatoid arthritis; a controlled autopsy study and review. *Archives of Internal Medicine*, **124**, 714–19.

Boyle, A.C. (1971). The rheumatoid neck. *Proceedings of the Royal Society of Medicine* **64**, 1161–5.

Bromley, L.M. and Hirsch, N.P. (1984). Cardiac problems and ankylosing spondylitis (letter). *Anaesthesia*, **39**, 723–4.

Bulkley, B.H., Ridolfi, R.L., Salyer, W.R. and Hutchins, G.M. (1976). Myocardial lesions of progressive systemic sclerosis. A cause of cardiac dysfunction. *Circulation*, **53**, 483–90.

Burry, H.C. (1972). Reduced glomerular function in rheumatoid arthritis. *Annals of the Rheumatic Diseases*, **31**, 65–8.

Calin, A. (1985). Ankylosing spondylitis. In: *Textbook of Rheumatology*. Second Edition, pp. 995–1007. Edited by Kelly, W.N., Harris, E.D., Ruddy, S. and Sledge, C.B. W.B. Saunders, Philadelphia.

Chia, B.L., Mah, E.P.K. and Feng, P.H. (1981) Cardiovascular abnormalities in systemic lupus erythematosis. *Journal of Clinical Ultrasound* **9**, 237–43.

Clements, P.J., Furst, D.E., Cabeen, W., Tashkin, D., Paulus, H.E. and Roberts, N. (1981). The relationship of arrhythmias and conduction disturbances to other manifestations of cardio-pulmonary disease in progressive systemic sclerosis (PSS). *American Journal of Medicine*, **71**, 38–46.

Colvard, D.M., Robertson, D.M. and O'Duffy J.D. (1977). The ocular manifestations of Behcet's disease. *Archives of Ophthalmology*, **95**, 1813–7.

D'Arcy, E.J., Fell, R.H., Ansell, B.M. and Arden, G.P. (1976). Ketamine and juvenile chronic polyarthritis (Still's disease). Anaesthetic problems in Still's disease and allied disorders. *Anaesthesia*, **31**, 624–32.

Davidson-Lamb, R.W. and Finlayson, M.C.K. (1977). Scleroderma. Complications encountered during dental anaesthesia. *Anaesthesia*, **32**, 893–5.

Deboard, J.W., Ghia, J.N. and Guilford, W.B. (1981). Caudal anaesthesia in a patient with ankylosing spondylitis for hip surgery. *Anesthesiology*, **54**, 164–6.

De Vere, R. and Bradley, W.G. (1975). Polymyositis: its

presentation, morbidity and mortality. *Brain*, **98**, 637-66.

Dubost, J.J., Sauvezie, B., Galtier, B., Bussiere, J.L. and Rampon, S. (1985). Behcet's syndrome and ankylosing spondylitis. *Review of Rheumatology*, **52**, 457-61.

Eisele, J.H. (1981). Connective tissue disease. In: *Anesthesia and Uncommon Diseases. Pathophysiological and Clinical Correlations.* Second Edition, pp. 508-29. Edited by Katz, J., Benumof, J. and Kadis, L.B., W.B. Saunders.

Eisele, J.H. and Reitan, J.A. (1971). Scleroderma, Raynaud's phenomenon and local anaesthetics. *Anesthesiology*, **34**, 386-7.

Ericson, S. and Lundberg, M. (1967). Alteration in the temporomandibular joint at various stages of rheumatoid arthritis. *Acta Rheumatologica Scandinavica*, **13**, 257-74.

Fauci, A.S. and Wolff, S.M. (1973). Wegener's granulomatosis: studies in 18 patients with a review of the literature. *Medicine* (Baltimore), **52**, 535-61.

Ferri, C., Bernini, L., Bongiorni, M.G., Levorato, D., Viegi, G., Bravi, P., Contini, C., Pasero, G. and Bombardieri, S. (1985). Non-invasive evaluation of cardiac dysrhythmias and their relationship to multisystem symptoms in progressive systemic sclerosis patients. *Arthritis and Rheumatism*, **28**, 1259-66.

Frohnert, P.P. and Sheps, S.G. (1967). Long-term follow-up study of periarteritis nodosa. *American Journal of Medicine*, **43**, 8-14.

Gardner, D.L. and Holmes, F. (1961). Anaesthetic and postoperative hazards in rheumatoid arthritis. *British Journal of Anaesthesia*, **33**, 258-64.

Ghose, M.K. (1975). Pericardial tamponade. A presenting manifestation of procainamide-induced lupus erythematosis. *American Journal of Medicine*, **58**, 581-5.

Goldberg, M.J., Husain, M., Wajszczuk, W.J. and Rubenfire, M. (1980). Procainamide-induced lupus erythematosis. Pericarditis encountered during coronary bypass surgery. *American Journal of Medicine*, 69, 159-62.

Gomar, C., Luis, M. and Nalda, M.A. (1984). Sacroiliitis in a heroin addict. A contra-indication to spinal anaesthesia. *Anaesthesia*, **39**, 167-70.

Greenstein, A.J., Janowitz, H.D. and Sachar, D.B. (1976). The extraintestinal complications of Crohn's disease and ulcerative colitis: a study of 700 patients. *Medicine* (Baltimore), **55**, 401-12.

Griffin, J.W. Jr and Harrison, H.B., Tedesco, F.J. and Mills, L.R. (1982). Behcet's disease with multiple sites of gastrointestinal involvement. *Southern Medical Journal*, **75**, 1405-8.

Haslock, I. and Wright, V. (1973). The musculo-skeletal complications of Crohn's disease. *Medicine*, **52**, 217-25.

Hepper, N.G., Ferguson, R.H. and Howard, F.M. Jr. (1964). Three types of pulmonary involvement in polymyositis. *Medical Clinics of North America*, **48**, 1031-42.

Hill, C.M. (1980). Death following dental clearance in a patient suffering from ankylosing spondylitis - a case report with discussion on management of such problems. *British Journal of Oral Surgery*, **18**, 73-6.

Hill, D.L. and Barrows, H.S. (1968). Identical skeletal and cardiac muscle involvement in a case of fatal polymyositis. *Archives of Neurology*, **19**, 545-51.

Hodgkinson, R. (1981). Anaesthetic management in a parturient with severe juvenile rheumatoid arthritis. *Anesthesia and Analgesia*, **60**, 611-12.

Holsinger, D.R. Osmundson, P.J. and Edwards, J.E. (1962). The heart in periarteritis nodosa. *Circulation*, **25**, 610-18.

Horvath, G. and Fajnor, K. (1968). Uveal changes in spondylitis ankylopoetica. *Acta Rheumatologica Scandinavica*, **14**, 141-7.

Jacobs, J.C. and Hui, R.M. (1977). Cricoaryteroid arthritis and airway obstruction in juvenile rheumatoid arthritis. *Pediatrics*, **59**, 292-4.

Jayson, M.I.V., Salmon, P.R. and Harrison, W. (1971). Amyloidosis in ankylosing spondylitis. *Rheumatology and Physical Medicine*, **11**, 78-82.

Kanard, R.R. (1977). Eosinophilic fasciitis. *Rocky Mountain Medical Journal*, **74**, 186-8.

Kassan, S.S., Hoover, R., Kimberly, R.P., Budman, D.R., Decker, J.L. and Chused, T.M. (1977). Increased incidence of malignancy in Sjogren's syndrome. *Arthritis and Rheumatism.* 20, 123.

Larheim, T.A., Dale, K. and Tveito, L. (1981). Radiographic abnormalities of the temperomandibular joint in children with juvenile rheumatoid arthritis. *Acta Radiologica*, **22**, 277-84.

Larheim, T.A., Haanaes, H.R. and Dale, K. (1981). Radiographic temporomandibular joint abnormality in adults with micrognathia and juvenile rheumatoid arthritis. *Acta Radiologica*, **22**, 495-504.

Lebowitz W.B. (1963). The heart in rheumatoid arthritis (rheumatoid disease). A clinical and pathological study of 62 cases. *Annals of Internal Medicine*, **58**, 102-23.

LeRoy, E.C. and Fleischmann, R.M. (1978). The management of renal scleroderma: experience with dialysis, nephrectomy and transplantation. *American Journal of Medicine*, **64**, 974-8.

Lewis, G.B.H. (1974). Prolonged regional analgesia in scleroderma. *Canadian Anaesthetists' Society Journal*, **21**, 495-7.

Lietman, P.S. and Bywaters, E.G. (1963). Pericarditis in juvenile rheumatoid arthritis. *Pediatrics*, **32**, 855-60.

Lloyd, E. (1984). Ankylosing spondylitis anaesthesia (letter). *Anaesthesia*, **39**, 722-3.

Lofgren, R.H. and Montgomery, W.W. (1962). Incidence of laryngeal involvement in rheumatoid arthritis. *New England Journal of Medicine*, **267**, 193-5.

MacDonald, W.J. Jr, Crawford, M.H., Klippel, J.H., Zvaifler, N.J. and O'Rourke, R.A. (1977). Echocardiographic assessment of cardiac structure and function in patients with rheumatoid arthritis. *American Journal of Medicine*, **63**, 890–6.

McGowan, B.L. (1967). Active temporal arteritis as a contraindication to elective surgery with general anaesthesia. *American Journal of Opthalmology*, **64**, 455–7.

Marks, J.S. and Sharp, J. (1981). Rheumatoid cervical myelopathy. *Quarterly Journal of Medicine*, **50**, 307–19.

Martin, T.H. (1969). Pharyngeal oedema associated with arteritis. A report of 2 cases. *Canadian Medical Association Journal*, **101**, 229–31.

Matthay, R.A., Schwartz, M.I. Petty, T.L., Stanford, R.E., Gupta, R.C., Sahn, S.A. and Steigerwald, J.C. (1975). Pulmonary manifestations of systemic lupus erythematosis: review of 12 cases of acute lupus pneumonitis. *Medicine*, **54**, 397–409.

Metheney, J.A. (1978). Dermatomyositis: a vocal and swallowing disease entity. *Laryngoscope*, **88**, 147–61.

Murray, G.C. and Persellin, R.H. (1981). Cervical fracture complicating ankylosing spondylitis: a report of 8 cases and review of the literature. *American Journal of Medicine*, **70**, 1033–41.

Neill, R.S. (1980). Progressive systemic sclerosis. Prolonged sensory blockade following regional anaesthesia in association with reduced response to systemic analgesics. *British Journal of Anaesthesia*, **52**, 623–5.

Orringer, M.B., Dabich, L., Zarafonetis, C.J. D. and Sloan, H. (1976). Gastro-oesophageal reflux in oesophageal scleroderma: diagnosis and implications. *Annals of Thoracic Surgery*, **295**, 120–30.

Radford, E.P., Doll, R. and Smith, P.G. (1977). Mortality among patients with ankylosing spondylitis not given X-ray therapy. *New England Journal of Medicine*, **297**, 572–6.

Resnick, D. (1974). Temporomandibular joint involvement in ankylosing spondylitis. Comparison of rheumatoid arthritis and psoriasis. *Radiology*, **112**, 587–91.

Roelofse, J.A. and Shipton, E.A. (1983). Difficult intubation in a patient with rheumatoid arthritis. *South African Medical Journal*, **64**, 679–80.

Scharf, J., Levy, J., Benderly, A. and Nahir, M. (1976). Pericardial tampanade in juvenile rheumatoid arthritis. *Arthritis and Rheumatism*, **19**, 760–62.

Schneider, P.D., Wise, R.A., Hochberg, M.C. and Wigley, F.M. (1982). Serial pulmonary function in systemic sclerosis. *American Journal of Medicine*, **73**, 385–94.

Schwartz, M.I., Matthay, R.A., Sahn, S.A., Stanford, R.E., Marmorstein, B.L. and Scheinhorn, D.J. (1976). Interstitial lung disease in polymyositis and dermatomyositis. Analysis of 6 cases and review of the literature. *Medicine*, **55**, 89–104.

Shaulian, E., Shoenfeld, Y., Berliner, S., Shaklai, M. and Pinkhas, J. (1981). Surgery in patients with circulating lupus anticoagulant. *International Surgery*, **66**, 157–9.

Sinclair, J.R. and Mason, R.A. (1984). Ankylosing spondylitis. The case for awake intubation. *Anaesthesia*, **39**, 3–11.

Smith, B.L. (1985). Anaesthesia and Still's disease (letter). *Anaesthesia*, **40**, 209.

Smith, G.B. and Shribman, A.J. (1984). Anaesthesia and severe skin disease. *Anaesthesia*, **39**, 443–55.

Steckel, R.J., Bein, M.E. and Kelly, P.M. (1975). Pulmonary arterial hypertension in progressive systemic sclerosis. *American Journal of Roentgenology, Radium Therapy and Nuclear Medicine*, **124**, 461–4.

Stevens, J.C., Cartlidge, N.E.F., Saunders M., Appleby A., Hall, M. and Shaw, D.A. (1971). Atlanto-axial subluxation and cervical myelopathy in rheumatoid arthritis. *Quarterly Journal of Medicine*, **159**, 391–408.

Strimlan, C.V., Rosenow, E.C., Divertie, M.B. and Harrison, E.G. (1976). Pulmonary manifestations of Sjogren's syndrome. *Chest*, **70**, 354–6!.

Svantesson, H., Marhaug, G. and Haeffner, F. (1981). Scoliosis in children with juvenile rheumatoid arthritis. *Scandinavian Journal of Rheumatology*, **10**, 65–8.

Sweeney, B. (1984). Anaesthesia and scleroderma. *Anaesthesia*, **39**, 1145.

Talal, N., Zisman, E. and Schur, P.H. (1968). Renal tubular acidosis, glomerulonephritis and immunologic factors in Sjogren's syndrome. *Arthritis and Rheumatism*, **11**, 774–86.

Taylor, R.C., Way, W.L. and Hendixson, R.A. (1968). Temporomandibular joint problems in relation to the administration of general anaesthesia. *Journal of Oral Surgery*, **26**, 327–9.

Thadani, U., Iveson, J.M.I. and Wright, V. (1975). Cardiac tampanade, constrictive pericarditis and pericardial resection in rheumatoid arthritis. *Medicine*, **54**, 261–70.

Thomas, D.J., Kendall, M.J. and Whitfield, A.G.W. (1974). Nervous system involvement in ankylosing spondylitis. *British Medical Journal*, **i**, 148–50.

Thompson, J. and Conklin, K.A. (1983). Anaesthetic management of a pregnant patient with scleroderma. *Anesthesiology*, **59**, 69–71.

Tucker, C.R., Fowles, R.E., Calin, A. and Popp, R.L. (1982). Aortitis in ankylosing spondylitis: early detection of aortic root abnormalities with 2 dimensional echocardiography. *American Journal of Cardiology*, **49**, 680–68.

Turner, M.E. (1972). Anaesthetic difficulties associated with Behcet's syndrome. Case report. *British Journal of Anaesthesia*, **44**, 100–102.

Wainwright, J. and Davson, J. (1950). The renal appearances in the microscopic form of periarteritis nodosa. *Journal of Pathology and Bacteriology*, **62**, 189–96.

Weisman, R.A. and Calcaterra, T.C. (1978). Head and neck manifestations of scleroderma. *Annals of Otology, Rhinology and Laryngology*, **87**, 332–9.

Windfield, J., Cook, D., Brook, A.S. and Corbett, M. (1981). A progressive study of the radiological changes in the cervical spine in early rheumatoid disease. *Annals of Rheumatic Disease*, **40**, 109–14.

Wortmann, D.W., Kelsch, R.C., Kuhns, L., Sullivan, D.B. and Cassidy, J.T. (1980). Renal papillary necrosis in juvenile rheumatoid arthritis. *Journal of Pediatrics*, **97**, 37–40.

Wright, V. and Watkinson, G. (1965). The arthritis of ulcerative colitis. *British Medical Journal*, **ii**, 670–75.

Index